an introduction to the
Principles of Disease

an introduction to the
Principles
of Disease

third edition

JOHN B. WALTER, M.D.

Departments of Pathology and Medicine
University of Toronto
Toronto, Ontario, Canada

Department of Pathology
Toronto General Division of the Toronto Hospital

Department of Medicine (Dermatology)
St. Michael's Hospital

W. B. SAUNDERS COMPANY
Harcourt Brace Jovanovich, Inc.
Philadelphia   London   Toronto   Montreal   Sydney   Tokyo

W. B. SAUNDERS COMPANY
Harcourt Brace Jovanovich, Inc.

The Curtis Center
Independence Square West
Philadelphia, Pennsylvania 19106

Library of Congress Cataloging-in-Publication Data

Walter, J. B. (John Brian)

An introduction to the principles of disease / John B. Walter. — 3rd
ed.

     p.   cm.

Includes bibliographical references and index.

ISBN 0–7216–9082–3

1. Pathology.   I. Title.

[DNLM: 1. Pathology.   QZ 4 W232i]

RB111.W15 1992

616.07—dc20

DNLM/DLC   91-20490

Editor: Selma Ozmat
Designer: Nina McDaid Ikeda
Production Manager: Linda R. Garber
Manuscript Editor: RoseMarie Klimowicz
Illustration Coordinator: Lisa Lambert
Indexer: Nancy Weaver
Cover Designer: Ellen Bodner-Zanolle

An Introduction to the Principles of Disease, 3rd edition   ISBN 0–7216–9082–3

Printed in the United States of America.

Last digit is the print number: 9   8   7   6   5   4   3   2   1

Preface to the Third Edition

The aim of *An Introduction to the Principles of Disease* is to initiate the student into clinical medicine via the study of pathology. No prior knowledge of medicine is assumed, but the reader ideally has received some instruction in biology, chemistry, human anatomy, and physiology.

Part I, "General Pathology," describes the general principles of disease and the disorders that affect the body as a whole. Part II, "Special Pathology," concentrates on diseases of individual organs or systems. The objective is to describe important pathologic mechanisms in considerable detail and to omit any reference to rare conditions unless they illustrate important points that have a wider implication. This book is not a synopsis of pathology; consequently, readers who are aiming for a degree in medicine will need to graduate to the larger texts of medicine and pathology before attaining their objective.

The complexity and ever-increasing cost of providing medical care have led to a reappraisal of the role of the medical doctor. In the past, it was expected that physicians would assume absolute responsibility for the diagnosis and management of their patients. No longer can this view be upheld. Physicians now rely on the competence of coworkers who are not trained as medical practitioners but whose specialized knowledge and skills are of vital importance in the prevention of disease and in the diagnosis and treatment of patients. Nurses, midwives, physical therapists, pharmacists, and medical laboratory technologists are the group of workers in the health sciences for whom this book has been written.

When studying medicine for the first time, the student meets many new words and concepts. An attempt has been made to define these items when they are first introduced, so that learning can proceed by a series of progressive steps. Little attempt has been made to avoid the specialized terminology of medicine, because this technical language is widely used in medical practice, and if used correctly, it acts as a type of shorthand by which medical personnel can express their ideas either by the spoken or the written word. Without exposure to the language of medicine, it is difficult for the untrained health worker to communicate with a physician or to comprehend the medical literature. The untrained health worker will forever be on the outside looking in on the medical scene and will never become a member of the team.

Ten years have elapsed since the second edition was published, and this has necessitated revision of the whole book. Nowhere is this more evident than in the sections related to immunology, carcinogenesis, and the newly emerging infections typified by the acquired immunodeficiency syndrome. So extensive have been the changes that the opportunity has been taken to reset the whole book. Double columns have replaced the single-column format to make for easier reading; subjects previously presented in separate chapters have been merged into single comprehensive units—for instance, tissue reaction to injury (Chapter 5) and the circulation (Chapter 19).

An outline of the contents precedes the objectives in each chapter, and a summary is appended at the end, followed by an updated list of selected readings.

JOHN B. WALTER

Acknowledgments

The production of this book would have been greatly delayed and extremely difficult without the cooperation of Churchill Livingstone of Edinburgh. Mr. Andrew Stevenson has generously allowed me to use material from their publication *General Pathology*, which I coauthored with Dr. Martin Israel. More than 30 illustrations have been taken from this source. Four illustrations are taken from *Principles of Pathology for Dental Students*, also published by Churchill Livingstone. I thank my other coauthors, Margaret Grundy (née Hamilton) and Martin Israel, for permitting me to use this material.

I am no less indebted to Lea & Febiger for generously allowing me to use material, including eight pictures, from their publication, *Pathology of Human Disease*, which I also authored.

I am once again grateful to those who have given me pictorial material or have allowed me to modify their original published work. The source of donated material is acknowledged in each caption.

A number of figures (also appearing in *General Pathology*) are of specimens from the Welcome Museum of Pathology, Royal College of Surgeons of England, London; I am grateful to the President and the Council of the Royal College of Surgeons of England for permission to reproduce these illustrations. In accordance with the wishes of the Council, each specimen is acknowledged at the end of each caption and the catalogue number of each is indicated. Some specimens are from the Boyd Museum, University of Toronto, and I thank Dr. M. D. Silver of that institution for permission to use these. I owe special gratitude to Mrs. Sonja Duda, librarian at the Banting Institute, Toronto, for valuable help in checking and obtaining new references, and to my secretary, Mrs. Elizabeth Forsythe, for expert typing and secretarial assistance.

As with many other authors, my greatest debt is to my wife, who suffered, not always in silence, during the arduous preparation of this revision.

JOHN B. WALTER

Contents

SPECIAL PATHOLOGY

General Pathology

Role of Pathology in Medicine

After studying this chapter, the student should be able to:

- Define the terms sign, symptom, lesion, etiology, pathogenesis, syndrome, idiopathic, biopsy, thoracotomy, and laparotomy.
- List the units of measurement used in microscopy.
- Compare and contrast the techniques and value of light microscopy with those of electron microscopy with respect to
  (a) resolution;
  (b) magnification;
  (c) ease of studying living cells;
  (d) thickness of tissue sections used;
  (e) methods of staining.
- Describe the major steps in the preparation of a paraffin wax section and the appearance of cells when stained with hematoxylin and eosin (H & E).
- Describe the main uses in pathology of phase contrast and dark ground illumination in microscopy.
- Discuss the advantages that the frozen section technique has over the paraffin wax technique.
- Describe the techniques of immunofluorescence and compare them with those of immunoperoxidase.
- Describe how monoclonal antibodies are prepared and indicate their value in pathology.
- Indicate the value of flow cytometry.
- Give examples of the use of radioactive isotopes in clinical medicine and in experimental pathology.
- Give an account of computed tomography, magnetic resonance imaging, and ultrasound imaging.

The majority of persons seeking medical help do so because of some abnormality causing them distress. Often such *symptoms* can be dispelled by simple remedies—quite often by reassurance. Much of medicine is an art, which its practitioners—whether they be doctors, dentists, nurses, or physical therapists—must learn. Nevertheless, there have always been individuals who were not content simply to observe disease and the effects of time-honored remedies upon it. They have attempted to describe and record the abnormalities in their patients in an objective manner; by introducing measurements, they initiated the science called *pathology*.

Disease itself is as difficult to define as is the normal, from which it is a departure. As generally used, the term "disease" is employed to describe a state in which there is a sufficient departure from the normal for *signs* or *symptoms* to be produced. A symptom is an abnormality noted by the patient. A sign is one noted by another observer. The objective variations from the normal are called *lesions,* and although the term generally refers to structural changes, it may also be used to describe functional abnormalities, such as *biochemical lesions* (Chapter 4). The theory of the cause of a disease is its *etiology,* and the development of the lesions is its *pathogenesis.* When used strictly, these two terms are quite separate entities, but in practice they are often used interchangeably. Thus, it is commonly said that the cause of a heart attack is blockage of an atherosclerotic coronary artery. Nevertheless, the cause of this may be some genetic defect or an abnormality in the diet. The coronary disease is merely part of the pathogenesis of the whole picture.

The great advances in bacteriology that started at the end of the nineteenth century fostered the concept that each disease had a single cause. To state that the common wart is always caused by a particular virus is true; nevertheless, this is an incomplete statement. It is known that some patients with multiple warts have a deficient immunity that either can be inherited or can be acquired by administration of drugs or the effects of disease. Which is the cause of the warts—the virus or the impaired immunity? Present doctrine would still favor the organism, but the genetic or acquired immunologic deficiency would be labeled a major predisposing factor. Multiple causes are probably much more common than we think. The doctrine of one cause for one disease has certainly failed to be a profitable concept in the search for the etiology of many common diseases such as cancer, atherosclerosis, emphysema, and chronic bronchitis. Nevertheless, the concept that each disease is an entity implies a specific cause for each.

To avoid the difficulty of defining disease, the term *syndrome* has been introduced. A syndrome is a condition having a defined collection of lesions, signs, or symptoms that are not necessarily always due to the same agent. Raynaud's syndrome is a condition in which the hands are unduly susceptible to cold and on exposure become pale, then blue, and finally red and painful. This syndrome can be found in patients with systemic sclerosis, it may be seen in workers who use pneumatic hammers, and finally it can occur for no apparent reason. When the cause is unknown, the condition is said to be *idiopathic.* Clearly, those conditions commonly labeled "diseases" in which the cause is not known are difficult to distinguish from syndromes. Indeed, the terms "syndrome" and "disease" are frequently used quite indiscriminately and interchangeably.

Pathology is the scientific study of disease. It describes the cause, course, and termination of disease as well as the nature of its lesions. In almost all diseases the lesions are of varying nature and may be structural, chemical, or functional. Nevertheless, anything that can be measured is within the domain of pathology. The height of the blood pressure, the rate of the heart beat, and the temperature of the patient are all valued measurements. If they are accurately recorded, they are as scientific as measurements of the size of a nucleus or of the amount of DNA that it contains. The remainder of this chapter is devoted to a brief account of the methods of investigation that can be employed.

MICROSCOPY

The application of the compound light microscope to the examination of biologic material was one of the most important steps ever taken in scientific medicine. From it stemmed the concept that all living organisms are composed of cells and cell products.

The Light Microscope

The light microscope is now routinely used in the examination of diseased tissue. The study of the changes seen is termed *histopathology.*

The ability to distinguish two closely placed points is called the *resolving power* of the microscope. When light is used, it is limited by the wavelength of the light beam used. With the light microscopes currently available, the resolving power is about 250 nm.* One of the great advantages of the electron microscope is that its resolution is much greater; in fact, it is about 0.5 nm. The maximum magnification obtainable with light microscopes of current design is about 1200. Further magnification is useless, because it merely produces a large image that is indistinct owing to the limited resolution obtainable.

Living tissue is transparent, and the homogeneity in optical density of its components hides its detailed structure. Staining techniques must therefore be employed. Unfortunately, staining almost invariably means that the cells must be dead. To obviate this difficulty, two special techniques, having limited specific uses, can be employed to visualize living cells.

Dark-field illumination relies on the fact that objects placed in a beam of light may be seen by the light they reflect in much the same way that dust particles are rendered visible by a shaft of sunlight. Using a special substage condenser, this method finds particular application in the demonstration of the organism responsible for syphilis, *Treponema pallidum*, that is regularly demonstrated in venereal disease clinics by this method.

Phase contrast microscopy takes advantage of the different refractive indices of various parts of the cell. These differences are converted into differences in optical density. In this way, living cells can be examined, and the method may be applied in virology where thin sheets of cells in culture can be seen and the effect of viruses on them examined (Figs. 9–7 and 9–8).

Routine Examination of Tissue by Microscopy. The material must be processed and then sectioned into thin slices. The two methods available, the *paraffin section technique* and the *frozen section technique*, are described in the following. Human tissue for histopathologic studies is obtained in two ways:

1. *Biopsy*. This entails the removal of a small

piece of living tissue for examination. With skin lesions, this can be done easily under the anesthesia produced by the local injection of 1 or 2 per cent lidocaine (Xylocaine) solution. Biopsy through an endoscope is an extension of this method, *e.g.*, bronchoscopy (lung lesions), mediastinoscopy, colonoscopy, and cystoscopy (bladder lesions). Solid organs like liver and kidney can be examined by needle biopsy; a core of tissue is obtained by this technique. By use of a fine needle, pancreas and lymph node specimens can be obtained for biopsy, the needle being so thin that it can pass through normal tissues without complications. Thoracotomy, opening the chest wall, is used to diagnose some diffuse lung lesions not readily examined by needle biopsy. *Laparotomy* (opening the peritoneal cavity) is a necessary prelude to the biopsy of abdominal lesions and is generally followed by some definitive treatment.

2. *Necropsy*. Necropsy provides abundant tissue for histopathologic study, but unfortunately, postmortem autolysis (Chapter 4) often limits detailed examination.

Paraffin Section Technique. This is the most commonly used routine method of examination. Fresh tissue is placed as soon as possible in *fixative*, generally a 10 per cent solution of formalin. It can remain in this solution for many months without deteriorating. Fixation renders many cell constituents insoluble, and it also inhibits enzymatic action. Blocks no thicker than 2 mm are prepared, *dehydrated* in graded alcohol, *cleared* in xylol, chloroform, or some other solvent that is miscible in both alcohol and wax, *impregnated* with molten paraffin wax, and finally, when cooled, blocked out or *embedded* in paraffin wax. From the block obtained in this way, 5-μm sections are *cut* on a microtome (Figs. 1–1 and 1–4).

When mounted on glass slides, the sections must be stained to render tissue components visible. The commonly used stains are *hematoxylin and eosin* (H & E). Hematoxylin is a blue basic dye obtained from the heartwood of a Central American tree. It is oxidized to hematein and mixed with an alum to form a lake. The dye so formed is taken up by acidic substances in the cell. Hence, the nucleus with its nucleic acid content is stained blue. Eosin is a red synthetic

---

*1 mm = 1000 μm (micrometers or microns); 1 μm = 1000 nm; 1 nm = 10 Å (Ångström units). The present tendency is to dispense with the Ångström unit and use the nanometer (nm) instead. It is useful to remember that most cocci (*e.g.*, *Staphylococcus aureus*) are about 1 μm in diameter, a normal red cell is about 7 μm in diameter, and most nuclei are 5 to 10 μm in diameter.

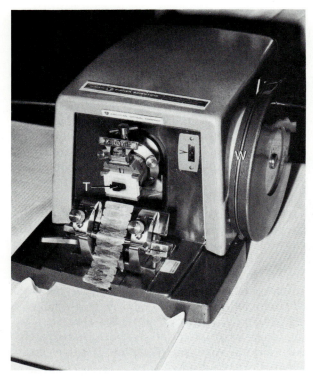

Figure 1–1 The rotary microtome. When the wheel (W) is rotated, the chuck holding the paraffin-embedded tissue (T) moves up and down against the knife. With each rotation, the tissue advances 5 to 7 μm, and a thin section is obtained. Each section adheres to the previous one so that a ribbon of sections forms.

acidic dye that binds to basic proteins found for the most part in cytoplasm. H & E stained sections are used routinely for diagnostic purposes.

Frozen Section Technique. The *cryostat* is an instrument consisting of a microtome within a refrigerator. Tissue is frozen and cut in this solid state when embedded in a block of ice. The technique has several advantages over the paraffin wax technique:

1. Frozen sections can be prepared and stained within 2 or 3 minutes. Hence, a diagnosis can be given rapidly during the course of a surgical procedure. Some hospital laboratories use this method routinely, so that all surgical material can be examined immediately and the surgeon advised as to the nature of the lesions he encounters and the extent of any disease process, *e.g.,* the extent of the spread of a cancer. The quality of frozen sections does not equal that of the routine paraffin sections, but the technique provides a rapid diagnosis and often saves the patient from having to be operated on a second time.

2. The paraffin wax technique removes lipids from cells and tissues. These substances are retained in the frozen section technique and can be stained specifically.

3. Frozen sections contain the active enzymes present in the cell, and these can be detected histochemically.

4. The frozen section technique causes little protein denaturation. Specific proteins, such as antigens and immunoglobulins, can be detected by immunologic procedures.

Histochemistry

H & E and many other staining techniques (*e.g.,* the Ziehl-Neelsen stain) used in histopathology have been discovered empirically. Others have been developed with the intention of demonstrating specific chemicals in the tissue. The technique is called *histochemistry*, and it depends on specific chemical interactions. A simple example of this technique is the Prussian blue reaction for hemosiderin (Fig. 1–2). Acid is applied to a section and releases Fe^{3+} from hemosiderin, a breakdown product of hemoglobin. Next potassium ferrocyanide is applied; this reacts with the Fe^{3+} to form bright blue insoluble ferric ferrocyanide.

Enzymes may be detected by applying a suitable substrate to a section and devising methods for visually demonstrating an end product of the reaction.

The highly specific property of antibodies can be utilized to detect specific proteins within a cell or tissue. Thus, in order to detect a bacterium or a bacterial antigen, an antibacterial IgG antibody is applied to the section. It forms a stable complex with the antigen. If the antibody has been labeled previously with fluorescein, examination of the section under ultraviolet microscopy will reveal brilliant fluorescence at the site of antigen-antibody interaction. In practice, a more complex technique is often used. *Unlabeled* antibacterial IgG (of human origin) may be applied to the section, and a second fluorescein-

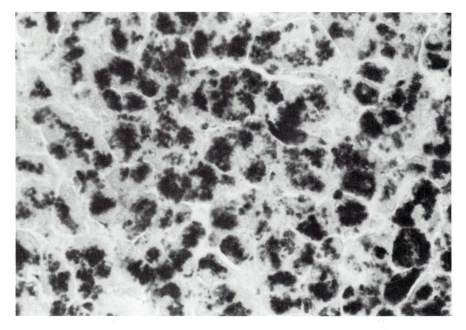

Figure 1–2 Section of liver stained for hemosiderin by the Prussian blue method. The pigment is stained brilliant blue but appears black in the photograph. The detailed structure of the liver cells is not well shown. This tissue was from a patient with hemochromatosis (×600).

labeled antihuman IgG antibody is then applied, thereby forming a type of sandwich. This modification, the multilayered or sandwich technique, has the effect of amplification of the fluorescence. A supply of labeled antihuman IgG is needed as well as unlabeled specific antibodies to each antigen that is to be investigated. The technique described is termed *immunofluorescence* and is widely used to detect microbial antigens, antibodies (see Fig. 31–9), and complement. A disadvantage of the method is that fresh tissue is generally required because frozen sections must be used. Also, the preparations are not perfect, their quality is often not good, and finally an ultraviolet microscope must be available.

A further development is the *immunoperoxidase technique*. The enzyme horseradish peroxidase is used as a label instead of fluorescein. The peroxidase itself is detected by applying a chromogen that is specifically acted upon by the enzyme to produce a stable, colored insoluble product. Diaminobenzidine, or DAB, is commonly used and produces a crisp brown color that does not fade. As with immunofluorescence, a variety of sandwich modifications are utilized (Fig. 1–3). The immunoperoxidase technique has several advantages over immunofluorescence. No special microscope is needed. Tissues embedded in

paraffin wax for routine H & E histology can be used for the demonstration of many antigens. Immunoglobulins, lysozyme, alpha-fetoglobulin, hormones, and many other antigens can be demonstrated by the use of specific antibodies and the immunoperoxidase technique; the method is now part of the routine examination of pathologic material, particularly in tumors. As an example, antibodies to a protein called S100 react with melanoma cells but not with those of a carcinoma. Frozen sections are still necessary for the demonstration of certain antigens (*e.g.,* surface immunoglobulins).

The Electron Microscope

Transmission Electron Microscope. This instrument resembles the ordinary microscope except that a stream of electrons is used instead of light, and electromagnetic fields replace the glass lenses. The theoretical resolving power is on the order of 0.005 nm. In practice, most instruments have a working resolving power of approximately 0.5 nm, and magnifications of up to 500,000 are possible. The electron microscope has revealed cell structure (*ultrastructure*) in minute detail, but it has many disadvantages. It is ex-

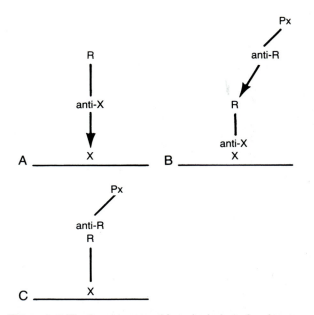

Figure 1–3 The immunoperoxidase technique for demonstrating cellular antigen. The antigen X on the cell surface is to be detected. *A*, Application of the rabbit anti-X antibody (R—anti-X) to the tissue results in the antibody's uniting with the antigen on the cell surface. *B*, The adherent antibody is itself detected by the addition of antibody to rabbit globulin labeled with peroxidase (anti-R—Px) as shown in *C*. Finally, diaminobenzidine solution is added, and a colored precipitate indicates the site of the antigen. More complex modifications of this technique are available. (Modified from Walter, J. B., and Israel, M. S.: General Pathology. 6th ed. Edinburgh, Churchill Livingstone, 1987.)

pensive and needs constant expert maintenance. Specimens for electron microscopy must be placed in special fixative, and one containing glutaraldehyde is routinely used as the initial fixative. Osmium tetroxide solution is commonly used as an additional fixative. It also acts as a "stain" because the metal brings out cellular detail. Lead and uranium salts are similarly employed. The blocks of tissue must be small (1 to 2 mm in size) so that the fixative penetrates rapidly. They are dehydrated and finally embedded in an epoxy resin (Fig. 1–4). Sections, 50 to 60 nm thick, are cut on a microtome with a glass or diamond knife. Finally, the sections are placed on a copper grid and examined in the vacuum of the column of the electron microscope (Fig. 1–5). The tremendous magnification available is impressive, but it does cut down the field of view by a similar dimension. In addition, although the image in the electron microscope can be seen on a fluorescent screen, any detailed examination must be done by taking photographic pictures. Electron microscopy therefore is a highly specialized technique that is very time-consuming. It can be used for specific research or diagnostic purposes, but not for routine tissue examination. It is now a common practice in large centers to fix and embed some routine surgical and necropsy tissue, but not to cut and examine it unless there is a particular need. This need may arise when the paraffin sections reveal a tumor to be poorly differentiated for definite diagnosis. Formalin-fixed tissue and even tissue in a paraffin block can be processed for electron microscopy, but the quality of the final pictures is not so good as that obtained in well-prepared tissue.

Viruses can be seen with ease by the electron microscope; it is in this field that the instrument has really great diagnostic capability. For example, in patients with recurrent ulceration of the genitalia, it is important to determine whether herpes simplex is the cause. An electron microscopist can demonstrate the presence of a virus within a few minutes of receiving a swab from a lesion. The precise identification of the virus is performed by culture.

The *high-voltage electron microscope* employs a voltage ten times that of the standard electron microscope. Whole cells suitably prepared can be examined, and this has the advantage over thin sections in that the internal structures of the cell are revealed in depth. However, the microscope is not only very expensive but also very large. Current versions are about 30 feet high and weigh 20 tons!

Scanning Electron Microscope. This instrument works on a different principle from that of the conventional transmission electron microscope: a very fine beam of electrons is focused to a point and made to scan the surface of a specimen. Secondary electrons scattered from the surface are collected and amplified. The current so generated is used to modulate the brightness of a television tube that is scanned in synchronicity with the electron beam scanning the object. With this method for examining the surfaces of objects, the pictures so obtained have a remarkable three-dimensional appearance (Fig. 1–6). Mi-

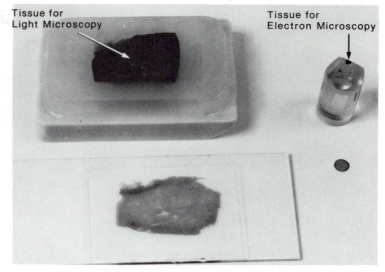

Figure 1–4 Comparison of the paraffin wax technique with that of electron microscopy. Top left shows tissue embedded in a paraffin wax block. A section cut on a microtome (see Fig. 1–1) has been mounted on a 3 × 1 inch glass slide and stained with hematoxylin and eosin (bottom left). Compare the size of the tissue with the 1-mm block taken for electron microscopy and embedded in epoxy resin (top right). After sectioning on a special microtome, a number of sections have been floated onto a circular copper grid that is 3.8 mm in diameter (bottom right). The mesh of the grid is so fine that it cannot be seen with the naked eye.

croorganisms, red and white cells, the lung, sinuses of the spleen, and the surface of the intestinal mucosa have all been studied with advantage by this technique (Fig. 23–14).

RADIOACTIVE ISOTOPES

Radioactive isotopes are treated by living cells in the same way as the normal elements. Their radiation can be detected by suitable counters, and they may usefully be employed as labels in a wide range of fields. Clinically, the greatest breakthrough in this area has been the introduction of the manmade element *technetium*. This element emits gamma radiation only, and it is therefore safer to use than are isotopes that emit other more damaging radiation. It has a half-life of 6 hours. When injected intravenously with pyrophosphate, technetium is selectively taken up by bone, probably by the osteoid tissue. With use of this technique, the whole skeleton can be surveyed, and the method now augments radiography in the detection of bone lesions, particularly tumors (Fig. 1–7). If the technetium is attached to aggregated albumin, it becomes concentrated in the lung; an estimate of blood flow through this organ is then obtained. By various techniques, it is now possible to scan many other organs. It is particularly useful in investigating lesions of the liver and thyroid. In the past,

thyroid function has been investigated by estimating the distribution of an administered dose of radioactive iodine, but this has now been replaced by the technetium technique. Many other radioactive techniques are used in medicine; for example, radioactive chromium can be attached to red cells and the length of their survival estimated. Elements that emit gamma rays or charged particles are termed *radionuclides*, and their widespread use in diagnostic techniques has resulted in the formation of a separate specialty, that of *nuclear medicine*.

Case History I

The patient was a 15-year-old boy who complained of pain and swelling of the right leg (see Fig. 1–7). About 1 year before seeking medical aid, he noticed aching of the leg after skiing or skating. He paid little attention to this, but he noticed the aching gradually became severe and continuous. About 3 months previously he first noticed a swelling. On examination, a slightly tender swelling over the midshaft of the right tibia was the only abnormality detected. A radiograph revealed a bony defect in the region; a provisional diagnosis of primary bone tumor was made. Secondary cancer could have produced a similar picture but is a very uncommon condition at this age. The figure shows a technetium bone scan; the increased activity in the region of the tumor is obvious. Note also the increased activity over the ends of the long bones, particularly at the knee, wrist, and upper ends of the humeri. This is due to epiphyseal bone growth in this 15-year-old boy. A chest radiograph and a liver scan revealed no evidence of metastatic tumor. A biopsy of

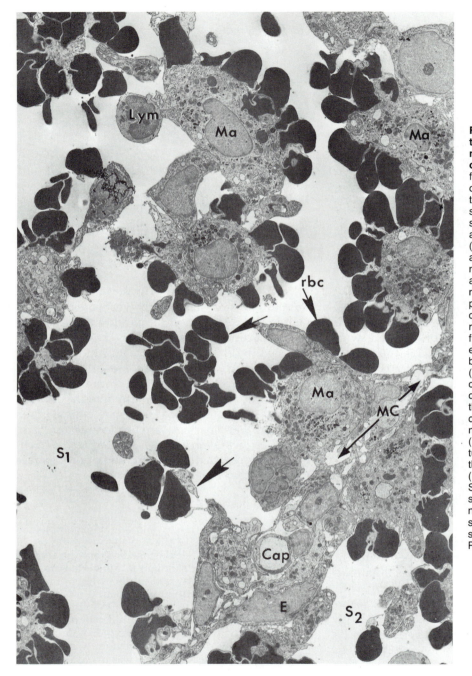

Figure 1–5 Transmission electron micrograph showing the medulla of a hemolymph node of a rat. Hemolymph nodes differ from the usual type of lymph node commonly present in humans in that red cells are present in the sinuses. This picture shows two sinuses, S_1 and S_2, which are separated by a thin medullary cord (MC) containing a capillary (Cap) and macrophages (Ma) to which many red blood cells (rbc) are adherent. In the cytoplasm of the macrophages there are many phagosomes representing degradation products of red cells. In S_1, red cells in groups appear to be free. On closer examination, however, they are partially surrounded by pseudopods of macrophages (large arrow). The medullary cords are covered by sinus endothelial cells (E) between which the macrophages push out pseudopodia to entrap red cells. The macrophages and lymphocyte (Lym) seen at the top of the picture are in one of the trabeculae that cross the sinus ($\times$2400). (From Nopajaroonsri, C., Luk, S. C., and Simon, G. T.: The structure of the hemolymph node—a light, transmission, and scanning electron microscopic study. Journal of Ultrastructure Research, *48*:325–341, 1974.)

the tumor revealed osteosarcoma. An above-knee amputation was performed. The boy adapted well to the procedure but shortly afterward developed a wound infection from *Staphylococcus aureus.* Three months after the amputation a sinus was excised, and a 2-inch section of femur was removed so that a better stump could be fashioned. The wound healed well, and the

patient was able to walk. He remains well 14 months after diagnosis. Nevertheless, the prognosis must be guarded, since less than 20 per cent of patients survive for more than 5 years following treatment. This case illustrates two other important features: (1) Noninvasive investigations such as a bone scan are carried out before invasive procedures such as biopsy. (2) Radical

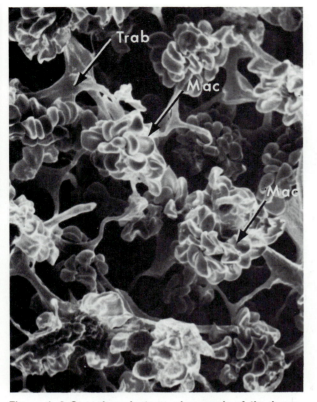

Figure 1–6 Scanning electron micrograph of the hemolymph node of the rat. Trabeculae (Trab) are seen crossing a sinus. Grapelike groups of red cells are present around macrophages in the medulla (Mac). Compare this picture with Figure 1–5, noting the difference in magnification (×1300). (From Luk, S. C., Nopajaroonsri, C., and Simon, G. T.: The architecture of the normal lymph node and hemolymph node. Laboratory Investigation, 29:258–265, 1973. © 1973 U.S.–Canadian Division of the International Academy of Pathology.)

surgery for malignant disease should never be undertaken without first obtaining a definite tissue diagnosis.

Autoradiography

Radioactive isotopes can be used at a microscopic level. If a section of tissue is placed on a photographic film for a suitable time, subsequent photographic development will reveal the site of isotope localization as a series of black grains. This principle is often applied in experimental pathology; for example, it is found that tritiated thymidine (thymidine containing tritium, the radioactive isotope of hydrogen) is incorporated

into DNA in the same way as ordinary thymidine. DNA synthesis and therefore mitotic activity can be investigated by this technique (Fig. 1–8).

TISSUE CULTURE

Tissues of various types can be cultured outside the body with comparative ease. Growth commonly occurs on the surface of glass or plastic, and tissues can be grown in test tubes, medicine-flat bottles, or the surface of a coverslip.

There are two types of tissue culture.

Cell Culture. If isolated cells of an organ or tissue (or portions of a tissue) are placed in a tissue culture medium, individual cells grow as a flat sheet on the surface of the container. This is an extremely important technique in virology, because viruses can be grown in the cultivated cells (Chapter 9). Its use for other purposes, such as in cancer research, is limited, because the cells are growing in a highly artificial medium and often do not carry out the specific functions of the organ from which they were isolated. Nevertheless, cell culture has found many uses. *Fetal cells from amniotic fluid* (obtained by amniocentesis, see Chapter 3) can be cultured in order to detect chromosomal abnormalities or specific enzyme defects, *e.g.,* that found in Tay-Sachs disease (Chapter 16). Likewise, cells from individuals with known inherited disease can be studied in the laboratory in order to unravel the biochemical defect responsible for their condition. Short-term *lymphocyte culture* is used extensively in chromosomal analyses (see Chapter 3).

Normal cells are difficult to maintain in culture because with repeated subculture they invariably die. Efforts to establish a permanent *cell line* consisting of a single *clone** are invariably unsuccessful, and even fibroblasts, which grow relatively easily, die out after 50 to 60 generations. Normal cells have a finite life span.

Sometimes a change occurs in a culture (termed *transformation*) after which the cells can be subcultured indefinitely. These potentially im-

---

*A clone is a group of cells of like hereditary constitution that has been produced asexually from a single cell. The word is derived from the Greek *klon,* meaning a cutting used for propagation.

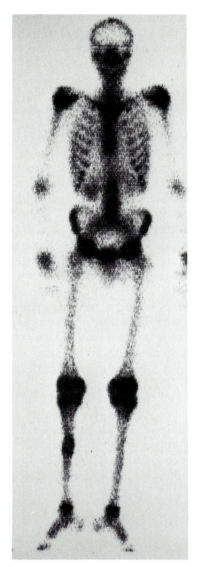

Figure 1–7 Bone scan showing tumor of the right tibia in a 15-year-old boy. See Case History I for details.

Lane, a patient after whom the cell line was named.

Somatic cell hybridization is a technique whereby two dissimilar cells are allowed to fuse

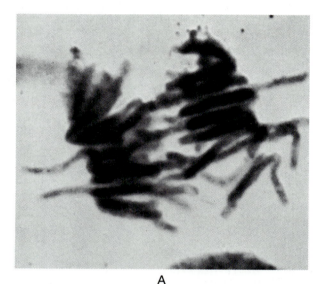

A

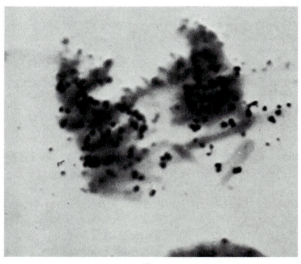

B

Figure 1–8 Autoradiograph of a mitotic figure. Tissue from the root tip of an onion was fed with tritiated thymidine. *A,* Photograph at the level of the section to show the chromosomes. *B,* The same cell photographed at the level of the photographic emulsion. The labeled thymidine has been taken up by the cells and incorporated into the cell's DNA. Note how the silver dots correspond to the chromosomes. This technique is used to indicate the sites of DNA synthesis during the period that the labeled thymidine was available ($\times$3200). (Courtesy of Dr. P. B. Gahan.)

mortal cells develop into malignant neoplasms if grafted into a suitable host. Transformation may occur spontaneously (presumably by mutation) or as a result of a viral infection. Thus, *lymphoblastoid cell lines* have been obtained by transforming human lymphocytes with the Epstein-Barr virus.

The best-known example of a permanent cell line is that of the *HeLa cell*. This was derived from a carcinoma of the uterine cervix of *Helen* to produce a single hybrid cell. The two cells may be from the same individual or from completely separated species, *e.g.*, man and mouse. This technique is used in the production of monoclonal antibodies. If a mouse is injected with a particular antigen, it manufactures specific antibodies. It is possible to take spleen cells from the animal and identify one lymphoid cell that makes this highly specific antibody. Such a cell will not grow indefinitely, but if it is made to fuse with a compatible mouse malignant cell (a myeloma cell), the resultant hybrid cell will grow indefinitely *in vitro*. Such a clone of cells is called a *hybridoma* and is used in the manufacture of the specific antibody. Commercially prepared monoclonal antibodies are now available against many antigens and are widely used in pathology. As noted previously, these antibodies, combined with the peroxidase method, can detect specific antigens on fixed tissue sections in diagnostic pathology.

The antibodies can be labeled with fluorochromes, which fluoresce in ultraviolet light. Antibodies to leukocyte cell markers have been particularly useful in the analysis of leukemic cells. The technique of *flow cytometry* has hastened progress in this area. In flow cytometric analysis, cells in suspension are passed in single file through a laser beam that activates the fluorochrome-labeled antibody attached to the cell. Different fluorochromes can be used as labels to different antibodies. Hence, if several specific labeled antibodies are added to a mixed population of cells, a count can be made of the number of cells that react to each labeled antibody. The technique can be adapted for actually separating the differently labeled cells.

Organ Culture. A fragment of tissue is grown on a grid, so that there is no cellular outgrowth, but histologically the organ is kept as normal as possible. Limb buds, eye rudiments, and bones have been studied while growing in an artificial medium, and their differentiation has been observed.

CHEMICAL AND PHYSICAL ANALYSIS OF BIOLOGIC MATERIALS

Chemical technology has now advanced to the stage at which it is possible to analyze large molecules such as myoglobin and insulin. Apart from these research applications, modern methods of chemical analysis combined with automation now make it possible to estimate a large number of chemical substances in the small quantity of body fluids, *e.g.*, blood. With the SMA-12 Auto Analyzer, which is routinely used, it is currently possible to estimate 12 substances from a single sample of blood, *e.g.*, sodium, potassium, chloride, blood urea nitrogen, glucose, and others.* In many centers, this biochemical analysis (*biochemical profile*) is now performed routinely in much the same way that the pulse has been taken and the blood pressure recorded for many years.

RADIOLOGY AND OTHER IMAGING TECHNIQUES

The methods of clinical investigation may seem out of place in a pathology book, but several techniques have evolved that enable physicians to see images of the internal organs of living patients in much the same way that their predecessors acquired knowledge at the traditional necropsy. Radiology has been at the forefront of these advances, and this section gives a brief account of the methods that are in use.

Conventional diagnostic radiology is too familiar to warrant a detailed description. As x-rays pass through the tissues, they cast an image that is recorded on a photographic film. The method has many modifications to enhance the image. Soft x-rays generated at 20 to 50 kV are used in mammography to detect breast cancer. Radiopaque contrast material can be introduced into cavities to outline them, taken by mouth or introduced into the rectum and colon to investigate the alimentary tract, or injected into blood vessels to delineate their course and appearance. Those chemicals injected intravenously are excreted by the kidneys, thus allowing the urinary tract to be visualized.

---

*The others usually estimated are aspartate aminotransferase, lactic dehydrogenase, alkaline phosphatase, bilirubin, calcium, phosphate, and uric acid.

Computed Tomography Scanning

Technological advancements involved rotating the x-ray tube around a selected focus in the patient, producing a tomogram (see Fig. 22–11). In computed tomography, multiple detectors (solid-state crystal chips coated with cesium iodide) are used to detect x-rays, and the electronic impulses produced are fed into a computer and displayed in visual form on a monitor. This *computed tomography* (CT) scan or CAT scan (for computerized axial tomography) reveals a two-dimensional "slice" through the patient that is of great value in detecting lesions that would remain undetected by conventional radiography (Fig. 1–9).

In an attempt to reduce the low risks from radiation exposure, new diagnostic technologies were developed that do not use x-rays.

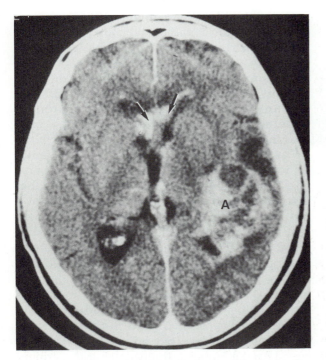

Figure 1–9 Computed tomography scan of the brain. The scan shows a large mass in the left side of the brain (A) and further extension of the tumor around the frontal horns of the lateral ventricles (arrows). The internal characteristics of the mass suggest the diagnosis of malignant astrocytoma. (Courtesy of Dr. M. A. Keller, Department of Radiology, Toronto General Division of the Toronto Hospital, Toronto.)

Magnetic Resonance Imaging

This latest imaging technology involves placing the patient in a powerful magnetic field so that the hydrogen molecules of the body line up. A radiofrequency signal is transmitted to upset their arrangement. When the signal is turned off, the hydrogen atoms (actually their protons) return to their lined-up state and, in doing so, emit a small electric current. By measuring this current, computer analysis can display an image on a monitor. Magnetic resonance imaging is complementary to computed tomography, allowing visualization of anatomic areas that are poorly seen by computed tomography, specifically the brain stem and spinal cord (Fig. 1–10). There are disadvantages to magnetic resonance imaging. Patients with pacemakers, intracranial ferromagnetic aneurysm clips, and metallic bodies in the orbits and patients who are claustrophobic cannot be scanned.

Ultrasound Imaging

This technique is noninvasive, harmless, and relatively inexpensive. It works on a principle also used in sonar and radar. A transducer (transmitter-receiver) is placed on the skin surface, and a signal of high frequency is transmitted into the body. The transducer passes in an arc over the area of the body to be investigated and records the signal reflected from the tissues in the body. The process is repeated line by line until the area has been covered. The time delay between sending the signal and receiving the reflected signal is measured and analyzed, and the result is displayed on a monitor (Fig. 1–11). The pictures are not easy to interpret but find many uses in medicine. The method is safe and can be used to investigate the fetus *in utero*.

As more and more complex techniques become available and adapted to medical use, there is a tendency to regard patients as objects for the academic exercise of investigation and scientific treatment. Batteries of investigations are ordered, and abnormalities are treated. This can lead to disastrous results, because every test has its limitations: experimental errors, biologic variations, and significance under particular circum-

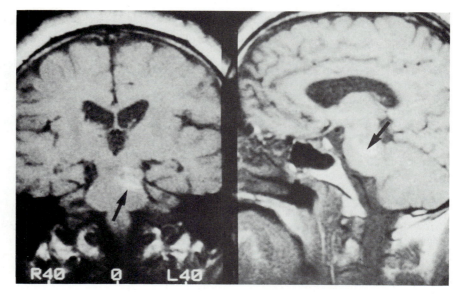

Figure 1–10 Magnetic resonance scan of the brain. Note the bright signal area in the brain stem (arrows). This area is particularly difficult to see well on a computed tomography scan. Magnetic resonance has the advantage of imaging the brain stem well. Additionally, the ability to image in multiple planes (coronal on the left, sagittal on the right) without altering the patient's head position from neutral is very advantageous. (Courtesy of Dr. M. A. Keller, Department of Radiology, Toronto General Division of the Toronto Hospital, Toronto.)

stances, all of which must be taken into consideration. The patient must be treated as an individual and not dehumanized by the modern medical center. Too often one hears of a patient failing to respond to treatment and then dying. The truth is that the wrong treatment was applied through miscalculations on the part of the medical attendants, or that no effective treatment was available. Blame the practice of medicine but not the patient!

Summary

- Light microscopy is limited by the resolving power of the microscope. It can be expanded by dark ground illumination and phase contrast microscopy. The paraffin wax method is routine; H & E and empirical histochemical stains are now augmented by specific immunostaining with use of either ultraviolet microscopy or the immunoperoxidase method.
- Frozen sections have the advantage of speed and are used for some immunostaining methods.

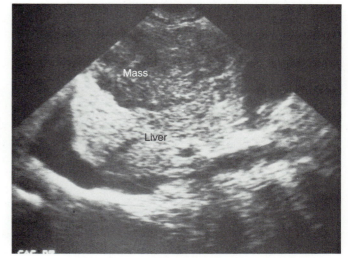

Figure 1–11 Ultrasonography of the liver. The scan shows a large mixed density mass with characteristics very different from the underlying normal liver. The histologic type of the tumor cannot be determined from the ultrasound scan. (Courtesy of Dr. M. A. Keller, Department of Radiology, Toronto General Division of the Toronto Hospital, Toronto.)

- Transmission electron microscopy uses special embedding and cutting techniques. Small specimens only can be examined.
- Radioactive isotopes are used as labels in the living patient or animal and combined with tissue culture in experimental pathology.
- Normal cells have a limited life span in culture but can be used for chromosomal and biochemical analysis.
- Permanent cell lines are malignant cells; the best known is the HeLa cell line.
- Fusion of a normal antibody-producing cell with a myeloma cell (malignant) produces a hybridoma that will grow indefinitely. This technique is used to produce large quantities of specific antibody.
- Radiology, magnetic resonance imaging, and ultrasound imaging can now detect structural abnormalities previously visible only at surgery or necropsy.

Selected Readings

Armstrong, P., and Keevil, S. F.: Magnetic resonance imaging. 1: Basic principles of image production. 2: Clinical uses. Br. Med. J. *303:*35 and 105, 1991.

Coon, J. S., Landay, A. L., and Weinstein, R. S.: Advances in flow cytometry for diagnostic pathology. Lab. Invest. *57:*453, 1987.

Doane, F. W., and Anderson, N.: Electron Microscopy in Diagnostic Virology. Cambridge, Cambridge University Press, 1987.

Falini, B., and Taylor, C. R.: New developments in immunoperoxidase techniques and their application. Arch. Pathol. Lab. Med. *107:*105, 1983.

Sochurek, H.: Medicine's New Vision. Easton, Pa., Mack Publishing Company, 1988.

Weakley, B. S.: A Beginner's Handbook in Biological Transmission Electron Microscopy. 2nd ed. Edinburgh, Churchill Livingstone, 1981.

Normal Structure and Function

**After studying this chapter, the student
should be able to:**

- Distinguish epithelial cells from mesenchymal cells
  with respect to their structure and function.
- Describe the structure of the plasma membrane and
  list its functions, particularly in relation to its
  receptors.
- Draw a diagram of a typical epithelial cell and
  include its nucleus, nucleolus, mitochondria,
  lysosomes, glycogen granules, endoplasmic
  reticulum, and Golgi apparatus. Indicate the
  functions of these cytoplasmic structures.
- Relate the structure of DNA to chromosomes and
  genes.

- Draw a diagram to show how the information of
  DNA is utilized in the formation of protein.
- List the information that can be learned about the
  chromosomes and their arrangement from an
  examination of
  (a) nuclear morphology;
  (b) the Barr body.
- Describe the two components of the endoplasmic
  reticulum and relate them to lysosomes and the
  Golgi apparatus in terms of both structure and
  function.
- Describe the distribution of cells of the mononuclear
  phagocyte system and their functions.
- Describe the components of the ground substance
  (interfibrillary matrix).
- Describe collagen fibers with respect to their
  (a) distribution in the body;
  (b) appearances under the light microscope and the
      transmission electron microscope;
  (c) relationship to reticulin;
  (d) chemical composition;
  (e) formation.
- Describe the cell cycle and the phases of mitosis.

The human body is formed from the division
of a single cell, the fertilized ovum. The process
of division, *mitosis*, is described later in this
chapter. It results in the formation of two daughter cells, each of which closely resembles the
original. Nevertheless, as division follows division, the daughter cells exhibit new or altered

structure and function. This process is called *differentiation* or *maturation*. The first evidence of differentiation in the mass of cells of the developing embryo is the formation of three distinct germ layers. An outer layer of cells forms the *ectoderm*; a tube develops within the mass, and the cells lining it form the *endoderm*. This tube forms the basis of the future alimentary canal and organs that bud from it—lungs, liver, pancreas, and others. The *mesoderm* consists of cells lying between the ectoderm and the endoderm.

The primitive cells of each germ layer can differentiate along two separate lines, forming either epithelium or mesenchyme (connective tissue).

Epithelial cells cover surfaces (*e.g.,* skin) or line cavities (*e.g.,* the mouth); in these situations they are essentially protective in function. Covering epithelia may also perform a secretory function: the intestinal and respiratory epithelia, for instance, secrete mucus (Figs. 2–1 and 2–2).

In addition to covering surfaces, the secretory type of epithelium may be arranged to form solid glands. During development, buds of endodermal cells form masses that subsequently differentiate into liver, pancreas, and salivary glands. Likewise, buds from the ectoderm form sweat glands and breast tissue. The secretory cells are arranged around a central cavity to form acini into which the secretion is poured (Fig. 2–3). From here, the secretion passes into collecting ducts and reaches the epithelial surface from which the gland originated. In some glands the connection with the epithelial surface is lost, the duct disappears, and secretion takes place directly into the blood stream. Such secreting organs are the *endocrine glands*; even in these, although no secretion is collected into ducts, acinar spaces may be formed. This configuration is clearly seen in the normal thyroid (Fig. 29–5). A feature common to all epithelial cells is that they are closely contiguous with one another. This structural feature is evident on light microscopy; even under the electron microscope, the cells appear to be separated by only a thin layer of electron-dense material that is about 15 nm in width.

Connective tissue, or *mesenchymal, cells* are the other cell type present in the body. They are usually widely separated from each other by a

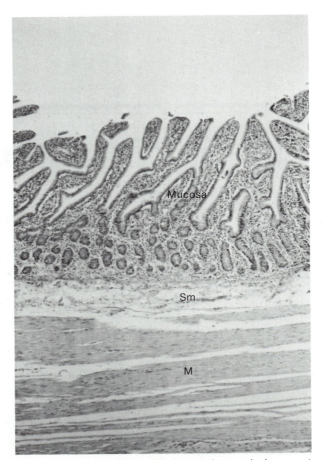

Figure 2–1 Small intestine. This photomicrograph shows part of the muscle coat (M) covered by the mucosa. Between the muscle coat and the mucosa there is a layer of loose connective tissue called the submucosa (Sm). The picture is typical of a slide prepared by the paraffin wax technique and stained with hematoxylin and eosin (×50).

zone containing ground substance in which fibers are embedded. *Collagen fibers* are the most abundant, but in some areas (*e.g.,* the walls of large arteries) *elastic fibers* are also present. This type of connective tissue—typified by tendon, bone, cartilage, and fibrous tissue—is primarily supportive in function. Other connective tissue cells have been endowed with specialized cytoplasm either for *contraction* (muscle fibers) or for *conduction* (nerve cells). It should be noted that whereas much of the body's connective tissue is derived from mesodermal cells, the mesoderm is also capable of differentiating into epithelium. The kidney and the gonads are mesodermal in

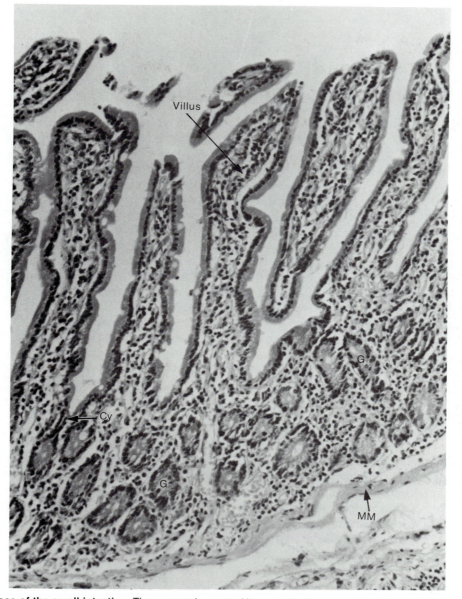

Figure 2–2 Mucosa of the small intestine. The mucosa is covered by an epithelium composed of a single layer of tall columnar cells, some of which secrete mucus. The absorptive surface is increased by the folds, or villi, that project into the lumen of the gut. Simple tubular glands (G) open into the crypts (Cy). Beneath the epithelium, the mucosa consists of connective tissue containing thin fibers of collagen, associated fibroblasts, and blood vessels. There is a sparse infiltration by small round cells, most of which are lymphocytes or plasma cells. It is not possible to identify individual cells at this magnification. The thin layer of muscle of the mucosa, the muscularis mucosae (MM), is seen in the lower part of the picture (×200).

origin, and yet they are epithelial in structure. The ectoderm and endoderm tend to differentiate into epithelia; even here, however, there are exceptions. Some of the muscle of the eye is of ectodermal origin. Most of the nervous system, including its glial connective tissue, is derived from ectoderm. Only the microglia are mesodermal.*

―――――――――――
*Because nervous tissue and muscle are so different from ordinary connective tissue, some authorities describe four basic tissues: epithelial, connective, nervous, and muscular. This further subdivision serves little purpose in pathology.

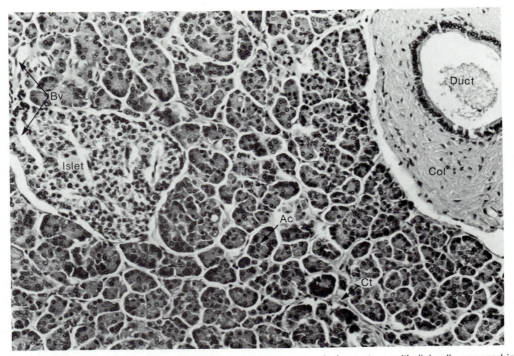

Figure 2–3 Normal pancreas. The exocrine portion of the gland is composed of secretory epithelial cells arranged in groups or acini (Ac), each of which has a central lumen into which the secretion is poured (the lumina cannot be seen at this magnification). Secretion is collected into small ducts, and these drain into larger ducts and finally into a main pancreatic duct. The endocrine portion of the gland forms a small portion of the pancreas and is represented in this figure by one islet of Langerhans, which has no acini or duct. The connective tissue of the gland is represented by small blood vessels (Bv) and a collagenous stroma (Ct), scanty between the acini but more obvious around the duct (Col) (×250).

The study of the embryologic origin of cells and tissues is of some importance in pathology in explaining certain curious phenomena. Thus, in some diseases of the breast, gland structures are found that closely resemble those of the apocrine sweat gland. Both sweat glands and breast tissue have a common ectodermal origin. Likewise, tumors can be found in the anterior lobe of the pituitary that closely resemble those found normally in the jaw or skin. The pituitary gland, teeth, and epidermis all have a common ectodermal origin.

The process of differentiation, by which cells become highly specialized, is sometimes accompanied by loss of ability to divide. Neurons are highly specialized and are quite incapable of mitosis as they become differentiated. Nevertheless, in other tissues—liver cells, for instance—the power to divide is never lost. What is lost during the process of maturation is the ability to differentiate along different lines. The fertilized ovum is *totipotent, i.e.,* capable of producing all the tissues of the body, and its immediate daughter cells have a similar capability. Separation of cells at this early stage results in multiple fetuses with consequent identical twins, triplets, and other such multiple births.

The cells of the body show considerable diversity of structure and function, yet each is remarkably independent. Each receives a supply of oxygen and foodstuff from the blood stream, with which it must produce its own structural components and secretions. Each cell must also release the energy required for mechanical, chemical, or electrical work. It is therefore not surprising that all cells are built upon a similar plan (Fig. 2–4).

The number of chemical reactions known to occur inside the cell is so great that it would be difficult to understand how these could proceed in a structure that appears, under the light microscope, to be so simple. The electron micro-

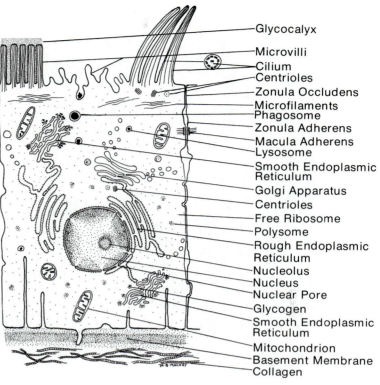

—Glycocalyx
—Microvilli
—Cilium
—Centrioles
—Zonula Occludens
—Microfilaments
—Phagosome
—Zonula Adherens
—Macula Adherens
—Lysosome
—Smooth Endoplasmic Reticulum
—Golgi Apparatus
—Centrioles
—Free Ribosome
—Polysome
—Rough Endoplasmic Reticulum
—Nucleolus
—Nucleus
—Nuclear Pore
—Glycogen
—Smooth Endoplasmic Reticulum
—Mitochondrion
—Basement Membrane
—Collagen

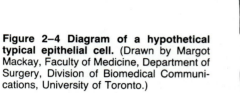

Figure 2–4 Diagram of a hypothetical typical epithelial cell. (Drawn by Margot Mackay, Faculty of Medicine, Department of Surgery, Division of Biomedical Communications, University of Toronto.)

scope has changed all this; the cell's appearance has been changed from a barren wilderness to that of a structure resembling a large industrial city with its factories, warehouses, streets, and powerhouses (Fig. 2–5).

STRUCTURE OF THE NORMAL CELL

The Cell or Plasma Membrane

Each cell is surrounded by a *cell or plasma membrane* that is composed of a complex protein-lipid combination (Fig. 2–6). The plasma membrane is not a rigid structure and its movement allows phagocytosis, a process whereby prolongations of the cell surround particles and envelop them to form a vacuole in which the contents are digested. Likewise, motility of cells is a function of plasma-membrane movement. This is well illustrated by the ameboid movement of the white blood cells.

At the ultrastructural level, small invaginations of the cell membrane can become nipped off to

form vesicles called phagosomes. In this way, small quantities of fluid may be imbibed by a process known as endocytosis.

The cell membrane has other important functions. It contains specific antigens by which the body is able to *recognize* its own cells and tolerate them. The cells from another genetically different individual are regarded as aliens and are attacked (see Chapter 6). The cell membrane is also concerned with *adhesiveness,* which is a factor that induces cells of like constitution to stick together. This property can be well demonstrated experimentally: if the cells of an embryo are separated from each other and then are allowed to come together again under suitable conditions, like cells tend to aggregate to re-form organs and tissues. This affinity that cells have for their own kind must be an important mechanism in the development and maintenance of the architecture of multicellular animals. But not all cells behave in this manner. The mature cells of the blood do not stick to each other, and the lack of adhesiveness exhibited by cancer cells allows them to wander off and infiltrate freely into the

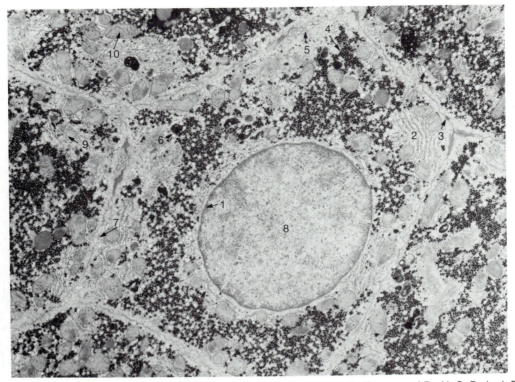

Figure 2–5 Survey of normal human liver. Parts of six cells are shown (×10,000). (Courtesy of Dr. Y. C. Bedard, Department of Pathology, Mount Sinai Hospital, Toronto.)

surrounding tissues. This characteristic allows cancer cells to spread and kill.

The cell membrane acts as an *exchange surface* across which cell constituents are interchanged with those of the extracellular fluids. Thus, the cell membrane acts as a chemical barrier as well as a mechanical one, and it is this function that is responsible for the maintenance of the characteristic chemical composition of the interior of the cell. Potassium, magnesium, and phosphate ions are present in high concentration in the cytoplasm. In contrast, the extracellular fluids are rich in sodium, chloride, and bicarbonate ions. The cell membrane is able to extrude sodium ions and thereby allows the potassium to accumulate within the cell. This mechanism, which is sometimes known as the *sodium pump*, requires energy. The integrity and normal functions of the cell membrane are therefore important factors in maintaining this special chemical composition of the cell substance.

Important components of the cell membrane are proteins, the exposed portion of which acts as a *cell or surface receptor*. Separate receptors exist

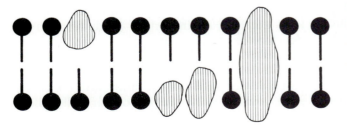

Figure 2–6 Diagrammatic representation of the plasma membrane. The membrane is shown as a double layer of phospholipid molecules with their hydrophilic (water-loving) ends pointing outward and their hydrophobic (water-hating) ends facing inward. Globular proteins are partially or completely embedded in the lipid. This concept of a fluid lipid bilayer with embedded protein was described by Singer and Nicolson (Science, *175:*720, 1972). (Drawn by Margot Mackay, Faculty of Medicine, Department of Surgery, Division of Biomedical Communications, University of Toronto.)

for drugs, toxins, hormones, growth factors, bacteria, viruses, and many other agents. One group of receptors (termed integrins) are specific for extracellular substances such as laminin. The number of receptors for any particular agent varies from cell type to cell type. This explains why hormones, for instance, act on particular target cells, *i.e.*, cells that have suitable receptors. Furthermore, the number of receptors on any cell type is not static and can vary according to many circumstances. A reduction of the number of receptors for a particular hormone renders the cell resistant to the action of that hormone. Thus, insulin resistance is a factor in some types of diabetes mellitus.

The attachment of an agent to its receptor sets in motion a series of chemical events that culminates in a specific response, *e.g.*, secretion of a hormone, mitosis of the cell, or the cell's differentiation. The events that follow attachment of an agent to its receptor vary from one instance to another. With many protein or polypeptide hormones, there is stimulation of the catalytic enzyme adenylate cyclase, the activity of which leads to the formation of adenosine 3':5'-cyclic monophosphate, widely known simply as cAMP (Fig. 2–7). This acts as a second messenger that stimulates the cell to appropriate activity. Not all cell membrane receptors are coupled to adenylate cyclase; their activity may involve systems that regulate intracellular calcium. With steroid hormones, the specific cell receptors are in the cytoplasm.

The *cytokines* are a group of polypeptides produced by one cell that acts locally on another cell. They have been most studied in relation to the immune response and inflammation (see Chapter 6). Cytokines produced by monocytes have been called monokines; those produced by lymphocytes have been termed lymphokines. The term *interleukins* is now preferred because they are produced by one type of white cell and act on another type. Nevertheless, the situation is now less clear as research has revealed that interleukins are also produced by other cell types (*e.g.*, keratinocytes) and act on many others (*e.g.*, interleukin-1 acts on the brain and induces fever).

One fascinating aspect of cell receptor function deserves mention. It has been found that opiate (morphine) receptors are present in certain areas of the central nervous system. It seems that the brain can manufacture substances (called *enkephalins*) that have a morphine-like action and are normal chemical transmitters within the brain. This helps explain how the appreciation of pain can vary according to circumstances. A cut finger in the kitchen can be extremely painful, and yet during the heat of battle a whole limb can be lost almost without notice.

The Cytoplasm

The *cytoplasm*, or *cytosol*, is that part of the protoplasm not included in the nucleus. It is subdivided into many compartments by membranes that closely resemble the cell membrane in structure. The major component is termed the *cytocavitary network*; it consists of a series of membrane-bound sacs, channels, and vesicles that are

Figure 2–7 The second-messenger concept. Many hormones act first by becoming attached to specific receptor sites on the membranes of target cells. Thus, adrenal cells have receptors that "recognize" adrenocorticotropin. The enzyme adenylate cyclase is activated in the cell membrane and passes into the cytoplasm, where it catalyzes the formation of cyclic AMP, which acts as a second messenger. In some cells it leads to enzyme activation. Thus, in the liver, phosphorylase is activated and leads to the formation of glucose from glycogen. This is a mechanism by which epinephrine causes the release of glucose from the liver cell. Cyclic AMP appears to act also by stimulating the expression of genetic information. It may therefore be regarded as a type of chemical switch that turns on the cell to perform specific functions.

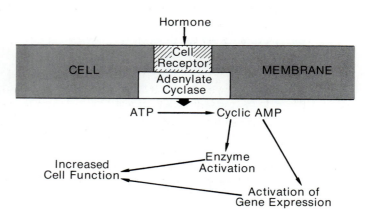

continuous with the outer layer of the nuclear membrane and the cell membrane, either directly or via vesicles that bud off and fuse with other components of the system. Its major components are the endoplasmic reticulum (rough and smooth) and the Golgi complex. *Mitochondria* are the other cytoplasmic membrane-bound structures.

Endoplasmic Reticulum

This consists of a series of membranes that enclose an intercommunicating series of tubes and vesicles (Fig. 2–8). In most areas, ribosomes are attached to the endoplasmic reticulum, which therefore appears rough; this part is known as the granular or *rough endoplasmic reticulum*. Ribosomes are granules 15 nm in diameter, contain ribonucleic acid (RNA), and play a very important part in cell metabolism; it is in relation to

them that protein synthesis occurs. Some of the ribosomes are not attached to endoplasmic reticulum but appear to be lying free in the cytoplasm to form small aggregates (*polysomes*). These polysomes are concerned with the formation of protein that is retained within the cell for its own requirements. Protein produced for export is synthesized in the rough endoplasmic reticulum, passes into the Golgi apparatus, and is packaged to form secretory granules.

The endoplasmic reticulum and its associated ribosomal granules cannot be distinguished in the ordinary "paraffin" sections used in routine pathology. The ribonucleoprotein content, however, can be distinguished by its basophilia (having an affinity for basic dyes) with hematoxylin. It follows that the cytoplasm of cells actively engaged in protein synthesis appears mauve or blue in hematoxylin and eosin (H & E) sections.

The other component of the endoplasmic reticulum forms a complex lattice of tubules that have

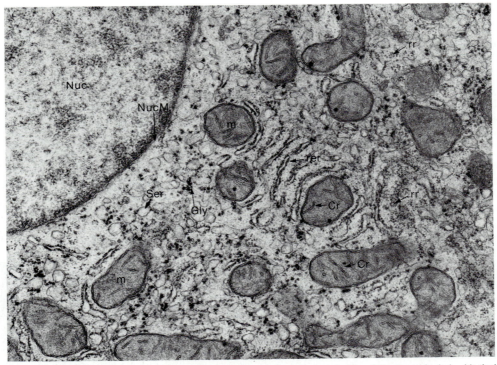

Figure 2–8 Liver cell showing part of its nucleus (Nuc) and cytoplasmic organelles. Mitochondria (m) with their cristae (Cr) are shown along with rough endoplasmic reticulum (rer) to which are attached ribosomes. Smooth endoplasmic reticulum (Ser) is associated with glycogen granules (Gly). Some ribosomes appear free in the cytoplasm and are forming rosettes (rr). Note also the nuclear membrane (NucM) surrounding the nucleus (×40,000). (Courtesy of Dr. Y. C. Bedard, Department of Pathology, Mount Sinai Hospital, Toronto.)

no attached ribosomes and therefore appear smooth. This is called the *smooth endoplasmic reticulum;* its functions involve many metabolic processes including conjugation of bilirubin, detoxification of drugs, lipoprotein synthesis, and steroid metabolism. In striated muscle, the smooth endoplasmic reticulum forms the sarcoplasmic reticulum that is involved in recapture of calcium during muscular activity.

The Golgi Complex

The Golgi complex is best developed in glandular cells and is usually situated close to the nucleus on the side nearest to the lumen. In routine paraffin sections, the Golgi complex is not stained and appears as a clear zone known as the "negative Golgi." On electron microscopy, the Golgi complex appears as a series of curved, flattened sacs arranged in stacks from which vesicles bud. Newly formed glycoproteins

formed in the sacs of the rough endoplasmic reticulum pass into the sacs of the Golgi complex and are modified there. For instance, a carbohydrate moiety may be added or removed, or lipid may be added. The finished product is then packaged into vesicles. Their fate depends on the type of cell involved. If the contents are protein for export, the vesicles (secretory granules) fuse with the cell membrane, and their contents are discharged by the process of *exocytosis;* the membrane component is added to that of the cell membrane. In this way, damaged membrane can be replaced. Other vesicles remain in the cell as *primary lysosomes* or in melanocytes as *melanosomes.*

Lysosomes

Lysosomes are round, membrane-bound vesicles containing lytic enzymes that act at a low pH (Figs. 2–9 and 2–10). The enzymes include

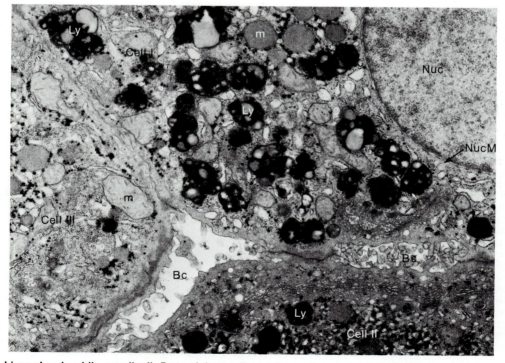

Figure 2–9 Liver showing bile canaliculi. Parts of three adjacent liver cells are shown; between them are the bile canaliculi (Bc), which ultimately drain into the bile duct. Short, irregular microvilli are seen projecting into the lumen. One liver cell contains numerous lysosomes (Ly). Also shown are parts of one nucleus (Nuc) with the double-layered nuclear membrane (NucM), and mitochondria (m) (×17,500). (Courtesy of Dr. Y. C. Bedard, Department of Pathology, Mount Sinai Hospital, Toronto.)

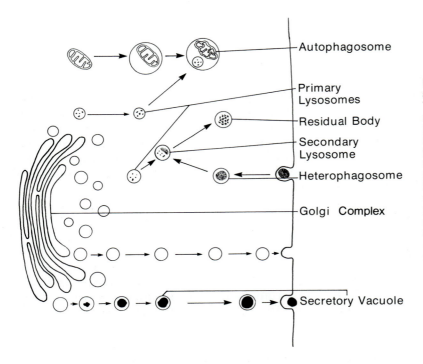

- Autophagosome
- Primary Lysosomes
- Residual Body
- Secondary Lysosome
- Heterophagosome
- Golgi Complex
- Secretory Vacuole

Figure 2–10 The Golgi complex (Golgi apparatus) and its possible functions. This diagram depicts the Golgi complex as a series of flattened sacs from which numerous vacuoles arise. Some vacuoles contain secretory material that has been synthesized in the endoplasmic reticulum. Some vacuoles appear to be empty and travel to the cell surface, where their membranes fuse with the cell membrane. Other vacuoles contain lytic enzymes and become primary lysosomes. These fuse with autophagosomes or heterophagosomes to form secondary lysosomes. Undigested material remains in residual bodies. (Drawn by Margot Mackay, Faculty of Medicine, Department of Surgery, Division of Biomedical Communications, University of Toronto.)

Figure 2–11 Outline of the metabolic pathways involved in energy production. The entire process in the oxidation of glycogen to CO_2 and H_2O can be considered as occurring in two phases. The first, which requires no oxygen (anaerobic), results in the formation of pyruvate and is known as *glycolysis*. If oxygen is not available, pyruvic acid is converted into lactic acid. The second phase, which requires oxygen (aerobic), is known as the *Krebs cycle.* Products of carbohydrate, fat, and protein metabolism are fed into the Krebs cycle, and the energy generated ultimately appears in the form of ATP. The hexose monophosphate shunt is shown on the right as an alternative pathway and results in the formation of ribulose 5-phosphate. This is an aerobic process and is important in the metabolism of white cells and red cells. Various genetic defects are known that result in hemolytic anemia or incompetent polymorphs, which are unable to destroy bacteria. NAD, nicotinamide adenine dinucleotide; NADH$_2$, dihydronicotinamide adenine dinucleotide; Pi, inorganic phosphate; ADP, adenosine diphosphate; ATP, adenosine triphosphate. (From Walter, J. B., and Israel, M. S.: General Pathology. 6th ed. Edinburgh, Churchill Livingstone, 1987.)

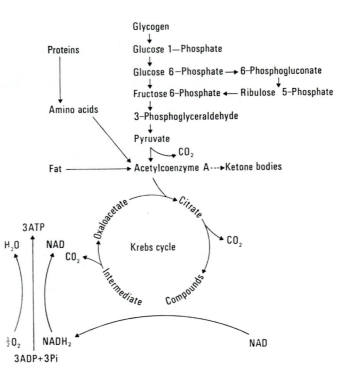

acid phosphatase and many proteolytic enzymes. They are formed from the Golgi complex and are termed *primary lysosomes* when they first enter the cytoplasm. They cannot normally be seen in paraffin sections, but in certain cells, polymorphonuclear leukocytes for instance, lysosomes are visible as the characteristic granules. Particles ingested by a cell during phagocytosis appear as membrane-bound vesicles, and fusion with a primary lysosome results in the formation of a *secondary lysosome*. In this way, the lysosomes are an important source of the enzymes necessary for the digestion of phagocytosed material.

Likewise, when parts of a cell wear out or are damaged, they also are enclosed in lysosomal bodies. Such lysosomes containing remnants of degenerate cell structure are called *cytolysosomes*, or *autophagocytic vacuoles.* Release of lysosomal enzymes from dead cells plays an important part in the digestion of dead material. The enzymes may also activate mediators of acute inflammation (Chapter 5). Under some circumstances, lysosomal enzymes, particularly those derived from neutrophils, can cause severe tissue damage (see Arthus reaction, Chapter 6).

Mitochondria

These rod-shaped bodies have a characteristic appearance (Fig. 2–8); their complex internal structure is a reflection of their function. They contain all the enzymes of the Krebs cycle and of the terminal electron transport system. The Krebs cycle, illustrated in Figure 2–11, is a system whereby the products of carbohydrate, fat, and protein metabolism are oxidized to produce energy. This process requires oxygen and is therefore called *aerobic respiration* or *oxidative phosphorylation,* since the energy is stored in the form of high-energy bonds of adenosine triphosphate (ATP). The energy can be released by the breakdown of ATP and utilized whenever the cell performs any kind of work. The mitochondria are therefore the powerhouses of the cell and are among the first structures to be affected when adverse conditions prevail. An interesting feature of mitochondrial structure is that these bodies also contain some DNA that appears to replicate during cell division. Some people have held it to

indicate that mitochondria originated from symbiotic bacteria.

The Cytoplasmic Matrix

The cytoplasmic matrix consists of the material not included within the nucleus, the cytocavitary system, or the mitochondria. It contains lipid, free ribosomes (producing protein for the cells' own use), and glycogen. Most important are the filaments and microtubules of the cytoskeletal and cytocontractile system.

Intracytoplasmic Filaments. The myofilaments consist of thick *myosin filaments* (12 to 15 nm in diameter), thin *actin filaments* (6 to 8 nm in diameter), and other filaments containing neither myosin nor actin. They are 8 to 11 nm in diameter and for this reason are called *intermediate filaments.* The myosin and actin filaments are best developed in muscle cells and are important in muscle contraction. They are, however, also present in other cell types and are involved in movement, *e.g.,* phagocytosis, pinocytosis, and mitosis.

Intermediate filaments have attracted much attention because their composition varies from one cell type to another. Their detection by the use of specific monoclonal antibodies, with the immunoperoxidase technique, can be used to identify cell types and tumors derived from them. *Cytokeratins* are largely confined to epithelial cells. Macromolecular cytokeratins are particularly characteristic of keratinizing squamous epithelium. *Vimentin* filaments are the predominant class found in mesenchymal cells other than muscle. *Desmin* is characteristic of muscle. *Neurofilaments* are found in nerve cells; *glial* filaments are found in astrocytes.

Microtubules. Microtubules are hollow noncontractile rods (diameter 24 nm) that form a *cytoskeleton.* They are an important component of cilia and the spindle formed during mitosis. The skeleton is not rigid, however, because the microtubules are composed of a protein called tubulin, and rapid polymerization and depolymerization of its components gives the structures their ability to involve movement, *e.g.,* during mitosis as the chromosomes separate.

The Nucleus

Situated within the cell and enclosed by a membrane is the nucleus, an important structure because it contains in chemical form the coded information that is handed down from one cell to its progeny and from one generation to the next. The chemical that performs this function is deoxyribonucleic acid (DNA). Like the RNA of the cytoplasm, this substance is basophilic in H & E–stained sections, and the nucleus invariably stains deep blue. This blue material was named *chromatin* before the discovery of DNA, and the term is still convenient and in common use.

Chemical Structure of DNA

The chemical structure of DNA is well known. The molecule is composed of a double helix formed by two polynucleotide chains, each chain consisting of monounits or nucleotides (Fig. 2–12). Each nucleotide consists of a base combined with deoxyribose sugar and phosphate. The common bases are either purines (adenine and guanine) or pyrimidines (cytosine and thymine). The two polynucleotide chains are united by their bases, with adenine pairing with thymidine and guanine pairing with cytosine (Fig. 2–12). When DNA replicates, the double helix unwinds, and each strand acts as a template for the formation of a new strand. Again, cytosine pairs with guanine, and adenine pairs with thymine.

Role of Nucleic Acids As Genetic Material

The DNA of the nucleus contains genetic information that is passed via RNA into the cytoplasm where it is used in the manufacture of proteins—often enzymes—of exact composition. The word *gene* is used to describe a hypothetical unit of heredity for any single characteristic. Genes are an expression of the information contained within the DNA molecule. The order of the bases in DNA constitutes the genetic code, a sequence of three bases designating a single

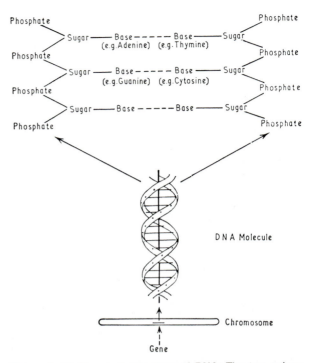

Figure 2–12 Chemical structure of DNA. The two polynucleotide chains are united by their bases, the order of which constitutes the genetic code. (After Watson, J. D., and Crick, F. H. C. Reprinted by permission of Nature, *171*:737. Copyright © 1953 Macmillan Magazines Ltd.)

amino acid. A type of RNA is manufactured in the nucleus in the presence of DNA-dependent RNA polymerase. This process is called *transcription,* and the RNA is modeled after one of the polynucleotide chains of DNA, which acts as a template. The base sequence of the RNA is complementary to that of DNA, *i.e.,* cytosine corresponds to guanine, but uracil rather than thymine corresponds to adenine. This RNA, the primary transcript, is modified by removal of unwanted segments (corresponding to introns) and passes as messenger RNA (mRNA) into the cytoplasm where it becomes associated with a group of ribosomes (a polysome) (Fig. 2–13). Here protein synthesis occurs. Each triplet, or codon, of the RNA base order codes for one amino acid. As the ribosomes "read along" the RNA molecule, successive amino acids are added to an ever-increasing polypeptide chain. In this way, a protein of exact composition is built up. The actual addition of each amino acid is effected

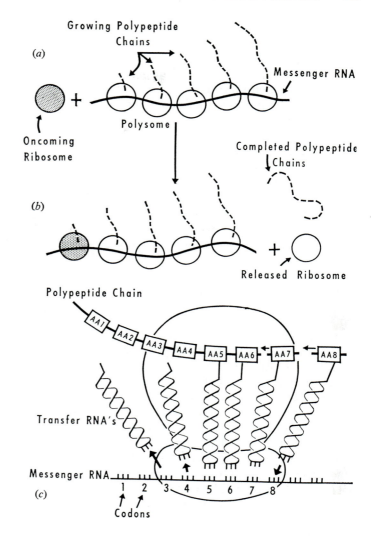

Figure 2–13 Schematic model of protein synthesis. In *(a)* and *(b)*, a long single-stranded molecule of messenger RNA (mRNA) is seen associated with a group of ribosomes to form a polysome. As each ribosome moves along the mRNA, an ever-growing polypeptide chain is produced. In *(c)*, a single ribosome is depicted as a combination of two particles of unequal size. The sequence of bases of the mRNA forms triplets, or codons, which for the sake of clarity are drawn as groups of three upright lines. Each molecule of transfer RNA (tRNA) is composed of a long thread bent on itself to form a helical structure. At one end of the molecule there is a particular amino acid (AA1, AA2, and so on), and at the other end, where it is bent on itself, there are three unpaired bases that form an anticodon. Each codon of the mRNA is "recognized" by a corresponding anticodon of a tRNA. In this way, specific amino acids are added to the polypeptide chain in a specific linear sequence determined by the mRNA, which is itself modeled on the nuclear DNA. (Drawn by the Department of Art as Applied to Medicine, University of Toronto, after Warner, J. R., and Soeiro, R.: Reprinted by permission of The New England Journal of Medicine, 276:613, 1967; and Nirenberg, M. W.: The Living Cell. San Francisco, W. H. Freeman & Company, 1965.)

by another type of RNA (transfer RNA, or tRNA), a separate form of which exists for each of the amino acids. This process is described as *translation*, for the code of the DNA finally appears legible in the form of a polypeptide chain (Fig. 2–13).

Thus, the genetic code of DNA consists of codons that determine the insertion of particular amino acids in the peptide chain. The sequence of the codons is collinear with the sequence of amino acids. Codons responsible for an entire peptide chain form a group called a *cistron*. It is believed that a number of cistrons are grouped together to form a larger unit, the *operon*.

Control of Gene Action

It is evident that each newly created cell of the body contains the necessary information for the manufacture of every protein of which the body is composed. That all cells do not do so at all times is evidence that there is some very adequate control mechanism. For example, erythroid cells manufacture hemoglobin, and plasma cells form immunoglobulin. Nevertheless, it is not surprising that under abnormal circumstances, cells produce substances that are alien to their accustomed products. It is for this reason that a tumor of the lung can produce hormones normally produced only by the pituitary. Many examples of this phenomenon will be seen later.

Some genes lead to the production of either enzymes or proteins used in the metabolism of the cell. These are termed *structural genes*. It has been found that a group of genes can be closely linked together and can either function together or be completely repressed, *i.e.*, no mRNA is produced. Gene expression can be regulated at many steps: transcription (the most important), RNA processing, RNA transfer to the cytoplasm, and translation. Cells contain specific DNA binding proteins, the function of which is to turn genes off or turn them on. In humans, there is much more DNA present in the chromosomes than appears to be necessary to encode for all the proteins that are present in the body. The length of DNA containing information for one protein is not continuous but is broken up into segments (called *exons*), which are separated by long stretches of other intervening DNA (called *introns*) (Fig. 2–14). The RNA transcribed in the nucleus may be ten times or more longer than is needed for translation in the cytoplasm. The cell removes this excess RNA and splices the remainder to form mRNA. The function of the excess nucleic acid is not known. Some of the excess RNA probably provides signals that say in effect "start here" or "stop here." What other messages, if any, there are in these silent areas of DNA is not known. The subject is of more than academic interest. Current research wherein human DNA is recombined with bacterial DNA requires detailed knowledge of the structure of the DNA that contains the necessary information for one gene together with its regulatory switches (see Chapter 3).

Chromosomes

The DNA molecules are not lying free in the nucleus but are contained in long threads called *chromosomes*. Each resting somatic cell contains a definite number of chromosomes, the diploid or 2N number. This corresponds to the normal amount of DNA. In humans, the diploid number is 46; of these, 23 are derived from each parent. Two chromosomes, which are related specifically to sex, are called the *sex chromosomes*. One is considerably larger than the other and is called an X chromosome, whereas the smaller one is the Y chromosome. In humans, females have two X chromosomes; males have one X and one Y. The remaining 22 pairs are identical in appearance in both sexes and are called the *autosomes*.

Each resting somatic nucleus contains a constant number of chromosomes (the diploid number, which is twice the haploid number). Certain exceptions to this condition are found. As a person ages, some cells of the liver contain more chromosomes than normal. When a cell contains three or more times the haploid number of chromosomes, the condition is termed *polyploidy*. Thus, some liver cells have large nuclei containing 92 chromosomes. A similar event occurs in tumor cells.

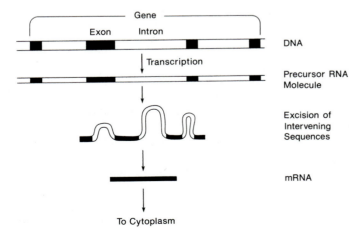

Figure 2–14 Transcription of genetic information. Diagrammatic representation of a gene, showing exons and introns. After the formation of a precursor RNA molecule, the intervening sequences coded by the introns are excised, and messenger RNA (mRNA) is assembled before being passed into the cytoplasm for translation. (Drawing by Rasa Skudra, Artlab Communication Inc., Toronto.)

During the period between cell divisions, the chromosomes are present in the nucleus as long, drawn-out threads. These are not visible as such when the light microscope is used, but in some areas along the thread there is sufficient coiling for the condensation of material to render these areas visible as basophilic chromatin dots in the nucleus. Such chromatin is thought to represent regions of the chromosomes that are condensed and relatively inert metabolically. The remainder of the nucleus is lightly stained, and the chromatin appears dispersed. The actual morphology of the nucleus varies considerably from one cell to another, and an assessment of function can be made from nuclear structure. Thus, in active cells, *e.g.,* cancer and nerve cells, the nucleus contains little condensed chromatin and is described as "vesicular." In inactive cells, such as small lymphocytes and spermatozoa, the condensed chromatin occupies much of the nucleus, which consequently is deeply basophilic and small.

Some very large cells, *e.g.,* megakaryocytes of the bone marrow, contain many nuclei and are called *multinucleate giant cells.*

Apart from DNA, the nucleus contains RNA, and some of this may appear as a separate structure called the *nucleolus.* This structure is particularly prominent in cells that are active metabolically. Nucleoli are therefore prominent features in the nerve cells and in many cancer cells.

The Barr Body. Dr. Murray Barr first noticed a discrete mass of chromatin in the nuclei of cells from a female animal, a mass that was not present in the nuclei of the male. This can be easily demonstrated in the human by examining suitably stained cells scraped from the buccal mucosa; it appears as a demilune on the nuclear membrane (Fig. 2–15). This chromatin can be shown to be formed by an X chromosome that is tightly condensed and mostly inactive. The normal female has two X chromosomes, and one of these is extended and active, whereas the other forms the Barr body. This hypothesis (now known as the *Lyon hypothesis*) was first proposed by Dr. Mary Lyon, and it appears that the inactivation of one of the X chromosomes is random and occurs in each cell in early embryonic life. Hence, in the normal female, about one half of

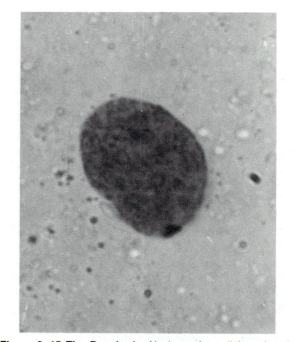

Figure 2–15 The Barr body. Nucleus of a cell from female buccal mucosal smear showing the sex chromatin mass on the nuclear membrane. (Courtesy of Dr. Nigel H. Kemp. From Walter, J. B., and Israel, M. S.: General Pathology. 6th ed. Edinburgh, Churchill Livingstone, 1987.)

the cells carry an active maternal X chromosome, whereas the other half carry an active paternal X chromosome. The inactive chromosome divides later than do other chromosomes during cell division, and its descendants follow the same pattern. It occasionally happens that an individual has more than two X chromosomes, and in these cases the number of Barr bodies seen in a cell is equal to the total number of X chromosomes less one. Examination of the buccal smear is an important investigation in cases of chromosomal abnormality. Cells possessing a Barr body are also called *chromatin positive.*

THE MONONUCLEAR PHAGOCYTE SYSTEM

The concept of a system of cells widely scattered throughout the body and having as its main obvious function the property of phagocytosis is not new. The term reticuloendothelial system was introduced by Aschoff. Its constituent cells have the ability to phagocytose particles and extract soluble dyes injected into the blood. It includes circulating monocytes and various fixed cells situated in many parts of the body. They line blood sinuses in the liver and spleen and therefore appear to be a type of endothelial cell. They are associated with lymphoid tissue and with the fine reticulin fibers that form the supporting framework of these structures. From these associations the term reticuloendothelial system was coined. However, the term is far from ideal because the system does not include the ordinary endothelial cells of the vascular system, nor do its cells produce reticulin. More recently, the alternative name *mononuclear phagocyte system* has been proposed. Its members are mononuclear cells derived from the bone marrow. They are phagocytic and include the blood monocytes, fixed tissue histiocytes, and certain cells that line sinusoids in various organs. When its members become phagocytic, they form the macrophages commonly encountered in many inflammatory and reparative processes (Fig. 2–

16). The majority of them are derived from blood monocytes. The term mononuclear phagocyte system has now come into common use. Nevertheless, it also is not ideal. Some of its members are not phagocytic in their resting phase (*e.g.*, histiocytes), whereas others are multinucleate. The system includes fixed cells and wandering or mobile cells.

Fixed Cells. These comprise cells that line the sinuses in liver (Kupffer cells), spleen, bone marrow, and lymph nodes (sinus-lining or littoral cells) and also resting histiocytes that lie in most connective tissues of the body. The histiocytes, also called histiocytic reticulum cells, do not form reticulin fibers but are capable of becoming macrophages. In the central nervous system, the equivalent cells are called microglia.

Wandering or Mobile Cells. These are the blood monocytes.

The cells of the mononuclear phagocyte system are intimately connected with lymphoid cells. Hence, it is convenient to group them together as the lymphoreticular system, with spleen and lymph nodes being the principal members.

THE EXTRACELLULAR MATRIX

The intercellular spaces contain fibers (collagen and elastic fibers), and an amorphous interfibrillary matrix, often called ground substance, made up of proteoglycans, noncollagenous glycoproteins, solutes such as electrolytes and glucose that are being conveyed to cells for metabolism or from cells for excretion, and water. It contains approximately one third of the body's water.

Collagen

Collagen as a whole forms about one third of the body's total protein; it is characterized by having a high content of glycine and hydroxyproline. Hydroxyproline is an amino acid that is not found to any extent in other proteins, and an estimate of the amount of it in hydrolysates of a tissue may therefore be used to measure the amount of collagen present. Collagen is not a single substance but consists rather of a group of fibrillar glycoproteins. Each molecule is composed of three coiled polypeptide chains, each

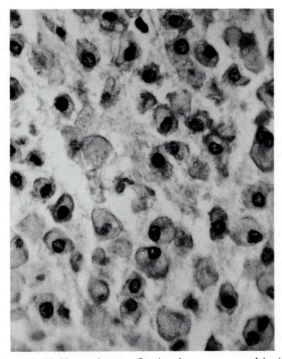

Figure 2–16 Macrophages. Section from an area of brain damage showing many macrophages that are engaged in removing dead brain tissue. The cells have abundant cytoplasm (×500).

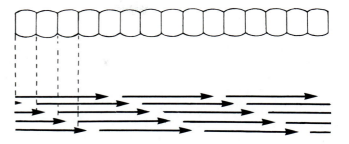

Figure 2–17 Formation of collagen fibril. Diagram to illustrate how the lateral arrangement of procollagen molecules, depicted as arrows, results in the formation of banded collagen fibril. (From Walter, J. B., and Israel, M. S.: General Pathology. 6th ed. Edinburgh, Churchill Livingstone, 1987.)

chain being formed separately under the influence of a particular mRNA. Collagen molecules are synthesized in fibroblasts and other cells, and after excretion into the intercellular space, the molecules polymerize with their neighbors (Fig.

2–17). In all, over 15 different types of collagen are known. There are many chemical steps in the synthesis of collagen, and an enzyme defect may lead to defective collagen formation. In addition, vitamin C is essential, so that collagen synthesis is impaired in scurvy.

Type I collagen is the most abundant and forms the major component of tough connective tissues such as dermis, tendon, cornea, and fascia. It also forms the major organic component of bone. It has a characteristic banded appearance on electron microscopy (Fig. 2–18). *Type II collagen* forms the major component of hyaline cartilage. *Type III collagen* forms the reticulin fibers of the stroma of many organs (*e.g.,* liver and lymph nodes, Fig. 2–19); it is also found in the early stage of granulation tissue formation. Reticulin fibers are commonly stained by a silver impregnation method.

Of the nonfibrillar collagens, type IV is the best known; it forms a major component of basement membranes.

Elastic Fibers

Elastic fibers are broader than are collagen fibers and consist of amorphous glycoprotein with embedded elastin; they give the tissue flexibility, *e.g.,* in the lung and aorta. On light microscopy, they stain deep red with eosin and can be specifically demonstrated by staining with orcein, which renders them black.

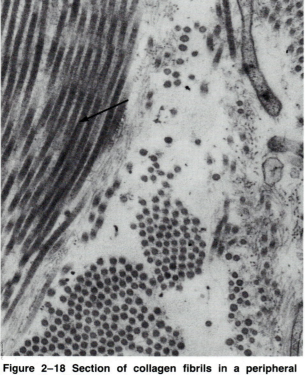

Figure 2–18 Section of collagen fibrils in a peripheral nerve. The fibrils show the characteristic cross-banding (arrow), which is best seen where the fibrils are cut longitudinally. Part of the cytoplasm of a Schwann cell (Sch) is also shown (×12,000). (Courtesy of Dr. N. B. Rewcastle, Department of Pathology, University of Calgary, Alberta, Canada.)

Proteoglycans

Proteoglycans (often called mucoproteins) consist of a core of protein with attached glucosa-

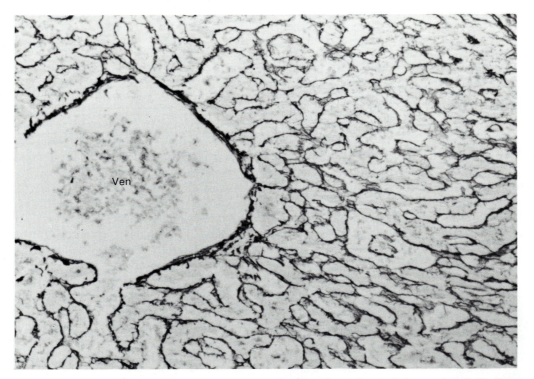

Figure 2–19 Reticulin fibers in liver. This section of liver has been stained by a silver technique; only reticulin fibers, which are stained black, can be seen clearly. The spaces between the reticulin fibers are occupied by hepatocytes and sinusoids that drain blood into a venule (Ven).

minoglycans (often called acid mucopolysaccharides). They are gelatinous, slimy substances and have water binding and lubricating functions. Genetic errors in glucosaminoglycan synthesis form a group of diseases known traditionally as the mucopolysaccharidoses.

Noncollagenous Glycoproteins

This is a heterogeneous group of proteins of which the *fibronectins* form an important component. They are a group of glycoproteins that have been described as forming a "molecular glue" because they are important in binding together the fibers of the intercellular spaces as well as being involved in many cell-to-cell interactions. They aid the adhesion of cells to fibers and perhaps guide migrating cells. They form cross links with fibrin in clot formation. *Laminin* is a similar protein found in basement membranes.

CELL DIVISION

Mitosis

Before cell division occurs, the DNA molecules unwind, and each half acts as a template for the manufacture of the corresponding half. In this way, the amount of DNA is doubled. The chromosomes divide and become double structures called *chromatids*; these are joined together by a single *centromere*. The chromosomes become coiled along their whole length, thereby becoming shorter, thicker, and therefore visible. The cell has now entered the first phase of mitosis, *prophase*. Meanwhile, two centrioles have migrated, one to each pole of the cell, and microtubules develop in association with them. Each centriole looks like an *aster*, or star (Fig. 2–20).

The nucleoli and the nuclear membrane disappear next, and the cell enters into *metaphase*. By this time, the centrioles are at opposite poles of the cell, and their associated microtubules

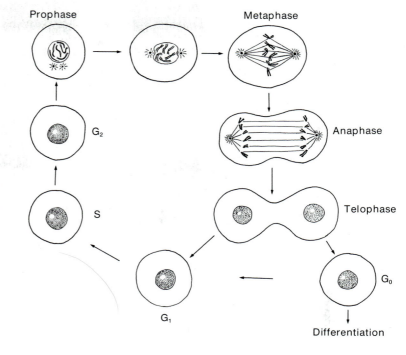

Figure 2–20 The cell cycle. DNA reduplication occurs during the synthesis (S stage). This is followed by a short resting stage (G_2) before the cell enters mitosis. After division, the daughter cells may enter the second resting stage (G_1) before recommencing DNA synthesis. Other daughter cells can pass into a resting phase (G_0) and after a period can either re-enter the cell cycle or become differentiated and cease to be capable of mitosis.

Prophase

Metaphase

G_2

Anaphase

S

Telophase

G_1

G_0

Differentiation

enter the nuclear region where the split chromosomes become arranged along an imaginary equatorial plate that bisects the cells. The microtubules are attached to the centromeres, and in this way the spindle is formed.

During the next phase, *anaphase,* each set of chromatids, now again called chromosomes, is pulled by the microtubules of the spindle to either pole of the cell. The final stage (*telophase*) involves division of the cytoplasm of the cell and reconstitution of the nuclear membrane of each daughter cell.

It can readily be understood how during mitosis each chromosome reduplicates itself exactly, and the two daughter cells contain an identical quota of nuclear material. Each DNA molecule is also reduplicated exactly. Should an error occur during mitosis such that an abnormality of the DNA is produced, the process is called a *somatic mutation.* Presumably, this is related to an abnormal sequence of the bases in the DNA molecule.

Meiosis

In the testis and ovary, the process of cell division is more complex and is called meiosis.

The process results in cells containing only half the number of chromosomes (the "N" or haploid number, *i.e.,* 23 in humans) and half the amount of DNA. These cells develop into gametes— either sperm or ova. With fertilization, the diploid number of chromosomes (46) is restored.

During meiosis, the chromosomes become paired off into 23 pairs, with one of each moving into each of the daughter cells. Which chromosome of each pair migrates into which daughter cell is random; thus, the total number of possible combinations is extremely great. Furthermore, during the complex process of meiosis, portions of one chromosome sometimes move and are replaced by corresponding portions of the homologous chromosome. This is termed *crossing over* and together with the random distribution of each of the pairs of chromosomes within a single gamete is responsible for the tremendous variation that is seen in the progeny of individuals produced by sexual reproduction.

It sometimes happens that during meiosis a pair of chromosomes fail to separate and both are drawn into one daughter cell. This is called *nondisjunction,* and it results in one gamete's having an extra chromosome while the other is deficient. Sometimes fragments of chromosomes are lost (by a process called *deletion*) or become attached to another chromosome (by a process called *translocation*). If two breaks occur in the same chromosome, the ends may join together to form a ring chromosome. Chromosomal breaks that result in deletion, translocation, or the formation of ring chromosomes can be induced by the action of ionizing radiation, by certain drugs, and by viruses. It is of interest that it is these same agents that are capable of causing cancer.

The next chapter deals with some of the effects of genetic errors and chromosomal abnormalities.

Summary

- Each of the three primitive germ layers (ectoderm, mesoderm, and endoderm) differentiates to form epithelial or mesenchymal (connective tissue) structures.
- The plasma membrane is an important exchange surface and contains numerous specific receptors; attachment of specific antigen, *e.g.*, a hormone, stimulates or modifies the function of the cell.
- The rough endoplasmic reticulum is concerned with protein synthesis; the Golgi complex packages the product for export.
- The smooth endoplasmic reticulum has many functions, including steroid metabolism and drug detoxification.
- Mitochondria are the site of energy production.
- Lysosomes contain lytic enzymes.
- Intermediate filaments are important intracytoplasmic filaments; detection of the various types helps identify cell type in tumors.
- Transcription of the nuclear DNA produces a primary transcript RNA that is processed to mRNA and passed to the cytoplasmic ribosomes for translation to protein.
- Chromosomes contain 22 pairs of autosomes and one pair of sex chromosomes: XX in the female, XY in the male. One X in the female is active in the interphase cell, the other is inactive and forms the Barr body. Which X is inactivated in each cell (and all its descendants) is determined early in development (the Lyon hypothesis).
- The cells of the mononuclear phagocyte system are all derived from bone marrow cells. Included are monocytes and histiocytes; macrophages are derived from them.
- The extracellular matrix contains fibers (collagen and elastic) and noncollagenous glycoproteins such as fibronectins.
- The collagens are coiled proteins formed by several types of cells. Type I, derived from fibroblast type cells, is banded and present in fibrous tissue, osteoid, and tissues in which strength is required. Type II collagen occurs in hyaline cartilage. Type III collagen forms reticulin. Other types of collagen are nonfibrillar and form basement membranes, being synthesized by endothelial and epithelial cells.
- Mitosis is seen in somatic cells and has four recognized morphologic stages: prophase, metaphase, anaphase, and telophase. Meiosis occurs in the gonads and is highly complex; errors in this process can be passed to the next generation.

Selected Readings

Cormack, D. H.: Ham's Histology. 9th ed. Philadelphia, J. B. Lippincott, 1987.

Fawcett, D. W.: Bloom & Fawcett: A Textbook of Histology. 11th ed. Philadelphia, W. B. Saunders Co., 1986.

Gall, J. G., Porter, K. R., and Siekevitz, P. (eds.): Discovery in cell biology. J. Cell Biol. *91* (3, Part 2, Supplement), 1981.

Ghadially, F. N.: Ultrastructural Pathology of the Cell and Matrix. 3rd ed. London, Butterworth, 1988.

Leeson, C. R., Leeson, T. S., and Paparo, A. A.: Textbook of Histology. 5th ed. Philadelphia, W. B. Saunders Co., 1985.

The Genetic Basis of Disease

After studying this chapter, the student should be able to:

- Draw diagrams to illustrate the mode of inheritance of a disease inherited as
  (a) an autosomal dominant;
  (b) an autosomal recessive;
  (c) an X-linked dominant;
  (d) an X-linked recessive.
- Give at least one example of each type of inheritance.
- Describe the steps involved in obtaining a preparation of human chromosomes for karyotypic analysis.
- Describe the chromosomal abnormality and the outstanding clinical features of each of the following:
  (a) the most common type of Down's syndrome;
  (b) Klinefelter's syndrome;
  (c) ovarian dysgenesis;
  (d) cri du chat syndrome.
- Describe the nature of plasmids and indicate their importance in relation to
  (a) bacterial resistance to antibiotics;
  (b) gene cloning.
- Describe the role of restriction endonucleases in gene cloning.
- Indicate the significance of restriction length polymorphism.
- List the investigations that can be performed on amniotic fluid to detect fetal abnormality. Give examples of the types of defects that may be found.

The study of medicine has largely revolved around the effects of adverse external agents. The great discoveries made in bacteriology, virology, and immunology at the end of the last century strengthened the belief that each disease had a specific cause and that often this cause was a particular external agent, frequently a living organism. As diseases of obviously infective origin have been recognized and brought under control, it has become clear that some diseases have no simple cause and are probably due to many agents acting simultaneously. Inherited diseases were certainly recognized in the past, but they were often regarded as being uncommon. Inherited traits were believed to result from a merging of parental traits, and in this climate of thought the discoveries of Gregor Mendel were passed over and ignored for 25 years. Mendel himself followed the course of many other successful yet frustrated investigators: he abandoned research and became an administrator.

Today we realize that disease has two major bases. It is the result of the interplay between inherited genetic constitution on the one hand and the environment on the other. This chapter is mainly concerned with the first of these components.

THE GENETIC BASIS OF DISEASE

Mendel's laws of inheritance have laid the foundations of the science of genetics and are of great importance in the understanding of many disease processes. He postulated that a particular characteristic is determined by a pair of factors, now called *genes*, each of which is situated at a particular site (or *locus*) on one of a pair of chromosomes. Such genes, forming a pair, are called *alleles*. An individual with a pair of similar genes is called *homozygous*, whereas if the genes are dissimilar, the individual is *heterozygous*. The genetic make-up of an individual is called the *genotype*, and the effect that is produced is called the *phenotype*.

It is basic in modern genetics to assume that genes occur in pairs, that one of each pair is received from each parent, and that the genes remain unchanged through many generations. The simplest approach to the mode of inheritance of a particular characteristic—for example, a disease—is to consider that the condition is due to a *single-gene disorder*. The gene may be either *dominant* or *recessive*. A dominant gene produces its effect both in the heterozygote and in the homozygote. Recessive genes, on the other hand, produce their effects only in the homozygous condition. Genes occupying an intermediate position are described later. Sometimes a particular locus on a chromosome can be occupied by one of many possible genes. An example of this type is illustrated in the following with the explanation of ABO blood grouping.

Dominant Genes

A simple example of inheritance of a dominant gene is shown by reference to the ABO blood grouping. The allelic genes that can occupy one locus are *A, B,* or *O.*

A homozygous individual who has two *A* genes (genotype *AA*) has on red blood cells the blood group substance A (phenotype group A). Likewise, the heterozygote *AO* is also phenotypically blood group A because the *A* gene is dominant, whereas *O* is recessive. The *B* gene, like the *A* gene, is dominant, and both are described as *codominant*. The possible blood groups in this system are shown.*

Genotype	Phenotype
AA	**A**
AO	**A**
OO	**O**
BB	**B**
BO	**B**
AB	**AB**

Thus, the six genotypes produce only four recognizable blood groups. A person of blood group A may be genotype *AA* or *AO*. It is not easy to distinguish between these two genotypes by an examination of the individual, but the genotype can be deduced from the family pedigree. It should be noted that the occurrence of two or more genetically different classes of individuals with respect to a single trait is known as *polymorphism*. The blood groups provide an excellent example of this, but many others are known. For example, there are many genetically determined variants of plasma proteins, hemoglobin, and enzymes.

The mode of inheritance of a dominant disease is illustrated in Figure 3–1. It should be noted that

1. The disease appears in every generation or else it dies out. The occasional instance of poor penetrance (discussed later in this chapter) and the occurrence of a new mutant, as is common in multiple neurofibromatosis, provide exceptions to this rule. If the disease greatly reduces

---

*The ABO blood groups are more complicated than this. For example, *O* is an amorph, and subgroups of A are known.

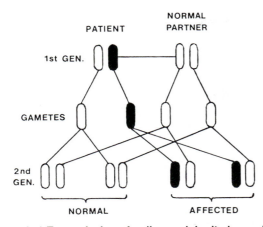

Figure 3–1 Transmission of a disease inherited as a dominant trait. One pair of chromosomes is shown for each individual, the black chromosome being the one carrying the defective gene. Each person inheriting the defective gene will have the disease. Each member of the next generation has a 50 per cent probability of inheriting the disease. (From Walter, J. B., and Israel, M. S.: General Pathology. 5th ed. Edinburgh, Churchill Livingstone, 1979.)

chances of additional members of the family being affected or passing on the trait can be calculated. Thus, the chances of the next child being affected are one in four. One half of the offspring will be heterozygous and carriers of the trait. If the affected individual mates with a normal partner, all of the progeny will be carriers.

3. The seriousness of producing carriers should not be overemphasized. It has been estimated that we all carry harmful genes that usually remain hidden for generations. A particular gene is liable to be more frequent in a particular family; the danger of close intermarriage is therefore evident. The incidence of defective offspring is much higher in consanguineous matings (those between close relatives) than when the parents are not related.

Some of the best-known diseases inherited as

the breeding potential of the affected person, it follows that most cases encountered will be sporadic and due to new mutations.

2. Unaffected members do not pass on the disease.

3. The affected members are usually heterozygous, and if the breeding partner is normal, the chances of the offspring being affected are 50 per cent.

4. Males and females are equally liable to be affected.

Huntington's chorea, achondroplasia, multiple neurofibromatosis (Fig. 3–2), and some types of osteogenesis imperfecta are examples of diseases inherited as dominant traits.

Recessive Traits

Frequently, these are severe and reduce the breeding potential of the affected person. The mode of transmission is shown diagrammatically in Figure 3–3. The following features should be noted.

1. The birth of an abnormal child is usually the first indication of the condition.

2. As with other mendelian characters, the

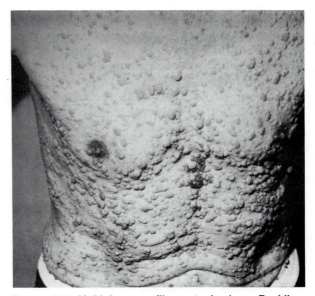

Figure 3–2 Multiple neurofibromatosis (von Recklinghausen's disease). This patient appeared normal at birth except for the presence of several irregularly shaped pigmented macules (café au lait spots). The skin lesions shown in the picture began to appear at about 13 years of age. The patient, who is now 60 years old, has thousands of soft skin nodules, many of which are pedunculated. These show neurofibromas on microscopic examination. The disease is named after von Recklinghausen, who gave the first good account of the disease in 1882. The patient was an orphan and has three children. One daughter is similarly affected, but the others apparently have escaped the disease.

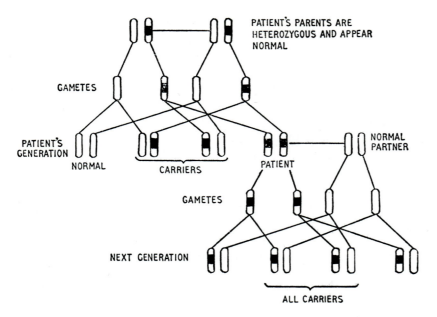

GAMETES

PATIENT'S PARENTS ARE HETEROZYGOUS AND APPEAR NORMAL

PATIENT'S GENERATION

NORMAL   CARRIERS   PATIENT

NORMAL PARTNER

GAMETES

NEXT GENERATION

ALL CARRIERS

Figure 3–3 Transmission of a disease inherited as a recessive factor. The patient is homozygous and therefore expresses the disease. Both parents are heterozygous and consequently appeared normal. All the patient's offspring are heterozygotes and thus carriers of the trait. (From Walter, J. B., and Israel, M. S.: General Pathology. 5th ed. Edinburgh, Churchill Livingstone, 1979.)

recessive traits are galactosemia, phenylketonuria, and cystic fibrosis of the pancreas.

Other Features of Gene Expression

Not all human inherited disease can be explained in terms of simple dominant or recessive gene action. There are many complicating factors.

It may happen that a trait, although apparently dominant, occasionally misses a generation. The trait is said to exhibit *reduced penetrance*. Another complication is seen in some families in which a dominant gene produces a variable effect. Some individuals who possess it have a severe disease, whereas others have a minor defect (known as *forme fruste*) of the disease. In this instance, the trait is said to exhibit *variable expressivity*. Clearly, penetrance and expressivity are closely related, but whereas penetrance is defined in terms of an all-or-none effect, expressivity is variable.

When the heterozygote differs from either homozygote, the inheritance is described as *intermediate*. A good example is sickle cell disease. The homozygote who has two sickle cell genes has the fully developed sickle cell anemia, whereas the heterozygote carrying one defective allele and one normal allele has the mild sickle cell trait—a state intermediate between the disease and the normal. This condition is described in more detail later in the chapter.

Genes are said to be *linked* when they are closely situated on the same chromosome; they tend to segregate together at meiosis and appear as a group in the next generation. The closer together they are on the chromosome, the more likely they are to behave as a unit. A good example is HLA genes of the major histocompatibility complex; they are so closely linked that they are inherited as a group, termed a haplotype. Certain HLA genes are associated with susceptibility to infection, arthritis, or other disease. It is not certain whether this effect is due directly to the HLA gene or other closely linked genes.

The genes that determine inherited diseases that are more common in one sex are said to be *sex-limited* or *sex-influenced*. Male-pattern baldness is one such example; although it is inherited as an autosomal dominant trait, a suitably high testosterone level is needed for it to be expressed. Therefore, it normally affects only males. Diseases that appear to be sex-influenced are open neural tube defects, which are more common in females, and pyloric stenosis and coarctation of the aorta, which are most common in males.

A gene is said to be *sex-linked* when it is localized on an X or Y chromosome. Usually the gene is recessive and is situated on the X chromosome. The most famous disease to be inherited as a sex-linked recessive is hemophilia A, which is illustrated in Figure 3–4.

Sex-linked dominant traits are recognized but are rare. Affected females convey the gene to half their sons and daughters, whereas affected males transmit it only to their daughters. Because there can be no male-to-male transmission, there is therefore an excess of female victims. Hemolytic anemia due to glucose-6-phosphate dehydrogenase deficiency is an example of this type of inheritance.

Different mutant genes may produce the same apparent effect or phenotype. Termed *genetic heterogeneity*, this occurs when the same phenotype results from a different mutant gene. A good example is congenital deafness, which may be inherited as an autosomal dominant, autosomal recessive, or X-linked trait. The most direct proof that different genes are involved is evidenced by two individuals with similar phenotypes who mate and produce a normal child. Furthermore, deafness may be due to an infection or the effects of a toxin. It is then called a *phenocopy*.

In some diseases, such as systemic hypertension and obesity, environmental factors appear to act in concert with genetic factors. The pathogenesis of these diseases is therefore said to be *multifactorial*.

Mode of Gene Action

Some genetic diseases are thought to arise as a point mutation, *i.e.*, the mutation occurs at a specific molecular site in the DNA of the genome. A good example is sickle cell anemia in which there is a defect in the DNA molecule such that there is substitution of valine for glutamine at a specific site in the two beta-polypeptide chains of the globin molecule. This amino acid substitution is a direct result of mutation in the nucleotide of the gene so that it codes for valine rather than glutamine. In this example, the abnormal hemoglobin leads to both a functional and a structural abnormality.

The point mutation of other inherited diseases can involve genes coding for metabolic enzymes, and the resulting diseases are known collectively as *inborn errors of metabolism*. Some examples are considered in Chapter 16.

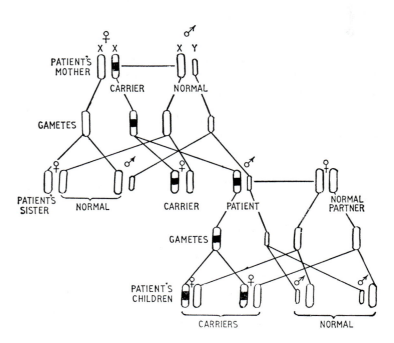

Figure 3–4 Mode of transmission of a disease inherited as an X-linked recessive mendelian factor. A common example of such a disease is hemophilia A. The abnormal gene is situated on an X chromosome and therefore produces its effect in the male but not in the female except in the very rare event of her being homozygous. The patient's daughters are all carriers of the disease, and his sons are all normal. There is never any direct male-to-male transmission; the disease is perpetuated by the females in the family. (From Walter, J. B., and Israel, M. S.: General Pathology. 5th ed. Edinburgh, Churchill Livingstone, 1979.)

RECOMBINANT DNA TECHNOLOGY

The blueprint for making an entire animal lies in its cell's DNA, and details of individual inherited traits lie in the exact chemical structure of DNA. Chemicals can be manipulated *in vitro,* and it is understandable that great efforts have been made to analyze the exact sequence of the nucleotides that constitute each gene. Great strides are being made toward deciphering the whole human genome. The subject is complex, and only a brief outline of the subject of recombinant DNA technology (popularly called genetic engineering) is presented.

Isolation of a gene, normal or abnormal, has many potential uses. Its detection can be used to diagnose disease both in a fetus and postnatally. Its products can be analyzed and used therapeutically. It may even be possible to replace abnormal, mutated genes with normal ones. A commonly used technique is to isolate fragments of DNA. The fragments are incorporated into the DNA molecule of a vector (*e.g.,* a plasmid), which is then introduced into a suitable host (*e.g., Escherichia coli*) and grown in culture to produce clones with multiple copies of the DNA fragment (Fig. 3–5). This can then be harvested.

One technique commonly used is to produce DNA fragments that contain specific genes of interest together with short nucleotide sequences containing suitable signals by the action of bacterial enzymes, termed *restriction endonucleases,* that cleave DNA at specific base sequence sites. Many enzymes are known, each cutting the DNA at a different point. Thus, the enzyme EcoRI cleaves the DNA molecule between the bases guanine and adenine in the sequence GAATTC (see illustration below).

The cleaved fragments of the DNA helix are

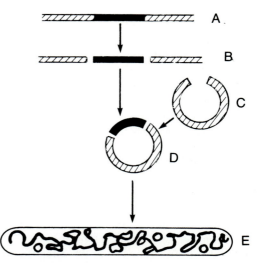

Figure 3–5 Gene cloning. *A,* Portion of foreign DNA with segment containing the gene depicted in solid black. *B,* DNA molecule cleaved by restrictive endonuclease. *C,* Circular DNA molecule of plasmid opened by the same restrictive endonuclease. *D,* Segment of foreign DNA inserted into the plasmid's DNA. *E,* Host *Escherichia coli* with plasmids. The plasmids may multiply independently of the bacterial DNA as shown here, or they may become incorporated into the single strand of DNA that constitutes the bacterial chromosome. (Drawing by Rasa Skudra, Artlab Communication Inc., Toronto.)

"sticky" and readily anneal by base pairing on the ends of other DNA molecules that have been cleaved by the same endonuclease and hence have complementary sticky ends. The *DNA polymerase chain reaction* allows the selected region of the genome to be amplified *in vitro* more than a millionfold by use of a DNA polymerase.

After a fragment of DNA containing the required gene has been obtained, it can be used to prepare a probe or inserted into a suitable vector so that it can be allowed to express itself *in vivo*. The common vectors in use are plasmids, bacteriophages, and cosmids. Phage vectors are de-

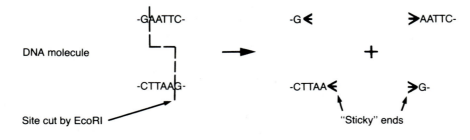

rived from *E. coli,* and cosmids are produced *in vitro* by packaging plasmid DNA into a phage particle. The types and properties of plasmids are described before this account of genetic engineering is continued.

Plasmids. Plasmids are small particles found in bacteria that consist of a circular double strand of DNA. They have no outer protein coat and therefore have a simpler structure than do viruses. Plasmids may exist in the bacterial cells as separate entities that replicate independently of the cell, or their DNA may become incorporated into the single molecule of DNA that constitutes the bacterial chromosome. In the latter event, the plasmid DNA becomes part of the genome of the bacterium and replicates when the cell divides. Plasmids are known to be of importance in several respects. It has been found that some bacteria undergo a process called *conjugation,* in which two cells closely approximate to each other and exchange genetic material. This is a primitive type of sexual reproduction. Only bacteria that contain a particular fertility factor (termed *F factor*) are able to undergo conjugation; this F factor is a plasmid. A second important role of plasmids (originally called *R factor*) is the transfer of bacterial resistance to antibiotics. Some plasmids contain DNA that so alters the host's metabolism that the organism is resistant to antibiotics; the effect may be brought about by excluding the antibiotic from the bacterium, by destroying the antibiotic, or by circumventing the effect that the antibiotic has on the cell's metabolism. Transfer of a plasmid from one bacterium to another is one way in which antibiotic resistance can develop. Thus, an antibiotic-resistant *E. coli* can have its information transferred to a pathogen such as one of the salmonellae. Furthermore, a plasmid may have many DNA components that render the bacterium resistant to a whole range of antibiotics. In this way, resistance to many antibiotics can develop quite suddenly. Although bacterial antibiotic resistance can occur by mutation of the bacterial chromosome itself, it is likely that plasmid transfer is a more common mechanism. In recombinant DNA research, plasmids play a major part (see later). Plasmids are not known to play any part in human disease as yet, but it is possible that similar agents exist and are responsible for extrachromosomal genetic mechanisms. It has been suggested that slow viruses are agents of this nature, but this is at the moment speculation. The presence of plasmids and other extrachromosomal genetic nucleic acids indicates that simple mendelian inheritance is by no means the only way by which a cell can acquire genetic information.

The vector plasmids used in recombinant DNA remain as structures separate from the bacterial chromosome. Replication occurs independently of the bacterial chromosomal replication. If the DNA of a plasmid is opened *in vitro* by a suitable restriction endonuclease, a portion of foreign DNA, *e.g.,* containing a human gene, can be inserted (Fig. 3–5). The molecular circle is then rejoined (annealed) with a suitable enzyme (ligase). The manipulated plasmids so formed are introduced into *E. coli,* where they replicate, producing high copy numbers. The host *E. coli* containing the gene of interest can be selectively grown if the plasmid chosen also confers on the organism resistance to a particular antibiotic.

The source of the DNA segment to be cloned can be obtained directly from the DNA of a mammalian cell. Alternatively, a specific mRNA product of the gene of interest is isolated from the cell. By use of a reverse transcriptase (isolated from an RNA tumor retrovirus), it is possible to use this mRNA as a template and synthesize *in vitro* a complementary single-stranded DNA molecule, called cDNA. A second complementary DNA strand can be synthesized by use of bacterial DNA polymerase. By this procedure, mRNA extracted from the cell can be used to prepare double-stranded cDNA for cloning.

After a section of DNA containing the gene for a particular protein has been cloned, the protein can be prepared in large quantities from bacterial cultures. Yeast cells are commonly used instead of bacteria because they are more suitable for the production of complex proteins. In this way, interferon, insulin, human growth hormone, and other valuable molecules can be mass-produced *in vitro.*

The isolated single- or double-stranded DNA can be used as a molecular probe, after having first been labeled with a radioactive isotope, *e.g.,* ^{32}P, or a fluorescent label. The action of a probe depends on the basic principle of the DNA double helix—complementary strands of nucleotides combine to form stable double-stranded molecules. mRNA probes can also be used, because mRNA will also hybridize with its corresponding DNA sequence; in practice, pure mRNA probes are less often used because they are more difficult to prepare.

If a nucleotide sequence or the amino acid sequence of a protein is known, it is possible to synthesize short stretches of DNA called oligonucleotides through commercially available automated techniques. This oligonucleotide can then be used as a probe.

One way of identifying a gene in a nucleated cell is to fragment the cell's DNA with a suitable endonuclease and then separate the fragments by electrophoresis on an agarose gel. Owing to the size of the DNA molecule, individual bands do not resolve separately, and a smearing effect is obtained. In the gel, the DNA is denatured to single-stranded fragments, and these are then transferred to a nitrocellulose filter by a process of blotting. The process is termed *Southern blotting*, after the name of the inventor of the process. The advantage of blotting is that the DNA becomes fixed onto the nitrocellulose. Next, a specific radioactive DNA probe is applied, and it hybridizes with its complementary DNA on the blot. Autoradiography will reveal the site or sites as distinct bands. These bands of DNA fragments can then be selected from an original agarose gel and used for further study. Northern blotting is a similar technique for RNA.

There are many uses for DNA probes. They can be used to detect viral DNA in a cell, for instance, hepatitis B virus or herpes simplex viruses. If a specific probe is available, it can be applied to a fixed metaphase chromosomal preparation, and the site of the individual gene can be localized to a particular region of a specific chromosome. In some diseases, DNA probes are available for the mutated gene as well as for the normal counterpart. These diseases include alpha$_1$-antitrypsin deficiency, hemophilia A, sickle cell anemia, and phenylketonuria. These diseases may therefore be diagnosed by direct gene analysis. For the majority of diseases, however, this technique cannot be used because the normal gene or its mutant has not been identified.

In human chromosomes, there are certain nucleotide sequence variations (known as *restriction fragment length polymorphism*) distributed in areas throughout the genome. These sequences are inherited and can be detected by suitable probes. Although they themselves are without obvious phenotypic effect, they may be closely linked to a specific disease-associated gene. Hence, specific probes can be used to detect the presence of the genes for a particular disease, *e.g.*, Huntington's chorea and polycystic kidney disease, even though the specific gene structure is not known. In the case of Duchenne's muscular dystrophy, markers are available that delineate each end of the DNA sequence that contains the gene, yet isolation of the gene itself has not been achieved until recently.

Isolation of a disease-producing gene and its normal counterpart has many intriguing possibilities. Study of the gene products can lead to a better understanding of the disease. The normal gene product can be prepared *in vitro* and possibly used in treatment. Perhaps permanent cure can be obtained because it may be possible to take cells from a patient with a genetic defect, remove a segment of DNA containing an abnormal gene, replace it with a normal gene, and finally return the cell to the patient.

Restriction Endonuclease Analysis

By use of restriction endonucleases to digest genomic DNA of organisms into discrete DNA fragments, different patterns are obtained so that one organism can be compared with another. This process, commonly referred to as fingerprinting, can assist the epidemiologist in tracing the sources and routes of transmission of infective agents. The method can replace previous techniques based on serologic or phage sensitivity.

CYTOGENETICS

The study of chromosomes is termed cytogenetics. It is a rapidly expanding specialty, and many of the recent advances are related to the discovery of methods whereby chromosomes can be examined in great detail. Before the abnormalities are described, a brief account of the methodology is given.

Cytogenetic Methods

In order to study chromosomes, cells in mitosis are required. Blood lymphocytes (treated with phytohemagglutinin), being easily obtainable, are most commonly used; amniotic and chorionic cells are cultured if the fetus is to be studied. Colcemid (a colchicine derivative) is added to the culture and has the effect of inhibiting spindle formation so that cells are halted at metaphase. Hypotonic solution is added to make the cells swell; the preparation is fixed, spread on a slide, and stained in such a way that each chromosome develops alternating regions of light and dark stain. The standard method is to pretreat the preparation with trypsin and stain with Giemsa (G-banding). This technique of "banding" allows the chromosomes to be more easily identified and abnormalities to be detected. A photograph of such a preparation is shown in Figure 3–6. The normal cell contains 46 autosomes and two sex chromosomes. Each chromosome in the picture can be cut out, matched with its homologue, and arranged in order of size. Such a preparation is called a karyotype, and its analysis may reveal abnormalities (Fig. 3–7).

Diseases Associated with Gross Chromosomal Abnormalities

Certain individuals have been found to have more than 46 chromosomes, whereas others have fewer. Abnormalities in the shape or form of individual chromosomes have also been noted. These abnormalities may be considered under two headings: (1) alteration in *number* of chromosomes and (2) alteration in *structure* of chromosomes.

Although the finding of chromosomal abnormality is regarded as uncommon, it is now apparent that those cases detected in postnatal life represent only the residue of a much larger group of abnormal zygotes. About one half of the fetuses spontaneously aborted in the first 3 months of pregnancy have chromosomal abnormalities, one of the commonest being *triploidy* (the cells having 69 chromosomes). It has been estimated that about one third of the results of conception

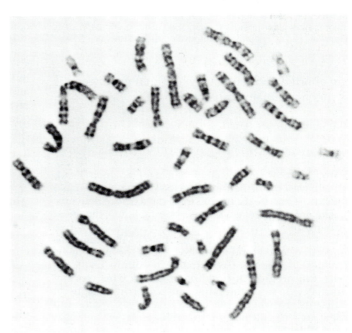

Figure 3–6 Human chromosomes at metaphase. The mitosis shown contains 46 chromosomes, each of which is a divided structure joined by a centromere. The individual chromosomes can be cut out with scissors and arranged in pairs as shown in Figure 3–7. Such an arrangement is called a karyotype. (Courtesy of Dr. H. A. Gardner, Director of Genetic Services, Oshawa General Hospital, Oshawa, Canada.)

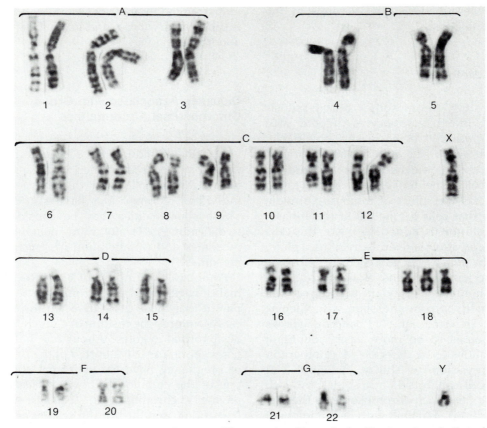

Figure 3–7 Karyotype showing trisomy 18 from a stillborn male with cyclopia. The karyotype is that of a cell with 47 chromosomes. It is evidently from a male, since there is a Y chromosome. The anomaly must therefore be of fetal origin, since the mother had a normal 46,XX karyotype. The additional chromosome 18 arose by nondisjunction; its manifestations were incompatible with postuterine life. For a more complete description, see Case History I. (From Lang, A. P., Schlager, M., and Gardner, H. A.: Trisomy 18 and cyclopia. Teratology, *14*:195–203, 1976. Reprinted by permission of John Wiley & Sons, Inc.)

are aborted spontaneously and that gross genetic errors are a major cause of this (Fig. 3–7).

Case History I

A 26-year-old woman gave birth to a stillborn male child at 41 weeks of gestation (see Fig. 3–7). Before birth, there was clinical evidence of a small head, which was confirmed at ultrasonic examination. No fetal heart was heard during the 3 days before delivery.

The infant showed many abnormalities, the most striking of which was a single eye, containing two lenses, in the center of the forehead. The brain was underdeveloped and exhibited many severe abnormalities. An attempt was made to culture fetal skin cells, but no growth could be obtained. This was not unexpected, since the fetus showed obvious signs of autolysis. However, placental tissue was viable and grew well in culture; photographs of several mitoses were obtained. One of these was arranged as shown in Figure 3–7. The chromosomes are arranged in pairs and are numbered 1 to 22 in order of length, position of the centromere, and banding characteristics. With good technique it is possible to identify each chromosome. When this identification is not possible, the pairs of chromosomes are then arranged into seven groups, A to G, excluding the X and Y chromosomes.

Alteration in Number of Chromosomes

Additional Chromosomes. The most common example of this abnormality is when there is one extra chromosome. This condition is called *trisomy*, and the best-known example is trisomy 21. The individual has 47 chromosomes and may be either male or female. The condition is *Down's syndrome*, otherwise known as mongolism (Fig.

3–8). This is always accompanied by mental defect, and the condition is quite common since such affected children are produced with an incidence of approximately 1 in every 600 live births. Trisomy of other autosomes is known but is much less common.

The presence of additional sex chromosomes is not uncommon. Certain individuals are found to have an extra X. Some are apparent males, have the genetic constitution 47,XXY, and have chromatin-positive cells. They have small testes that fail to develop at puberty; there is little facial

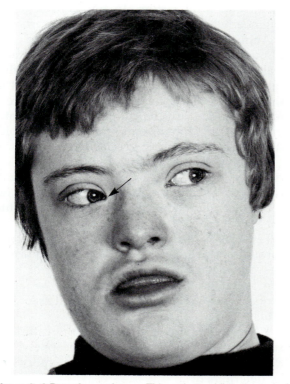

Figure 3–8 Down's syndrome. This patient exhibits the typical facial appearance of persons having the syndrome. Note the large tongue protruding from the mouth. Particularly characteristic is the presence of an epicanthal fold, which is best seen on the right side (arrow). This is a fold of skin that covers the medial angle of the palpebral fissure and gives the eyes an appearance that superficially resembles that of an Oriental. Down's syndrome can generally be recognized at birth, with the diagnosis being confirmed by chromosomal analysis. The mortality is high during the first few years of life, death being related to respiratory infection, congenital heart disease, or leukemia. Dwarfism is common and mental deficiency invariable. Mothers over the age of 35 years are more likely to give birth to an affected child than are younger women. (Courtesy of Dr. Margaret C. Grundy and the Department of Clinical Illustration, University of Birmingham, Birmingham, England.)

hair; they may have a female type of breast development (gynecomastia); and they are sterile. These features become evident at puberty; the condition is known as *Klinefelter's syndrome.* Another group of patients have the karyotype 47,XXX and are females, usually with normal secondary sex characters and sometimes with mental defect.

In the 47,XYY syndrome, the patients appear as normal males, but in some instances the subject is abnormally tall and exhibits a criminally aggressive temperament. Nevertheless, other individuals with this anomaly appear normal.

Reduction in the Number of Chromosomes. The loss of an autosome is incompatible with postuterine life. In those cases in which such a state has been described, a small chromosome is involved, and it seems likely that the chromosome is in fact present but has become attached to some other chromosome, *i.e.,* it has been translocated.

The sex chromosomes are less vital for survival, and deletion of one is quite compatible with life. In about 1 in every 3000 births, a female is produced with the karyotype 45,XO. The condition, which is known as *ovarian dysgenesis,* becomes obvious at adolescence when the ovaries fail to function normally, ovulation does not occur, and menstruation is absent (primary amenorrhea). Such individuals tend to be short because of stunted growth and are sterile. Often they have a number of other abnormalities such as webbing of the neck and a shieldlike chest with widely spaced nipples. Abnormalities of the cardiovascular system are common—in particular, coarctation of the aorta—and the eponym *Turner's syndrome* is applied. These unfortunate females are chromatin-negative, since only one X chromosome is present.

Other Chromosomal Abnormalities

It is now realized that there are many types of chromosomal abnormality that can easily escape detection. There may be deletions of part of a chromosome, or part of a chromosome may be translocated to another chromosome. An example of a deletion is seen in the cri du chat syndrome. Affected infants exhibit mental deficiency and cry with a whimpering noise resembling that of a cat in distress. There is deletion of the short arm of chromosome 5.

An additional chromosome or part of a chromosome may be attached to another; hence, an individual can be trisomeric for a small chromosome even if the total number of chromosomes is normal. Furthermore, some individuals are mosaics, *i.e.,* their body is composed of two populations of cells, each with a different karyotype, *e.g.,* XX and XY. These various syndromes may be associated with chromosomal changes more subtle than is indicated, and their investigation by a specialized cytogenetic laboratory is essential.

Chromosomes may be abnormal in ways that do not involve their apparent structure. Some conditions have been recognized in which the chromosomes are fragile and readily break in culture. One of the best known is xeroderma pigmentosum. The chromosomes show undue fragility on exposure to ultraviolet light. This is because the cells lack an enzyme necessary to repair damage to the DNA. The patients are very sensitive to sunlight and develop multiple skin cancers unless they are protected from an early age. An example of greater importance is the fragile X syndrome. This is an inherited condition that affects about 0.1 per cent of the population, males more frequently than females. It is a marker for an X-linked type of mental retardation and is second only to Down's syndrome as a cause of mental retardation.

The first acquired disease to be found to have any consistent chromosomal abnormality was chronic myeloid leukemia. The abnormal white cells have a short or abnormal chromosome 22 (called the Philadelphia chromosome) due to the reciprocal balanced translocation between chromosomes 9 and 22. Other similar abnormalities have been found in tumors, *e.g.,* there is a translocation between chromosomes 8 and 14 in Burkitt's lymphoma.

AVOIDANCE OF GENETIC DEFECTS

Genetic counseling will dissuade some high-risk couples from procreation, but once conception has occurred, the only available course may be the induction of abortion. Therefore, it is essential to be able to detect the presence of fetal abnormality as early in pregnancy as possible. This is particularly important if there is a known familial disease or if the patient has previously given birth to a child with a chromosomal disorder. Also, women over the age of 35 years are advised to be tested because there is an increased risk of chromosomal disorder, particularly Down's syndrome. Several methods of investigation are available. If a defect is found, an abortion can be performed safely at this time. Whether to adopt this course also depends on moral and legal factors. In the future, genetic engineering may offer an alternative approach.

Amniocentesis. Removal of amniotic fluid through a needle passed through the abdominal wall is a simple and safe procedure. The fluid can be examined biochemically and checked for the presence of virus. The amniotic cells are of fetal origin and can be cultured for biochemical investigation, chromosomal analysis, and molecular studies, *e.g.,* using specific DNA probes.

Chorionic Villus Sampling. A small sample of chorionic villi can be biopsied through a small catheter passed through the cervix uteri. They can be used for cytogenetic and molecular studies.

Fetoscopy. The fetus can be seen directly through a small endoscope. Obvious abnormalities can be seen, and samples of skin or blood can be taken. Of the three methods so far described, this test involves the greatest risk to the fetus.

Ultrasonography. Ultrasonography can detect some anatomic defects, *e.g.,* anencephaly, and defects of bone. Often the sex of the embryo can be determined.

ACQUIRED DISEASE

Many human diseases are acquired in postnatal life as a result of the action of external factors. The effects of physical and chemical agents, living organisms, and dietary deficiencies are the common causes of these *acquired diseases*. It should be remembered that the developing fetus is also sensitive to environmental factors, and the tragedies that followed administration of thalidomide to pregnant women bear witness to the extreme sensitivity of the fetus under some circumstances. Intrauterine events may produce defects that are present at birth (*congenital*) but are not inherited, since no genetic mechanism is involved. Inherited diseases may be congenital, *e.g.,* achondroplasia, but they may also appear later in life, *e.g.,* familial polyposis coli (Chapter 23). The time of onset of a disease gives no indication as to whether the cause is environmental or genetic.

Summary

- Mendelian principles of inheritance describe the features of dominant, recessive, intermediate, sex-limited, and sex-linked traits.
- The restrictive endonucleases allow DNA to be cleaved into fragments that contain a gene of interest or adjacent nucleotide sequences; subsequently, the fragment is inserted into the DNA of a vector, usually a plasmid. This is grown in a bacterium or yeast, thereby allowing the gene to multiply and be expressed to produce its specific product. The DNA containing the gene can also be constructed *in vitro* by use of specific mRNA. Isolated genes can also be used to fashion probes.
- A karyotype is obtained by preparing a stained smear of suitably cultured cells. Chromosomes are counted, and individual chromosomes are analyzed for abnormalities.
- Abnormalities in the sex chromosomes are relatively common and compatible with life; in Klinefelter's syndrome, there is an extra X chromosome; in ovarian dysgenesis, one X is missing; the fragile X syndrome is associated with mental retardation.
- Abnormalities in the autosomes are less well tolerated and are responsible for many spontaneous abortions. Minor defects cause severe disease, *e.g.,* Down's syndrome and xeroderma pigmentosum.
- Prenatal diagnosis of genetic defects involves examining fetal cells by amniocentesis or chorionic villus sampling, direct vision by fetoscopy, and ultrasonography.

Selected Readings

Antonarakis, S. E.: Diagnosis of genetic disorders at the DNA level. N. Engl. J. Med. *320:*153, 1989.

Stent, G. S., and Calendar, R.: Molecular Genetics. 2nd ed. San Francisco, W. H. Freeman and Company, 1978.

Thompson, J. S., and Thompson, M. W.: Genetics in Medicine. 4th ed. Philadelphia, W. B. Saunders Co., 1986.

Weinberg, R. A.: The molecules of life. Sci. Am. *253:*48, 1985.

4

Cell and Tissue Damage

**After studying this chapter, the student
should be able to:**

- Describe the concept of a biochemical lesion as a
  cause of cell damage, and give examples of such
  lesions.
- Differentiate cell death, autolysis, apoptosis, and
  necrosis.
- List the events that can lead to cell damage.
- Define the terms ischemia, hypoxia, and infarction.
- Describe the effects of hypoxia on a cell.
- Describe the pathogenesis of fatty change in the
  liver.
- Give examples of the value of serum enzyme
  determinations in the diagnosis of
  (a) liver disease;
  (b) heart disease.
- Define the term gangrene.
- Describe the pathogenesis of gangrene in the
  (a) intestine;
  (b) mouth;
  (c) limbs.
- Describe hyaline degeneration and elastosis as
  applied to connective tissue.
- Contrast necrobiosis with hyaline degeneration.
- Describe the concept of clonal aging in relation to
  aging.

    The importance of the cell as the basic unit of
the body has been recognized since the microscope was first applied to the analysis of biologic
material. This is scarcely surprising, because simple forms of life like the ameba consist entirely
of one cell. Our concept of many diseases now
centers on abnormalities in cellular behavior or
appearance. The cells of any particular organ or
tissue usually closely resemble each other, and it
is not surprising that a sick cell such as one from
the liver is the essential component of a sick liver;
likewise, this "sickness" at the cellular level pro-

duces a particular clinical syndrome called liver failure. The advent of electron microscopy has greatly increased our knowledge of cellular changes in disease and has further strengthened the concept that abnormalities in cellular appearance and behavior are the building blocks from which disease entities are built. Nevertheless, a morphologic view of cellular behavior has its limitations. The application of chemical techniques has considerably widened our views. At a cellular level, the techniques of histochemistry allow us to identify particular chemicals within cells. Furthermore, chemists have exerted a quite different influence on the study of disease by adopting another approach. Instead of concentrating on the individual cell or its organelles, they have turned their attention to specific chemical reactions. Thus, with respect to the metabolism of galactose, most cells can be regarded as behaving in a standard way. The disease *galactosemia* is characterized by a defect in an enzyme involved in the conversion of galactose to glucose (Chapter 16). Deficiency of this enzyme produces a disease leading to microscopic changes in cells that are particularly dependent on this chemical reaction during development. The brain, the lens of the eye, and the liver are most severely affected. This second approach to the study of a pathologic condition has been of immense value both in the delineation of disease processes and in the treatment of individual patients. Ultimately, the broad concept of "biochemical disorder" must be reduced to a cellular level. In some instances this has already occurred. Cells may be injured in many ways, and it is convenient to list them here.

CAUSES OF CELL DAMAGE

Cells may be damaged by events that occur within the body (internal events) or by agents that act from the outside (external events).

Internal Events

Genetic error—enzyme defects (see galactosemia).

Deprivation of essential chemicals such as hormones, vitamins, and oxygen.

Loss of blood supply. Deficient blood flow through a part is described as *ischemia*. This causes *hypoxia* in all organs except the lung.

Immunologically mediated damage involving both immunoglobulin-mediated events and the effects of delayed type hypersensitivity (DTH) T lymphocytes.

External Events

Physical—heat, cold, trauma, ultraviolet light, and ionizing radiation.

Chemical—poisons and lack of oxygen.

Microbial—microbial invasion and the effects of toxins.

The mechanism of cell injury and its effects vary greatly according to the causative agent. Some of these mechanisms are examined in greater detail.

Most agents, it may be assumed, affect cells by upsetting some important chemical reaction. In this event, a *biochemical lesion* is the first change; in turn, this produces secondary results. The concept of a biochemical lesion causing cell dysfunction was first advanced by Sir Rudolph Peters; he observed that thiamine-deficient birds developed a severe neurologic disease characterized by convulsions and eventual death. In spite of the severity of the disease, no abnormality could be detected by histologic examination of the brain. Thiamine is a necessary cofactor for the conversion of pyruvate to acetylcoenzyme A used in the Krebs cycle. Hence, the cerebral damage results from impaired energy production in the nerve cells—cells that have a high energy requirement.

After a biochemical lesion, structural changes often take place within the cell, and these are usually described as *degenerative*, although *adaptive* is a better term because the changes sometimes indicate that the cell is countering the effects of the damage and may well recover. However, if the damage is severe, there is reached a *point of no return* from which recovery is impossible, and the cell dies. Death is accompanied by many changes including increased permeability of the outer cell membrane, fragmentation of membranes of the cytocavitary network (endoplasmic reticulum and others), swelling of mitochondria, and nuclear changes. At some point the cell must be regarded as being "dead," but there is no morphologic or biochemical marker by which this event may be pinpointed. After death, two types of change may occur.

Apoptosis. This is an energy-dependent process whereby the nucleus breaks up into fragments and the cytoplasm becomes condensed and homogeneous. The apoptotic bodies so produced are well exemplified by the Councilman bodies in the liver in yellow fever and similar acidophilic bodies in viral hepatitis. Apoptosis affects single cells, no inflammatory reaction is stimulated, and the apoptotic bodies are usually phagocytosed by macrophages; the loss of cells that ensues can lead to atrophy of a tissue. Apoptosis is also a physiologic phenomenon whereby surplus cells are removed during development.

Necrosis. This is the more common result of cell death. It generally affects wide areas of tissue rather than isolated cells. After cell death, the lytic lysosomal enzymes act on cell components, and the process of *self-digestion* or *autolysis* takes place. If this happens after the death of the whole individual, the term *postmortem change* is used. When, however, a group of cells dies in continuity with the living, similar changes occur, and it is by noting them that cell death can itself be recognized; to this process the term *necrosis* is applied. Unlike apoptosis, necrosis generally excites an inflammatory reaction in the adjacent viable tissue.

Hypoxic Cell Damage

Hypoxic tissue damage secondary to ischemia is a major cause of morbidity (cerebral and renal ischemic disease) and of death (myocardial ischemia often with infarction). In hypoxic cells there is a reduction of ATP production due to a reduction in aerobic respiration (oxidative phosphorylation). There are many consequences:

1. Active cells cease to function, *e.g.*, heart muscle ceases to contract.

2. Anaerobic glycolysis leads to the production of pyruvate and lactic acid. If there is widespread ischemia of tissue, as in shock, a metabolic acidosis may ensue.

3. The sodium pump is impaired. Sodium is retained in the cell, potassium escapes from it, and the cell undergoes acute swelling as fluid accumulates in the sacs of the endoplasmic reticulum. Indeed, the cell becomes water-logged.

4. Ribosomes become detached from the rough endoplasmic reticulum, and protein synthesis is reduced or modified.

Although total deprivation of oxygen eventually causes cell death, it is likely that a substantial part of the injury occurs not during the initial phase of hypoxia but during a later phase when the tissue is reoxygenated as it again becomes perfused with blood. During this phase, there is set in motion a train of biochemical events that lead to the *formation of powerful oxidants:* one of these is the superoxide radical O_2^-. Such powerful, damaging oxidants have many effects. One is on lipids (*lipid peroxidation*), and this may be the cause of cell membrane damage. The pretreatment of experimental animals with drugs that inhibit superoxide formation lessens the damage caused by ischemia.

Damage by Chemicals

Chemicals can produce damage in a variety of ways. Some act directly, whereas others produce subtle biochemical lesions. Some chemicals are not directly toxic but are metabolized, usually in the smooth endoplasmic reticulum, to highly reactive derivatives. This production of toxic metabolites generally takes place in the liver; the metabolites may act on other tissues or may cause liver damage. Sometimes free oxidant radicals are formed, and these can be neutralized by sulfhydryl compounds such as cysteine and glutathionine. Hence, increasing the supply of glutathionine protects the liver against the effect of some toxic compounds. This has found practical application: patients who take an overdose of the analgesic drug acetaminophen (Tylenol) may develop severe liver damage. *N*-acetylcysteine, a glutathionine substitute that is less toxic than cysteine, is an effective antidote.

Chemicals may produce damage by the process of lethal synthesis. Some chemotherapeutic agents are used with the deliberate intention of producing a biochemical lesion in microorganisms. This mechanism provides the basis for the action of the sulfonamides and some antibiotics, *e.g.*, penicillin, which blocks cell wall synthesis. Cells mistake 5-fluorouracil for uracil, but the abnormal end product blocks other essential metabolic processes. Hence, this drug finds use in the treatment of malignant disease.

EFFECTS OF CELL DAMAGE

The effects of a biochemical lesion vary considerably. The cell's metabolism may be gravely disturbed and cause marked alteration in behavior without any structural change being apparent; thus, cholera toxin acts on the intestinal epithelium and causes a disturbance of the sodium pump that results in a tremendous outpouring of fluid into the lumen of the gut. There is severe watery diarrhea characteristic of cholera; dehydration is the major cause of death in this disease. Another example is the effect of ischemia on the myocardium; within 3 minutes of the onset of ischemia, the myocardium shows no structural change but loses its ability to contract normally. This is due to lack of energy release and an impairment of the calcium transport within the cell that is necessary for contraction.

Damage to cells may produce morphologic changes, which by tradition are classified as degenerative. The concepts of cellular degeneration were evolved during the past 100 years by pathologists using the relatively crude methods available for the study of cells. Three types of change have been described; they are purely descriptive terms applied to the appearance of cells by light microscopy of sections from paraffin wax–embedded tissue. The changes are, first, *cloudy swelling* and *hydropic degeneration,* each of which is associated with accumulation of water in the cell. Second, there is *fatty change.* Finally there is a heterogeneous group in which eosinophilic material appears in the cell either as droplets or as ill-defined masses. This group is termed *hyaline degeneration* or *hyaline-droplet change.*

Changes Associated with Accumulation of Water in the Cell

These changes are described as cloudy swelling and hydropic or vacuolar degeneration.

Cloudy Swelling. The changes of cloudy swelling are encountered in parenchymatous cells such as those of liver and kidney when the organ is subjected to ischemia, hypoxia, or the effects of a poison. The cells are swollen, and the cytoplasm is granular. These changes closely resemble those of postmortem autolysis, but experimentally it has been shown that they can develop in the living cell. In gross appearance the affected organ is swollen; its cut surface bulges and has a gray parboiled appearance. The consistency is soft.

Hydropic Degeneration. The cells show great swelling due to an accumulation of fluid. The condition is reversible, but this is the most severe form of this group of degenerations and may terminate in cell death. The formation of balloon cells in the epidermis of early lesions of herpes simplex and chickenpox is an example of this type of degeneration.

The mechanism whereby cells become waterlogged is explained in Figure 4–1. Diminished ATP production impairs the sodium pump so that both sodium and water accumulate in the cell.

Fatty Change

Normally no stainable neutral fat can be seen in cells except for fat cells in the adipose tissue. Excessive accumulations of fat are found in response to many adverse conditions, *e.g.*, hypoxia and poisoning. This occurs readily in the liver, and the lipid accumulations appear in the rough endoplasmic reticulum and sacs of the Golgi complex. Such membrane-bound lipid droplets are termed *liposomes.* Later, if the adverse conditions persist, much larger, non–membrane-bound lipid droplets appear, and these can be seen by light microscopy as small droplets that stain with Sudan IV in frozen sections. In due course, the small droplets fuse together until one large droplet comes to occupy most of the cell cytoplasm (Fig. 4–2). The process is termed fatty change; the excess fat is derived from the fat deposits of adipose tissue. When fat is mobilized from these stores, free fatty acids are released into the blood stream, transported in combination with albumin, and subsequently taken up

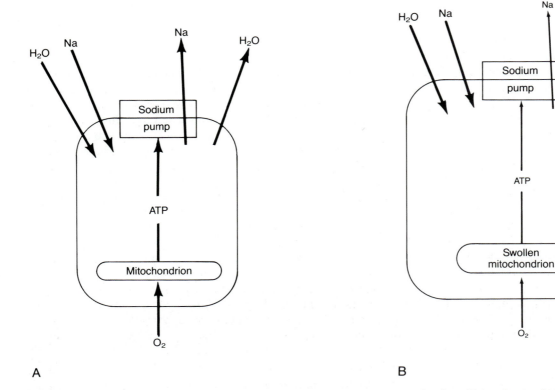

A

B

Figure 4–1 Mechanism of cell waterlogging. *A*, In the normal cell, the amount of sodium (Na) and water (H_2O) that enter a cell are counterbalanced by the Na extruded by the sodium pump. An equivalent amount of water accompanies it. Adenosine triphosphate (ATP) produced by mitochondria provides the energy. *B*, In a cell that is damaged, there is mitochondrial swelling, impaired ATP production, and decreased extrusion of sodium. The cell therefore swells.

by cells, particularly in the liver, where the fatty acids are utilized for metabolic purposes including the production of phospholipids and the production of lipoprotein, which is returned to the blood. If liver cells are damaged, protein synthesis is impaired, and lipoprotein manufacture is impeded. Therefore, fat accumulates as droplets of neutral fat. This, then, is the explanation of fatty change in the liver under some circumstances such as poisoning with phosphorus or ethanol (Fig. 4–3).

Fat may also accumulate in the liver if the supply of fatty acids is increased above the liver's ability to metabolize them. This occurs in starvation (see kwashiorkor) as fat in the adipose tissue is metabolized. An absolute or relative lack of choline, used in the synthesis of lipoproteins, is an additional factor (Fig. 4–3).

A fatty liver is enlarged; its cut surface is pale and in severe cases yellow. Fatty change is also encountered in other organs, *e.g.*, in the heart muscle in patients with severe untreated anemia. In practice, this is rarely encountered.

Hyaline Degeneration

The term "hyaline" is applied to any homogeneous eosinophilic substance. Hyaline degeneration is used to describe a change in cells in which either the whole cell or part of it becomes eosinophilic and homogeneous. *Alcoholic hyaline* (Mallory bodies) in liver cells is one example (Chapter 24). The *hyaline droplets* seen in the proximal tubular cells of the kidney in the nephrotic syndrome are composed of reabsorbed protein that the cells are unable to metabolize because they are so overloaded by the massive proteinuria. It is evident that the term hyaline is purely descriptive and does not signify a single

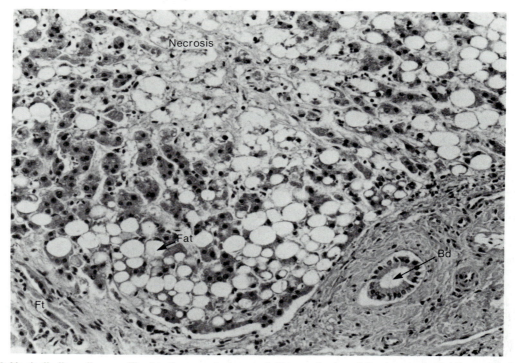

Figure 4–2 Alcoholic liver disease. The liver is severely damaged. Some cells show fatty change, the lipid in each cell appearing as a clear intracellular globule (Fat). Other cells are necrotic, and the structure of the liver lobule has collapsed. In the area of necrosis, the reticulin fibers will be replaced by collagen fibers. Such a change to fibrous tissue (Ft) has already occurred in another area as a result of a previous episode of necrosis. The amount of fibrous tissue around a bile duct (Bd) is increased (×250).

substance. Hyalinization is also described in dense collagenous tissue and effete glomeruli because each has a homogeneous eosinophilic structure.

Other Changes

The classic changes seen in damaged cells have been discussed, and it is appropriate now to describe other changes that have been observed.

Damage to the cell frequently causes an alteration in the permeability of the cell membrane such that it becomes more permeable. This may be detected *in vitro* by exposing the cell to a solution of a dye such as trypan blue. Entry of the dye into the cell indicates that it is dead. This type of test is used to detect the cytotoxic effect of T lymphocytes.

One of the earliest of the nuclear changes in damaged cells is condensation of the chromatin adjacent to the nuclear membrane and loss of nucleolar granular component suggesting impaired synthesis of ribosomal material and mRNA. In damaged liver cells, the rough endoplasmic reticulum shows dilation of its sacs and loss of attached ribosomes. Polysomes are reduced in number; there is reduced RNA synthesis and a reduction of protein synthesis. These changes are particularly associated with hydropic degeneration.

Ultraviolet light has the specific effect of causing damage to the bases of the DNA molecule without causing a break of the polynucleotide chain. This damage can be repaired; first the chain is opened and the damaged segment is excised. A replacement segment is synthesized on the template provided by the undamaged chain. Finally the new chain is inserted into the chain by the action of a polynucleotide ligase. It follows that after the application of ultraviolet light to a tissue, there is a burst of DNA synthesis that is not

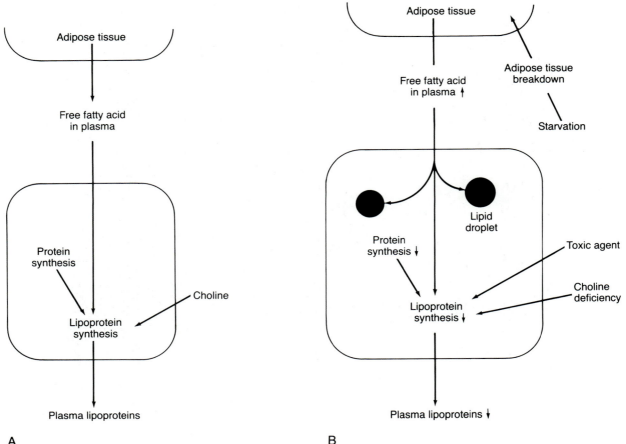

A   B

Figure 4–3 Pathogenesis of fatty change in liver cell. *A,* In the normal cell, free fatty acid derived from the adipose tissues is taken up by the cell and metabolized. Much is excreted as lipoprotein into the blood. Protein and other substances such as choline are required. *B,* If lipoprotein synthesis is impaired (by the effects of a toxin on protein synthesis or the lack of choline in starvation), or if the supply of fatty acid is increased (as in starvation), neutral fat accumulates in the cytoplasm.

related to mitosis. This is termed *unscheduled DNA synthesis.*

Ionizing radiation also causes DNA damage. If one strand of the double helix is broken, the lesion can be repaired by a process similar to that described for ultraviolet light–induced damage. Chromosomal breaks and cell death occur if both chains of the molecule are broken.

Cytoplasmic cellular components may proliferate or reorganize in a manner that suggests a state of hyperfunction. Thus, in response to certain poisons and drugs (*e.g.,* phenobarbital), the smooth endoplasmic reticulum becomes more abundant and forms complex whorls (Fig. 4–4); this is regarded as an adaptive mechanism,

for it parallels the cell's ability to detoxify the drug and is the morphologic expression of drug-induced enzyme induction. The increased glucuronidation induced by phenobarbital increases the rate of detoxification and rate of excretion of the drug. Bilirubin is treated similarly, and the effect can be used therapeutically in icterus gravis neonatorum. The drug increases the rate of detoxification and excretion of the bilirubin that accumulates in the blood in this condition. Some agents, including some carcinogens, cause a proliferation of smooth endoplasmic reticulum that is not accompanied by increased enzyme activity; indeed, it is actually reduced. Form and function do not always go hand in hand.

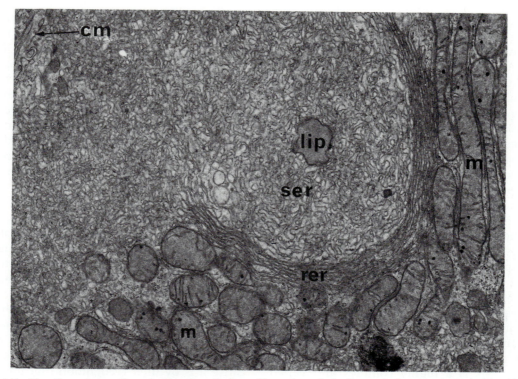

Figure 4–4 Proliferation of smooth endoplasmic reticulum. Shown is part of a liver cell of a rat poisoned with ethionine. The tightly packed proliferated vesicles of smooth endoplasmic reticulum (ser) have formed around a lipid droplet (lip) and contrast with the rough endoplasmic reticulum (rer) that can be identified by the ribosomes studded on its membranes. Mitochondria (m) are elongated. The cell membrane (cm) is shown on the left. Tissue was stained by lead hydroxide (x15,750). (Courtesy of Dr. Katsumi Miyai, Department of Pathology, University of California at San Diego. From Walter, J. B., and Israel, M. S.: General Pathology. 6th ed. Edinburgh, Churchill Livingstone, 1987.)

Mitochondrial changes are common in damaged cells. These organelles may become swollen with fluid and the cristae become shortened, unfolded, and reduced in number. Impaired function results in reduced oxidative phosphorylation and reduced ATP production. Since this substance forms the main immediately available source of energy, it is not surprising that many cell functions are impaired. Thus, the sodium pump is impeded so that sodium and water accumulate in the cell, which in this way becomes progressively more water-logged (Fig. 4–1).

Abnormal Accumulation of Substances in the Cell. Lipid is an example of this and has already been described. There are many diseases in which there is an accumulation of some material within a cell owing to a specific enzyme defect. For instance, absence of an enzyme necessary for glycogen metabolism results in accumulation of glycogen (glycogen storage disease). Also there are other conditions in which lipid or mucopolysaccharide accumulates within the cells. These conditions are all rare and are generally inherited as autosomal recessive traits.

Degenerative Changes. The term "focal cytoplasmic degeneration" is applied when localized areas of the cell become degenerate and are cast off. As an example, damaged renal tubular cells can show loss of the brush border and adjacent cytoplasm. Sometimes cytoplasmic components, *e.g.,* endoplasmic reticulum and mitochondria, are seen within vacuoles containing lysosomal enzymes. These are called *autophagocytic vacuoles, autophagosomes,* or *cytolysosomes,* and an increase in their number is an indication of cell injury. Thus, large numbers of autophagocytic vacuoles are seen in the cells of an organ undergoing atrophy. Material that resists digestion in an autophagosome or in a vacuole formed by endocytosis may remain as a residual body; *lipofuscin, an oxidation product of lipid,* is often a component of this.

Myelin Figures. It is not uncommon to find intracellular whorls of laminated lipid material resembling the myelin of nerves. These are called *myeloid bodies,* or *myelinoid bodies,* and are present whenever the secondary lysosomes are overloaded with lipid as occurs in autophagosomes. This effect may be induced by poisons and is also encountered with genetic defects with impairment of lysosomal lipid degradation; a good example is the abundant myelinoid bodies found in the affected cells in Tay-Sachs disease.

It is evident that a damaged cell is not an inactive passive cell, and its reaction to injury may end in recovery. Parts injured beyond recovery are lysed or extruded, and the remaining structures re-form the lost components. The cell may return to normal, but some alterations may persist and form the basis for metaplasia and perhaps also neoplasia. Thus, the reaction of damaged cells is a highly complex and varied affair.

CELL DEATH AND NECROSIS

Cell death is difficult to define in precise terms, but in practice it may be regarded as having occurred whenever a cell is incapable of further division or of continuing its normal synthetic functions.

The appearance of the dead cells varies according to the cause of the injury. If the cells are killed suddenly as a result of physical or chemical trauma, they show no changes initially other than those directly attributable to the agent concerned, *e.g.,* disruption in electrical injuries and the effects of freezing or burning.

Cells less severely damaged—for instance, by poisons—may develop biochemical lesions that first progress to changes associated with waterlogging and fatty change. As noted previously, these changes as detected by light microscopy are cytoplasmic and in themselves do not indicate cell death.

In a dead cell, respiration ceases, but glycolysis proceeds for a while; as a result, there is the production of lactic acid and a drop in the pH. The synthetic activities of the cell stop, but the lytic destructive processes resulting from released lysosomal enzymes continue. As a result of this, the cell undergoes a process of self-digestion (*autolysis*) and within a few hours shows morphologic changes by which cell death can be recognized. This process is called *necrosis,* which may be defined as the *circumscribed death of cells or tissues with structural evidence of their death. Necrosis and cell death are therefore not synonymous.*

The microscopic changes of necrosis affect the whole cell. The cytoplasm generally becomes homogeneous—often brightly eosinophilic. At the same time, the nucleus shows changes that are pathognomonic of necrosis. Sometimes the nucleus becomes intensely dense-staining, and this is known as *pyknosis.* The pyknotic nucleus either breaks up into fragments (*karyorrhexis*) or becomes indistinct as the nuclear material is digested (*karyolysis*). The importance of these nuclear changes cannot be overemphasized, because it is by their recognition that the pathologist can diagnose necrosis. Autolysis also occurs after the death of the whole individual, and the term *postmortem change* is applied to this process. The microscopic changes can closely mimic those of necrosis, but of course there is no accompanying vital reaction such as inflammation (see discussion later in this chapter).

Diagnosis of Necrosis by Biochemical Means

A diagnosis of the occurrence of necrosis is frequently of great clinical importance. When areas of heart muscle, pancreas, liver, or brain are dying, the patient's life is often in jeopardy. As necrosis occurs, various soluble substances such as enzymes diffuse out of the cells and are absorbed into the blood stream, where their detection is an aid to clinical diagnosis. Some important examples of this response may be listed. The aspartate aminotransferase, hydroxybutyrate dehydrogenase, and lactate dehydrogenase are all raised after myocardial infarction, since these enzymes are found in high concentrations in heart muscle. An elevation of alanine aminotransferase and lactic dehydrogenase is found after liver cell necrosis, such as in viral hepatitis.

Creatine phosphokinase is present in high concentration in skeletal muscle, and an increased blood level occurs after muscle damage, *e.g.,* in polymyositis, alcoholic myopathy, and malignant hyperpyrexia, after strenuous exercise, and even following intramuscular injections. The highest levels are found in the muscular dystrophies.

Some enzymes can be separated into fractions by electrophoresis. These separate fractions, each having a similar biochemical activity, are termed *isoenzymes,* and specific isoenzymes sometimes occur in particular organs (Fig. 4–5). This refinement in the study of serum enzymes has been most rewarding in the diagnosis of myocardial infarction; an appreciable rise in the blood level of the MB fraction of creatine phosphokinase is virtually diagnostic of myocardial damage. In the case of lactic dehydrogenase (LDH), LDH1 and LDH2 are released from the heart muscle, whereas LDH5 is of hepatic origin (Fig. 4–5).

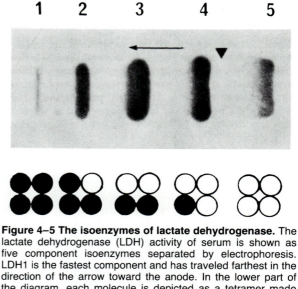

Figure 4–5 The isoenzymes of lactate dehydrogenase. The lactate dehydrogenase (LDH) activity of serum is shown as five component isoenzymes separated by electrophoresis. LDH1 is the fastest component and has traveled farthest in the direction of the arrow toward the anode. In the lower part of the diagram, each molecule is depicted as a tetramer made up of varying combinations of either H polypeptides (closed circles) or M polypeptides (open circles). The H and M chains are determined by separate genes. (After Latner, A. L.: Journal of Clinical Pathology [Association of Clinical Pathology], 4[Suppl. 24]:8–13, 1970.)

Types of Necrosis

Coagulative Necrosis. In most tissues the process of necrosis entails the denaturation of cytoplasmic proteins, causing the tissue to become firm and somewhat opaque. The process resembles the change seen in the white of an egg on boiling.

Denaturation often releases active side-chains of the molecules, which are then available for binding to dyes such as eosin. As noted previously, eosinophilia is a useful sign of cell death, and this is particularly helpful when one is looking for early signs of tissue necrosis. Thus, the patient who dies of a heart attack may show increased eosinophilia of the heart muscle fibers, indicating the early changes of an infarct (see later). Likewise, in patients suffering a cardiac arrest, the detection of eosinophilia in brain cells is a useful, reliable indication of permanent cerebral damage. In practice, of course, these changes are seen only at necropsy.

The increased binding capacity of necrotic tissue is also a factor in causing calcification. Necrotic tissue sometimes takes up calcium salts and becomes calcified. This response, which is termed *dystrophic calcification,* is quite frequently seen in necrotic tumor tissue. Since calcium can be detected easily by radiography, its detection has been utilized in diagnosis. In some cancers of the breast, characteristic flecks of calcium deposition can be seen even before the tumor can be palpated. The degenerate tissue of tuberculous lesions also commonly calcifies, as does the material found in atherosclerosis.

A common cause of necrosis is sudden deprivation of the blood supply to the part. The process is called *infarction* and is common in the heart, kidneys, and spleen. These infarcts show the typical changes of coagulative necrosis. In addition to nuclear changes of pyknosis, karyorrhexis, or karyolysis, another feature is noteworthy on microscopic examination. The general architecture of the tissue may still be recognizable, even though its constituent cells are dead and their nuclei have disappeared. This is called *structured necrosis,* and the appearance has been likened to that of a city of the dead. In other examples of coagulative necrosis, in which there may be no residual structure at all, the effect is called *structureless necrosis*. *Caseation* provides an example of structureless necrosis; it is a particular type of coagulative necrosis in which the dead tissue has a firm, dry, cheesy consistency and contains much lipid material. Although this type of change may occur in other conditions, the term caseation is by convention usually restricted to the necrosis of tuberculosis.

Colliquative Necrosis. Necrosis with softening (colliquative necrosis) rarely occurs as a primary event except in the central nervous system, where necrosis (usually due to infarction) results in softening.

Liquefaction may occur in an area of coagulative necrosis as a result of secondary changes such as suppuration, *e.g.*, in a septic infarct.

Fat Necrosis. Necrosis may occur in the adipose tissue of the peritoneum after the liberation of lipases from an injured or inflamed pancreas (*pancreatic fat necrosis*). The neutral fat is split: glycerol is removed, while the fatty acid remains and gives the damaged cells a cloudy appearance. Macroscopic areas of necrosis appear as opaque, white plaques. The lesions excite an inflammatory response and may be removed within a week or two. Sometimes calcification ensues and, when extensive, may lead to hypocalcemia.

Traumatic fat necrosis is generally encountered in the breast; the changes are similar to those of pancreatic fat necrosis, but the foreign-body giant cell reaction is particularly marked. The lesion may clinically resemble a carcinoma.

Further Changes in Necrotic Tissue

Acute Inflammation. Necrotic tissue excites an inflammatory response, which is followed by a phase of demolition and healing. The appearance of the acute inflammatory response, including an infiltration of polymorphs, is an important feature of most necrotic tissues and is a useful microscopic change that helps distinguish necrosis from postmortem change. Thus, if an area of apparently necrotic cardiac muscle is surrounded by a zone of acute inflammation, the lesion may be safely diagnosed as an infarct. Likewise, the appearance of degenerate renal tubules associated with much edema and separation of tubules

indicates premortem tubular necrosis, not a postmortem change. The acute inflammatory reaction is followed by a phase of demolition, as evidenced by the presence of many macrophages. If much lipid is present in the tissue, or if adipose tissue becomes necrotic, these macrophages contain multiple fine fat droplets and are called *foam cells*. This is a striking feature when necrosis affects brain or fatty tissue, such as in the breast. Sometimes macrophages fuse to form giant cells; these are described later in the section on granulomas (see Chapter 5). An important clinical effect of the acute inflammatory response is fever. This is caused by the release of interleukin-1 from macrophages (see Chapter 14). Thus, fever is encountered in patients with myocardial or pulmonary infarction, and its presence does not necessarily indicate infection.

Gangrene. Sometimes the dead tissue is invaded by saprophytic protein-splitting anaerobic bacteria, which cause its decomposition with the production of hydrogen sulfide and other foul-smelling substances. There is blackening of the area because of the formation of iron sulfide from the iron of decomposed hemoglobin. This *necrosis with superadded putrefaction is called gangrene*, which is an old clinical term that was applied to any black, foul-smelling area in continuity with living tissue.

Clostridial Gangrene. The putrefactive bacteria are usually the clostridia of intestinal origin. Therefore, necrosis of the bowel, particularly of the large intestine, is often followed by gangrene. These putrefactive bacteria are of little importance in themselves, because they live on dead tissue and do not invade or harm the living tissues. Nevertheless, gangrenous lesions always contain pathogenic bacteria that invade tissues and cause further destruction. It follows that gangrene is a very serious condition and is fatal unless treated expeditiously.

Gangrene Due to Other Organisms. Some putrefactive bacteria are also pathogenic, *e.g.*, certain strains of anaerobic streptococci and members of the family Bacteroidaceae, which includes the well-known member *Fusobacterium fusiforme* that is often found in company with a spirochete (*Borrelia vincentii*).

These putrefactive organisms are frequently found in the mouth and are the cause of ulcerative gingivitis, which is often seen following neglect; it is known as "Vincent's infection" or "trench mouth." A more serious gangrenous lesion occasionally affects the soft parts of the face and leads to great tissue destruction. It tends to occur in debilitated children, particularly following measles, but it is now extremely rare in developed countries.

This same group of anaerobic putrefactive organisms is also found in the vagina and is occasionally responsible for gangrene of the uterus after badly conducted labor or ill-performed abortion.

Gangrene of the Limbs. All the examples of gangrene so far mentioned are "wet." There is progressive tissue destruction, and unless effective treatment is instituted without delay, death results. A similar type of wet gangrene occurs in the limbs. It is usually due to sudden blockage of the main arterial supply and is not infrequently a complication of diabetes mellitus. Generally the legs are affected, rather than the arms.

Dry Gangrene. If the blood supply to a limb is slowly occluded, the tips of the digits become black and necrotic and at the same time undergo desiccation. This drying of the part greatly impedes bacterial growth, and infection with pathogenic organisms is minimal. The condition therefore slowly extends until a point is reached at which the blood supply to the limb is adequate. A line of demarcation develops, and the dead tissue is discarded by a process of spontaneous amputation. This condition is called *dry gangrene,* but since the amount of putrefaction is minimal, the term is somewhat of a misnomer. The process is, in fact, mummification of an infarcted portion of a limb.

Gas Gangrene. This condition is due to invasion by pathogenic clostridia and is described in more detail in Chapter 8.

DEGENERATION OF THE EXTRACELLULAR MATRIX

Changes loosely described as degenerative may occur in the interfibrillary matrix or in the fibers themselves, either collagen or elastic.

Changes in the Interfibrillary Matrix

An increased accumulation of water and proteoglycans in the interfibrillary matrix of the dermis occurs in myxedema. The associated fibroblasts tend to become stellate in shape, and the change is usually described as *myxomatous.* A similar change can also occur in other situations, *e.g.,* in the aortic wall in patients with dissecting aneurysm. Because there appears to be degeneration of the tissue involved, the term *myxomatous degeneration* is used. A similar change is seen in the stroma of some epithelial tumors and in some mesenchymal tumors themselves; when marked, the tumor can be called a myxoma.

Changes in Collagen

Fibrosis. In those organs in which collagen formation stops at the reticulin stage, damage seems to stimulate the maturation of the fibers to ordinary fibrous tissue. The term *fibrosis* is used to describe this response. Good examples are the fibrosis seen in cirrhosis of the liver and the fibrosis of lymph nodes draining areas of chronic infection.

Hyalinization. "Hyaline" is a term used to describe any glassy, eosinophilic, acellular tissue. Intracellular hyaline has been described previously. Amyloid may be described as hyaline until its true nature is recognized. As generally used, however, the term hyalinization is applied to a change in collagenous tissue when it becomes acellular and homogeneous. The changes are seen in the collagen of old scars, in the fibrous tissue of chronic inflammatory lesions, in the walls of small blood vessels in hypertension, in atheroma, and in "fibroid" tumors of the uterus. Hyalinized collagen has the normal staining properties of collagen, and it appears very inert and stable.

Necrobiosis. Sometimes collagen becomes eosinophilic and weak and breaks up. This is a characteristic feature of rheumatoid arthritis, and the degenerate collagen excites a chronic inflammatory reaction (see Chapter 30). Necrobiosis in collagen is sometimes described as "fibrinoid necrosis," but this term is also used in other contexts. Thus, the blood vessel walls in malignant hypertension show necrosis and marked eosinophilia. This latter change is probably different from the necrobiosis of rheumatoid arthritis and represents degeneration of the vessel wall as well as infiltration with fibrin.

Changes in Elastic

Changes occur in the elastic tissue in many rare conditions and these are not described. By contrast, a very common condition is *solar elastosis,* in which there is a marked increase in elastic tissue in the dermis; this occurs in skin after prolonged exposure to ultraviolet light. It gives the skin the familiar wrinkled, aged look in those fair-skinned individuals whose occupation or pleasures have resulted in excessive sun exposure.

The genetic disorders of the interfibrillary matrix and of the collagen and elastic fibers are mentioned in Chapter 16.

CELL AGING

The apparent inevitability of death has spurred much research into the process of aging. In tissue culture, it has been found that normal somatic cells will live only for a limited time before they all die. This is termed *clonal aging.* The cell's life span depends on the source of the cells, in particular the age of the subject and the species; so far as human cells are concerned, embryonic fibroblasts divide about 50 times before dying. Malignant cell lines (*e.g.,* HeLa cells), on the other hand, can be grown indefinitely and do not show clonal aging. The mechanisms involved are not understood, but it seems that living cells are programmed to die.

Summary

- Cell damage may be caused by internal events (genetic error, deprivation of blood supply or essential chemicals, or immunologic mechanisms) or external events (heat, cold, radiations, poisons, or microbial effects). A biochemical lesion is often the first event. Later, changes occur in the cell membrane, endoplasmic reticulum, and mitochondria. Abnormal substances (fat, glycogen, mucopolysaccharide) may accumulate.
- Proliferation of the smooth endoplasmic reticulum is an effect of some drugs and can indicate drug-induced enzyme induction.
- Hypoxic damage causes waterlogging (cloudy swelling and hydropic degeneration) and may be mediated by superoxide radical formation.
- Chemical damage is often indirect after metabolism of the agent in the smooth endoplasmic reticulum.
- Fatty change has many causes and is best seen in the liver.
- Hyaline degeneration is a descriptive term; it may be intracellular (alcoholic hyaline) or affect connective tissue.
- Unscheduled DNA synthesis follows damage by ultraviolet light and ionizing radiation damage.
- Cell death is followed by autolysis. It is indicated by nuclear changes. Apoptosis or necrosis follows.
- Necrotic cells release enzymes into the blood, which can be of diagnostic value.
- Necrosis is usually coagulative; if it is due to ischemia, it is called infarction. Other types include colliquative necrosis and caseation.
- Gangrene is necrosis with superadded putrefaction. Descriptive types include infective (clostridial and others), wet, and dry.
- Myxomatous degeneration, fibrosis, hyalinization, and necrobiosis are changes that can occur in the extracellular matrix. Solar elastosis is a common change in the skin caused by excessive sun exposure.

Selected Readings

Alberts, B., Bray, D., Lewis, J., Raff, M., Roberts, K., and Watson, J. D.: Molecular Biology of the Cell. 2nd ed. New York, Garland Publishing, 1989.

Dormandy, T. L.: An approach to free radicals. Lancet 2:1010, 1983.

Finch, C. E., and Schneider, E. L. (eds.): Handbook of the Biology of Aging. New York, Van Nostrand Reinhold, 1985.

Goldstein, S., et al.: Some aspects of cellular aging. J. Chron. Dis. *36:*103, 1983.

Halliwell, B., and Gutteridge, J. M. C.: Lipid peroxidation, oxygen radicals, cell damage, and antioxident therapy. Lancet *1:*1396, 1984.

McCord, J. M.: Oxygen-derived free radicals in postischemic tissue injury. N. Engl. J. Med. *312:*159, 1985.

Searle, J., et al.: Necrosis and apoptosis: Distinct modes of cell death with fundamentally different significance. Pathol. Annu. *17:*229, 1982.

Tissue Reaction to Injury: Inflammation and Healing

After studying this chapter, the student should be able to:

- Describe the vascular changes of acute inflammation and relate these to the formation and composition of inflammatory edema.
- Describe the cellular components of the inflammatory exudate, outline the mechanisms involved in their accumulation, and indicate the role of each type of cell.
- List the variations of the acute inflammatory reaction and give examples of each.
- List the possible local sequelae of an acute inflammation.
- Describe the process of suppuration.
- Describe the triple response.
- List the important chemical mediators of acute inflammation and indicate their probable role.
- Compare the process of axial regeneration in amphibians with that of healing in humans.
- Compare wound contraction with cicatrization.
- Describe the mode of formation and the components of granulation tissue.
- Describe how an incised skin wound heals and compare it with the healing of a skin wound with separated edges.
- List the important complications of wound healing.
- Describe the main features of healing in liver, kidney, tendon, and muscle.
- Compare and contrast healing in the peripheral nervous system with healing in the central nervous system.
- Describe the physical and chemical factors that are involved in the control of cell movement and cell division in wound healing.
- Enumerate the causes of chronic inflammation.
- Give examples of chronic suppurative inflammation and describe the microscopic appearance of a pyogenic membrane.
- Define the term granuloma and describe the three types of the tuberculoid variety.
- Discuss the role of the immune response in relation

to the cause of chronic inflammation and in terms of the tissue response seen.
- Discuss the general effects of chronic inflammation and relate these to the mononuclear phagocyte system.

The body's reaction to injury is complex, for it involves not only a generalized response, which is described in Chapter 19, but also a localized response that is described in this chapter. This response has several components. The initial local reaction is concerned mainly with changes in the connective tissues. The blood vessels dilate and, by becoming more permeable, allow white cells and plasma to leak into the affected area. This exudative reaction is termed *acute inflammation*. Acute inflammation continues as long as tissue damage continues. If the cause of the injury is removed or becomes dissipated, large phagocytic scavenger cells of the mononuclear phagocyte system (macrophages) enter the area from the blood stream and by a process termed *demolition* remove cellular debris and damaged tissue. If little damage has been inflicted on the tissue, the part returns to normal; the process is termed *resolution*. If, on the other hand, there has been structural damage to the part, a process ensues in which new tissue is made for restoration of the defect. This process of *healing* involves repair and regeneration as described later. It sometimes happens that the cause of the damage (*e.g.*, a bacterial infection) is not removed. In this event there is a prolonged tissue response in which acute inflammation is combined with demolition and attempts at healing. This process is termed *chronic inflammation*. An outline of this local reaction to injury is shown in Figure 5–1, and each of its components is described in this chapter.

ACUTE INFLAMMATION

Acute inflammation is familiar to anyone who has ever experienced a boil or suffered from a pustule of acne. It is characterized by four cardinal signs that were originally described by Celsus in the first century A.D. These are *rubor, tumor, calor,* and *dolor,* which indicate that the area is *red, swollen, warmer* than the surrounding tissues (this applies only to skin), and *painful.* Because an inflamed part is often held still, *loss of function* has been added as a fifth sign.

Inflammation is extremely common in clinical practice, and it is convenient to use the suffix *-itis* to denote its presence as in tonsill*itis* for inflammation of the tonsils. In itself, this is not a complete diagnosis, for it does not indicate the cause. There can be tonsillitis due to streptococcal infection or tonsillitis due to infectious mononucleosis or to other viral infections.

Definition

Acute inflammation may best be described as *a reaction of the vascular and supporting elements of the tissue to injury; it results in the formation of a protein-rich exudate, providing the injury has not been so severe as to destroy the area.*

Acute inflammation is mainly a vascular phenomenon and cannot occur in an avascular tissue like the cornea. The reaction is usually beneficial but may not be so under all conditions. The inflammatory cells, particularly macrophages, can themselves spread infection; this is a feature of tuberculosis. Furthermore, inflammatory edema may in some situations endanger life. Thus, in acute laryngitis, the patient, particularly if it is a young child, may asphyxiate. Inflammation must be regarded as a mechanism that has evolved to protect the individual from a wide range of hazards. On the whole it is a beneficial reaction, but under certain circumstances the reaction itself becomes a hazard.

Causes of Acute Inflammation

The causes are the same as those of tissue injury and have been described in Chapter 4.

Changes in Acute Inflammation

Inflammation can be studied in the living animal by observations of thin tissues. The mesentery of the rat and the stretched-thin tongue of

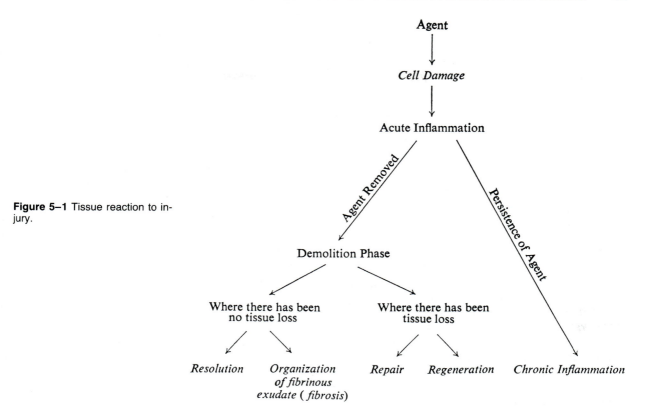

Figure 5–1 Tissue reaction to injury.

the frog have all been used to observe the changing events of inflammation.

The Vascular Response

Although most tissues are liberally provided with capillaries, the limited supply of blood that normally reaches the part is carefully distributed so that at any one time only some vessels contain a stream of blood. Indeed, there is a central or *thoroughfare channel,* and during inactivity much blood passes through it directly from the arterioles to the venules (Fig. 5–2). During activity, the thoroughfare channel closes, and blood is diverted to perfuse the tissues in response to their increased metabolism. In addition, there is arteriolar dilation, which increases the total volume of blood available. In acute inflammation, the response is similar. There is arteriolar dilation so that more blood passes into the part. The precapillary sphincters open, so that the capillaries become distended and blood ceases to flow

through the preferential channel (Fig. 5–2*B*). This increased content of blood is termed *hyperemia* and is the reason the inflamed part appears red. The skin, being normally cooler than the arterial blood, becomes warmer because of the increased flow. Dilation of blood vessels (*vasodilation*) is thus a characteristic feature of acute inflammation.

Changes in Blood Flow. In a normal tissue, blood in the arterioles travels so fast that one cannot discern individual cells. In the large tortuous venules, on the other hand, the cells can be seen to occupy the central or axial part of the stream and are separated from the endothelial lining by a clear zone of plasma (*plasmatic zone*). This arrangement is dictated by physical laws and has the advantage of reducing the viscosity of blood. In acute inflammation, plasma leaks from the vessels, and the blood consequently becomes more viscid; the lubricating action of the plasmatic zone is impaired, and the stream slows down. This process is termed *stasis.* Meanwhile, two other important changes occur. The

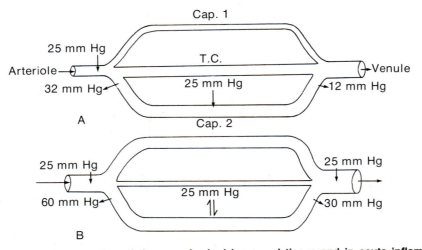

Figure 5–2 Diagrammatic representation of the vascular bed in normal tissue and in acute inflamed tissue. *A,* In the normal resting tissue, much of the blood passes directly through the thoroughfare channel (T.C.) from the arteriole to the venule. One capillary is closed (Cap. 1), whereas some blood passes through the other capillary (Cap. 2). The hydrostatic pressure at the arteriolar end of the capillary is 32 mm Hg and at the venous end 12 mm Hg. These forces tend to drive fluid out of the vessel and are countered by the osmotic pressure of the plasma proteins—about 25 mm Hg. The interstitial extravascular fluid normally contains very little protein. Hence, fluid tends to leave the vessel at the arteriolar end and to be reabsorbed at the venous end.

B, In an inflamed tissue, the arteriole is dilated, the thoroughfare channel is closed, and both capillaries are dilated by the increased blood flow. The hydrostatic pressure throughout the capillary is shown. Plasma proteins have leaked from the vessel so that their concentration in the interstitial fluid approximates that of the plasma. The osmotic effect of the plasma proteins tending to drive fluid into the vessels is thereby neutralized. Fluid exudes along the entire length of the capillary and is ultimately halted by a rise in tissue tension. (Drawing by Margot Mackay, Faculty of Medicine, Department of Surgery, Division of Biomedical Communications, University of Toronto.)

endothelial cells contract, and the spaces between adjacent cells become widened, thereby permitting plasma and cells to pass between them. At the same time, white cells move into the plasmatic zone and stick to the altered vessel wall. This adhesion is highly characteristic of acute inflammation and is best seen in the venules. At first, the cells adhere for a short time, and then they either roll gently along the endothelial lining or get swept back into the blood stream. Later, however, the cells become more firmly adherent and line the endothelium, forming masses that may even block the lumen. This phenomenon is known as *margination of the leukocytes,* or *pavementation of the endothelium,* and is the prelude to the emigration of the white cells from the blood stream into the interstitial tissue spaces (Fig. 5–3).

The mechanism whereby white cells adhere to the endothelium involves the presence of adhesion molecules on the cell membrane of leukocytes and endothelium. For instance, leukocytes have several such molecules, one of which is termed LAF-1. An adhesion molecule on endothelium, termed intracellular adhesion molecule-1 (ICAM-1), serves as a receptor for LAF-1. In inflammation, the various chemical mediators (such as interleukin-1 and complement fractions) promote the expression of these adhesion molecules on the surface of leukocytes, endothelial cells, or both and promote leukocyte adhesion.

Formation of the Exudate

The most characteristic feature of acute inflammation is the formation of an exudate that has both a fluid and a cellular component (Fig. 5–4).

The Fluid Exudate. Under normal conditions, the vascular endothelium is virtually impermeable to the plasma proteins, and the fluid that escapes from the vessels has a low protein content; on reaching the interstitial tissues, it either returns to the venules or is gathered by the lymphatics and returned to the circulation. In acute inflammation, the increased vascular permeability allows the plasma proteins to leak through the vessel wall, causing the osmotic

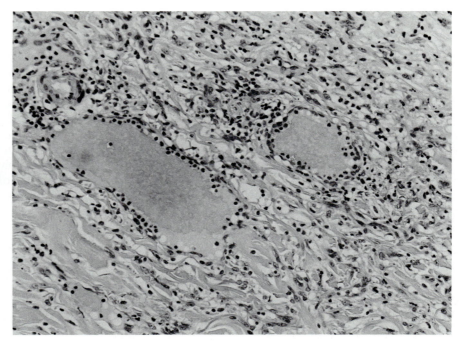

Figure 5–3 Pavementation of the endothelium. The two large vessels are venules. Their lining is covered by adherent white cells, mainly neutrophils.

pressure effect of the plasma proteins to be lost. An increased volume of fluid therefore leaves the vessels, and this forms the inflammatory exudate (Fig. 5–2*B*). A useful method of investigating this phenomenon is to tag the blood albumin either with a dye such as trypan blue or with a radioactive isotope of iodine. The accumulation of tagged albumin in the interstitial tissues of an area of inflammation then becomes an index of the change in vascular permeability.

This type of investigation indicates that increased permeability occurs in three phases.

Immediate Transient Phase. This lasts about 30 minutes, affects venules, and is largely mediated by histamine.

Immediate Prolonged Phase. The exudation starts immediately and persists for days. It appears to be due to direct damage to vessels.

Delayed Prolonged Phase. In this phase, which peaks 4 to 24 hours after injury, it is thought that

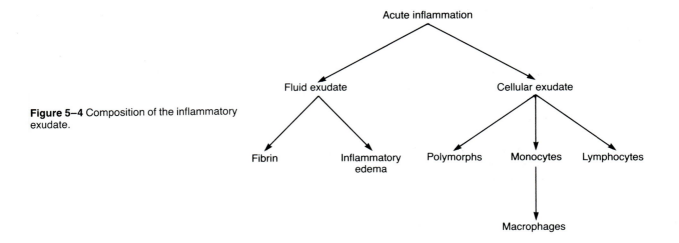

Figure 5–4 Composition of the inflammatory exudate.

both capillaries and venules are affected both by direct injury and by chemical mediators. The swelling and erythema of sunburn is a good example.

There is another factor that plays an important part in the formation of the inflammatory exudate: one of the first detectable changes in experimental lesions is an alteration in the ground substance, causing it to become more fluid. The effect of this increased fluidity is to allow the exudate to diffuse into surrounding tissues more readily and thereby to prevent an immediate rise in tissue tension. Nevertheless, the tissue tension eventually increases, thereby limiting the amount of exudate formed, because it tends to drive fluid back into the venules. The increased tissue tension is one important factor in the causation of pain. It follows that inflammation in a densely compact tissue or in an enclosed space causes severe pain. This is well illustrated by the pain that is experienced in infections of the pulp of a finger, an acne pustule on the nose, and acute osteomyelitis in which the marrow is encased in unyielding bone.

The fluid leaving the blood vessels in acute inflammation has almost the same composition as plasma, and it contains antibacterial substances (such as complement) as well as specific antibodies. If present in the plasma, drugs and antibiotics also appear in the exudate. The importance of the early administration of therapeutic agents is obvious when one recalls that these agents are merely carried to the inflamed area in the exudate and are in no way concentrated there. Furthermore, the fluid in the exudate is in a state of flux, since it is in equilibrium with the circulating plasma. Therapeutic agents must therefore be administered continuously if their concentration is to remain at a therapeutic level in the area of inflammation.

The fluid of the exudate has additional effects. It dilutes any irritating chemicals and bacterial toxins that might be present. The fibrinogen in it is converted into fibrin by the action of tissue factor (Chapter 18), and a *fibrin clot* forms. This fibrin forms a fine network of fibers and has three main functions:

1. It forms a *union* between severed tissues.
2. It forms a *barrier* against bacterial invasion (Chapter 7).

3. It aids *phagocytosis* (discussed later in this chapter).

The Cellular Exudate. The white cells adhering to the endothelium of blood vessels soon push pseudopodia between adjacent endothelial cells, penetrate the basement membrane, and emerge on the external surface of the vessel. This remarkable process is called *emigration of the white cells*; for the most part, neutrophil polymorphonuclear leukocytes* predominate during the early phases of an acute inflammatory response. The gap that is left by the emigrating white cell soon closes behind it, although sometimes a few red cells escape at the same time. A variable number of lymphocytes and monocytes also leave the blood vessels. Figure 5–5 shows the typical appearance of an acutely inflamed tissue. The fixed tissue cells are separated by edema, and fibrin threads can be seen bathed in the edema fluid. Numerous white cells—for the most part polymorphs—are seen lying within the fluid exudate.

The movement of white cells into the interstitial tissues of an inflamed part appears to be a purposeful event, but it is obvious that the cells are not capable of independent, thoughtful action and that there must be some mechanism by which they are enticed from the vessels into the area of damage. It is generally believed that the attraction is of a chemical nature. Directional movement of cells in response to a chemical gradient is well known in biology and is called *chemotaxis*. An example of this movement is seen in the reproduction of the fern. The spermatozoids of the male are attracted by malic acid produced by the female germ cells.

The mechanism whereby white cells sense the presence of a chemotactic agent is believed to involve the activation of specific membrane receptors for the particular agent. With use of the Boyden chamber, a number of such chemotactic agents have been identified (Fig. 5–6); these include starch and certain bacterial products, particularly those containing formyl peptides. Antigen-antibody complexes and dead tissue are chemotactic, but only if complement is present and activated. Several separate components are

---

*These cells are commonly called "PMNs," "polys," or "polymorphs." The abbreviation *polymorph* is used frequently in this book.

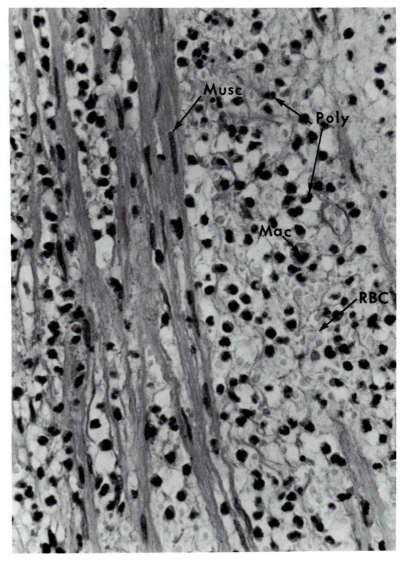

Figure 5–5 Acute appendicitis. This section was taken through the wall of an acutely inflamed appendix. The smooth muscle cells (Musc) are separated by inflammatory edema, and the whole of the area is heavily infiltrated by inflammatory cells, mostly polymorphs (Poly). Macrophages (Mac) and red cells (RBC) are also present in the exudate (×600).

involved; the most important is C5a. Other chemotactic agents are leukotriene B4 and platelet-activating factor. Present evidence suggests that polymorphs are attracted to a site of inflammation by chemotactic agents, but the relative importance of the various factors is not known. It probably varies according to the cause of the inflammation.

One of the characteristic features of the inflammatory exudate is that in the initial stages, polymorphs predominate; but as time goes by, these are replaced by monocytes. One explanation of this phenomenon is that polymorphs, having a very limited life span (probably a few hours), soon die off, leaving the long-lived mononuclear cells to replace them. Until recently, it was thought that all agents attracting polymorphs also attract monocytes and that the change in population of the inflammatory exudate could be explained on the basis of a slow, steady recruitment of monocytes in the face of rapid destruction of polymorphs. It is now

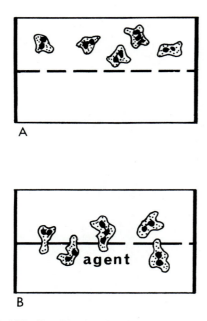

Figure 5–6 The Boyden chamber for detecting chemotactic activity. The Boyden chamber consists of two tissue culture chambers placed one on top of the other and separated by a membrane of 3 μm pore size (*A*). A suspension of polymorphs is placed in the upper chamber, and the test substance is placed in the lower. The number of cells that migrate to the lower surface of the filter is a measure of the chemotactic effect (*B*). (From Walter, J. B., and Israel, M. S.: General Pathology. 6th ed. Edinburgh, Churchill Livingstone, 1987.)

known that this is an oversimplification of the process and that some chemotactic agents can act on different types of leukocytes.

The immune response plays a part. The reaction of antigen with IgE bound to mast cells causes the release of a chemotactic factor (ECF-A) that specifically acts on eosinophils, cells that are prominent in certain allergic inflammations. Another important source of chemotactic agents is derived from T lymphocytes with receptors for the particular antigen. When these cells are acted upon by the antigen, they release *lymphokines,* some of which appear to have specific chemotactic effect on neutrophils, eosinophils, monocytes, or lymphocytes.

Lymphocytes are found in areas of inflammation, particularly during the healing process. In certain instances, they are the predominant cell in the early phase of acute inflammation; viral infections and acute dermatitis are good examples in which this occurs. The mechanism of

their accumulation is less well understood. As noted before, lymphocytes can release lymphokines; they may therefore play several roles in acute inflammation.

Functions of Cellular Exudate: Phagocytosis

Polymorphonuclear Leukocytes. The main function of these cells is *phagocytosis.* They ingest bacteria and other foreign particles (Fig. 5–7). Phagocytosis is aided by two mechanisms.

1. Opsonization. Opsonins are proteins present in the plasma that coat organisms and cause them to be more easily phagocytosed. Some opsonins appear to be quite *nonspecific* and are present in all normal individuals, whereas others (*immune opsonins*) are antibodies that are *specific* for the particular organisms that excited their formation. It follows that phagocytosis is more marked in the inflammation of an individual who has been immunized against the particular infecting organism. Phagocytes possess Fc and C3b receptors that enable them to recognize and adhere to organisms coated with antibody or complement (Chapter 6).

2. Surface phagocytosis. The fibrin clot of the inflammatory exudate provides a network on which polymorphs can trap organisms. This method of phagocytosis can occur in the absence of opsonins and is presumably of value to the individual who is not immune.

Fibronectins aid attachment of monocytes to particles, and this plays a part in initiating phagocytosis by these cells.

Polymorphs show loss of their granules after phagocytosis. The granules are, in fact, lysosomes; they fuse with phagocytic vesicles, and their lytic enzymes enter the common sac where digestion proceeds (Fig. 5–7).

Polymorphs release various chemicals after phagocytosis. These include *lysosomal enzymes,* which play a part in the digestion of dead tissue during the phase of healing.

Another factor released by phagocytes, particularly macrophages, is interleukin-1, previously called endogenous pyrogen. It acts on the hypothalamic heat-regulating center and leads to fever. It also increases catabolism in skeletal muscle. This is probably the mechanism of fever and muscle pains with wasting that often accompany many acute infections (see Chapter 14).

The way in which organisms are killed by

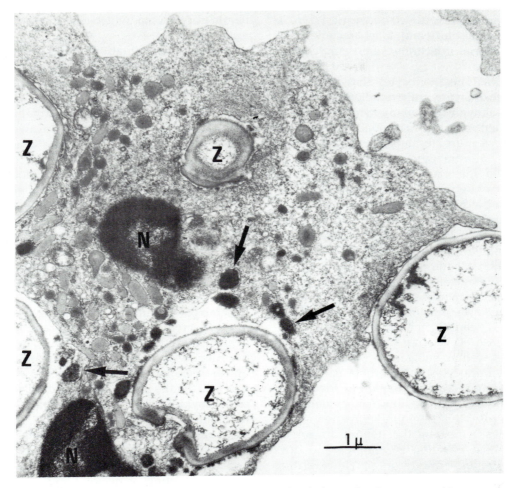

Figure 5–7 Phagocytosis. A human peripheral blood polymorphonuclear leukocyte has been exposed to zymogen particles (Z). Two lobes of its nucleus are seen (N), but they are not seen to be connected in this section. At the right is a particle that has been bound to the cell wall but has not yet been phagocytosed. In the lower portion of this picture are zymogen particles in phagocytic vacuoles. Lysosomes surround the particles and have degranulated into the vacuoles (arrows). Bacteria are treated in a similar manner and may later be destroyed (×21,500). (Courtesy of Dr. Sylvia Hoffstein and Dr. Gerald Weissmann, New York University Medical Center. From Walter, J. B., and Israel, M. S.: General Pathology. 6th ed. Edinburgh, Churchill Livingstone, 1987.)

polymorphs and macrophages is complex and incompletely understood. The energy for phagocytosis is derived from glycolysis, and the lactic acid produced by this anaerobic process is bactericidal. Nevertheless, bactericidal activity is dependent mainly on oxidative reactions, with glucose being oxidized via the hexose monophosphate shunt (see Fig. 2–11). Hydrogen peroxide appears to be one of the vital bactericidal agents produced as a result of this.

The details of polymorph activity in acute inflammation have been stressed because these cells play a vital role in the body's defenses against many infections. Patients with a low neutrophil count (*e.g.*, due to bone marrow aplasia or acute leukemia) often develop severe gingivitis or pharyngitis and subsequently die of overwhelming infection. Furthermore, there are a number of rare but interesting diseases in which polymorph function is defective. In the "lazy leukocyte syndrome," there are defective movement and chemotaxis. In the more common *chronic granulomatous disease*, there is defective bactericidal activity after normal phagocytosis of bacteria. The disease affects boys (it is an X-linked recessive trait) and is characterized by repeated bacterial infections, often staphylococcal.

Macrophages. The monocytes that accumulate in the area of acute inflammation are highly phagocytic; as with the polymorphs, their ingestion of virulent organisms is aided by opsonins. The monocytes are termed *macrophages* when they show morphologic evidence of having phagocytosed material within them. Thus, the monocyte may be regarded as a resting cell that circulates in the blood. Once it enters an area of inflammation, it enlarges, becomes highly phagocytic, and is then termed "a macrophage." Another important function of the macrophage is its role in the immune response (Chapter 6).

The macrophage also acts as a secretory cell in that it releases many substances, particularly when engaged in phagocytosis. These include interleukin-1, complement components, lysozyme, elastase, collagenase, and plasminogen activator, as well as substances (*monokines*) that stimulate lymphocytes and fibroblasts. The importance of the secretory function of the macrophage is not fully known, but it is evident that this cell plays a vital role in inflammation and in the processes of healing that follow. Its role in defense against infection is complex and does not appear to rest entirely on activities relating to scavenger function.

Variations of the Acute Inflammatory Reaction

Although all examples of acute inflammation have many features in common, some types have been categorized on the basis of some particular gross or microscopic feature—often the type of exudate. The categories are useful for descriptive purposes and are commonly used, but the differences are of no fundamental importance.

Serous Inflammation. In inflammation of serous sacs and loose tissues such as the subcutaneous tissues around the vulva, scrotum, and eyes, the fluid component of an inflammatory exudate exceeds the cellular one, because the limiting factor of increased tissue tension is absent. There results a large accumulation of inflammatory edema, which is termed *serous inflammation.*

Fibrinous Inflammation. Fibrin formation is an obvious feature of inflammation in the lungs and on the surface of the serous membranes. Thus, it forms a well-marked feature of pericarditis and peritonitis (Fig. 5–8). Fibrinous inflammation of this type is often accompanied by an accumulation of serous fluid; thus, the term "serofibrinous inflammation" is an apt one.

Hemorrhagic Inflammation. The blood-stained exudate indicates severe vascular damage and bleeding. It is seen in the lungs after phosgene poisoning and in acute influenzal pneumonia. Hemorrhagic inflammation is encountered in vasculitic lesions, *e.g.*, those of gonococcal septicemia (Fig. 8–3) and the Arthus reaction (Chapter 6). Acute hemorrhagic pancreatitis provides another example (Chapter 24).

Catarrhal Inflammation. This is seen when a mucus-secreting mucous membrane is involved in an acute inflammatory reaction. There is some destruction of the epithelial cells and a profuse mucus secretion from those cells that remain as well as from the underlying glands. The common cold provides an excellent example of this type of inflammation.

Pseudomembranous Inflammation. This type of reaction is encountered on mucosal surfaces and describes the formation of a pseudomembrane, consisting of necrotic epithelium and inflammatory exudate, that covers the surface and is tightly adherent to it in the initial stages of its formation. The reaction is characteristic of diphtheritic lesions of the tonsils or pharynx. If an attempt is made to remove the gray membrane, bleeding results. Pseudomembranous colitis is described in Chapter 23.

Gangrenous Inflammation. Gangrene occurs in inflammation when the dead tissue is invaded by putrefactive organisms (Chapters 4 and 8).

Suppurative Inflammation. Inflammation resulting in the formation of pus is described later in this chapter.

Variability of the Cellular Exudate

Certain inflammations do not show the usual neutrophil polymorph response. Sometimes *eo-*

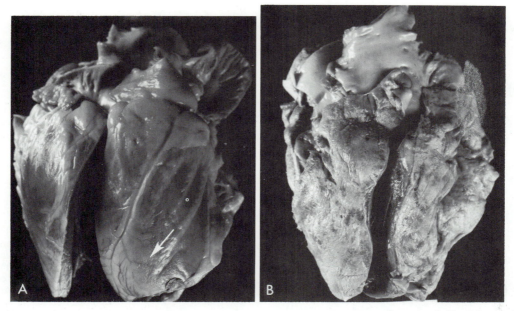

Figure 5–8 Acute pericarditis. Two hearts have each been opened in the routine way at necropsy. *A,* Heart from a 24-year-old woman who had been diagnosed as having systemic lupus erythematosus. In spite of treatment, the patient developed the nephrotic syndrome and died of renal failure. At necropsy, the pericardial sac contained 60 ml of straw-colored clear fluid; in some areas overlying the left ventricle, the pericardium was covered by a thin layer of fibrinous exudate (arrow). Elsewhere the pericardium is thin, shiny, and normal-appearing. This is an example of serofibrinous inflammation. *B,* Heart from a patient who had been operated on for cancer of the stomach but in whom the area of surgery had become infected. At necropsy, pus was present in the left pleural space (thoracic empyema or pyothorax). Infection had spread to the pericardial sac, which also contained thick pus. The pericardial surface of the heart is seen to be covered by a thick, shaggy inflammatory exudate. Compare with *A.*

sinophils are plentiful—particularly with inflammations produced by parasitic worms and with some allergic conditions, such as hay fever. *Lymphocytic infiltration* is frequent in inflammatory lesions produced by viruses, even in the early stages. It is also a feature of acute inflammation in many skin diseases. Occasionally *macrophages* are the predominant cell in the inflammatory response (see Pathogenesis of Typhoid Fever, Chapter 7). This variation in cellular response is probably brought about by the actions of various chemotactic agents.

Local Sequelae of Acute Inflammation

The changes that follow acute inflammation are shown in Figure 5–1 and depend on two major factors: (1) the amount of tissue damage sustained and (2) whether the causative agent remains in the body.

Resolution. In acutely inflamed tissues in which cellular damage has been relatively slight and reversible, necrosis does not occur. If the causative agent is eliminated by the inflammatory reaction—for instance, the pneumococcus in lobar pneumonia—or if the agent itself acts only once, such as in acute sunburn, the acute inflammatory reaction terminates by resolution (Fig. 5–9). The polymorph cellular infiltrate is replaced by macrophages that engulf degenerate fibrin, red cells, polymorphs, and any other dead tissue that remains. Some of the fluid exudate returns to the blood in the venules, but most of it is carried away by the lymphatics to the regional lymph nodes, where mononuclear phagocytes remove cellular debris before the fluid is returned to the circulation. With the removal of the inflammatory exudate and subsequent return of the macrophages to the lymphatics, the tissue is restored to its normal, previous state. *Resolution is the term applied to the process by which the tissue returns to normal after acute inflammation.*

Organization of Exudate. Occasionally the in-

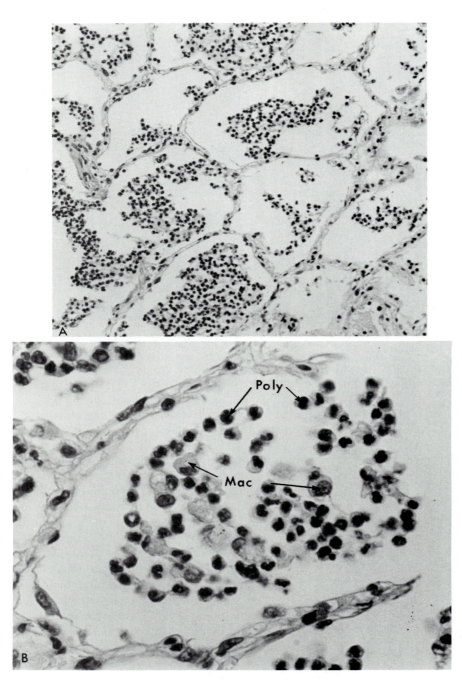

Figure 5–9 Bronchopneumonia. *A,* Instead of containing air, the alveoli are filled with inflammatory exudate, the cellular component of which is obvious. An inflamed lung such as this is airless (*consolidated*); the condition is called pneumonia (×250). *B,* Higher magnification of one alveolus from the same case as *A.* The cellular exudate contains many macrophages (Mac) in addition to the polymorphs (Poly). The pneumonia is beginning to resolve (×600).

flammatory exudate is not removed expeditiously enough, and it becomes invaded by granulation tissue and converted into scar tissue. It is a very common event to find fibrous adhesions between the visceral and parietal layers of the pleura. These are the organized remnants of some previous pleurisy. Likewise, fibrous adhesions are very common in the abdomen. They may occur around a site of previous inflammation such as an inflamed appendix, or they can follow surgery. Such adhesions make subsequent surgery more difficult; they can render it impossible to undertake sterilization by ligating the fallopian tubes through a peritoneoscope.

Suppuration. When the noxious agent produces much necrosis of the tissue involved, resolution is impossible. If the exudate contains many polymorphs, the center of the inflammatory lesion becomes a cavity filled with a liquid containing dead tissue and numerous polymorphs, which are now called *pus cells*. The fluid is referred to as *pus*, and an inflammation with this type of response is termed *suppurative*. An agent causing this type of reaction is termed *pyogenic*, and a typical example of such an infection is a boil caused by *Staphylococcus aureus*. The hair follicle and adjacent dermis undergo necrosis, and a small sac of pus is formed. The necrotic tissue in an area of suppuration softens by virtue of the proteolytic lysosomal enzymes of the polymorphs as well as by autolysis mediated by the tissue's own enzymes. The creamy fluid is contained in a cavity called an *abscess* (see Fig. 33–4), and surrounding this there is a *pyogenic membrane*, which at this stage consists of inflamed and necrotic tissue with much fibrinous exudate and polymorph infiltration. The pus itself is composed of (a) leukocytes, some of which are dead; (b) other components of the inflammatory exudate, such as edema fluid with fibrin; (c) organisms, many of which are alive and can be cultured; and (d) tissue debris, such as nucleic acids and lipids. The pus tends not to remain at the site of its formation but rather to track in the line of least resistance until a free surface is reached. Then the abscess bursts and discharges its contents spontaneously. In clinical practice this is usually anticipated by surgical drainage, because until the pus has been evacuated, healing is much delayed. If drained, an abscess heals by granulation tissue, but if the causative agent persists, chronic inflammation ensues. This response is considered later in this chapter.

If, as occasionally happens, the abscess is not drained and remains localized or sequestered in the tissues, its walls become organized into dense fibrous tissue, and the pus undergoes thickening, or *inspissation*. It develops a porridgelike consistency and eventually calcifies.

When an acute suppurative inflammation involves an epithelial surface, the covering is destroyed and an ulcer is formed (Fig. 5–10). An *ulcer* is a term used to describe a localized defect of a covering or a lining epithelium. In the first instance, the floor of the ulcer is covered by necrotic tissue and acute inflammatory exudate; this layer is called a *slough* and is at first adherent, because the dead tissue has not yet become liquefied. Eventually, however, the slough becomes detached, and the ulcer heals by the processes of repair and regeneration. Alternatively, the ulceration may persist and become chronic (see Fig. 5–16).

Chronic Inflammation. This is described later in the chapter.

The Chemical Mediators of Acute Inflammation

The apparent uniformity of the acute inflammatory response—regardless of its cause—has led many investigators to presume that the changes are mediated by chemical agents that are formed when the tissue is damaged, rather than being caused directly by the injury itself. The search for these mediators has a practical as well as a theoretical objective. If these chemical substances could be identified, antagonistic drugs might be designed and administered to prevent or modify the acute inflammatory response. The mediators are listed in Table 5–1.

Histamine

At first, it appeared that the major mediator in acute inflammation was histamine. This is a simple amine of the amino acid histidine; if it is

Table 5–1 CHEMICAL MEDIATORS OF ACUTE INFLAMMATION

Histamine
Kinins—bradykinin
Products of complement
Polymorph products
Arachidonic acid derivatives
    Prostaglandins
    Leukotrienes
Other possible mediators

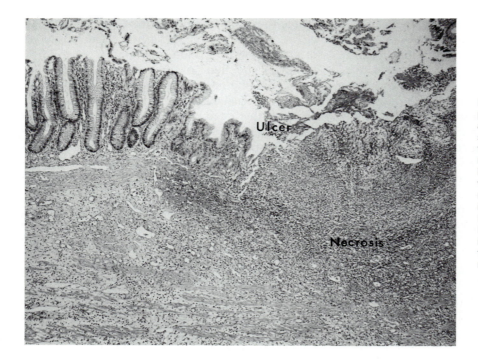

Figure 5–10 Suppurative appendicitis with mucosal ulceration. The wall of the appendix shows the changes of acute inflammation. Edema separates the muscle fibers, and there is a heavy infiltration by polymorphs, which cannot be identified at this magnification. On the right there is necrosis. The overlying epithelium has been cast off, thereby leaving an area of ulceration. This is an example of suppurative inflammation with ulceration of the mucous membrane ($\times$60).

injected into the skin, it produces a reaction that is very similar to that produced by injuring the skin mechanically.

The Triple Response. Shortly after a firm stroking of the skin, a *red line* appears that is due to capillary dilation. Soon after this, a more diffuse and widespread *flare* appears surrounding the red line. This results from arteriolar dilation. Finally, a swelling or a *wheal* appears at the site of the red line, and this is due to exudation of fluid through the altered vascular wall (Fig. 5–11). This triple response of the red line, flare, and wheal was first noted by Sir Thomas Lewis to be very similar to the local changes that follow an injection of histamine. Indeed, there is little doubt that injury to the skin releases histamine from mast cells and that histamine is responsible for the phenomenon of the triple response. It now appears that histamine is the important mediator of the early phase of acute inflammation. Antihistaminic drugs have been developed, and their administration, while blocking the early phase of exudation, is without effect on the prolonged phases. Histamine is especially important in inflammation having a type I allergic basis (Chapter 6), and antihistaminic drugs are of some value in the treatment of hay fever. Nevertheless, in the acute response to most infections, histamine appears to play little part. Antihistamines are therefore of limited value in practice.

The Kinins

The blood contains an enzyme called *kallikrein*, which exists as a precursor (*prekallikrein*) and can be activated under certain circumstances (Fig. 5–12). The kallikrein acts on a plasma protein (*kininogen*) and produces a polypeptide called *bradykinin*. This was so named because it causes a slow contraction of guinea pig small intestine *in vitro* as opposed to the kick produced by histamine. Bradykinin is an extremely potent chemical that causes an increase in vascular permeability and is chemotactic to white cells. It causes pain and clearly is a good candidate for being a mediator of acute inflammation. There is good evidence that bradykinin is formed after injury; as with histamine, however, it seems that its role is limited strictly to the early phase of acute inflammation. Tissues become refractory to the prolonged action of both bradykinin and histamine; therefore, neither can be mediators of the prolonged phases.

Products of Complement Activation

Complement can be activated not only by antigen-antibody interaction but also by tissue damage. A number of fragments of complement, *e.g.*, C5a and C3a, can release histamine from mast cells (Chapter 6).

Components of Polymorphs

Although inflammation can occur in the absence of polymorphs, these cells can release vasoactive compounds that may play a part in the inflammatory reaction. Among these are lysosomal enzymes that can activate kallikrein and indirectly can lead to the formation of bradykinin. In addition, they can lead to local tissue destruction and activate complement. This is an important mechanism in the pathogenesis of immune-complex reactions.

Arachidonic Acid Derivatives

Arachidonic acid, a long-chain polyunsaturated fatty acid, is released by the action of phospholipase A2 from lipids released from the cell membranes when they are disturbed. It can be converted into either prostaglandins or leukotrienes by the action of separate pathways (Fig. 5–13). This transformation can occur in many cell types, but mast cells and platelets have been most intensively studied.

Prostaglandins. The action of cyclo-oxygenase on arachidonic acid leads to the formation of a variety of prostaglandins. Some, *e.g.*, PGE1 and PGE2, produce vasodilation, increase vascular permeability, and cause pain. It is believed that these also potentiate the actions of kinins in increasing vascular permeability. Hence, their action in inflammation is in part direct and in part due to a modulating action on the effect of other mediators. *Thromboxane A2* causes platelet aggregation so that more platelet-derived factors are available at a site of damage. Aspirin and other nonsteroidal anti-inflammatory drugs inhibit the enzyme cyclo-oxygenase and thereby prevent prostaglandin formation. In part, this explains the popularity of these drugs in the management of acute inflammatory lesions and

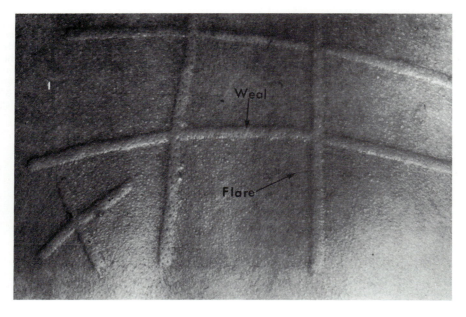

Figure 5–11 The triple response. This game of tick-tack-toe was started on the skin of the back about 3 minutes before the photograph was taken. Red lines developed and were soon replaced by well-marked wheals. The response is more marked in this subject than in the average person, but the ability to write on the skin in this way is not uncommon and is termed *dermatographism.* It is generally asymptomatic as in this 21-year-old female.

pain. The action of the glucocorticoids is different—they inhibit phospholipase A.

Leukotrienes. Metabolism of arachidonic acid via the 5-lipoxygenase pathway leads to the formation of a variety of leukotrienes. The slow-reacting substance of anaphylaxis (SRS-A) is a mixture of LTC4, LTD4 and LTE4. Another leukotriene, LTB4, is a potent chemotactic agent affecting neutrophils, eosinophils, and mono-

cytes. The leukotrienes are regarded as secondary mediators, being generated by mast cells rather than being released from a storage form in granules.

Platelet-Activating Factor

This substance is released from IgE-sensitized mast cells when they are acted upon by the

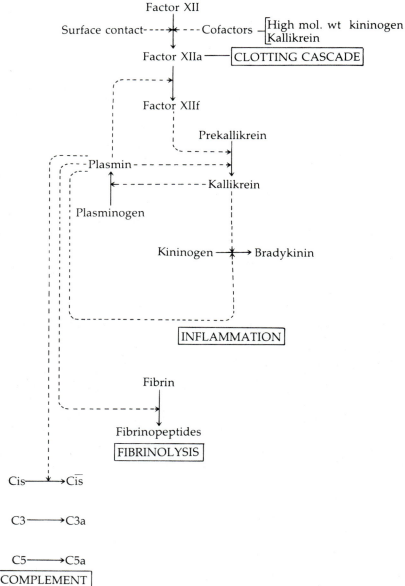

Figure 5–12 The kinin system. The Hageman factor (factor XII) plays a central role in initiating clotting, fibrinolysis, and kinin formation. When activated, it forms factor XIIa and factor XIIf. Factor XIIa has a major role in initiating the clotting cascade but a minor one in activating prekallikrein. Conversely, factor XIIf has as its major action the activation of prekallikrein to kallikrein, the enzyme that activated kininogen to kinin. Transformations are depicted as solid lines, whereas enzymatic actions are shown as interrupted lines. Inhibitors are not shown. (Modified from Walter, J. B.: Pathology of Human Disease. Philadelphia, Lea & Febiger, 1989. Courtesy of Dr. B. K. Fisher, Wellesley Hospital, Toronto.)

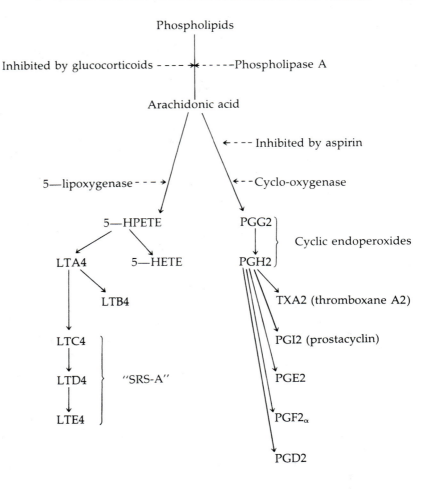

Figure 5–13 Arachidonic acid derivatives. Cyclo-oxygenase acts on arachidonic acid to form the two cyclic endoperoxides PGG2 and PGH2. From these are formed a variety of prostaglandins including PGI2 (prostacyclin) and TxA2 (thromboxane A2). The enzyme 5-lipoxygenase generates 5-hydroperoxyeicosatetraenoic acid (5-HPETE). From this can be formed the leukotrienes LTC4, LTD4, and LTE4, which together have been called the slow reactive substance of anaphylaxis (SRS-A). LTB4 is a powerful chemotactic agent. The product actually formed, whether along the 5-lipoxygenase or cyclo-oxygenase pathway, depends on the cell type, the species, and the stimulus applied to the cell. (From Lewis, R. A., and Austen, K. F.: Mediators of local homeostasis and inflammation by leukotrienes and other mast cell–dependent compounds. Nature *293*:103, 1981. Copyright © 1981, Macmillan Magazines Ltd.)

appropriate antigen. In addition to its effect on platelets (causing aggregation and release of histamine), it is chemotactic to white cells and causes vasodilation and increased vascular permeability.

Cytokines

Cytokines are polypeptides produced by one cell that act on the same cell (an autocrine action), an adjacent cell (a paracrine effect), or a distant cell (an endocrine effect). The best known are the *lymphokines* produced by lymphoid cells and the *monokines* produced by monocytes. These terms in fact refer to groups of cytokines, and more recently individual members have been categorized. Interleukin-1 (IL-1) and tumor necrosis factor (TNF) are two such agents. They

have similar actions; these include promotion of the expression of adhesion molecules responsible for white cell adhesion to endothelium, and induction of the release of PGI2 and platelet-activating factor. When released into the blood, they lead to fever, increased protein catabolism in muscle, and other manifestations of the acute phase response (see Chapters 14 and 19). This is probably the mechanism of fever and muscle pains with wasting that often accompany many severe infections (see Chapter 17).

Conclusion

Although many agents are known that can simulate the changes encountered in the acute inflammatory response to trauma and infection, their actual role and relative importance are not known. Indeed, the number of chemicals that have been suggested as mediators of acute inflammation is now so large, and their interrelationship is so complex, that it is not possible to give any clear account of their role in acute inflammation. One cannot but agree with Ryan and Majno—the inflammatory "soup" is so complicated that no single individual can claim to know how the dozens of components relate to each other or how they change during the evolution of the inflammatory response. There has been a tendency to stress the uniformity of the inflammatory reaction regardless of its cause, but this uniformity may be more apparent than real. There can be little doubt that bacterial toxins can also initiate or modify the inflammatory response; in particular, clostridia produce toxins that are capable of acting directly on blood vessels and increasing their permeability. Recent observations of the details of the vascular response to injury have revealed that it is a multiphased response with both early and delayed components affecting capillaries and venules. The precise changes vary according to the type of injury and the species of animal involved. It is therefore hardly surprising that no single common chemical mediator is involved. So far, much research has been directed to the vasodilation and increased vascular permeability of acute inflammation caused by trauma and chemical agents. The much more complex cellular changes and the intricacies of infection have been largely neglected.

HEALING: REPAIR AND REGENERATION

Healing is one of the fundamental processes in pathology. It follows obvious traumatic damage, such as that caused by a surgical incision or a stab wound, as well as damage produced by heat, freezing, radiation, infection, chemical toxin, and ischemia or as a result of a damaging immune reaction. The process of healing has obvious survival value for the individual and has therefore been highly developed in all forms of life. Nevertheless, it differs from one species to another as well as from one tissue to another within the same individual.

In insects, amphibians, and crustaceans, the ability to replace lost parts has long been known and is truly remarkable. For example, if the lens of the eye of a salamander is removed, a new lens develops from the adjacent iris. Other well-known examples of regeneration are the regrowth of the amputated limbs of insects and newts and of the claws of lobsters. The process whereby whole limbs are re-formed is well developed in lower forms of life; it is complex and resembles embryonic development or asexual reproduction. The process is termed *axial regeneration* by zoologists and has been intensively studied in the hope that it might provide some clues to our understanding of healing in humans. After the amputation of the arm of a newt, the stump rapidly becomes covered by a layer of epidermal cells while the underlying connective tissue cells dedifferentiate to form a mass of primitive cells that form a *blastema*. Its cells multiply rapidly in an avascular field in the first instance. Later there is vascularization and differentiation: bone, muscle, tendon, nerves, and blood vessels are produced in a coordinated manner such that there is accurate replacement of the limb that was lost. No matter what the level of the original amputation, only the distal parts are replaced. Hence, after a forearm amputation, the wrist and hand are re-formed, but never an elbow. This rule of *distal transformation* has been summed up by the trite description "hands from elbows, but never elbows from hands."

In humans, the cells adjacent to the area of damage fail to dedifferentiate, and no blastema comparable to that described in the preceding is formed. The healing process has several aspects (Fig. 5–14).

Contraction. This is the process whereby the size of the wound decreases during the first few days following the infliction of the wound.

Replacement of Lost Tissue. In this process, migration of cells as well as division of adjacent cells provides extra tissue to fill the defect. This can be accomplished in two ways:

*Repair.** This is a process by which the lost

---

*The term repair is also used in pathology to describe the process whereby damaged molecules are restored to normal. Thus, a section of a DNA molecule damaged by ultraviolet light can be excised and replaced by a normal segment by a process of repair.

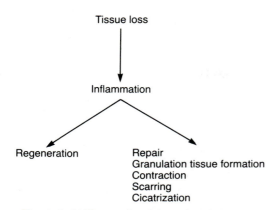

Figure 5–14 The results of tissue loss in humans.

specialized tissue is replaced by granulation tissue, which later matures to form scar tissue. It is an inevitable end result when the surviving specialized cells do not possess the ability to proliferate. Such cells are termed permanent.

Regeneration. This term is applied to the process by which the lost tissue is replaced by a tissue similar in type. This is illustrated by the healing of a damaged liver when the destroyed liver cells are replaced by liver tissue produced by proliferation of the surrounding undamaged specialized cells. Regeneration occurs when the damaged tissue is composed of labile or stable cells. *Labile cells*, also called continuous replicators, undergo division throughout life to replace those that are lost through differentiation or desquamation. Most protective or covering epithelia fall into this group. *Stable cells*, also called discontinuous replicators, rarely divide under normal cir-

cumstances but are able to proliferate if suitably stimulated. Glandular tissue such as liver, kidney, and endocrine glands falls into this category.

It should be noted that there is no dedifferentiation of cells as occurs in the axial regeneration of amphibians. Indeed, the only human counterpart to this situation is seen in the healing of bone fractures. Here connective tissue cells—osteoblasts, fibroblasts, and others—do dedifferentiate to form a blastema that is capable of redifferentiating to form fibrous tissue, cartilage, or bone (see Chapter 30).

Before the coordinated process that occurs during simple skin wound healing is described, it is convenient to describe *wound contraction* and *granulation tissue formation*. These are two components of the process that can be studied experimentally and can be quantitated.

Wound Contraction

This is a dynamic process that can be studied in the experimental animal by excising a circular, full-thickness disk of skin from the back or flank. Figure 5–15 shows the result of such an experiment. The size of the wound is measured at regular intervals; after an initial period of 2 to 3 days, there follows a phase of rapid contraction, which is largely completed by the fourteenth day. It can be seen that with good contraction a small scar is produced, whereas with inadequate contraction a large scar results, with all the cosmetic and functional complications that follow.

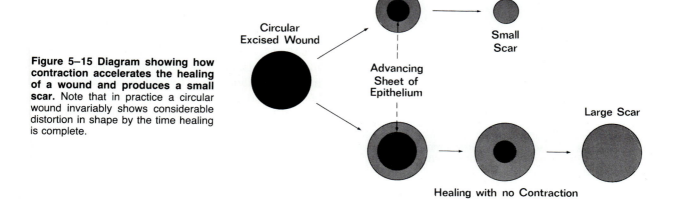

Figure 5–15 Diagram showing how contraction accelerates the healing of a wound and produces a small scar. Note that in practice a circular wound invariably shows considerable distortion in shape by the time healing is complete.

Much experimental work has been carried out with a view to understanding the process of wound contraction so that it may be brought under control when necessary. It is generally agreed that the contractile force is generated by the myofibroblasts in the new granulation tissue around the circumference, or picture frame area, of the healing wound.

Wound contraction can be inhibited by the systemic administration of glucocorticoids and by the local application of ionizing radiation. Mechanical factors, such as tethering of the wound edges, are also effective in preventing contraction. This is well illustrated by the large chronic ulcers that occur around the ankle in patients with venous stasis (Fig. 5–16). Dense, fibrous tissue fixes the wound edges to the periosteum of the tibia, and healing results in very extensive scar tissue formation. The scar is covered by thin (atrophic) epidermis and is liable to ulcerate with subsequent injury—even quite trivial injury.

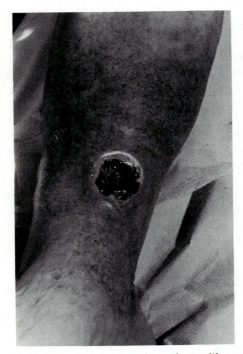

Figure 5–16 Chronic leg ulcer in patient with varicose veins. The ulcer is almost circular and is covered by a dark, blood-stained slough. A thin layer of regenerating epidermis is beginning to grow across the ulcer bed. The surrounding skin is thickened as a result of edema and fibrosis of the dermis. Because it is tethered to the underlying muscle sheaths and bone, there can be no contraction in such an ulcer. The discoloration of the skin is due to the deposition of blood and hemoglobin-derived pigment (hemosiderin). There is also increased melanin pigmentation of the epidermis.

Granulation Tissue Formation

The initial response to an injury is an acute inflammatory reaction. The exudation and neutrophil infiltration is soon followed by a macrophage response. These scavenger cells remove necrotic tissue and inflammatory debris. This phase of demolition is followed by ingrowth of granulation tissue formed by the proliferation and migration of surrounding connective tissue elements. Buds of endothelial cells grow out from existing blood vessels at the wound margin, undergo canalization, and form a series of vascular arcades by joining with their neighbors (Fig. 5–17). The stimulus for this vascular proliferation is an *angiogenic factor* probably produced by macrophages. At first, the new-formed vessels all appear similar and have a thin wall consisting of only endothelium. These vessels leak protein readily, so that the fluid bathing the area consists virtually of plasma and forms an admirable nutrient medium. Very soon, differentiation occurs: some vessels acquire a muscular coat and become arterioles, whereas others form thin-walled large venules. Some persist as part of the capillary bed; the remainder disappear as the granulation tissue steadily becomes modified.

As the vessels grow into the clot, fibroblast-like cells around the wound margin multiply and accompany the vascular invasion. Thus, the clot is converted into a living vascular granulation tissue, and the process is called *organization*. The cells have in the past been termed "fibroblasts," but they differ from the fibroblasts seen in other situations. The cells have contractile elements in their cytoplasm and have therefore been renamed *myofibroblasts*. These cells can contract and by doing so cause wound contraction. At first, the cells are large and plump and have in their cytoplasm the endoplasmic reticulum necessary for the formation of collagen. Hence, collagen fibrils steadily form around cells that become thin and elongated and finally resemble the inert fibrocytes of adult tissue. The myofibroblasts are

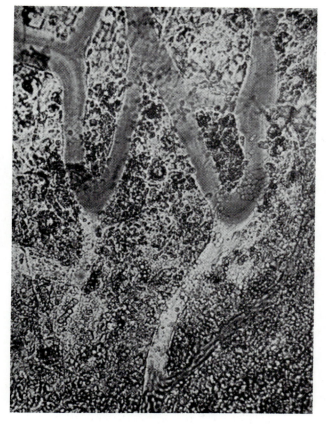

Figure 5–17 Granulation tissue at the edge of a healing wound in a living animal. The capillary loops at the top of the photograph contain streaming blood so that individual red cells cannot be identified. The pale globules are white cells adherent to the vessel walls. There is little flow in the advancing hollow buds in the lower part of the field. The vessels are largely filled with plasma, but some individual red cells can be distinguished. (From Walter, J. B., and Israel, M. S.: General Pathology. 6th ed. Edinburgh, Churchill Livingstone, 1987.)

also responsible for the formation of *proteogly-cans*, which contribute to the ground substance, and *fibronectin*, which acts as a cellular glue. Fibronectin plays a part in the migration of cells and their subsequent adhesion to other cells and to connective tissue fibers.

Lymphatic vessels grow into the maturing granulation tissue in much the same way the blood vessels do. The two sets of vessels do not anastomose, and the lymphatics form blind-ended channels. At the same time, there is an ingrowth of nerve fibers so that not only do blood vessels acquire an autonomic nerve supply but also the tissue regains sensation.

As maturation proceeds, there is a general remodeling of granulation tissue. Some vessels undergo atrophy and disappear, whereas others exhibit thickening of their coats and eventual obliteration of the lumen. This process of devascularization and collagen formation eventually results in the formation of an avascular scar.

Granulation tissue forms under a variety of circumstances. It is formed not only in a healing wound but also when dead tissue has to be demolished and replaced by living tissue. After *acute inflammation,* the fibrinous exudate, unless it is rapidly removed, can be invaded by granulation tissue that matures to fibrous tissue. Likewise, fibrosis is a prominent feature of *chronic inflammation.* Organization is often encountered in a *thrombus,* a *hematoma,* and an *infarct.* In tumors, granulation tissue formation is stimulated by an angiogenic factor secreted by the tumor cells. The formation of stromal collagen is particularly marked in certain tumors, *e.g.,* desmoplastic carcinoma of the stomach or breast.

Healing of Skin Wounds

Skin wounds are so common that one takes it for granted that they will heal. Nevertheless, the process by which this occurs is by no means well understood. Following is a description of the healing of two separate types of wound, the factors that influence healing, and some of its complications.

Healing of a Clean, Incised Wound with Apposed Edges. This process, described as *healing by primary intention,* is the desired result in all healing surgical incisions. Little tissue is lost, and the separated skin edges are brought together by the use of sutures, clips, or tape.

Bleeding occurs immediately after injury, and a small amount of blood clot forms in the wound area. An acute inflammatory reaction follows, and the fibrinous exudate helps to join the cut margins of the wound together.

Epithelial Changes. Within 24 hours of injury, the epithelial cells from the adjacent epidermis migrate into the wound and slide between the inert dermis and the overlying clot (Fig. 5–18). A continuous layer of epidermal cells soon covers the surface, and overlying this is a crust or scab of dried clot. During the next 24 hours, these epidermal cells invade the space where connective tissue will eventually develop. In this way, spurs of epidermal cells are formed not only in

the area of incision but also along the tracts of any sutures that have been inserted. These epidermal cells are derived from the cut epidermis and from any severed hair follicle or sweat gland cells.

Connective Tissue Changes. After the initial acute inflammatory reaction, the edema subsides and the polymorphs are replaced by monocytes. These cells, which become phagocytic and perform a scavenger function, are then called *macrophages.* This *demolition phase* is an essential prelude to the organization that follows.

Organization. By about the third day, the area of the wound is invaded by granulation tissue from the adjacent subepithelial layers. The major part of this ingrowth occurs from the subcutaneous tissues, since there is little or no contribution from the dense, inert reticular dermis.

Soon after the granulation tissue appears, collagen formation commences. At first this consists of type III collagen that can be demonstrated by silver impregnation methods and is termed *reticulin.* Later, thick bundles of type I collagen are produced. This mature collagen is of vital importance to the wound because it forms the main connecting tissue between the originally divided skin. The amount of collagen can be assessed subjectively by examining sections of wounds. A more accurate method is to measure the amount of hydroxyproline in hydrolysates of wound tissues. By this technique, it can be shown that the *tensile strength* of a wound during the first month is proportional to the amount of collagen formed. The tensile strength can be measured experimentally by excising the entire wound area and applying a disrupting force across the wound. The force needed to cause separation of the wound edges is measured, and from this information it is possible to calculate the amount of energy necessary to disrupt the wound. Such measurements are not of purely academic interest, because the strength of a wound is of prime importance when one considers the way in which surgical incisions heal. Were it not for the tensile strength of a laparotomy wound, this common surgical incision could burst open and the abdominal contents would spill out to the exterior. This is an occasional catastrophe after surgery; it is often fatal. A remarkable experimental finding is the fact that the tensile strength of a wound

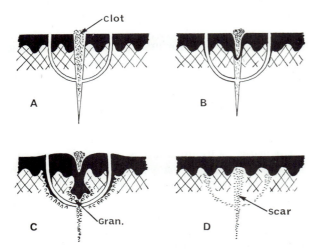

Figure 5–18 Diagrammatic representation of the healing of an incised wound held together by a suture of which the track alone is shown. *A,* The wound rapidly fills with clot. *B,* Shortly afterward, the epithelium migrates into the wound and down the suture tracks. *C,* Epithelial spurs are formed, and granulation tissue (Gran.) formulation proceeds. *D,* The suture has been removed, and scar tissue remains to mark the site of the incision and the suture tracks. The epithelial ingrowths have degenerated. (From Walter, J. B., and Israel, M. S.: General Pathology. 6th ed. Edinburgh, Churchill Livingstone, 1987.)

continues to increase for many months, long after the total amount of collagen has ceased to increase. It is thought that the formation of new bonds between adjacent collagen bundles accounts for this phenomenon.

The granulation tissue formed in a healing wound appears to prevent excessive epithelial migration into the wound. The epithelial spurs noted previously soon undergo degeneration and are replaced by granulation tissue. Only the surface epithelial cells persist, and these divide and differentiate so that a multilayered covering of epidermis is re-formed. It first covers a vascular granulation tissue, so that the wound has a pink color. Gradually, devascularization occurs; the scar shrinks in size and changes in color from red to white.

In the healing of a simple incised wound, it therefore appears that the epithelial cells are first stimulated to divide, and they then migrate into the wound. The stimulus for the epithelial growth and migration is not known. Experimentally it has been noted that cells in tissue culture continue to divide until they have established contact with similar cells, at which point mitosis stops. This process is termed *contact inhibition.* The epithelial cells appear to excite a connective tissue response; this results in the formation of granulation tissue, which in its turn prevents excessive epithelial migration into the wound. The presence of epithelial ingrowths along a suture tract explains why granulation tissue is formed in this situation. It is a common finding that if stitches remain *in situ* for 3 days or more, their site is marked subsequently by small punctate areas of scarring that remain permanently. It is to avoid these ugly punctate marks that surgeons often use tapes to hold skin edges together. A subcuticular stitch is used to hold the wound together while healing proceeds. It should be noted that puncture wounds due to injections do not form such scars, because the wound is not held open, and therefore no epithelial invasion occurs.

Healing of a Wound with Separated Edges. When the edges of a wound are not approximated or when there is extensive tissue loss, either by direct trauma or following infection, a large defect is present that has to be corrected. This type of healing is traditionally known as

healing by secondary intention. It is also known as healing by granulation. The term, however, is a poor one because it wrongly implies that granulations are not formed in a simple incised wound. The difference between primary and secondary intention healing is quantitative, not qualitative.

In healing by secondary intention, the wound edges are widely separated so that healing has to proceed from the base outward as well as from the edges inward. From a practical point of view, healing of a well-approximated incised wound is fast and leaves a small, neat, linear scar. Healing of a wound with separated edges is slow and results in a large distorted scar. The difference lies in the type of wound and not in the type of healing. The following account of the healing of a large uninfected wound is illustrated in Figure 5–19.

1. There is an initial inflammatory reaction affecting the surrounding tissues, and the wound area is filled with a coagulum consisting in part of inflammatory exudate and in part of blood clot. This coagulum dries on its surface and forms a scab or crust.

2. The wound contracts, as has already been fully described. This process is important, because it reduces the size of the wound and the

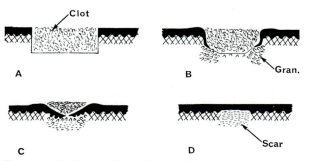

Figure 5–19 Diagram illustrating the healing of an excised wound. The wound is rapidly filled with clot. *A,* Epithelium soon migrates in from the margins to undermine the clot, which dries to form a crust. *B,* Granulation tissue (Gran.) grows into the wounded area and is most profuse around the circumference, where it is derived from the subcutaneous fat. *C,* Epithelial ingrowth continues, and spurs are produced; these, however, do not persist. *D,* The end result is a scar covered by epidermis that lacks rete ridges. During the healing process, contraction has taken place so that the final scar is considerably smaller than the original wound. (From Walter, J. B., and Israel, M. S.: General Pathology. 6th ed. Edinburgh, Churchill Livingstone, 1987.)

amount of tissue that has to be produced to fill in the gap.

3. There is mitotic activity of the epidermis adjacent to the wound, and the epithelial cells migrate into the wound as a thin tongue that grows between the pre-existing viable connective tissue and the central area of coagulum, which includes some necrotic epithelium and connective tissue. The epithelial cells secrete a fibrinolytic enzyme that aids their penetration between the fibrinous crust and the viable connective tissue.

4. Demolition follows acute inflammation, and the clot in the center of the wound is invaded and replaced by granulation tissue. This grows from the subcutaneous tissues at the edge of the wound; it is believed that this zone is responsible for wound contraction. Granulation tissue is also formed in the base of the wound, the amount depending on the vascularity of the area.

When the wound is viewed with a magnifying glass, the surface (under the scab, if one is present) is deep-red and granular, the capillary loops forming elevated mounds. It is very fragile, the slightest injury causing bleeding. It is this granularity that is responsible for the name *granulation tissue*. The covering of a wound by granulation tissue serves an important protective role because it has the ability to withstand bacterial infection. Under experimental conditions, organisms introduced into a recent wound are likely to cause infection. However, if the wound is first allowed to granulate, infection does not occur. Thus, granulation tissue forms a temporary protective layer until the surface is finally covered by epithelium.

5. The migrating epidermis covers the granulation tissue. A mushroom-shaped scab is thereby formed with a central attachment that finally becomes nipped off.

6. The regenerating epidermis becomes thicker and re-forms the multicellular layer of epidermis. Initially there are pointed epidermal spurs that project into the dermis (Fig. 5–20), but these structures disappear and ultimately the epidermis is thin and lacks rete ridges.

Although cells from hair follicles and sweat glands can contribute to the re-formation of epidermis, these structures themselves are not re-formed. The healing of epidermis falls into the category of regeneration, but the regeneration is imperfect, because in humans none of the appendages are replaced.

A scar differs from normal skin in many respects. The epidermis is thin and lacks hair follicles and sweat glands. Melanocytes are not re-formed in normal numbers, and the area therefore appears hypopigmented. The underlying scar tissue consists mainly of collagen, but its arrangement is quite different from that of the structured dermis.

Factors Influencing Wound Healing

The ability of wounds to heal is of fundamental interest in the practice of surgery. Surgeons must pay great attention to anything that could influence the healing process. It would be desirable to analyze the factors that influence repair according to whether they affect granulation tissue formation, collagen production, contraction, or some other process. Unfortunately, this is rarely possible because we are ignorant about many of these fundamental processes. In practice, the factors affecting wound healing may be divided into two groups: those that act locally, and those whose influence is general.

Local Factors

Blood Supply. The normal blood supply varies greatly from one part of the body to another. The scalp and face have an excellent blood supply, and wounds there heal quickly. It is possible to remove stitches on the third day without having the wound gape, provided undue traction is not applied. The skin of the leg has a poor blood supply, and wounds there heal much more slowly.

Pathologic changes affecting the blood vessels have an enormous effect on wound healing. Patients with poor circulation in the leg vessels due to varicose veins or atherosclerosis show very slow healing: trivial injuries can lead to ulceration, which takes many months to heal. Other causes of poor blood supply are local pressure and chronic inflammation. *Bed sores* are caused by local pressure, which is also a factor in their poor healing. Likewise, *chronic inflammation* is liable to be accompanied by endarteritis

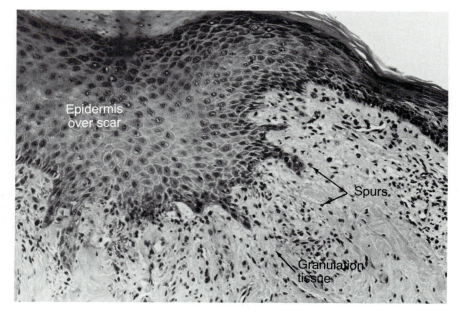

Figure 5–20 Healing wound. A dysplastic nevus had been excised from a patient, and 12 days later the wound was re-excised. The epidermis has completely covered the original wound and is now thicker than normal. Note the presence of pointed epidermal spurs that project into the dermis and are associated with underlying granulation tissue formation; these are temporary structures and will soon disappear, leaving the epidermis atrophic. The stage of healing is slightly more advanced than is depicted in Figure 5–19C.

obliterans, ischemia, and slow healing. An excellent example of this is x-ray dermatitis, in which ulceration is notoriously slow to heal. Finally, the slow wound healing of old age is in part related to a poor circulation.

Continued Tissue Breakdown and Inflammation. Any condition causing continued tissue breakdown leads to persistent inflammation and delay in healing. Important examples are *infection,* the presence of a *foreign body* or irritant chemical, and *excessive movement.*

If a simple incised wound becomes infected, the two edges do not become adherent, and the wound tends to gape. Furthermore, the infection may result in tissue destruction, causing healing to proceed, in effect, by secondary intention.

The presence of a foreign body in a wound may delay healing, either as a result of its direct irritant properties or by encouraging infection. The overenthusiastic use of irritating antiseptics can cause considerable damage and delay healing. The use of potent antiseptic and antibiotic agents was once popular in the local treatment of wounds, but it is now appreciated that they frequently did more harm than good. Sometimes hypersensitivity develops and leads to extensive inflammation. A good example of this is the acute allergic contact dermatitis that can follow the use of ointments containing neomycin.

It is a time-honored dictum that injured parts should be kept at rest. Movement delays healing because the edges of the wound are continually disrupted, and this damages the delicate granulation tissue, leading to repeated injury and consequently to inflammation.

Adhesion to an Underlying Bony Surface. By anchoring the wound edges, this adhesion prevents contraction.

Direction of the Wound. Skin wounds made parallel to or in the crease lines of the skin heal faster than those made at right angles to them, and the scars are less visible. Skin incisions made across the lines tend to gape, and their healing is delayed. Therefore, when one plans a surgical incision, these lines should be taken into consideration.

The Presence of a Large Hematoma. Some blood clot is always present in a wound, but a large hematoma should be avoided. Its presence favors infection, and in any case the space caused by its presence leads to delayed healing and to the formation of a large scar.

General Factors

Age. Wound healing is fast in the young and

is generally of normal rate in old age unless there is some associated debilitating disease or ischemia.

Nutrition. Animals starved of protein show poor wound healing and defective collagen formation. This abnormality can be corrected by the administration of proteins containing methionine and cystine.

Vitamin C Deficiency. Vitamin C is essential for the formation of collagen and animals deficient in this vitamin therefore show poor wound healing. Wound contraction is normal and so are epithelial regeneration and granulation tissue formation. The abnormality is in the absence of normal collagen formation, and the wound is therefore very weak. Capillaries are unduly fragile and bleeding occurs. Although overt scurvy is uncommon in Western countries, minor degrees of vitamin C deficiency are not infrequent in patients on a marginal intake of the substance and in those who are stressed.

The Role of Zinc. The addition of zinc salts to the diet of rats has been shown to promote wound healing. The mechanism of this is not known, but the oral administration of zinc sulfate has been tried in humans and claimed to accelerate wound healing. These claims have not been substantiated by all workers, and the role of zinc in healing of human wounds remains problematic.

Glucocorticoids. The administration of excessive amounts of these steroids delays wound contraction and the formation of granulation tissue.

Complications of Wound Healing

Infection. Wounds form a ready avenue for the invasion of pathogenic bacteria. All the techniques of aseptic surgery are devoted to preventing infection of surgical wounds.

Delayed Healing. Any of the factors mentioned, either local or general, may produce delayed healing.

Wound Dehiscence. The bursting open of a wound is described as *dehiscence.* It occurs when stress is applied before the wound has healed sufficiently. It is a particularly serious complica-

tion of an abdominal incision because it results in the exposure of the abdominal contents to the outside atmosphere. Quite apart from delayed healing due to infection and the other factors just considered, another important contributing element is increased intra-abdominal pressure, such as is caused by heaving coughing.

Cicatrization. Scar tissue tends to contract in an erratic way such that the wound becomes greatly distorted. This process is quite different from contraction, because it occurs as a late event and appears to be due to some change in the dense avascular collagenous scar tissue. The mechanism is not understood. Cicatrization is a frequent complication in the healing of skin after extensive burning. It produces great deformity and can immobilize joints in the affected area. Cicatrization involving hollow viscera such as intestine, esophagus, or urethra is an important cause of stenosis.

Excessive Granulation Tissue Formation. Sometimes there is excessive granulation tissue formation such that a mass of tissue, by tradition called proud flesh, protrudes from a wound and hinders epithelialization and normal healing.

Keloid Formation. Occasionally, an excessive amount of collagen results in the appearance of a raised nodule of scar tissue called a *keloid* (Fig. 5–21). The precise cause of this is not known, but keloid formation is particularly common in young women (particularly if they are pregnant) and in blacks. Keloids are found most frequently in the region of the neck and shoulders. They are especially frequent after burns. One should be particularly wary of performing nonessential surgery on patients who are prone to develop keloids. Thus, the removal of a small nevus for cosmetic purposes can result in the formation of a large ugly keloid, far more disfiguring than was the original lesion. The treatment is quite unsatisfactory, because removal is followed by even more keloid formation. Postoperative intralesional injections of glucocorticosteroids can be given in an effort to prevent this.

Weak Scars. If the scar tissue is subjected to continuous strain, it may stretch. Incisional wounds may therefore bulge and, in the abdomen, produce incisional hernias.

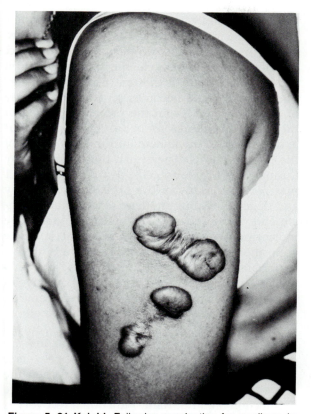

Figure 5–21 Keloid. Following vaccination for smallpox, keloids developed at both sites of vaccination in this dark-skinned patient. The firm fibrous nodules involve the adjacent skin as well as the scarred area where the vaccination was performed. (Courtesy of Dr. B. K. Fisher, Wellesley Hospital, Toronto. From Walter, J. B.: Pathology of Human Disease. Philadelphia, Lea & Febiger, 1989.)

Healing in Specialized Tissues

It is generally stated that the greater the degree of specialization of a tissue, the less well developed are its powers of regeneration. Certainly, nerve cells are highly specialized and are incapable of division, but degrees of specialization in the cells are as difficult to define as are degrees of specialization among human beings. Is a liver cell more or less specialized than a simple smooth (unstriated) muscle fiber? Liver cells show remarkable powers of proliferation and yet perform functions of which they alone are capable. Similarly, it is impossible to compare the degree of specialization of the different types of epithelium, each of which has its own particular characteristics. It seems likely that the power of regeneration is best developed in those organs and tissues that are most liable to injury and the replacement of which has survival value for the individual and for the species.

Regeneration in Epithelial Tissues

All covering epithelia show good regeneration power. They are repeatedly subjected to trauma, and the integrity of the surface therefore depends on the ability of the cells to regenerate. The reformation of the squamous epithelium of epidermis has already been described in the healing of skin wounds, and a similar regeneration is seen in the mucosa of the mouth, the intestine, the respiratory tract, and the urinary tract.

The solid epithelial organs show varying regenerative capacity. In the liver it is quite remarkable; if three quarters of the liver of a rat is resected, there is such active division of the remaining cells that within a few weeks the organ is restored to its original weight. Its anatomic shape is different, but normal liver lobules are formed in relationship to new blood vessels and bile ducts. In humans, regeneration of liver cells is seen after any type of necrosis, provided the patient survives. The end result of this regeneration varies widely, depending on the type of necrosis (see Chapter 24 for a consideration of this important subject). Kidney tubules show excellent regenerative capacity; in patients with extensive tubular necrosis (as occurs in shock), it is common for regeneration to result in complete recovery, provided the patient does not die in the acute phase. This type of renal disease is therefore most eligible for treatment by dialysis (artificial kidney), since the ultimate prognosis is good. If entire nephrons or glomeruli are destroyed, there is no replacement.

Regeneration in Connective Tissues

As a general rule, specialized connective tissues show good regeneration if circumstances are favorable. The *mesothelial lining* of the peritoneum and other serous cavities is readily reformed from exposed underlying connective tissue cells, which take on the form and function of flattened mesothelium. Were it not for this, abdominal surgery would be hazardous. One can leave extensive areas of tissue exposed in the abdominal cavity, and they will be rapidly covered by newly formed mesothelium: adhesions do not form, unless healing is complicated by infection or by the presence of irritants such as suture material or the talc or starch in glove powder. Likewise, synovial cells are readily re-formed. With cut *tendons* regeneration is good, provided the severed ends are carefully approximated and are held in good position. It is important that the ends be meticulously sewn together; otherwise, the space between them becomes organized, and ultimately union is by scar tissue. Since scar tissue is relatively weak, it will stretch. *Unstriated muscle* shows little regenerative capacity, and destroyed muscle tissue is replaced by scar tissue. For example, with a deep penetrating gastric ulcer, even though it may heal, scar tissue remains for life to indicate the site of the previous ulceration. *Heart muscle*, unfortunately, shows no regenerative capacity either, and patients who suffer extensive myocardial necrosis are forever destined to have a scar replacing the pre-existing muscle. With *striated voluntary muscle*, the situation is somewhat more variable; under good conditions, striated muscle can regenerate so that a clean surgical incision through a voluntary muscle will ultimately unite, and no scar tissue will remain to indicate the site of previous surgery.

Healing in Nervous Tissue. Adult nerve cells are unable to divide; therefore, when part of the brain or spinal cord is destroyed, no new neurons are produced. The common "stroke," therefore, inevitably results in the formation of scar tissue (Chapter 33). When the axons of the nerve cells are damaged, the situation is quite different, because the body of the cell itself is not directly affected. The effects vary according to whether the axon is in the peripheral or central nervous system.

Peripheral Nervous System. After the section of a nerve fiber, the corresponding nerve cell shows degenerative changes. Sometimes the cell dies, but more usually it recovers. The severed axis cylinder itself becomes irregular in shape and by 48 hours has broken up. With myelinated nerves, the surrounding myelin shows fragmentation, and the Schwann cells enlarge, proliferate, and become phagocytic. These changes are known as *wallerian degeneration*, and they affect the nerve fiber distally to the point of section and proximally up to the first node of Ranvier. The original nerve becomes replaced by a mass of Schwann cells. From the proximal portion of the cut axon, numerous neurofibrils sprout out and are seen to invaginate into the cytoplasm of the Schwann cells. They push their way distally through the Schwann cells at a rate of about 1 mm per day. Many of the fibrils lose their way and degenerate, but one may reach an appropriate end organ and persist to form the definitive replacement axon. It is evident that accurate apposition of the cut ends of the nerve is of vital importance in facilitating this process. The final process involves the re-formation of the myelin sheath by the Schwann cells as the regenerating nerve axon matures and increases in diameter.

The functional end result of nerve damage depends on various factors. If the axons are damaged but the nerve trunk itself is not severed, an excellent result may be expected. When the nerve is severed, careful suturing and avoidance of infection are important. Functional recovery is more complete when a pure motor or a pure sensory nerve is cut. Recovery from section of a mixed nerve—like the median nerve—is often poor, and this is presumably because motor nerves often find themselves arriving at sensory nerve endings and vice versa.

Central Nervous System. In the central nervous system, the oligodendroglia takes on the functions of the Schwann cells in relation to the axons. For reasons that are not clear, regeneration of long axon tracts does not occur. In some experiments on mammals, a limited degree of regeneration has been reported; but with humans, when long tracts such as the corticospinal and spinothalamic tracts have been destroyed, no effective regeneration occurs. Degenerating tissue is phagocytosed by macrophages, and the area becomes replaced by a type of granulation tissue. Unlike the granulation tissue of ordinary connective tissue, the proliferating cells are astrocytes rather than fibroblasts. The end result is a glial scar containing astrocytes with their matted processes but with relatively little collagen and few fibrocytes.

Mechanisms of Repair and Regeneration

Experimental work has provided some insight into the mechanisms involved in repair and regeneration. A number of polypeptide growth factors have been identified that stimulate proliferation of cells (particularly fibroblasts, smooth muscle cells, and endothelial cells) and may also have a chemotactic effect on them. *Epidermal growth factor* is a polypeptide that is mitogenic for both epidermal cells and fibroblasts. *Fibroblast growth factors* are derived from macrophages, stimulate fibroblastic proliferation, and induce new blood vessel formation. This angiogenic activity is probably important in granulation tissue formation. *Platelet-derived growth factor* stimulates migration and proliferation of fibroblasts and smooth muscle cells. *Transforming growth factors (TGF-α and TGF-β)* were originally extracted from tumor cells. TGF-α has properties similar to epidermal growth factor; TGF-β is a growth inhibitor but is chemotactic to fibroblasts and promotes collagen formation. *Interleukin-1* and *tumor necrosis factor* also promote collagen formation and are chemotactic to fibroblasts. Interferon and some prostaglandins have growth-inhibiting activity. The term *chalone* was originally used to describe a group of growth-inhibiting factors; they have never been categorized and probably represented mixtures of inhibiting factors that are now being recognized and named separately.

Another approach to the explanation of wound healing focuses on the part played by mechanical physical factors. It has been noted that cells in tissue culture continue to divide and move on a surface until they establish contact with similar cells, at which point movement stops. This is called *contact inhibition*. Also, in tissue culture, growth tends to stop when a certain mass of tissue is produced. This appears to be dependent on the density of cells present and has been termed *density-dependent regulation of growth*. These effects are thought to be related to complex cell-to-cell or cell-to-matrix interaction. *In vitro*, the behavior of connective tissue cells is influenced by the extracellular matrix. For example, cells in contact with laminin behave differently from ones in contact with collagen or fibronectin. The cells are thought to have special receptors (termed *integrins*) for these extracellular components. Possibly fibrin plays a similar role in the early stages of granulation tissue formation.

It is evident that our knowledge of the phenomenon of healing is fragmentary. A number of mechanisms have been investigated, but how they are controlled and so integrated that division, migration, and differentiation of cells proceed in orderly fashion is not understood. It is to be hoped that future research will clarify the position, because some oncogene products are very similar to growth factors and there is every hope that an understanding of wound healing will shed new light on malignant disease; this is the major disorder of cell division, migration, and differentiation.

CHRONIC INFLAMMATION

When a substance causing tissue damage and acute inflammation persists locally, it leads to chronic inflammation, which may be defined as *a prolonged process in which tissue damage and inflammation are proceeding at the same time as attempts at healing.*

Causes of Chronic Inflammation

Any cause of tissue damage can, if it persists, lead to chronic inflammation. Three main groups can be recognized.

Infections. The body has a limited ability to destroy certain organisms, *e.g.,* the tubercle bacillus and *Treponema pallidum.* Infection with these agents therefore commonly leads to chronic inflammation (Fig. 5–22). Moreover, if local or general conditions impair the body's defenses, an organism that usually produces a self-limiting acute inflammation may persist to cause a chronic one. For example, *Staphylococcus aureus,* which can produce a boil that generally heals rapidly, can also produce chronic inflammation in some situations, such as in the bone marrow (see Chronic Suppurative Osteomyelitis, Chapter 30). Any of the causes of delayed healing may so turn the scales against the host that there develops the "frustrated healing" that chronic inflammation has so aptly been called.

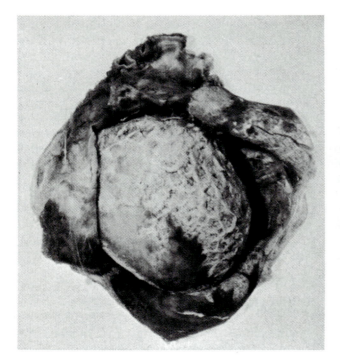

Figure 5–22 Tuberculous pericarditis. The pericardial sac has been opened to show the heart covered by thick fibrinous exudate. Over the apex there is a layer of blood clot due to recent hemorrhage. The parietal pericardium is greatly thickened and is also covered by fibrinous exudate. The patient was a 22-year-old man who had pulmonary tuberculosis for 5 years. (Reproduced by kind permission of the President and Council of the Royal College of Surgeons of England. Hunterian Museum specimen EC 12.1. From Walter, J. B., and Israel, M. S.: General Pathology. 6th ed. Edinburgh, Churchill Livingstone, 1987.)

Insoluble Particulate Irritants. Silica and asbestos are examples of irritant particles that the body cannot easily remove. Inhalation of such substances leads to persistent chronic inflammation of the lungs (see Pneumoconioses, Chapter 22).

Hypersensitivity. The development of hypersensitivity is an important factor in chronic infective diseases, of which tuberculosis is the prototype. Much of the continuing damage produced by persisting tubercle bacilli is mediated immunologically. There is also a group of diseases in which damage is produced by an autoimmune mechanism; rheumatoid arthritis is a typical example.

Types of Chronic Inflammation

Chronic inflammation is encountered in all organs of the body; many examples will be described later. These inflammations share certain pathologic features. All consist of varying mixtures of the basic pathologic reactions previously described as acute inflammation, demolition, and healing (Table 5–2). The reaction encountered under any particular circumstance consists of varying mixtures of these three basic ingredients. Cells involved in an immune response are often added to this mixture and contribute to the variety of the tissue response to chronic irritation.

Chronic Suppurative Inflammation. Suppura-

Table 5–2 COMPONENTS OF CHRONIC INFLAMMATION

Component	Tissue Response
Acute inflammation	Polymorph infiltration
	Edema
	Fibrin
Demolition	Macrophage formation
	Epithelioid cell formation
	Giant cell formation
Healing	
Repair	Granulation tissue
	Blood vessels
	Fibroblasts
	Collagen
	Neuroglia in CNS
Regeneration	Epithelial overgrowth
	Specialized connective tissue overgrowth
Immune response	Lymphocytes
	Plasma cells
	Eosinophils

tion is frequently followed by chronic inflammation if the causative agent is not removed or if the pus is not adequately drained. A chronic abscess consists of a central cavity filled with pus and lined by a pyogenic membrane. The pyogenic membrane consists of granulation tissue heavily infiltrated with neutrophils and a variable number of lymphocytes, plasma cells, and macrophages (Fig. 5–23). Examples of this type of lesion are seen in the lung after bronchopneumonia, in chronic osteomyelitis, and in a chronic brain abscess (Fig. 33–4). The term *empyema* denotes a collection of pus in a cavity. In *empyema thoracis*, there is pus in the pleural cavity. This condition often becomes chronic, especially if the pus is inadequately drained. Empyema thoracis follows the rupture of a lung abscess into the pleural cavity; in preantibiotic days, it was high on the list of the complications of pneumonia.

Granulomatous Inflammation. In some types of chronic inflammation, the predominant cell is the macrophage. By tradition, an inflammation showing a heavy macrophage infiltration is called *proliferative*, in contrast to the exudative lesions of suppuration. This concept was based on the supposition that the macrophages were derived from local histiocytes by mitosis. In fact, most of them are derived from blood monocytes, but the term "proliferative" is still retained. The accumulation of macrophages and cells derived from them can produce a tumorlike swelling; this type of inflammation is traditionally called "granulomatous." In the past, the term has been used to describe a tumorlike mass composed of inflamed granulation tissue, but it is not now used in this context. In fact, granulomatous inflammation is now used to denote a particular microscopic appearance, namely, an inflammatory reaction in which there is a predominance of macrophages or cells derived from them.

Two main types of granulomatous inflammation are recognized: diffuse and tuberculoid.

Diffuse Type. Under some circumstances, the macrophage infiltration is diffuse, causing a nearly uniform enlargement of the tissue, perhaps with some areas of nodularity. This type of reaction is uncommon, but it is seen typically in lepromatous leprosy.

Tuberculoid Type. Under certain circumstances, macrophages enlarge, lose their phagocytic activity, develop eosinophilic cytoplasm, and are so closely applied to their neighbors that individual cell borders cannot be defined other than by electron microscopy. The cells then somewhat resemble the epithelial cells of the epidermis and are therefore called *epithelioid cells*.

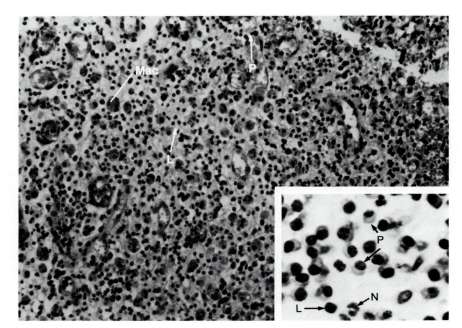

Figure 5–23 Inflammatory granulation tissue. The granulation tissue is edematous and its vessels are dilated. There is a heavy cellular infiltrate of inflammatory cells, among which can be recognized macrophages (Mac) with abundant granular cytoplasm containing phagocytosed material; neutrophils (N) with their lobed nuclei; and lymphocytes (L) with only the nuclei recognizable. (From Walter, J. B.: Pathology of Human Disease. Philadelphia, Lea & Febiger, 1989.) The inset shows the lymphocytes and neutrophils more clearly and also plasma cells (P) with their eccentric nucleus and a clear zone in the cytoplasm. This is the Golgi complex.

Epithelioid cell formation is accompanied by a tendency for the cells to be arranged in groups rather than in diffuse sheets. The formation of groups of epithelioid cells is characteristic of the reaction to the tubercle bacillus. An inflammation characterized by the formation of groups of epithelioid cells is traditionally called a *tuberculoid reaction* (see Fig. 8–3).

When macrophages encounter insoluble material, they frequently coalesce to form giant cells (Fig. 5–24). This response is seen around exogenous foreign bodies, *e.g.,* catgut, silk, and talc. Coalescing macrophages are also seen around endogenous debris such as dead bone, cholesterol crystals, keratin, and uric acid crystals. They are formed in response to the tubercle bacillus, to fungi, and to many other organisms that cause chronic inflammation. It frequently happens, therefore, that in a tuberculoid reaction, in addition to epithelioid cells, a considerable number of giant cells is also present.

The reason that macrophages predominate in certain chronic inflammations and change to epithelioid cells under some circumstances is not well understood. Experimentally it has been found that macrophages develop into epithelioid cells when they have not undertaken phagocytosis, have completely digested phagocytosed material, or have successfully extruded phagocytosed material by exocytosis. It follows that epithelioid cells contain few if any bacteria in an infection (*e.g.,* tuberculoid leprosy), whereas the undifferentiated macrophages in such an infection are stuffed with bacilli (see Lepromatous Leprosy, Chapter 8).

The development of hypersensitivity is thought to be another factor in the development of a granulomatous reaction. Certainly, the hypersensitivity can lead to necrosis, which is often a feature of tuberculoid granulomatous inflammation. Indeed, three variants of this are recognized: (1) *noncaseating tuberculoid granuloma,* as seen in sarcoidosis, tuberculoid leprosy, and early lesions of tuberculosis (Fig. 8–3); (2) *caseating tuberculoid reaction,* as commonly seen in tuberculosis and also in some of the deep mycoses (Fig. 8–4); and (3) *suppurative tuberculoid reaction,* in which small abscesses filled with polymorphs are found and surrounded by a mantle of epithe-

lioid cells. The commonest example of this is cat-scratch disease.*

Although the macrophage is traditionally regarded as a phagocytic scavenger cell, it has other important functions. It acts as a *secretor cell,* and its products play a part in the production of fever as well as influencing the healing process that follows inflammation. Its role in the immune response is indicated later in this chapter and is described in more detail in Chapter 6.

Chronic Inflammation with Features of Healing (Chronic Nonspecific Inflammation). The formation of granulation tissue is a feature of many types of chronic inflammation. The tissue consists of endothelial cells forming blood vessels and lymphatics, fibroblasts forming collagen, and an infiltration by numerous lymphocytes and plasma cells. In hematoxylin and eosin sections, it is often difficult to identify each cell as either lymphocyte or plasma cell; therefore, the term *small round cell* is often used to encompass both groups. A heavy infiltration by such cells is a common finding in chronic inflammation.

Inflammatory granulation tissue is seen in the pyogenic membrane surrounding a chronic abscess and in the chronic inflammatory tissue in the base of an ulcer. Since the vascularity of the tissue can result in easy bleeding, chronic peptic ulcers are associated with intestinal bleeding. Likewise, chronic inflammation of the bronchial tubes leads to hemoptysis (coughing up of blood).

Fibroblasts are prominent in most chronic inflammation; since they lay down collagen, the end result is fibrosis. This scar formation is characteristic of many chronic inflammatory lesions. It is seen in fibroid tuberculosis, in the base of a chronic peptic ulcer, and in the wall of an abscess. If fibrin is the hallmark of acute inflammation, fibrosis can be considered the salient feature of chronic inflammation. As scarring proceeds, the lumina of small arteries and arterioles are gradually obliterated by the thickening of the

---

*This curious disease is probably caused by a small as yet unnamed bacterium that has yet to be cultured. The appearance of an ulcerated nodule at the site of a cat scratch is followed by enlargement of the regional lymph nodes. These nodules suppurate, and the overlying skin may ulcerate so that the pus drains spontaneously. The pattern of infection and tissue response in the nodes closely resembles the changes seen in lymphogranuloma venereum (Chapter 9).

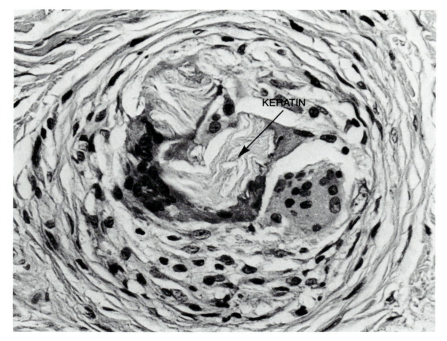

KERATIN

Figure 5–24 Keratin granuloma. The section was taken from the wall of a ruptured epidermoid cyst. Extravasated keratin flakes from the cyst contents have spilled into the tissues and caused an inflammatory reaction. The keratin is being engulfed by a large foreign body type giant cell, adjacent to which are a number of macrophages and spindle-shaped fibroblasts. (From Walter, J. B.: Pathology of Human Disease. Philadelphia, Lea & Febiger, 1989.)

tunica intima; this process is called *endarteritis obliterans.* The end result is a mass of dense avascular scar tissue. *Contracture* or *cicatrization* follows, and this leads to many important complications of chronic inflammation. Thus, chronic inflammation of the heart valves leads to stenosis and distortion of the valves; chronic gastric ulcers proceed to pyloric stenosis; and a chronic arthritis, such as rheumatoid arthritis, results in fibrous adhesions in the synovium and around joints.

In chronic inflammatory lesions involving specialized tissue, there is sometimes evidence of regeneration. This is usually seen in covering or lining epithelia; at times, the regeneration is followed by definite hyperplasia and even tumor formation. One of the best examples of this event is found in ulcerative colitis, which can proceed to polypoid overgrowth of epithelium and ultimately to the development of cancer. In general, however, chronic inflammation in most organs is an infrequent precursor of cancer.

Chronic Inflammation with Evidence of an Immune Reaction. Although a few lymphocytes and plasma cells are found in uninflamed granulation tissue, many examples of chronic inflammation are characterized by a heavy infiltration

of these cells (Fig. 5–23). Together with macrophages they are engaged in the processing of antigen and in the manufacture of immunoglobulins or formation of effector T cells. An infiltration by eosinophils is found in some examples of chronic inflammation in which hypersensitivity plays a part, *e.g.,* some parasitic infections.

General Effects of Chronic Inflammation

The general effects of chronic inflammation depend on the nature and extent of the responsible agent. In a localized foreign body reaction or in a chronic ulcer of the leg, there is no noteworthy general response at all. On the other hand, in chronic infective diseases like tuberculosis, there may be widespread changes in the lymphoreticular system and in the blood stream.

Changes in the Mononuclear Phagocyte System. Most chronic inflammatory reactions lead to hyperplasia of the mononuclear phagocyte system. The local accumulation of macrophages in some types has already been described; in addition, the lymph nodes draining a chronic inflammatory lesion generally show hyperplasia of the cells of the mononuclear phagocyte system and sometimes of the germinal centers and medullary cords.

If organisms gain access to the blood stream, they are taken up by the other members of the mononuclear phagocyte system. These cells may destroy the organism or may themselves become parasitized. Proliferation of the cells of the mononuclear phagocyte system can lead to enlargement of the lymphoreticular organs: of clinical importance is the enlargement of the spleen and lymph nodes, since they can be detected readily. This lymphoreticular hyperplasia is also a component of the immune response.

The Immune Response. Antibody production is a feature of most chronic inflammatory diseases, and the demonstration of specific antibodies is often a useful diagnostic procedure. Likewise, the detection of cell-mediated hypersensitivity is available as a diagnostic test.

The immune response is sometimes reflected in generalized enlargement of the lymphoreticular system. Enlargement of lymph nodes, the spleen, and—at times—the liver is a manifestation of this response.

Finally, the long-continued stress on the antibody-producing mechanism may be associated with amyloid disease (see Chapter 17).

Summary

- Acute inflammation is a tissue response to injury characterized by vasodilation, increase in vascular permeability, and the formation of an exudate that has a fluid and a cellular component.
- The cellular component of acute inflammation consists largely of neutrophil polymorphs and macrophages (derived from blood monocytes). Both are phagocytic, but macrophages have an important secretory function. Lymphocytes play an immunologic role; eosinophils are plentiful in parasitic infections and some allergic reactions. Adhesion molecules (*e.g.*, LAF-1 and ICAM-1) and chemotactic agents (*e.g.*, C5a, leukotriene B4, and platelet-activating factor) are important factors in the movement of white cells from the circulation to the area of damage.
- Suppuration denotes inflammation with tissue necrosis and pus formation.
- The changes of acute inflammation are caused partly by the direct effects of vascular damage and partly by the action of chemical mediators including histamine, kinins, lysosomal enzymes, arachidonic acid derivatives (prostaglandins and leukotrienes), platelet-activating factor, and cytokines.
- Repair denotes the formation of granulation tissue that matures to collagenous scar tissue; it follows tissue loss; the process of its formation is termed organization.
- Regeneration occurs when specialized tissue is replaced by similar specialized tissue. It is a feature of most covering epithelia and some glandular tissues, *e.g.*, liver. Neurons never regenerate.
- Wound contraction is due to the contraction of fibromyoblasts in granulation tissue; it is most obvious in skin wounds.
- Skin wound may heal by primary or secondary intention.
- Local factors influencing wound healing in skin include blood supply, inflammation, adhesion to underlying tissues, the presence of a large hematoma, and the direction of the wound. General factors include age, general nutrition, and adequate vitamin C.
- Growth factors are polypeptides derived from macrophages, platelets, and other cells that stimulate cell movement and division in healing. Inhibiting factors include TGF-beta. Physical factors also play a part as seen in contact inhibition and density-dependent regulation of growth. Receptors termed integrins are involved.
- Chronic inflammation occurs when continued tissue damage is accompanied by acute inflammation and attempts at healing.
- Chronic suppurative inflammation results in the formation of pus often contained within an abscess.
- Granulomatous inflammation is characterized by an abundance of macrophages or cells derived from them. It may be diffuse but is more commonly focal and called tuberculoid because it is characteristic of tuberculosis.
- Tuberculoid granulomas are composed of epithelioid cells and giant cells. A central area of caseation, or rarely suppuration, can occur.
- Chronic nonspecific inflammation is characterized by the presence of lymphocytes, plasma cells, granulation tissue, and ultimately scar tissue.

Selected Readings

Boxer, G. J., et al.: Polymorphonuclear leukocyte function. Hosp. Pract. *20*:69, 1985.

Demers, L. M.: Prostaglandins in human disease. Clin. Lab. Med. *4*:889, 1984.

Epstein, W. L.: Granuloma formation in man. Pathol. Annu. *7*:1, 1977.

Folkman, J., and Klagsburn, M.: Angiogenic factors. Science *235*:442, 1987.

Ford-Hutchinson, A. W.: Leukotrienes: Their formation and role as inflammatory mediators. Fed. Proc. *44*:25, 1985.

Forrester, L.: Current concepts in soft connective tissue wound healing. Br. J. Surg. *70*:133, 1983.

Gallin, J. I., et al. (eds.): Inflammation: Basic Principles and Clinical Correlates. New York, Raven Press, 1988.

Gelich, G. J.: Current understanding of eosinophil function. Hosp. Pract. 23:137, 1988.

Hunt, T. K. (ed.): Wound Healing and Wound Infection. New York, Appleton-Century-Crofts, 1980.

Hurley, J.: Acute Inflammation. 2nd ed. New York, Churchill Livingstone, 1983.

Johnson, R. B., Jr.: Monocytes and macrophages. N. Engl. J. Med. 318:747, 1988.

Karnovsky, M. L.: Steps towards an understanding of chronic granulomatous disease. N. Engl. J. Med. 308:274, 1983.

Kerr, J. F. R., Wyllie, A. H., and Currie, A. R.: Apoptosis: A basic biological phenomenon with wide-ranging implications in tissue kinetics. Br. J. Cancer 26:239, 1972.

King, G. D., and Salzman, F. A.: Keloid scars. Surg. Clin. North Am. 50:595, 1970.

Leading article: Polypeptide growth factors: A clinical perspective. Lancet 2:251, 1985.

Leading article: The myofibroblast. Lancet 2:1290, 1978.

Lewis, G. P.: Mediators of Inflammation. Bristol, John Wright, 1986.

Majno, G., and Cotran, R. S. (eds.): Current Topics in Inflammation and Infection. Baltimore, Williams & Wilkins, 1982.

Nathan, C. F.: Secretory products of macrophages. J. Clin. Invest. 79:319, 1987.

Peacock, E. E.: Wound Repair. 3rd ed. Philadelphia, W. B. Saunders Co., 1984.

Rytomaa, T.: The chalone concept. Int. Rev. Exp. Pathol. 16:155, 1976.

Samuelsson, B., et al.: Leukotrienes and lipotoxins: Structures, biosynthesis and biological effects. Science 237:1171, 1987.

Walter, J. B., and Israel, M. S.: In General Pathology. 6th ed. Chapters 6, 9, 10, 11. Edinburgh, Churchill Livingstone, 1987.

6

The Immune Response and Disease

**After studying this chapter, the student
should be able to:**

- Define the terms antigen, allergen, epitope, a
  positive response to an antigen, a negative
  response to an antigen, active immunity, and
  passive immunity.
- Describe the development of the lymphoid tissues of
  the body and distinguish between the B-cell system
  and the T-cell system.
- Discuss the concept of clonal selection in relation to
  the immune response.
- Describe how antigen presentation initiates a B-cell
  and T-cell response.
- Compare the primary response to antigen with the
  secondary response.
- Describe the chemical nature of the five classes of
  immunoglobulin and indicate how this is related to
  their properties and specificity.
- List the *in vitro* antigen-antibody reactions.
- Describe how complement can be activated and the
  effects of this activation in the intact animal.

- Describe and give examples of the cytokines, monokines, lymphokines, and interleukins.
- Describe the effector and regulator T cells and illustrate their role in immune mechanisms, in particular the body's reaction to bacteria and viruses.
- Describe specific immunologic tolerance; indicate how it may be induced and the possible mechanisms involved.
- Describe how the immune response leads to immunity to infection by bacteria, viruses, and helminths.
- Classify the immunologic deficiency diseases.
- Describe the acquired immunodeficiency syndrome.
- Describe the major histocompatibility complex and list its importance in the immune response and disease.
- Define the terms autograft, isograft, and allograft.
- Discuss the types of allograft rejection, the mechanisms involved, and the steps that can be taken to combat rejection.
- Describe the manifestations of the graft versus host reaction.
- Distinguish between type I, type II, type III, and type IV reactions and give examples of each type.
- Describe the pathogenesis, symptoms, and treatment of acute anaphylaxis in humans.
- Define atopy and describe its main manifestations.
- Describe the Koch phenomenon.
- List the circumstances under which an autoimmune reaction can occur, and discuss the role of this reaction in disease.
- Describe the main features of lupus erythematosus, mixed connective tissue disease, dermatomyositis, scleroderma, and polyarteritis nodosa.

The immune system has developed steadily during evolution to its present complex state in humans. It is involved in many pathologic processes, in particular as a defense against infection; its importance is evident in AIDS when the immune system is severely impaired and infections are devastating. However, the immune system has a much wider role in the pathogenesis of disease; sometimes it causes an excessive reaction to an abnormal substance, whether of external origin or an altered body substance. This is termed hypersensitivity. The immune system comes into play to reject foreign grafts, and on occasions it attacks the individual's own tissue.

GENERAL FEATURES OF THE IMMUNE RESPONSE

The essential feature of the immune response is self-recognition and its ability to reject foreign material. The body accepts its own normal constituents as "self"; others, such as altered self-constituents, microorganisms, and foreign substances, are recognized as "non-self" and provoke an immune response. The components recognized by the cells responsible for the immune response are termed *antigens*. They are generally proteins of high molecular weight, and their specificity is determined by specific sites called *antigenic determinants* or *epitopes*. New epitopes, called *haptens*, can be attached to a protein, which therefore acts as a carrier. The concept of haptens is important because it explains how a simple chemical, not necessarily antigenic itself, can cause an immune response by becoming attached to a normal body protein. Many drugs (*e.g.*, penicillin) can act as haptens, and the immune reaction that results is manifest as a drug rash. Likewise, acute "allergic" contact dermatitis caused by poison ivy is due to a component of the plant leaf acting as a hapten.

The immune response is the function of the lymphoreticular system, with lymphocytes playing the dominant role. These cells have specific receptors (termed T- and B-cell receptors) to which antigens become attached. This attachment stimulates the lymphocyte to produce an immune response. In order to understand how lymphocytes carry out this complex function, their origin and maturation must first be understood.

Lymphocytes originate during fetal life by maturation from a precursor cell in the bone marrow. These undifferentiated lymphoid precursor cells have the potential to manufacture a vast number of different antibodies. Some of these cells migrate to the thymus; others migrate in birds to the bursa of Fabricius, an organ situated near the cloaca that resembles the thymus. In humans, this second group is believed to remain in the marrow because no bursa or obvious bursal equivalent has been identified (Fig. 6–1).

In the special environment of the thymus and under the influence of locally produced hormones, the lymphocytes proliferate rapidly and mature. During maturation, each cell undergoes mutation and irreversible gene arrangement of the part of its genetic material that determines the type of antigen receptor expressed on the cell membrane. Each cell so produced has a

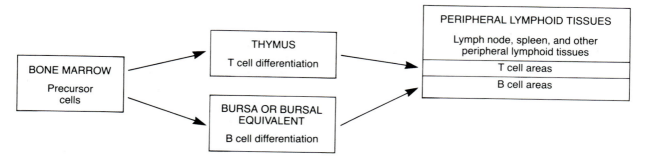

Figure 6–1 Development of T and B lymphocytes. Diagram shows the postulated development of the lymphoid tissue. Stem cells derived from the bone marrow migrate to the thymus, mature (involving gene rearrangement and clonal proliferation), and migrate to populate the lymph nodes and other peripheral lymphoid tissues. Similarly, B lymphocytes mature under the influence of the bursa or its equivalent and also migrate to complete the population of the peripheral lymphoid tissues.

unique DNA arrangement that encodes for a unique receptor; this genetic rearrangement occurs in the absence of the antigen to which the cell will become specific. These cells further divide to produce a clone, with each member having the same antigen receptor. Finally, the cells, now called *T lymphocytes,* migrate from the thymus to populate the T-cell areas of the peripheral lymphoid tissues—lymphoid aggregates, lymph nodes, and spleen (Fig. 6–2).

The cells that migrate to the bursa (or remain in the marrow in humans) undergo similar proliferation, maturation, irreversible gene rearrangement, and clonal expansion. The *B lymphocytes* so produced migrate to the peripheral lymphoid tissues and populate the B-cell zones

(Fig. 6–2). The apparent simplicity of the structure of the peripheral lymphoid system is therefore deceptive; the lymphocytes that all look alike are made up of members of many thousands of unique clones.

An antigen is recognized only by members of a clone of lymphocytes that have a specific antigen-combining receptor site with which it can bind. The process is termed *clonal selection* and is the basis for the specificity of the immune response.

THE B-CELL SYSTEM

The B cells produce the conventional immunoglobulin antibodies. The antigen receptor itself is

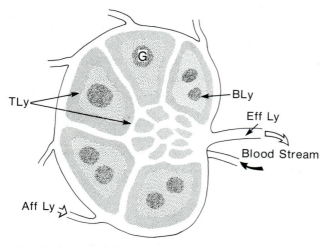

Figure 6–2 Diagram of a lymph node. Lymph enters the node through several afferent lymphatic vessels (Aff Ly) and percolates through a meshwork formed by reticulum cells and their reticulin fibers. In the medulla, the fluid is collected into sinuses lined by phagocytic sinus-lining cells that are members of the mononuclear phagocyte system. The cortex contains collections of B lymphocytes (BLy), some of which have one or more germinal centers (G). Surrounding these areas, there is a mantle of T lymphocytes (TLy); this is designated the *paracortical zone.* In the medulla there are groups, or cords, of B cells—both lymphocytes and cells that have differentiated into plasma cells. The B cells tend to remain in the node and are therefore described as being sessile. T cells, on the other hand, leave the node via the solitary efferent lymphatic vessel (Eff Ly), enter the blood via the thoracic duct, and finally return to a lymph node. They leave the blood stream by passing through the walls of the postcapillary venules in the paracortical zone. Lymph containing lymphocytes from tissues or other lymph nodes also enters the lymph node through one of the afferent lymphatics (Aff Ly). (Drawn by Margot Mackay, Faculty of Medicine, Department of Surgery, Division of Biomedical Communications, University of Toronto.)

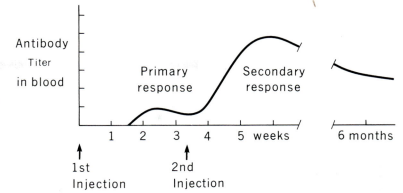

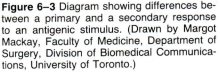

Figure 6–3 Diagram showing differences between a primary and a secondary response to an antigenic stimulus. (Drawn by Margot Mackay, Faculty of Medicine, Department of Surgery, Division of Biomedical Communications, University of Toronto.)

part of an immunoglobulin molecule. When an antigen is introduced into the body, it becomes attached to those lymphocytes that possess the appropriate receptor. The union acts as a signal and stimulates the cell; it enlarges, its cytoplasm becomes more abundant, and its nucleolus enlarges. This is called *blast transformation* and is followed by cell division, maturation into plasma cells, and formation of immunoglobulin. The number of functioning daughter cells rapidly increases as the clone expands. Initially IgM is produced, but under optimal conditions other classes are produced, *e.g.,* IgG or IgA. This change is termed the *class switch.*

When antigen is encountered for the first time, there is a delay of 7 to 10 days before antibodies appear in the blood. This is termed the *primary response* (Fig. 6–3). The antibodies are predominantly IgM, and their titer is low and soon wanes. Not all stimulated B lymphocytes mature to antibody-secreting cells. Some remain as memory cells, so that when an antigen is given on a subsequent occasion, there is a more rapid and vigorous antibody production. IgG is the predominant antibody. This is termed the *secondary response* (Fig. 6–3). The persistence of antibody and of the ability to generate a rapid antibody response to a second exposure to the antigen is of great importance in providing immunity to infection and explains the reason for administering two or more doses of toxoid or vaccine.

Although B-cell stimulation and antibody production can occur after the attachment of antigen to the specific B-cell receptor, for most B-cell responses a second signal derived from T cells, *e.g.,* interleukin-2 (IL-2) and interferon-gamma,

is usually required. It may be that a sequence of signals (*e.g.,* IL-4, IL-5, and IL-6) is required.

Structure of Immunoglobulins

Immunoglobulins are composed of four polypeptide chains: a pair of light (L) chains and a pair of heavy (H) chains held together by disulfide bonds as explained in Figure 6–4. There are two types of L chains, lambda (λ) and kappa (κ). Each monomeric antibody molecule contains two L chains or two K chains, never one of each. Each molecule has two antigen-combining sites (Figs. 6–4 and 6–5). There are five classes of immunoglobulin, depending on the type of heavy chain present: gamma (γ), alpha (α), mu (μ), delta (δ), or epsilon (ϵ) (Fig. 6–4). Each B cell makes only one type of L chain and one type of H chain at a time and makes antibody of only one specificity. Each chain consists of a series of globular, folded areas (called *domains*) separated by unfolded regions of the chain. Each chain has one variable domain and one or more constant domains; within each variable domain there are regions of the chain that are much more variable than the others, known as the *hypervariable regions.* It is the exact amino acid sequence (determined by the rearranged genetic DNA) in the hypervariable regions that determines the antigen-binding specificity of the molecule. The immunoglobulin molecule (Fig. 6–6) can be digested by papain, an enzyme that cleaves the heavy chains above the interchain disulfide bonds, to create two antigen-binding fragments (Fab) and

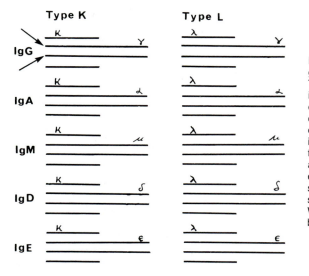

Figure 6-4 Structure of the immunoglobulins. Each immunoglobulin has two identical heavy chains and two identical light chains. There are five classes—IgG, IgA, IgM, IgD, and IgE—each differing in their heavy chains, which are γ, α, μ, δ, or ε, respectively. Of each class there are two types, type K and type L; the type depends on whether the light chain is κ (kappa) or λ (lambda). The specificity of each molecule is related to the two binding sites, which are indicated by the two arrows on the IgG type κ. Antibodies are therefore divalent. Note that following immunization by a single antigen, ten distinct types of immunoglobulin can be formed. They each have the same antibody specificity but differ in other respects, such as in chemical structure, physical properties, and ability to sensitize, to fix complement, and to cross the placenta. (From Walter, J. B., and Israel, M. S.: General Pathology. 5th ed. Edinburgh, Churchill Livingstone, 1979.)

one fragment that crystallizes readily (the crystallizing or Fc fragment).

Properties of the Immunoglobulin Classes

IgG. This immunoglobulin is characteristic of a secondary response and is the most abundant immunoglobulin in the serum; it is the only one to cross the placenta.

IgA. The IgA monomer is the second most abundant immunoglobulin class in serum but is the predominant immunoglobulin in secretions such as saliva. In the production of secretory IgA, the plasma cells in the submucosa produce IgA monomers plus a J chain, which are assembled to form IgA dimers. The dimers bind to *secretory component* before being transported through the epithelial cells, such as those of the salivary glands (Fig. 6–7). The secretory component appears to protect IgA from enzymatic digestion so that it can perform its protective role on epithelial surfaces, such as in the mouth, gut, or bronchi.

IgM. The IgM molecule is a pentamer of five IgM monomers joined together by a J chain (Fig. 6–7). Because of its size, IgM is largely restricted to the intravascular compartment.

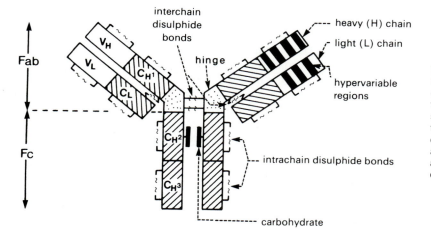

Figure 6–5 The structure of IgG. The molecule consists of two identical heavy chains and two identical light chains. The variable and hypervariable regions are shown. Cleavage by papain occurs above the disulfide bonds joining the heavy chains, thereby forming two Fab fragments and one Fc fragment. (From Walter, J. B., and Israel, M. S.: General Pathology. 6th ed. Edinburgh, Churchill Livingstone, 1987.)

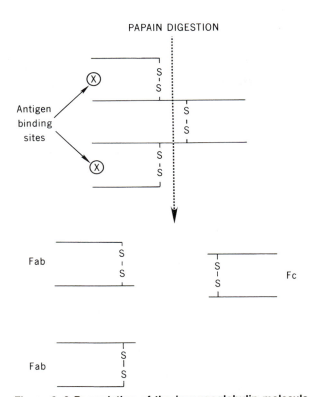

PAPAIN DIGESTION

Figure 6–6 Degradation of the immunoglobulin molecule by papain. The immunoglobulin molecule is represented as two heavy chains and two light chains joined together by disulfide groups. The antigen-combining sites are indicated by ⊗. Digestion with papain produces three fragments. Two are the Fab fragments, each with one antigen-combining site and composed of a light chain and part of a heavy chain. The third fragment has no power to combine with antigen and is termed the Fc fragment (fragment crystallizable). The structure of the Fc fragment determines whether the antibody will fix complement or cross the placenta. (Drawing by Rasa Skudra, Artlab Communication Inc., Toronto.)

IgD. Little is known about the role of IgD in the immune response.

IgE. This important immunoglobulin exists in serum in only trivial amounts but is the mediator of anaphylaxis and other type I reactions. When it is bound to mast cells, addition of antigen triggers the release of histamine and other products from their granules.

Antigen-Antibody Interactions

The receptor sites of the immunoglobulin are determined by the amino acid composition of the hypervariable regions of the adjacent light and heavy chains. Together the two chains create a three-dimensional site, which may be likened to a "lock" into which an antigen acting as a "key" will fit. When the lock and key fit well, the antigen binds to the combining site. The result of this binding may be a direct effect on the antigen, or it may cause effects indirectly by initiating the activation of complement or involvement of platelets, polymorphs, or macrophages.

Direct Effects of Antibody on Antigen

The principal direct effects of antibody on antigen are precipitation, agglutination, and neutralization. *Precipitation* of an insoluble antigen-antibody precipitate occurs when an antibody interacts with a soluble antigen (Fig. 6–8). *Agglutination* occurs when antibody causes the clumping together of antigen-bearing particles such as bacteria, erythrocytes, or latex particles artificially coated with antigen (Fig. 6–9). Both precipitation and agglutination are dependent on the ability of one antibody molecule (which has at least two antigen-binding sites, depending on the class) to link two antigen molecules or antigen-bearing particles together. *Neutralization* is an important function of antibody in the host defense against microorganisms. Antitoxins neutralize bacterial

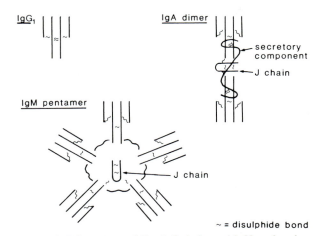

Figure 6–7 Structure of the IgG, IgA, and IgM molecules. The IgA molecule is a dimer around which is the secretory component. The IgM molecule is a pentamer with its five components joined by a J chain. (From Walter, J. B., and Israel, M. S.: General Pathology. 6th ed. Edinburgh, Churchill Livingstone, 1987.)

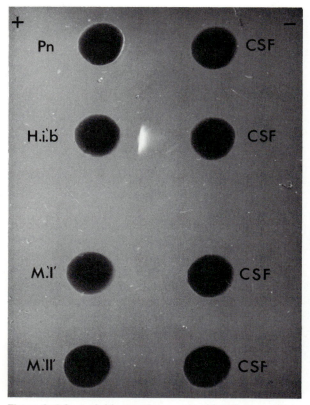

Figure 6–8 A precipitin reaction used to identify an antigen. A young child developed signs of meningitis and was admitted to a hospital after having received an antibiotic. A sample of cerebrospinal fluid (CSF) was obtained by lumbar puncture; although it contained many polymorphs, no bacteria could be cultured. Nevertheless, bacterial antigen was demonstrated by the technique of *countercurrent immunoelectrophoresis,* which is illustrated. The test is carried out in a sheet of agarose gel. CSF is placed in the four wells on the right, and specific antisera are placed in separate wells on the left. The meaning of each abbreviation is as follows: Pn, antipneumococcal serum; H.i.'b', antihaemophilus influenzae B serum; M'I', antimeningococcal type I serum; M'II', antimeningococcal type II serum. A current is passed through the gel, and bacterial antigen, which has a strong negative charge, is driven toward the anode (+). Under the conditions of the test, antibody moves toward the cathode (−). Hence, antigen and antibody move toward each other, and a precipitate is formed in which specific antibody meets antigen in optimal proportions. The well-marked precipitin line that is shown indicates that the CSF contains *Haemophilus influenzae* antigen. This test is useful in demonstrating antigen when bacteria cannot be cultured because of previous antibiotic therapy. The test is also used in identifying bacterial antigens in urine, blood, and body fluids.

Precipitin reactions can be obtained by allowing antigen and antibody to diffuse toward each other from separate wells in an agar sheet. However, the test is less sensitive, because diffusion occurs all around the periphery of the wells and the reagents are thereby diluted. Application of an electric field drives the two agents toward each other and thereby makes the test more sensitive. (Courtesy of Dr. C. Krishnan, Central Public Health Laboratory, Toronto.)

toxins, and antiviral antibody can prevent viruses from binding to and invading cells. Likewise, antibacterial antibody can prevent bacterial adherence to a surface—a step that precedes invasion. Precipitin and agglutination reactions are widely used in pathology. The test can be adapted to estimate antibody titer (using a standardized antigen preparation) or to measure antigen (using a standardized antibody preparation). Agar gel diffusion, radioimmunoassay (RIA), enzyme-linked immunosorbent assay (ELISA), immunofluorescence, and immunoperoxidase tests are other more specialized methods.

Indirect Effects of Antibody on Antigen

Complement activation and antibody-dependent cell-mediated cytotoxicity are considered.

The Complement System. The complement system consists of a set of soluble serum proteins (termed C1 through C9) that have an important role in host defense, both directly by their intrinsic ability to attack organisms and indirectly as an effector mechanism of the specific humoral immune response. When activated, the complement system can lyse organisms, bind them to important host cells, or release active peptides that contribute to an inflammatory response. As would be expected, there are a number of inhibitors that prevent excessive complement activation.

Activation of Complement by the Classic Pathway. Antigen-antibody interaction activates the components of C1, and then in turn C4, and C2 to form C4b2a (Fig. 6–10). This is the C3 convertase of the classic pathway. By its action on C3, C3b is formed. There is a natural inhibitor of C1 called C1 esterase inhibitor or C1–INA.

Activation of Complement via the Alternative Pathway. This pathway can be activated in a variety of ways that do not involve an immunologic reaction. These include the action of microbial polysaccharides and aggregated IgA or IgG. The activation results in the formation of the C3 convertase, C3bBb. This substance is normally inhibited by properdin (a naturally occurring inhibitor).

The Amplification Loop. C3b can itself become a C3 convertase, thus triggering more C3b for-

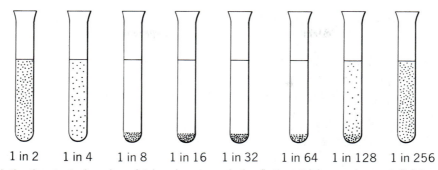

1 in 2 1 in 4 1 in 8 1 in 16 1 in 32 1 in 64 1 in 128 1 in 256

Figure 6–9 Agglutination test. A series of tubes is prepared, the first containing neat serum (left-hand tube), with each subsequent tube containing serum diluted with saline in proportions of ½, ¼, ⅛, and so on (*i.e.,* doubling the dilution). To each tube is added an equal volume of suspension of particles—bacteria, red cells, or latex particles coated with antigen. The tubes are incubated at 37°C for a suitable time. The final dilution of the serum in the last tube to show definite agglutination is described as the *titer of the antibody.* In this illustration, the titer is 1 in 128. Sometimes the left-hand tube, which contains the highest concentration of antibody, fails to show agglutination. Such a situation is described as the *prozone phenomenon.* Examples of this type of agglutination test are the Widal (for typhoid fever), the Weil-Felix (for typhus fever), and the Paul-Bunnell (for infectious mononucleosis). (From Walter, J. B., and Israel, M. S.: General Pathology. 6th ed. Edinburgh, Churchill Livingstone, 1987.)

mation. This causes amplification in both pathways.

Further Steps in the Complement Cascade. C3 convertase (C4b2a in the classic pathway and C3Bb in the alternative pathway) can combine with C3b to become a C5 convertase. The sequential activation of the remaining complement components leads to the formation of the *membrane attack complex* C5b–9, so named because, when membrane bound, it leads to cell membrane damage and lysis.

Effects of Complement Activation. Complement activation has many effects.

Assembly of the Membrane Attack Complex. This leads to cell lysis.

Adherence of Complement Components (e.g., C3b) to Cells (e.g., bacteria). Polymorphs and macrophages have C3b receptors and bind to C3b-coated cells. This opsonic effect encourages phagocytosis. Complement activation involves the *release of active peptides.* These include C2b kinin and the anaphylatoxins C3a and C5a, so called because they cause the release of histamine and other products from mast cell granules. C3a and C5a also act as chemotactic mediators of inflammation.

Figure 6–10 The complement system. This simplified diagram of complement shows how C3 is converted into C3b by a C3 convertase formed via either the classic pathway (involving C1, C4, and C5) or the alternative pathway. In either event, the amplification loop can augment the formation of C3b. (From Walter, J. B.: Pathology of Human Disease. Philadelphia, Lea & Febiger, 1989.)

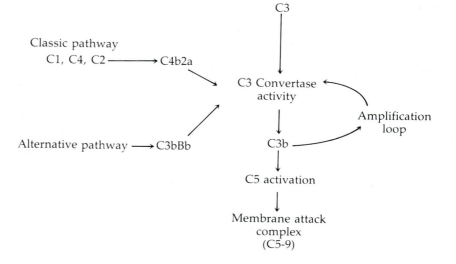

Antibody-Dependent Cell-Mediated Cytotoxicity. Effector host cells with Fc receptors adhere to and kill antibody-coated cells and microorganisms by means other than phagocytosis. The best known effector cell in antibody-dependent cell killing is the K cell, a type of lymphocyte that can kill IgG-coated nucleated cells very actively.* Neutrophils can also kill IgG-coated cells. Eosinophils can kill IgE-coated parasites, *e.g.*, schistosomes. The exact killing mechanism in each case probably varies according to the cell involved.

THE T-CELL RESPONSE

When pre–T cells mature in the thymus, there is genetic rearrangement, as with B-cell maturation, and a large number of T-cell clones are formed, each with a specific receptor. The T-cell antigen-specific receptor is not immunoglobulin but consists of a dimer of two nonidentical glycoprotein chains.

T-cell recognition is more complex than is B-cell recognition. T cells do not respond to antigen-binding to the specific antigen-combining site but respond when antigen is presented to them by an antigen-presenting cell, generally a macrophage. Much of the antigen is first taken up and degraded to short polypeptides by cells of the mononuclear phagocyte system. This is termed *antigen processing*. The processed antigen is then expressed on the surface of specialized cells, usually macrophages of the mononuclear phagocyte system or similar marrow-derived cells, for T-cell recognition (*antigen presentation*). Furthermore, T cells do not recognize antigen presented as such, but only when it is associated with antigens of the *major histocompatibility complex* (MHC) on the surface of the presenting cells. This phenomenon is known as the *MHC restriction of T-cell recognition* (see later in this chapter for a description of the MHC).

Other signals are usually required, *e.g.*, interleukin-1 or interleukin-2. Then T-cell activation, clonal expansion, and differentiation begin. This leads to the emergence of *effector cells* (*delayed type*

---

*K cells are probably the same as NK cells but differ in that in this context they kill cells that are coated with immunoglobulin.

hypersensitivity T cells and *cytotoxic T cells*) and *regulator cells* (either *helper T cells* or *suppressor T cells*).

Cytotoxic T Cells

Cytotoxic T lymphocytes kill cells by some direct cell-to-cell contact. Their most likely role is to destroy virus-infected cells and thereby limit an infection.

Delayed Type Hypersensitivity

In a delayed type hypersensitivity reaction, encounter with an antigen leads to an inflammatory reaction within 48 to 72 hours. The tuberculin or Mantoux reaction is a typical example. The pathogenesis is as follows. After the injection of tuberculin into the skin, T cells with the specific receptor encounter antigen on the surface of a macrophage or other antigen-presenting cell in the tissues, in association with class II HLA products. The T cell responds by activation, clonal expansion, and differentiation. T cells release many active compounds that are collectively called *lymphokines*. These include *interferon-gamma, lymphotoxin* (which can nonspecifically kill certain cells), and chemotactic factors (*macrophage chemotactic factor*) that attract macrophages. The macrophages that accumulate are immobilized by *macrophage migration inhibition factor* and then activated by *macrophage-activating factors*. The macrophage releases other factors that are responsible for such characteristic changes of the delayed type hypersensitivity reaction as vascular damage, edema, and activation of the coagulation system with fibrin formation. Another effect of T-cell activation is activation of *natural killer* (NK) *cells*, which are a type of lymphocyte that can kill cells nonspecifically.

The initiation of the delayed type hypersensitivity is highly specific, involving T-cell interaction with specific antigen properly presented. The damage, caused by macrophages and activated NK cells, that results is nonspecifically mediated.

Regulator T Cells

The regulator cells are either helper T cells or suppressor T cells.

Helper T Cells. Helper T lymphocytes produce agents (*e.g.*, interleukin-2) that promote the proliferation and differentiation of B and T cells in an immune reaction. They possess the CD4 marker and are called CD4$^+$ T lymphocytes, or T4 lymphocytes for short.

Suppressor T Cells. Likewise, other T cells possess the CD8 marker and are called CD8$^+$ T lymphocytes, or T8 lymphocytes for short. Called suppressor T cells, they inhibit the proliferation and differentiation of other cells, *e.g.*, macrophages, effector T cells, or helper T cells.

Cytokines

The term *cytokine* is now used to refer to a group of polypeptides produced by one cell that act locally on another cell. The lymphokines and interleukins are examples and were so named because they were initially found to be secreted by one white cell and to act on other white cells.

Lymphokines. Lymphokines were originally described as soluble factors produced by lymphocytes and released after lymphocyte stimulation. Many were poorly categorized and were named according to their biologic activity. Those that act on macrophages are described in the following.

Macrophage Inhibition Factor. Macrophage inhibition factor inhibits the migration of macrophages, an effect that can easily be assessed *in vitro* and used as an assay method for specific lymphocyte responsiveness to an antigen (Fig. 6–11).

Macrophage-Activating Factor. This substance is released by activated helper T cells. It acts on macrophages in such a way as to increase their ability to kill ingested bacteria and to kill tumor cells. The relationship between this factor and interferon-gamma is uncertain; possibly they are identical.

Interferon-gamma. This protein is produced by antigen-stimulated T cells. It induces an increased production and expression of class I and class II products of the MHC in macrophages, fibroblasts, and many types of epithelial cells. It induces differentiation and inhibits proliferation of many cell types and activates macrophages. It increases the cytotoxicity of NK cells.

Interleukins. The interleukins are better defined. The gene that codes for them can be isolated, cloned in bacteria, and used in their *in vitro* manufacture. *Interleukin-1* (IL-1) is a T-cell growth factor produced by cells of the mononuclear phagocyte system. It stimulates other cells to produce other interleukins and is chemotactic to white cells. It also acts on the hypothalamus to induce pyrexia (Chapter 14), and its action on the liver leads to the acute phase reaction (Chapter 19).

Interleukin-2 (IL-2) is a product of helper T cells and is essential for cell division in many clones of T cells after they have been stimulated by antigen. IL-2 enhances the tumoricidal action of cytotoxic T cells and NK cells. It is therefore being tested in the treatment of malignant disease. Other interleukins are known; they generally act as growth factors, but their actions are less well defined.

REGULATION OF THE IMMUNE RESPONSE

Much is known about the circumstances and mechanisms whereby the immune response is initiated, but less attention has been paid to the mechanisms that regulate and finally stop the process. One concept is that of an *idiotype–anti-idiotype reaction*. Each B-cell receptor (antibody) or T-cell receptor is unique and called an *idiotype*. In the unstimulated state, there are so few cells of each clone that the animal does not develop tolerance for the receptors. When an immune response occurs, there is rapid proliferation of the stimulated clones and with them the specific idiotype receptors. This provokes an anti-idiotype (antireceptor) response. This, in turn, rapidly expands the reciprocal clones, with anti-idiotype specificity, provoking an anti–anti-idiotype response. This sequence can theoretically continue indefinitely. Various models have been proposed whereby this mechanism might regulate the immune response.

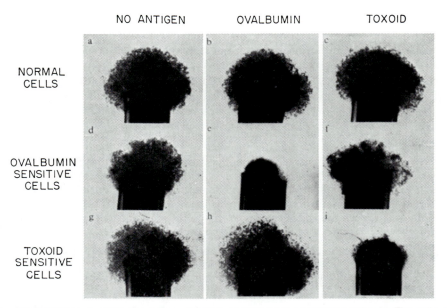

NO ANTIGEN   OVALBUMIN   TOXOID

NORMAL
CELLS

OVALBUMIN
SENSITIVE
CELLS

TOXOID
SENSITIVE
CELLS

Figure 6–11 Specific inhibition by antigen of the migration of cells from sensitized animals. The cells, mostly macrophages and lymphocytes from a peritoneal exudate, are placed in capillary tubes and incubated in a microchamber. Normally, the macrophages migrate from the open end and produce a tufted appearance. The cells derived from animals with delayed hypersensitivity show no migration in the presence of specific antibody. (From David, J. R., al-Askari, S., Lawrence, H. S., and Thomas, L.: Delayed hypersensitivity in vitro. Journal of Immunology, *93:*264–273, 1964.)

SPECIFIC IMMUNOLOGIC TOLERANCE

The type of immune response that follows the introduction of an antigen so far described is a *positive response* in which cells and antibodies are formed that tend to facilitate the elimination of the antigen. However, there may be a *negative response* for that particular antigen—neither immunoglobulins nor specific T cells are produced; instead, the body becomes less responsive to that particular antigen and indeed may never give a positive response. The phenomenon is termed *specific immunologic tolerance* and has been evolved to prevent rejection of self-proteins.

Specific immunologic tolerance was first noticed by Medawar when embryo mice were injected with donor allogeneic cells, *i.e.,* from a mouse of different genetic constitution. When the injected embryonic mice were born and reared, they were found to accept skin grafts from the original donor strain but not from those of any other strain (Fig. 6–12). The tolerance was therefore specific and not due to a generalized depression of the immune response.

Each individual has unique self-markers, particularly the highly polymorphic MHC molecules, which means that one animal's definition of self is another's definition of non-self or foreign. Specific immunologic tolerance is the mechanism whereby clones of T or B lymphocytes that could react against self-antigens are either destroyed or inhibited. Antigens present during fetal life, and to a lesser extent in neonatal life, usually promote tolerance in the individual rather than a positive response. Hence, as organs are formed and develop new antigens, the body does not attack them immunologically. Experimentally, very large doses of antigen or very small doses are especially likely to produce tolerance.

The mechanisms of tolerance are not well understood but probably involve several mechanisms. Self-reactive clones may be prevented from maturing (*clonal abortion*), or they may be destroyed (*clonal elimination*). Excessive activity of suppressor T cells can prevent self-reactive clones from responding even though they exist. The role of each of these mechanisms in tolerance

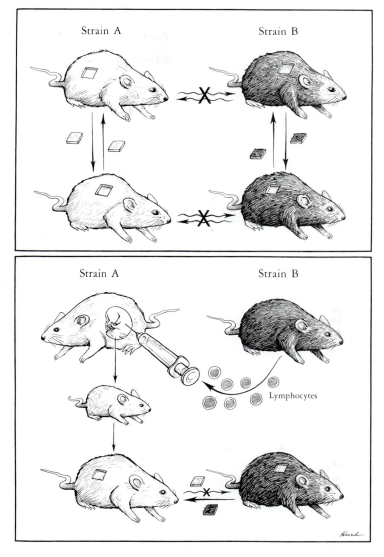

Figure 6–12 Representation of Medawar's experiment illustrating the fetal induction of tolerance in the mouse. Note that skin grafts can be exchanged between any two untreated mice of strain A or strain B but cannot be exchanged between mice of strain A and strain B. Injection of strain B cells into fetal strain A mice induces tolerance such that the strain A mice will accept a skin graft from a strain B mouse.

If the injected cells consist of adult lymphocytes (immunologically competent cells), they may react against the host. This is called a *graft versus host* (GVH) reaction. If it is severe enough, the baby mice are stunted and may die. Such a condition is called *runt disease.* The severity of the GVH reaction depends on the number and strength of tissue antigens present in the host (*i.e.,* strain A) and not present in the donor lymphocytes.

(From Bellanti, J. A.: Immunology. Philadelphia, W. B. Saunders Company, 1971.)

varies with the antigen, with the maturity of the lymphocytes and of the individual, and with the nature of antigen exposure.

IMMUNOSUPPRESSION

A particular immunologic reaction is sometimes detrimental to a patient, and it would be desirable to suppress it specifically; this has been accomplished in few instances. One example is the administration of anti-Rh antibody to Rh-negative women who have just given birth to, or aborted, an Rh-positive infant. This prevents the woman from manufacturing rhesus antibodies that could harm the next Rh-positive child. Transfusion of donor blood before living-donor renal transplantation is another example of an attempt to produce antigen-specific immunosuppression.

Nonspecific Immunosuppression. Nonspecific immunosuppression is widely used. The administration of *glucocorticoids* (particularly prednisone) and *cytotoxic drugs* (such as the alkylating agent cyclophosphamide and the antimetabolite azathioprine) is widely used. Unfortunately, these drugs have many side effects; in particular, they lay the patient open to infection. Irradiation of the whole body, and more recently of lymphocyte-bearing areas (total lymphoid irradiation), is a potent immunosuppressive, but its effects are irreversible. Another approach is to inject human lymphocytes into animals, harvest their serum (antilymphocytic serum) or separated globulin, and inject it into a patient to suppress the immune response. The precise mechanism of the action is unknown.

Cyclosporine. Cyclosporine, derived from a fungus, prevents IL-2 production and is a potent immunosuppressive agent, particularly for T cell–mediated responses. The drug must be given on a permanent basis because on withdrawal there is a rapid return of the undesired immune response. The relationship between immunosuppression and malignancy or opportunistic infections is considered elsewhere.

THE IMMUNE RESPONSE IN RELATION TO IMMUNITY TO INFECTION

Immunity to diseases caused by toxin-producing bacteria is due to the presence of antitoxins. Immunity to infection by a specific organism is associated with the presence of antibodies or effector T cells; it may be classified as outlined in Figure 6–13. When the host produces its own antibodies or effector T cells, the immunity is called active. When the immunoglobulins or T cells are donated from another individual, human or animal, the immunity is described as being passive.

Antitoxic Immunity

Some bacteria produce their major effect by secreting potent, highly antigenic exotoxins. The host responds by making antitoxins that protect the individual against future disease. Diphtheria is a typical example. The antitoxin provides immunity by neutralizing toxin and aiding its elimination. Hence, an individual who has had diphtheria, or even a subclinical infection, is invariably immune for life. If the individual is infected, a secondary immune response will en-sure rapid antibody production. This antitoxic immune state can be produced artificially by injecting diphtheria toxoid. Toxoids are toxins that have been rendered less toxic by addition of formaldehyde but are nevertheless still highly antigenic. It is now a common practice to give a series of injections of diphtheria and tetanus toxoid to induce active immunity. Active immunity means that the subjects produce their own antibodies and contrasts with passive immunity in which the subject is injected with antibody from another source, either a human or an animal donor. Passive immunity is a useful method of treating a patient with the disease because it provides immediate immunity. It is of temporary nature, however, and the antibodies are soon catabolized and immunity is lost. Also, there is a danger of anaphylaxis or serum sickness if the serum is from an animal source.

Antibacterial Immunity

Antibacterial immunity is much more complex than is antitoxic immunity. The reason for this is the antigenic complexity of organisms; many of their antigens are not related to the pathogenic action of the organism. Hence, the antibacterial antibodies formed against an invasive organism are not necessarily protective.

Invading bacteria may be killed directly by the mechanism of antibody-dependent cytotoxicity, in the cytoplasm of phagocytes (polymorphs or macrophages) after phagocytosis promoted by opsonins, or they may be lysed by the activation of complement. Often these mechanisms work hand in hand because complement activation results in the formation of potent mediators (C3a and C5a) that augment the inflammatory reaction. C3a and C5a also act as opsonins. Antibacterial antibodies play an important role in these antibacterial activities. One important aspect of immunity to bacterial infection of epithelial surfaces is the action of secretory IgA in preventing bacterial adherence.

Although many of the antibodies formed during an infection play no part in providing immunity, their presence can be of great diagnostic help, *e.g.,* the VDRL reaction of syphilis. With some infections, *e.g.,* viral infections, a rising

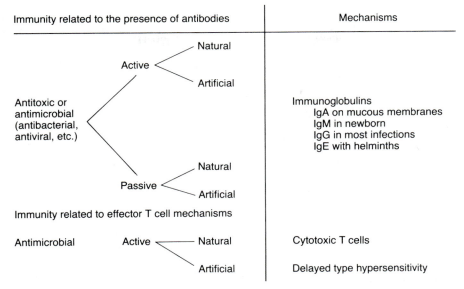

Figure 6–13 Immunity to infection. Immunity may be active if the animal produces its own antibodies or specific T lymphocytes. This occurs naturally after an infection and may be induced artificially by the administration of toxoids or vaccines. Passive immunity occurs naturally when antibodies are transferred by the mother to her child. It can be induced artificially by the injection of immunoglobulins derived from another individual. Passive cell-mediated immunity is not at present possible.

titer is especially convincing evidence of an infection.

Cell-Mediated Immunity in Bacterial Disease. The T-cell immune response is an important defense mechanism. Macrophages in the inflammatory response are activated and become more phagocytic and better able to destroy the organism. This applies particularly to intracellular organisms such as mycobacteria. Another mechanism is delayed type hypersensitivity that results in extensive destruction and inflammation.

Active Immunity. Natural active immunity follows an attack of the disease, either overt or subclinical. Active immunity can be produced artificially by injecting vaccines. A vaccine is a suspension of whole organisms; the precise preparation used is one that has been found to be effective in practice. Dead vaccines are effective for some diseases (typhoid and pertussis); for other diseases, a suspension of live attenuated organisms is required (*e.g.,* bacille Calmette-Guérin for tuberculosis, Sabin vaccine for poliomyelitis).

Natural Passive Immunity. Although at birth the body is poorly equipped for making antibodies, the infant nevertheless has IgG antibodies of

maternal origin that have crossed the placenta selectively from the maternal circulation. They confer good protection to the newborn child against some diseases, *e.g.,* diphtheria, but not others, *e.g.,* staphylococcal infections and whooping cough.

Passive Immunity by Grafting Cells of the Immune System. Bone marrow grafts are used to reconstitute the immune system that is absent through inherited defect or impaired by disease or its treatment (*e.g.,* leukemia).

Immunity to Viral Infection

Antiviral IgA antibodies in the secretions covering a mucous membrane prevent viral attachment and infection, whereas IgG neutralizing antibody in the plasma limits dissemination should infection occur; for example, in the presence of an adequate level of specific antibody, poliomyelitis remains an enteric infection, and central nervous system involvement does not occur. The T-cell response to viral infection is directed against the products of genes encoded by the virus in combination with a product of the HLA complex of the cell. Specific cytotoxic T cells destroy the virus-infected cells. Activated natural killer cells play a part, and other effector T cells produce a classic delayed type hypersensitivity reaction with macrophage infiltration, endothelial cell damage, and widespread tissue injury. Release of immune interferon (interferon-gamma) is another defense mechanism (see also Chapter 9).

Some viral infections directly affect the immune response. For example, in measles there is a period during which the immune response is suppressed; this is nonspecific, affects the immune response as a whole, and is termed anergy; this is the mechanism whereby measles can reactivate an old tuberculous focus. In AIDS, the virus is responsible for destruction of the helper T cell population, and the infections that ensue are devastating.

Immunologic Complications of Viral Infection. Some complications of viral illnesses are immunologically mediated. Thus, an encephalomyelitis can follow influenza or administration of influenza vaccine. Acute hemolytic anemia can accompany Epstein-Barr virus infection (infectious mononucleosis), and the formation of immune complexes in virus B hepatitis causes glomerulonephritis and urticaria.

Immunity to Fungal Infection

Immunity to fungi is mainly T cell–mediated by the delayed type hypersensitivity mechanism. With impairment of T-cell function, mucocutaneous *Candida albicans* infection and later systemic infections with *Candida, Aspergillus, Cryptococcus,* and many other fungi can occur.

Immunity to Protozoal and Helminthic Infection

The effect of the immune response on different parasites is very variable. Antibodies can damage parasites by acting as opsonins, by activating complement, and via antibody-dependent cell-mediated cytotoxicity. A striking feature of some helminthic infections is the production of IgE antibody, and this is responsible for some type I hypersensitivity reactions such as urticaria. Release of the eosinophil chemotactic factor of anaphylaxis is probably responsible for the heavy eosinophil accumulation around many helminths, but not around protozoa. Eosinophils appear to be able to attack and destroy some parasites, perhaps by IgE-dependent cell-mediated cytotoxicity.

Some parasites (*e.g., Trypanosoma cruzi,* causing Chagas' disease) do not stimulate an effective immune response, and the disease tends to be progressive and fatal.

IMMUNOLOGIC DEFICIENCY DISEASES

The primary immunodeficiency states first attracted attention when Bruton in 1952 described a young boy with a marked susceptibility to infection associated with low plasma immunoglobulin level. The immunodeficiency states may be classified into those with predominantly antibody deficiencies and those with predominantly T-cell immunity deficiencies. The situation is, however, more complex than would at first appear, for although there are examples in each group of diseases in which there is a defect in either immunoglobulin production or T-cell function, there are many cases in which both arms of the immune response are abnormal.

As a generalization, antibody defects are associated with recurrent pyogenic infections but also at times with unusual viral infections, giardiasis, or *Pneumocystis carinii* pneumonia. The T-cell defects tend to be associated with viral infections (such as overwhelming varicella, herpes simplex, and cytomegalovirus infections), candidiasis and other systemic fungal infections, *Pneumocystis* pneumonia, and mycobacterial infections.

Immunodeficiencies with Predominantly Immunoglobulin Defects

The best example is *Bruton's congenital sex-linked agammaglobulinemia.* There is marked lymphoid hypoplasia with lack of B lymphocytes and plasma cells associated with virtual absence of the three main classes of immunoglobulins. T-cell structure and functions are normal.

Selective IgA Deficiency. About 1 in 700 apparently normal persons have selective IgA deficiency. Some cases are associated with recurrent, generally mild, upper respiratory tract infections. People with IgA deficiency can have severe hypersensitivity reactions to blood transfusion due to the presence of anti-IgA antibodies after previous exposure to blood containing IgA.

Immunodeficiencies with Predominantly T Cell–Mediated Defects

Severe Combined Immunodeficiency. There are at least five varieties of this disease; affected infants have severe lymphopenia, particularly affecting T cells. Immunoglobulin levels are low, indicating a defect in B-cell function also. The principal manifestations are failure to thrive, skin eruption (due to graft versus host disease, as the mother's lymphocytes attack the infant's tissues), and a variety of severe fungal and viral infections, including slow-virus infections of the central nervous system.

The treatment of severe combined immunodeficiency is a bone marrow transplant, ideally from an HLA-identical sibling.

Acquired Immunodeficiency Syndrome (AIDS)

The acquired immunodeficiency syndrome was first noticed when previously fit young men became ill with *Pneumocystis carinii* pneumonia and an aggressive form of Kaposi's sarcoma. The number of cases has risen dramatically, and the disease has become worldwide. In North America, male homosexuals, drug addicts, Haitians, and hemophiliacs were first noted to be affected, but the disease has also spread to the female consorts of infected men as well as to newborn infants.

A new retrovirus was first isolated from a patient with lymphadenopathy in 1983 by Montagnier and colleagues at the Pasteur Institute in Paris. It was named the lymphadenopathy associated virus (LAV). The following year, Gallo and colleagues at the National Institutes of Health, Bethesda, isolated a similar retrovirus from a patient with AIDS. It was named the human T-cell lymphotropic virus, type 3 (HTLV-3). The viruses proved to be identical, and for avoidance of international tension, the organism is called the human immunodeficiency virus (HIV-I). A related strain (HIV-II) has subsequently been recovered from cases of AIDS in Africa.

The origin of the disease is debatable; it probably originated in Africa as a mutant of a simian virus. The disease spread via migrant workers to Haiti, a popular holiday resort for American homosexual males who spread the virus to the United States. It has now been recognized in most countries.

HIV is carried in the semen, blood, and other body fluids. The virus appears to be able to penetrate a mucosal surface even in the absence of obvious trauma. Thus, some cases of infection have followed artificial insemination. Nevertheless, approximately 70 to 75 per cent of cases of AIDS in the United States are male homosexual or bisexual males; passive anal intercourse appears to be the major hazard. Twenty per cent of cases of AIDS are intravenous drug addicts who acquire their infection from shared needles and intravenous equipment. The remaining cases are wives of infected bisexual males, customers of infected prostitutes, and infants of infected mothers. The most unfortunate group is patients who have had transfusions with contaminated blood or who have had a bleeding disease treated by injections of clotting factors. The screening of blood donors and the heat treatment of factor VIII preparations has virtually eliminated the last group. However, it has been estimated that up to 70 per cent of hemophiliacs who were treated previously are infected with the AIDS virus. There is no evidence that the disease can be acquired by casual contact with patients, even with close household contact.

Pathogenesis of AIDS. The virion of HIV is spherical, has a core containing RNA and reverse transcriptase, and has an outer lipid envelope derived from the host cell membrane during budding of the virus from the cell. The envelope contains two proteins designated gp120 and gp41; gp120 is especially important because it has affinity with the CD4 molecule. Hence, $CD4^+$

T cells (T4 lymphocytes) are the primary target for the virus. Macrophages also express the CD molecule and also form a target for the virus.

Once within the cell, the proviral DNA becomes incorporated into the nuclear DNA. Here it may remain dormant for an indeterminate period, but if the cell is active, as following antigenic stimulation, the virus replicates until ultimately mature virions bud from the cell surface. The infected cell dies, but the precise mechanism is unclear. The result is depletion of T4 lymphocytes, and the immunodeficiency state that ensues leaves the subject vulnerable to a wide array of infections and other effects including malignancy.

After infection, a number of syndromes can be recognized, but they do not affect all subjects. About 7 to 14 days after infection, a mild illness ensues with sore throat, fever, rash, and myalgia. The picture can resemble influenza or infectious mononucleosis. Next there may be persistent generalized lymphadenopathy (*PGL syndrome*). The AIDS-related complex (*ARC*) consists of diarrhea, weight loss, fatigue, fever, night sweats, lymphadenopathy, and hypergammaglobulinemia. Lymphopenia occurs with a decreased T4 lymphocyte count, so the T4 to T8 ratio is reversed. Opportunistic infections are not a feature of this stage. Finally, *AIDS* develops. It is characterized by the presence of immunodeficiency in the absence of other causes, opportunistic infections as described in the following, and the presence of antibodies indicative of HIV infection. As the disease develops, the antibody level decreases, and antigenemia increases. Weight loss is a striking feature and becomes extreme in the later stages of the disease ("slim disease"). Strict criteria have been laid down for national reporting purposes.

Clinical Features of AIDS. The clinical picture is dominated by the effects of a low T4 lymphocyte deficiency. There are repeated infections, often of unusual type. Widespread disseminated infection is common. Many types of organism have been encountered, but atypical mycobacteria, in particular *Mycobacterium avium-intracellulare*, and cytomegalovirus infection are common. Generalized infection with the helminth *Strongyloides stercoralis* is another hazard. Sixty per cent of cases present with pneumonia, the

great majority being due to *P. carinii*. Progressive fever, dyspnea, and a nonproductive cough are the main features. This is the major cause of death. *Candida* infection of the mouth (*thrush*) is almost universal, and an esophagitis (causing dysphagia) is common. It may also be due to *herpes simplex*, an organism that also causes persistent perianal infection producing chronic ulceration and blistering. Chronic and severe diarrhea are characteristic; many infective agents contribute to this, including cryptosporidiosis and infection with *Isospora belli, Entamoeba histolytica, Giardia lamblia*, atypical mycobacteria, *Salmonella, Shigella*, and cytomegalovirus. Perforation of the colon is a recognized hazard. Involvement of the central nervous system is encountered in over three quarters of the cases; dementia is common and may be the presenting feature with subtle loss of short-term memory. It may be due to HIV infection (AIDS encephalopathy), other infections (cryptococcosis, toxoplasmosis), progressive multifocal leukoencephalopathy, or lymphoma.

Malignant Disease. At the onset of the epidemic of AIDS, widespread purple papules of Kaposi's sarcoma were common in the skin. Often they were the first manifestations of the illness; the hard palate is a common site, and tumors also involve internal organs, being particularly common in the gut. For reasons that are not apparent, Kaposi's sarcoma is now less common in AIDS. Other malignant tumors are also common, *e.g.*, non-Hodgkin's B-cell lymphoma and, as noted previously, a diffuse lymphoma of the central nervous system.

In children, AIDS has some features not commonly encountered in adults. These include interstitial pneumonitis due to Epstein-Barr virus infection, parotid enlargement, and a terminal gram-negative septicemia.

Epidemiology, Treatment, and Prognosis. The presence of antibodies to HIV is considered to be good evidence of infection and infectivity. The evidence suggests that once infected, the individual remains infective for life. Furthermore, it is probable that AIDS eventually develops in all such people, but the incubation period is long; in one group, AIDS developed in only 34 per cent of homosexuals with HIV-positive serum within 3 years.

The incidence of infection in the general population varies greatly from one part of the world to another. In United States and Europe, the figure ranges from 0.005 to 0.52 per cent. In parts of Africa, where transmission appears to be heterosexual contact, 12 per cent of the population are seropositive. In these regions, prostitutes have shown a seropositivity rate of 50 to 88 per cent, and presumably they form an important source of infection.

There is no curative treatment available for AIDS, but supportive and antimicrobial agents can prolong life. Currently, the antiviral drug zidovudine (AZT) is being used, and the results are encouraging. The drug halts DNA synthesis, especially that associated with viral RNA-dependent DNA polymerase. The overall prognosis of AIDS is about 49 per cent survival at 1 year and 15 per cent at 2 years. Few patients live beyond 3 years.

Other Acquired Immunologic Deficiency States

The immune response is frequently impaired in patients with lymphoma, a state that is often aggravated by treatment. High dosage of glucocorticosteroids and cytotoxic drugs causes a severe depression of the immune response that is often complicated by opportunistic infection. There is depression of cell-mediated reactions in certain infections—measles and rubella provide examples.

TISSUE TRANSPLANTATION

In addition to its practical value in surgery, the transplantation of tissue has greatly extended our knowledge of the body's response to foreign tissue. The factors determining the fate of grafted tissue depend to a large extent on its origin; they may be summarized as follows.

1. Tissue transferred from a donor to a genetically identical recipient survives (*isografts survive*).

2. Tissue transferred from a donor to a genetically nonidentical individual of the same species is rejected (*allografts are rejected*).

3. Tissue transferred from a donor to a genetically nonidentical individual of a different species is rejected (*xenografts are rejected*).

The genes that encode for the transplantation antigens are codominant, that is, both alleles can be detected in each individual. Individuals who possess a particular antigen are tolerant of that antigen and do not recognize it in a graft.

It is evident that the fate of a graft is dependent on the genetic compatibility between donor tissue and the host.

Before the fate of grafts is discussed, some details of the major histocompatibility complex are described.

The Major Histocompatibility Complex

An important antigen responsible for stimulating tissue rejection in mice was discovered in 1936 by Gorer, who found that an antigen (termed histocompatibility 2 or *H-2 antigen*) was the target for rejection of allografts. Other antigens, determined by other genes, are also involved, but the H-2 locus determined the strongest antigens and for this reason is called the *major histocompatibility complex* or MHC. The human equivalent of the H-2 complex was discovered by Jean Dausset, who found that some human sera had antibody against allogeneic white cells. The human MHC therefore came to be known as the *human leukocyte antigen* or *HLA complex*. It consists of a set of closely linked genes on the short arm of chromosome 6. The MHC is important in transplantation and in many immunologic diseases.

Products of the MHC

The genes of the MHC code for transmembrane glycoproteins, which have an external region that is the portion of the molecule available for identification by tissue typing and for identification by other cells. They are of four main types termed A, B, and C (termed class I products) and DR, a class II product.

The external portions of these proteins are highly polymorphic and genetically determined.

There may be one of as many as 40 possible antigenic variants, each determined by separate alleles at one locus. The MHC products function as the targets of T-cell recognition of antigen and help determine the individual's T-cell responses.

Tissue typing consists of identifying the MHC allele products on an individual's cells by using specific antisera and the phenomenon of complement-dependent cytotoxicity. Specific antibody together with complement is mixed with a suspension of cells to be tested. If antibody has been bound, the complement is fixed to the cell surface, the membrane attack complex is assembled, and the cell dies. This is detected by adding a dye that readily enters cells whose membrane has been damaged.

Other techniques can be used for typing certain MHC products. The *mixed lymphocyte culture* (MLC) test is the best known. It is based on the principle that if immunocompetent T cells of one individual are incubated with cells bearing the MHC products of another genetically different individual, the T cells of the first individual proliferate. Such proliferation can be detected by the incorporation of radioactive nucleic acid precursors. The MLC test takes several days to perform and is not suitable for routine typing purposes.

Tissue Distribution of HLA Antigens

Class I molecules are widely distributed, being found in most tissues but in varying amounts. They are most strongly expressed on endothelial cells and those of the lymphoid and mononuclear phagocyte system. By contrast, the class II molecules are present on B lymphocytes and macrophages, but not under normal circumstances on most other types of cell.

The expression of both classes of antigen is greatly increased during an immune response, and this is most evident with the class II products because normally they have such a restricted distribution.

The Genetics of the Major Histocompatibility Complex

The individual genes are tightly linked, being organized into one complex called a haplotype. This tends to be inherited as a single unit so that within a family the inherited haplotypes follow the usual pattern for single codominant genes. Thus, if the one parent's haplotypes are designated (1 and 2) and the other parent's haplotypes are designated (3 and 4), then their children can have the following combination of haplotypes: (1 and 3), (1 and 4), (2 and 3), and (2 and 4). The chance of two children inheriting the same two haplotypes is 25 per cent. Each parent will always be one haplotype identical with each child, but never two haplotypes identical, unless the parents share one or two haplotypes.

The MHC and Disease

Patients with ankylosing spondylitis have a high incidence of the class I antigen HLA B27, compared with the general population. This event is not a unique one, for there are many other associations of a particular disease with one or more HLA antigens. For example, type I diabetes mellitus is associated with HLA DR3 or HLA DR4.

The MHC products are antigen-presenting structures; in particular, the products of the class II alleles are important in the presentation of antigens to T cells. Furthermore, the different allele products have differing abilities to present a particular antigen to T cells. The intensity of an immune response to a particular antigen is therefore determined by inherited factors. This may explain the association of a particular disease with certain HLA types.

The evolutionary value of this association is not clear. The polymorphism of HLA alleles may be of some advantage in the event of an epidemic. A heterozygous individual may have a greater chance of responding and overcoming an infection, and a heterogeneous community (with individuals having many different HLA genes) will have a better chance of surviving an epidemic caused by a new infectious agent.

Fate of Grafts

The fate of a graft depends largely on its origin and genetic compatibility with the host. Isografts and allografts are considered separately.

Isografts. Tissue from one part of an individual that is transferred to another area on the same individual (termed an *autograft*) or to an identical twin constitutes an *isograft* and does not provoke an immune reaction. Provided local conditions are satisfactory, such grafts survive.

Autografts have found extensive use in plastic surgery. Whole-thickness flaps of skin may be used as pedicle grafts and swung from one part of the body to another area. With such a procedure, part of the original blood supply is maintained until the graft has acquired a new blood supply at its new site. When the blood supply is thought to be adequate, the original connection with the donor site is divided. Alternatively, free grafts may be applied to a raw surface, *e.g.*, skin after a burn. Bone grafts are useful adjuncts to immobilization in the treatment of fractures. The bone fragments are steadily vascularized, and although much of the graft dies, it is steadily invaded by granulation tissue containing osteoblasts and replaced by new living bone; the process is called *creeping substitution*. Cartilage grafts, being avascular, do not require vascularization.

Allografts. Allografts are usually rejected unless the immune response is circumvented or blocked. Free allografts become vascularized in much the same way as isografts do, but the graft remains viable for a limited period only and becomes infiltrated by host T cells that lead to its rejection. Likewise, kidney grafts show deterioration of function and without immunosuppressive treatment are rejected. The reaction is mainly T cell–mediated.

If the recipient has previously been immunized against the donor (*e.g.*, by the receipt of a previous graft), the rejection occurs much earlier (by day 2 or 3). This is called the *"second-set" rejection* and is analogous to the secondary immune response that follows antigenic stimulation. In a highly sensitized individual and if antibodies are present, the graft never becomes vascularized. With a graft such as a kidney transplant connected by vascular anastomosis, the vessels become thrombosed and there is infarction. This type of reaction is termed a *hyperacute rejection*. It is mediated by antibodies.

Sometimes the graft appears to be accepted, but its vessels gradually become obstructed by intimal thickening. This *chronic rejection* has been most studied in patients with renal and heart transplants and can occur months to years after transplantation. It is mediated by T cells and antibodies.

Although allografts are usually rejected as described, certain tissues are found to behave differently and are capable of long survival. The cornea provides the best example, probably because acceptance does not involve vascularization. The graft remains clear and functional for a long time, and corneal grafts are widely used clinically.

The antigenic compatibility between the graft and the host is the single most important factor determining the fate of a graft. The HLA antigens are most concerned; because they are determined by histocompatibility genes, it follows that the genetic compatibility between graft and host is important.

Theories of Graft Rejection

When a graft of foreign tissue is transplanted to an allogeneic host, the host encounters the antigens, and an immune response is stimulated. The antigen is encountered either by host cells passing through the donor tissues or by antigen or cells from the graft being released and carried to the lymphoid organs of the host. The relative importance of the two alternatives is debatable. Two other factors must be considered: (1) passenger leukocytes in the graft and (2) changing immunogenicity of the graft.

Passenger Leukocytes in the Graft. Cells of the mononuclear phagocyte system (monocytes and tissue histiocytes) are strongly positive for class II antigens of the MHC; these antigens are efficient in stimulating T cells and therefore of evoking an allogeneic response. Possibly donor cells of the mononuclear phagocyte system in the graft provide a strong stimulus for an immune response. This may explain why pretreatment of a graft by radiation to destroy white cells can reduce its immunogenicity.

Changing Immunogenicity of the Graft. As noted, many cell types express little class II antigen under normal conditions but become strongly positive when exposed to an immunologic reaction. Interferon-gamma and other products of lymphocytes are important in this change. A vicious circle may ensue—the immune response increases the antigenic stimulus, and this in turn can evoke a stronger response.

Enhancement. Enhancement is the phenomenon whereby a host previously immunized to graft antigens accepts the graft and allows it to survive for a long period. The mechanism is believed to be mediated by the presence of anti-graft immunoglobulins. These antibodies destroy passenger leukocytes in the graft and therefore reduce its immunogenicity. Blood transfusion from a proposed donor is used in human transplantation work in an attempt to utilize this phenomenon.

The Status of Transplantation in Clinical Medicine

Kidney transplantation is now commonplace and has completely changed the prognosis of patients with end stage renal disease. The major limiting factor is the lack of donor material. In living-donor transplantation, HLA identity or one haplotype identity, as well as blood group compatibility, is required. Furthermore, the phenomenon of enhancement can be utilized by previous infusion of donor blood.

In cadaver-donor transplantation, using kidneys from *unrelated* individuals, HLA matching is not as important and indeed is sometimes ignored. Perhaps a "good match" *in vitro* is not a good match to a lymphocyte. Perhaps other non-HLA antigens are involved. Closely related individuals who are matched at several HLA types are likely to be identical in respect to many other loci because they share some haplotypes.

Bone Marrow. Bone marrow cells are now being used for several conditions. They are used in aplastic anemia and in patients with genetic defects involving stem cells. In leukemia, the leukemic cells of the patient's bone marrow are first destroyed by total body radiation or large doses of cyclophosphamide. Marrow grafts include large numbers of immunocompetent cells that are capable of recognizing alloantigens in the recipient. The result of this is a *graft versus host reaction*; it is characterized by skin eruptions

that initially resemble lupus erythematosus and later thickening of the dermis, producing a picture similar to scleroderma. Other features are lung infiltrations, marrow failure, diarrhea, and eventually death. Because of the severity of the graft versus host reaction, only HLA-identical sibling donors have been used successfully, but perhaps newer immunosuppressive methods will change this.

Liver. Cadaveric liver transplantation has been performed many times. With the advent of cyclosporine, the results are nearing 75 per cent 1-year survival.

Heart, Heart-Lung, and Lung. Heart transplantation and heart-lung transplantation have been used with considerable success. Isolated lung transplants have limited application because of the complex surgical problems related to anastomosis of donor bronchus to recipient.

The Fetus As a Graft

The fetus has one set of paternal haplotypes and expresses these paternal HLA antigens. The fetus can therefore be regarded as an allograft and yet does not stimulate an allograft rejection response. Why this is so remains a mystery because multiparous females frequently have antibodies against the HLA antigens of their husbands. Explanations offered include a barrier function of the placenta, poor antigenicity of the fetal trophoblast, and a mild state of immunosuppression induced in the mother by pregnancy.

DISEASES MEDIATED BY IMMUNOLOGIC MECHANISMS

Immunologically mediated tissue injury includes a group of reactions termed hypersensitivity in which an individual responds in an excessive way to an antigen; one way of classifying these reactions is into immediate and delayed. Other types of reaction, *e.g.*, glomerulonephritis following streptococcal sore throat, do not fit into this classification. Another classification of immunologic damage revolves around the specific mechanisms that predominate (*e.g.*, IgE-mediated versus immune complex–mediated) or the mediators involved (*e.g.,* complement, K cells, or mast cells). Unfortunately, no single system is satisfactory because the pathogenesis of many immunologically mediated diseases remains unknown. The most popular system is that of Gell and Coombs, who divide the mechanisms of immunologic tissue injury into four groups:

Type I: IgE-mediated, "immediate hypersensitivity."

Type II: mediated by direct binding of antibody (usually IgG or IgM) to a membrane antigen, where it activates complement.

Type III: mediated by deposition of immune complexes in the tissues.

Type IV: mediated by delayed type hypersensitivity.

Direct lysis of target cells by cytotoxic T cells is not included in this classification.

Type I IgE-Mediated Reactions

This type of hypersensitivity is mediated by immunoglobulins of the IgE type. The IgE molecules become bound to mast cells, and if two of these molecules are bridged by an antigen molecule, the mast cell is triggered to release the contents of its granules. The principal mediators are

1. *Histamine.*
2. *Slow-reacting substance of anaphylaxis (SRS-A).* This substance was so named because it causes a slow contraction of smooth muscle in *in vitro* experiments; this is in contrast to the kick produced by histamine. Actually, SRS-A is a mixture of leukotrienes C4, D4, and E4.
3. *Other factors,* including eosinophil chemotactic factor, neutrophil chemotactic factor, and heparin.

The IgE-mediated conditions are generalized anaphylaxis and allergy.

Generalized Anaphylaxis

Anaphylaxis can be demonstrated experimentally in the guinea pig. If an animal is given an injection of an antigen such as egg albumin, it shows no obvious discomfort. About 2 weeks later, specific immunoglobulin is present in the blood, and if a second injection of the same antigen is given intravenously, the animal rapidly develops difficulty in breathing, becomes unconscious, convulses, and dies. Richet, who first demonstrated this reaction in the dog, called it "anaphylaxis" because it seemed to represent the antithesis of immunity (Gr. *ana,* against, *phylaxis,* protection). A similar reaction can occur in humans.

The pathogenesis of anaphylaxis involves the production of IgE antibodies in response to the first antigenic stimulus. The antibody adheres to mast cells, which are thereby sensitized. The second encounter with antigen causes a severe reaction owing to the sudden release of mediators contained in the mast cell granules; histamine and SRS-A are the principal agents.

The clinical features in humans are the sudden onset of hypotension, bronchospasm, and edema of the larynx or skin. The danger of anaphylaxis should always be kept in mind by anyone administering animal sera or drugs by injection. A 1:1000 solution of epinephrine should always be available. At the first sign of anaphylaxis, 0.5 to 1.0 ml is given intramuscularly. The drug causes peripheral vasoconstriction and bronchodilation. Antihistamine drugs, glucocorticoids, intravenous fluids, and cardiopulmonary life support measures may also be necessary.

Anaphylactic shock is encountered in humans after the injection of foreign serum, the bite of a bee or wasp, or the injection of a drug, *e.g.,* penicillin, in which event this drug or one of its metabolites acts as a hapten. The tendency is more marked in atopic individuals, but not all subjects who have a history of anaphylaxis are atopic.

Detection of IgE Hypersensitivity. If a minute quantity of antigen is injected into the skin of a sensitized subject, an immediate local wheal and flare develop. This test has been used clinically to detect IgE sensitivity before a large therapeutic dose of foreign serum is given, but the skin test does not reliably indicate the possible sensitization to anaphylaxis. If foreign serum must be given, the safest procedure is to give a small dose subcutaneously and watch for any mild general reaction.

Allergy and Atopy

The term allergy has been used in many contexts, *e.g.*, drug allergy, allergic contact dermatitis, and bacterial allergy, but the current trend is to restrict its use to any clinical disorder caused by inappropriate IgE responses. Atopy is a variety of allergy that encompasses diseases with a hereditary tendency toward development of IgE-mediated illness in response to antigens. The hereditary nature of atopy is probably related to the fact that IgE production is dependent on T-cell recognition, and this itself is related to HLA type. The antigens involved in allergic states are often called *allergens.*

Although allergic reactions are mediated by antigen acting on IgE-sensitized mast cells, IgE regulation itself may not be primarily at fault. Inadequate IgG or IgA may allow antigen to reach sensitized mast cells. Likewise, excess IgG may block the reaction by preventing excess antigen from reaching the mast cells. This effect of blocking antibodies forms the basis of desensitization in atopic diseases.

Atopy. This term includes a variety of IgE-mediated clinical syndromes: allergic rhinitis (hay fever), extrinsic bronchial asthma (see Chapter 22), some types of urticaria and angioedema, and some gastrointestinal allergies. These conditions have in common a familial incidence. The exact mode of inheritance is not known, but one or more atopic diseases may occur scattered apparently randomly among different family members. Infantile eczema and atopic dermatitis (see Chapter 31) occur in atopic families, but neither appear to be IgE-mediated.

Allergic rhinitis tends to be seasonal and related to exposure to a particular allergen such as ragweed pollen. Characteristic are nasal congestion, sneezing, and a nasal discharge containing numerous eosinophils. The reaction is of the immediate type, and histamine is the principal mediator.

Mast Cell Degranulation by Non–IgE-Mediated Mechanisms

Not every syndrome described under the heading of atopy is caused by IgE-mediated mechanisms. Mast cells can be degranulated by other mechanisms. Thus, wasp venom peptides degranulate mast cells and cause a urticarial response. Angioedema can occur in patients with a deficiency of C1-esterase inhibitor, and urticaria is frequently idiopathic with no clear relationship to allergens.

Type II Hypersensitivity

Type II reactions are mediated by antibodies that become attached to antigenic determinants on cells and indirectly damage the cells by a variety of mechanisms. Activation of complement can cause lysis. Phagocytes, by becoming attached because of their Fc or C3b receptors, can destroy cells by phagocytosis. White cells can become attached to the antibody-coated cells and cause cell lysis without phagocytosis. This is termed *antibody-dependent cell-mediated cytotoxicity.* The precise mechanism is not clear. Most examples of type II reaction seen in human pathology concern the destruction of red cells. Occasionally during penicillin therapy, the drug, by acting as a hapten, can become attached to the red cell membrane and lead to the formation of destructive antibodies that cause hemolysis by complement activation. Similarly, autoimmune hemolytic anemia and autoimmune thrombocytopenia fall into this group. Likewise, the hemolysis that occurs after a mismatched transfusion or in hemolytic disease of the newborn can be included under this heading. In Goodpasture's syndrome, the autoantibodies damage kidney and lung. Graves' disease has been included in this group, but because the autoantibody stimulates the thyroid cells rather than destroying them, some workers prefer to classify it separately as a "type V reaction."

Type III Hypersensitivity: Immune-Complex Reactions

Some types of antibodies have the property of combining with their respective antigen to form complexes that can activate complement. Chemotactic factors are liberated, and polymorphs, which are attracted to the complexes, release damaging lysosomal enzymes. Four examples in which damaging immune complexes produce disease are described in the following.

The Arthus Phenomenon. Repeated weekly subcutaneous injections of antigen given to an animal lead to progressively more severe local reactions. Swelling and redness appear within 1 hour; over the next few hours, hemorrhage and necrosis develop. The pathogenesis is as follows. The injected antigen diffuses into vessel walls and encounters the specific precipitating type IgG that is present in the blood. Antigen-antibody complexes form in the vessel wall and activate complement. Polymorphs accumulate and release their lysosomal enzymes. The vessel wall is damaged, and thrombosis follows (Fig. 6–14).

Serum Sickness. Serum sickness occurs after the injection of a single large dose of foreign protein such as serum. Fever, a generalized itchy urticarial or morbilliform (measles-like) rash, joint pains, edema of the eyelids and dependent parts, proteinuria, and lymphadenopathy develop within 7 to 14 days. The reaction may be accelerated, appearing within 3 or 4 days, in patients who have encountered the same antigen previously.

On the basis of experimental observations, the following mechanism is postulated (Fig. 6–15). Immediately after a single administration of a large dose of antigen, free antigen is present in the blood in high titer. The titer steadily declines but drops rapidly with the onset of the immune response. As antibody enters the blood, antigen-antibody complexes form, and most are rapidly eliminated from the circulation by the activity of the mononuclear phagocyte system. It is during the period of circulating immune complexes that the illness of serum sickness occurs. The com-

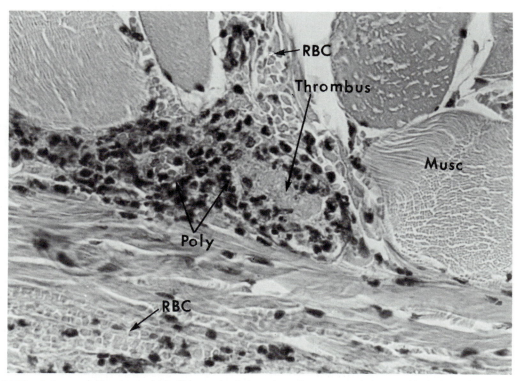

Figure 6–14 The Arthus reaction in a rabbit. This section is from the subcutaneous tissues and includes striated muscle (Musc). The blood vessel in the center is sectioned obliquely and shows occlusion of its lumen by a thrombus. Its walls are heavily infiltrated by polymorphs (Poly), many of which are degenerating. Free red cells (RBC) in the tissues bear witness to the severity of the vascular damage (×550).

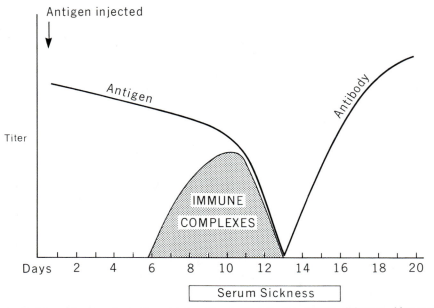

Figure 6–15 Graph indicating changes in antigen and antibody titer during serum sickness. After a single injection of a large dose of antigen, free antigen is present in the blood in high titer. The titer drops rapidly with the onset of the immune response. As antibody enters the blood, antigen-antibody complexes form and are rapidly eliminated from the circulation by the activity of the mononuclear phagocyte system. It is during the period of circulating immune complexes that the illness of serum sickness occurs. The complexes are deposited in the kidney, skin, and joints. Complement is activated, polymorphs accumulate, lysosomal enzymes are released, and damage is done. It is not known why the lesions tend to be restricted to those three sites. As the immune complexes are catabolized, the symptoms of the illness subside, and free antibody appears in the blood. This illustrates how the immune response results in elimination of foreign protein from the body. (Drawn by Margot Mackay, Faculty of Medicine, Department of Surgery, Division of Biomedical Communications, University of Toronto.)

plexes are deposited in vessels in the kidney, skin, and joints. As in the Arthus reaction, complement is activated, polymorphs accumulate, lysosomal enzymes are released, and damage is done. An acute vasculitis is a characteristic lesion and is seen in many organs, for instance, the skin and heart. Increased vascular permeability accounts for the proteinuria. In the kidney, a proliferative glomerulonephritis develops, and immune complexes form granular deposits in the glomerular basement membrane. It is not known why the lesions tend to be restricted to these three sites. As the immune complexes are catabolized, the symptoms of the illness subside, and free antibody appears in the blood.

Chronic Immune-Complex Disease. If daily injections of antigen are given to animals in doses such that antigen-antibody complexes are formed in the blood, a chronic glomerulonephritis develops. The pathogenesis is similar to that of acute serum sickness, but the dominant lesion is

renal—a localization that is not explained. The kidneys are readily damaged by circulating immune complexes, and this is the explanation of the renal component of many diseases, particularly those associated with a chronic infection (often viral) and in lupus erythematosus.

Some Clinical Examples of Hypersensitivity Mediated by Immunoglobulins. In clinical practice it sometimes happens that hypersensitivity reactions are mediated by several mechanisms, commonly a combination of type I and type III responses. Three examples are described: acute vasculitis, drug hypersensitivity, and immunologic lung disease.

Acute Vasculitis. Many forms of acute vasculitis resembling that seen in the Arthus reaction are examples of immune-complex disease. These include the vasculitis (palpable purpura) seen in the skin as a component of some drug eruptions, in *Streptococcus viridans* endocarditis, in meningococcal septicemia, and in gonococcal septicemia. On histologic examination, the lesions closely resemble those of the Arthus reaction.

Drug Hypersensitivity. Hypersensitivity to drugs is a common clinical event and is due to the drug, or one of its degradation products, acting as a hapten and stimulating the formation of sensitizing antibodies. Virtually any drug can produce a reaction, but common offenders are penicillin derivatives, cephalosporins, diazepam, thiazides, sulfonamides, furosemide, phenytoin, and quinidine.

Types of Drug Reaction. Drug reactions may be immediate and mediated by IgE; if the drug is given by injection, a reaction can occur within a few minutes. Urticaria is common; in severe cases, the features are those of acute anaphylactic shock with laryngeal edema, asthma, hypotension, and death.

Later drug reactions begin several days after the administration of the drug and are due to the formation of IgG or IgM, which form damaging immune complexes. The pathogenesis and symptoms resemble those of serum sickness. Urticarial, morbilliform, petechial, and other types of skin eruptions are common; arthralgia, renal damage, and fever may be present. In other cases, individual features may occur alone, *e.g.,* renal damage, drug fever, or acute vasculitis of the skin.

Late drug effects are thrombocytopenia, hemolytic anemia, erythema multiforme, cholestatic jaundice, and a syndrome resembling systemic lupus erythematosus. Methicillin is responsible for some cases of interstitial nephritis and is accompanied by anti–renal tubule basement membrane antibodies. The pathogenesis of many of these effects is obscure. In some instances, *e.g.,* hemolytic anemia, cytotoxic antibodies are present (type II reaction); they may be directed against the drug, as in penicillin-induced hemolytic anemia, or against the red cell surface antigens, an effect induced by alpha-methyldopa.

Immunologic Lung Disease. Lung tissue is a common site for immune-mediated disease. Several patterns of reaction can be found (see also Chapter 22).

Extrinsic Bronchial Asthma. This is an IgE-mediated disorder.

Extrinsic Allergic Alveolitis. The best known example is farmer's lung, an immune-complex reaction in the alveoli (type III reaction).

Goodpasture's disease. This is a type II reaction.

Type IV Reactions

Type IV reactions are mediated by specific effector T cells.

The Koch Phenomenon. Tubercle bacilli injected into a normal guinea pig lead to the appearance of a nodule at the site of the injection in about 14 days. Ulceration follows; the bacilli spread to the local lymph nodes, reach the blood stream, and produce generalized miliary tuberculosis and death. The injection of tubercle bacilli into the skin of a previously infected animal evokes a different type of response. A nodule appears in 1 to 2 days, ulcerates, and then heals. There is little tendency to spread to the local lymph nodes. This second type of response was described by Koch, and it should be noted that the reaction of a tuberculous animal to tubercle bacilli differs from that of a normal one in several important respects. The incubation period is greatly shortened—this may be described as hypersensitivity. The lesion heals quickly and there is no spread, suggesting that there is immunity to the infection.

The heightened tissue response of the tuberculous animal can be demonstrated not only to the living tubercle bacillus but also to dead organisms and extracts of organisms. Koch originally used "old tuberculin," but more recently a purified protein derivative (PPD) has been introduced.

The intradermal injection of a small quantity of PPD into a normal animal results in a negligible inflammatory response. In a tuberculous animal, however, an indurated erythematous lesion appears within 24 hours and reaches a peak by 72 hours. This is the Mantoux or tuberculin test, and a positive result indicates the existence of hypersensitivity to tuberculoprotein. The delay in the appearance of the reaction contrasts with the rapid appearance of the wheal and flare effect of IgE-mediated reactions. The injection of a larger quantity of PPD into a tuberculous animal may result in a flare-up of the local tuberculous lesion. Indeed, large doses of PPD can lead to fever, prostration, and death. Early attempts to "immunize" patients, therefore, often did more harm than good.

Under natural conditions, a type IV reaction to an organism or its products follows infection. A conversion from tuberculin-negative to a positive reaction during the course of an undiagnosed illness is therefore good evidence of its tuberculous etiology. If the infection is completely eradicated, the test may, over a period of years, revert to negative. Hence, the tuberculin test is of great importance clinically because a positive reaction indicates a past or present tuberculous infection. Indeed, in North America where tuberculosis is uncommon, a strongly positive tuberculin test is highly suggestive of active tuberculosis.

Hypersensitivity reactions akin to the Mantoux test are of diagnostic value in other infections. The following tests may be cited: Frei (lymphogranuloma venereum), coccidioidin, histoplasmin, blastomycin, and lepromin (Fernandez reaction).

Role of Type IV Reactions in Disease

Delayed type hypersensitivity reactions are responsible not only for the necrosis (*e.g.*, caseation) that occurs in some infections, but also for the continued tissue destruction that contributes to the chronicity of mycobacterial, fungal, and some other infections.

"Allergic" Contact Dermatitis. "Allergic" contact dermatitis,* typified by poison ivy and nickle dermatitis, is also mediated by a type IV hypersensitivity reaction (see Chapter 31).

Other Diseases Mediated by Aberrant Immune Mechanisms. Although it has been convenient to describe the four types of hypersensitivity and the human diseases in which they play a dominant role, it must be admitted that in many instances the reactions are more complex. Immune complexes may form *in situ* rather than be formed in the circulation as in the classic type III reaction. In some diseases, several types of reaction combine to produce complex lesions.

---

*The term "allergic" is used by convention. It does not imply an IgE-mediated reaction.

Sometimes the antigen involved is a self-protein, and the disease is labeled autoimmune. Lupus erythematosus is a typical example.

AUTOIMMUNE DISEASE: THE CONCEPT OF AUTOIMMUNITY

The concept of autoimmunity due to the host's defense system attacking and destroying the host's own tissues became popular with the discovery of autoantibodies in certain types of hemolytic anemia and Hashimoto's disease of the thyroid. It became fashionable to call any disease autoimmune if there was no known etiology and autoantibodies were present in the serum. This concept is too vague to be of great value. Antibodies to heart muscle are present in syphilis but are not the cause of the disease. They are of diagnostic value, however, in the VDRL.

Autoimmunity can be defined as a condition in which a major effector mechanism—humoral or cellular—reacts specifically with a self-component that is not altered by foreign antigen. It must be appreciated that the concept of autoimmunity is merely a facet of the pathogenesis of some diseases; in some, this component is a major factor in producing the lesions characteristic of the disease. In other diseases, the autoimmune component is an incidental factor and described as an *epiphenomenon*. In neither case does it indicate the cause. In some diseases, the cause is an infection, trauma, or the administration of a drug.

It will be remembered that T cells recognize antigens in association with HLA antigens, and it should occasion no surprise to find that genetic susceptibility also plays a role.

There are several suggestions as to how external agents (*e.g.*, a virus) can trigger an autoimmune reaction. One mechanism is presented in Figure 6–16. In the normal state, it is assumed that there are host B cells that can make an autoantibody but fail to do so because T cells are tolerant of the antigen and therefore fail to provide a stimulus. A foreign protein may carry the antigenic site recognizable by B cells and also one that is recognized by T cells in association with a determinant that triggers helper T cells.

A second popular theory suggests how viruses

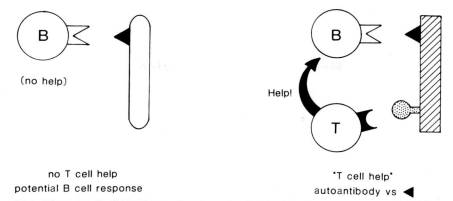

no T cell help
potential B cell response

'T cell help'
autoantibody vs ◄

Figure 6–16 Possible pathogenesis of autoimmunity. A mechanism is illustrated for explaining the ability of a foreign antigen (*e.g.*, an infectious agent) to trigger autoantibody formation. In the normal state (left), potentially autoreactive B cells exist but are not stimulated, because T cells have been made tolerant and helper cells are not formed. A foreign protein (right) may carry the determinant recognizable by B cells in association with a determinant that also triggers the formation of helper T cells. (From Walter, J. B., and Israel, M. S.: General Pathology. 6th ed. Edinburgh, Churchill Livingstone, 1987.)

could trigger autoimmunity. The virus stimulates the formation of antiviral immunoglobulin; this antibody has sites that combine specifically with the virus. However, cells attacked by the virus also have specific receptors, which in this respect resemble specific antiviral antibody. If the body makes anti–anti-virus antibody (an anti-idiotype reaction), this new antibody will be specific for the cell receptor. In other words, it is an autantibody. A third possible mechanism is that an event such as a virus infection could encourage expression of class II HLA antigen on cells that do not normally express them, so that reactive T cells can be stimulated and in turn lead to antibody production or the formation of effector T cells.

Renal Disease. The role of autoimmunity in the various types of glomerulonephritis is described in Chapter 25.

Liver Disease. There is little doubt that an immune mechanism is responsible for liver cell necrosis in acute viral hepatitis, but the precise pathogenesis is not clear. In several types of chronic liver disease, non–organ-specific auto-antibodies are found: chronic active hepatitis, primary biliary cirrhosis, and some cases of cirrhosis of unknown cause (cryptogenic cirrhosis). These have been grouped as "autoimmune liver disease," but the relationship between the antibodies and the pathogenesis of the disease is unknown. Rheumatoid factor and antinuclear antibodies may be found, but the most frequent

are anti–smooth muscle antibody (in chronic active hepatitis) and anti-mitochondrial antibody (in primary biliary cirrhosis).

Skin Disease. Antibodies to skin components occur in pemphigus vulgaris, bullous pemphigoid, and dermatitis herpetiformis.

Hemolytic Anemias and Other Autoimmune Cytopenias. Autoimmune hemolytic anemia, thrombocytopenia, and agranulocytosis are described in Chapter 18.

Endocrine Disease. Hashimoto's disease, Graves' disease, and some cases of myxedema and Addison's disease are associated with an autoimmune process (see Chapter 29).

Diabetes Mellitus. See type I diabetes mellitus in Chapter 16.

Other Diseases. Many other diseases appear to have a strong autoimmune component (see myasthenia gravis and pernicious anemia). The collagen vascular diseases are described in the following.

The Collagen Vascular Diseases

The term "diffuse collagen disease" was coined to describe a group of disorders in which the primary lesion appeared to be damage to collagen. *Lupus erythematosus, dermatomyositis,* and *progressive systemic sclerosis* are described in this chapter. *Polyarteritis, acute rheumatic fever,* and *rheumatoid arthritis* can also be included in this group, but they are described elsewhere.

The evidence for these diseases being primary disorders is no longer accepted, but because they share certain features it is convenient to group them together. Because blood vessel involvement is as constant a feature as is collagen damage, the term *collagen vascular disease* is currently used.

Lupus Erythematosus

Lupus erythematosus is more common in black than in white people and affects the 20- to 40-year-old age group; females predominate. The disease may occur as localized skin lesions or as a more serious multisystem disease.

Some patients with chronic discoid lupus erythematosus of the skin develop a systemic variety. The figures given for this event vary, but it is probably less than 5 per cent. The diseases therefore appear to be distinct entities. Nevertheless, lesions of discoid lupus erythematosus can occur in patients with systemic lupus erythematosus, and the precise relationship between the two diseases is not understood.

Chronic Discoid Lupus Erythematosus. This type of lupus erythematosus has been recognized for many years by dermatologists as a skin condition that occurs particularly on the face and other exposed areas of the body and is worsened by exposure to sunlight. The lesions consist of well-defined erythematous, scaly papules and plaque. As the lesions heal, there is dermal scarring and disturbance of pigmentation, with hypopigmentation being particularly noticeable in blacks. In addition, there is telangiectasia, and the combination is termed poikiloderma. When the scalp is involved, there is loss of hair (*alopecia*). Indeed, lupus erythematosus is an important cause of scarring alopecia.

Systemic Lupus Erythematosus. In systemic lupus erythematosus (SLE), there is widespread involvement of many organs, typically the skin, joints, pericardium, pleura, endocardium, and kidney. The skin may show lesions identical to those of chronic discoid lupus erythematosus, or it may merely show redness (erythema) and edema of the sun-exposed areas. Typically, it affects the nose and both cheeks, thereby giving the classic "butterfly rash." The disease varies considerably in severity. The onset may be acute with fever, malaise, weight loss, leukopenia, elevated erythrocyte sedimentation rate, joint pains, lymphadenopathy, and skin rashes. The onset of the disease may be insidious, starting with the development of a skin rash that is later followed by evidence of other organ involvement. Raynaud's phenomenon is common in SLE; when the brain is involved, there can be severe psychotic disturbances, and indeed this may be the presenting symptom. This should not be confused with the psychosis that is sometimes induced by corticosteroid administered as treatment of the disease.

A prominent feature of SLE is the presence of many autoantibodies in the serum. Antibodies to phospholipid include anticardiolipin, which is responsible for the positive VDRL sometimes noted in SLE; another antiphospholipid acts as an anticoagulant, since it is directed against platelet and endothelial cell membranes. These antiphospholipid antibodies are associated with the thrombosis and abortion noted in patients with SLE. Acute hemolytic anemia may occur, and the Coombs test is sometimes positive. Circulating anticoagulants may be present, and platelet antibodies can lead to thrombocytopenic purpura. The rheumatoid factor is present in about a third of the cases.

The most important antibodies in SLE from a diagnostic point of view are those that are active against nuclear components (*antinuclear antibodies*). These can be detected by immunofluorescent techniques. Suitable test cells are incubated with the patient's serum, thoroughly washed, and then incubated with fluorescein-labeled anti-IgG. Examination of the cells under ultraviolet light reveals the site of antibody deposition in the nuclei. Many patterns (diffuse, perinuclear or peripheral, speckled, and nucleolar) have been described. These have some diagnostic significance; for instance, the perinuclear or peripheral pattern is commonly seen in SLE, and the speckled pattern is seen in mixed connective tissue disease.

A less sensitive method of detecting these antibodies is to search for the LE cell phenomenon. This was the first specific laboratory test described in the diagnosis of SLE. When normal human leukocytes are incubated for about 2 hours with the serum of a patient with SLE, some neutrophils are found to contain a homogeneous basophilic mass of nuclear material. Such neutrophils are called *LE cells.* The mass is derived from a necrotic leukocyte nucleus that has been acted upon by antinuclear antibody. Its subsequent phagocytosis by a polymorph produces the LE cell.

The wide range of antibodies present in SLE react with widely distributed antigen and are non–organ-specific. There is no evidence that the antibodies against intracellular fractions are active against living cells. It is interesting that the relatives of patients with SLE show an increased incidence of autoantibodies and related diseases.

Pathogenesis of SLE. Some of the lesions in SLE are due to the deposition of damaging immune complexes. Thus, in lupus glomerulonephritis, there are deposits of soluble complexes of nuclear antigen (double-stranded DNA) and antinuclear antibody in the glomeruli. The initiating cause of lupus erythematosus is not known. Viral infection, administration of a drug, or exposure to sunlight have been suggested. An RNA virus has been implicated in the pathogenesis of a disease resembling SLE in New Zealand black (NZB) mice, but claims to have isolated a virus as the cause of human lupus erythematosus have never been substantiated. Whether the immunologic abnormalities noted in SLE are related to the pathogenesis of the disease or are merely epiphenomena is undecided.

Mixed Connective Tissue Disease

A syndrome having features of systemic lupus erythematosus, progressive systemic sclerosis, and dermatomyositis has been termed mixed connective tissue disease. Raynaud's syndrome is common; the condition has a good prognosis, since renal complications are uncommon and the response to prednisone is good.

Dermatomyositis

The combination of muscle inflammation (myositis) causing progressive weakness of the prox-
imal limb muscles and a variety of skin rashes constitutes this extraordinary disease. The occurrence of edema and erythema, giving a heliotrope discoloration, particularly around the eyes, is characteristic. Skin and muscle biopsies help establish the diagnosis. The disease may run a fulminating, fatal course, or it may be chronic. In patients over the age of 40 years, dermatomyositis is often associated with a malignant tumor of some internal organ. Hence, a thorough search for carcinoma should be undertaken. Specific signs or symptoms may indicate where this might be; the common sites, however (*e.g.,* lung, gastrointestinal tract, and kidney), should always be investigated.

Scleroderma

Like lupus erythematosus, scleroderma can occur in two forms. The purely cutaneous disease is called *morphea.* The skin becomes thickened and ultimately densely fibrous. Small plaques may occur at any site, or the disease can be widespread and affect many areas of skin.

In the systemic variety of scleroderma, called *progressive systemic sclerosis,* not only is the skin involved, but so also are the internal organs. Particularly involved are the esophagus and other parts of the gastrointestinal tract, which show fibrosis and impaired peristalsis, thereby leading to obstruction. Fibrosis can occur in the lungs, and the effects of aspiration are added to this. Systemic sclerosis is often associated with Raynaud's syndrome; indeed, some authorities maintain that in most instances, idiopathic "Raynaud's disease" is but an early manifestation of systemic sclerosis and that, given time, other manifestations of the disease will appear. Vascular involvement is usually not a feature except in the kidney; in this organ, progressive vascular obstruction leads to renal failure in a considerable number of patients.

Polyarteritis Nodosa

Classic Polyarteritis Nodosa. This type of polyarteritis, first described in the last century, usually affects middle-aged males and is characterized by an arteritis involving many organs. The inflamed arterial walls become necrotic and infiltrated with both inflammatory cells and fibrin, which gives the appearance of *fibrinoid necrosis.* The weakened vessel wall bulges, and the aneurysms so formed are responsible for the designation "nodosa." The lumen of the affected vessels becomes obstructed by thrombus, and the disease is characterized by ischemia and infarction affecting many organs, particularly nerves, spleen, and kidney. Renal failure, often with hypertension, is a common end result of this fatal disease.

Variants of Polyarteritis Nodosa. The classic polyarteritis nodosa is relatively uncommon, but many variants have been described. When the vessels affected are small, the term *microscopic polyarteritis* has been applied to these lesions. In some of them, the precipitating cause appears to be an infection; in others, hypersensitivity to a drug has been implicated. In none of them is the pathogenesis at all clear; an immune complex type of vasculitis has been postulated, however. Two of the recognized syndromes are as follows.

Progressive Allergic Granulomatosis. This variant usually commences with asthmatic attacks and pneumonia. Infarcted areas, which are found in the lung, excite a granulomatous reaction that closely resembles tuberculosis histologically.

Wegener's Granulomatosis. This disease is defined as a microscopic polyarteritis affecting kidneys, lungs, and upper respiratory tract. Death is usually due to renal failure.

It is not clear whether these variants of polyarteritis represent a single disease or are completely separate entities sharing one morphologic component, namely, a necrotizing vasculitis. Certainly necrotizing vasculitis can occur in other conditions. Thus, it is a prominent component of septicemia due to *Pseudomonas aeruginosa* and gonococcal septicemia. It is also a feature of the Arthus reaction, and it is encountered in rheumatoid arthritis, lupus erythematosus, and systemic sclerosis.

The validity of grouping these diseases under the heading of collagen vascular disease is dubious. Mixed cases occur, and patients appear who exhibit features of several diseases. Thus, some have lesions of scleroderma with vasculitis, or lupus erythematosus with rheumatoid arthritis. The occurrence of these mixed connective tissue diseases suggests that there is a common mechanism, but it does not prove a common cause. The presence of non–organ-specific autoantibodies is another feature that these diseases have in common, being the most striking in lupus erythematosus and the least evident in polyarteritis. Until the origin and pathogenesis of these diseases are discovered, it is convenient to refer to the group collectively as the "collagen vascular diseases" because they share many features. Thus, they are all *multisystem diseases,* since they produce widespread lesions affecting many organs, and often they exhibit marked constitutional effects such as fever, raised erythrocyte sedimentation rate, and hypergammaglobulinemia. This tendency is least marked in systemic sclerosis. All the diseases respond to glucocorticosteroid therapy as well as to other immunosuppressants such as azathioprine. Presumably, these act by suppressing autoantibody formation, thereby inhibiting the formation of new lesions. Once again, progressive systemic sclerosis is the exception and is least responsive to therapy.

Summary

- During development, lymphocytes undergo gene rearrangement and mature (in the bone marrow and thymus) into B and T cells; these migrate to populate the peripheral lymphoid areas.
- Antigens, with their specific epitopes, initiate a T-cell immune response first by being processed by macrophages and then, in association with HLA antigens, by combining with specific receptors on appropriate T cells. Clonal expansion and differentiation result in the formation of effector T cells (cytotoxic and delayed hypersensitivity T cells) and regulator T cells (helper and suppressor T cells). Interleukins are released by the regulator T cells.
- Delayed type hypersensitivity is initiated by specific T cells, but the subsequent release of lymphokines causes nonspecific changes.
- With a B-cell response, the B lymphocytes recognize antigen directly and, after clonal expansion and differentiation into plasma cells, secrete specific immunoglobulin. Helper T cells may be required.
- The primary response is characterized by IgM formation; the secondary response is more rapid and, following a class switch, leads to the formation of IgG and IgA.
- Immunoglobulins are detected *in vitro* by precipitation, agglutination and neutralization tests, and more spe-

cialized techniques. *In vitro,* they cause complement activation via the classic route and antibody-dependent cell-mediated cytotoxicity.

- Specific immunologic tolerance prevents rejection of self-protein.
- Immunity to bacterial infection may be antitoxic or antibacterial. Toxoids and vaccines are used to stimulate it artificially.
- Immunity to viral infection involves IgA, IgG, and a T-cell response with cytotoxic effect; delayed type hypersensitivity and interferon release are other factors.
- Immunity to fungi is T cell–mediated; in immunity to protozoa and helminths, various mechanisms are involved, *e.g.,* T cells and IgE.
- Immune deficiency states may be genetic, produced by drugs, or a result of irradiation or they may accompany other diseases. The outstanding disease is AIDS, which is the result of infection by the retroviruses HIV-I or HIV-II. Initial symptoms after infection are an influenza-like illness followed by persistent lymphadenopathy and finally the AIDS complex with severe opportunistic infections and Kaposi's sarcoma.
- Isografts survive; allografts are rejected by immunoglobulins and T-cell mechanisms. Differences in MHC alleles are most important. The MHC products are antigen-presenting structures, and this helps explain their association with particular diseases and plays a part in autoimmune disease.
- A complication of bone marrow grafts is graft versus host disease.
- Immunologic disease can be mediated by four mechanisms: type I is IgE-mediated and includes anaphylaxis and atopic diseases; type II is cytotoxic; type III is immune complex–mediated and includes the Arthus phenomenon, serum sickness, and vasculitis; type IV is delayed type hypersensitivity as seen in the Koch phenomenon.
- Autoimmune diseases are seen in kidney, liver, skin, thyroid, and other organs. Autoantibody formation is characteristic of the collagen vascular diseases, particularly lupus erythematosus, but is also encountered in the other members—mixed connective tissue disease, dermatomyositis, and scleroderma (systemic sclerosis).

Selected Readings

Chapel, H., and Heaney, M.: Essentials of Clinical Immunology. 2nd ed. Oxford, Blackwell, 1988.

Cohen, S., and Warren, K. S. (eds.): Immunology of Parasitic Infections. Oxford, Blackwell, 1982.

Halloran, P.: *In* Walter, J. B., and Israel, M. S. (eds.): General Pathology. 6th ed. Chapters 12 to 16. Edinburgh, Churchill Livingstone, 1987.

Harawi, S. J., and O'Hara, C. J.: Pathology and Pathophysiology of AIDS and HIV-Related Diseases. St. Louis, C. V. Mosby, 1989.

Klein, J.: Immunology: The Science of Self-Nonself Discrimination. New York, Wiley, 1982.

Morris, P.: Kidney Transplantation. London, Academic Press, 1985.

Paul, W. E.: Fundamental Immunology. 2nd ed. New York, Raven Press, 1989.

Roitt, I. M.: Essential Immunology. Oxford, Blackwell, 1988.

Snell, G. D., Dausset, J., and Nathenson, S.: Histocompatibility. New York, Academic Press, 1976.

Stites, D. P., et al.: Basic and Clinical Immunology. 6th ed. Los Altos, Calif., Lange Medical, 1987.

Infectious Diseases: General Considerations

After studying this chapter, the student should be able to:

- Distinguish between an endogenous infection and an exogenous infection.
- Describe how organisms are transmitted to the body.
- Define what is meant by a zoonosis and give some examples of the condition.
- Discuss the role of arthropod vectors in the spread of human infections.
- Discuss the importance of hospital infections.
- Describe the body's defenses against infection by using the skin, the intestine, and one other mucosal surface as examples.
- Discuss the three major patterns of infection, using as examples infection by

   (a) *Staphylococcus aureus;*
   (b) *Corynebacterium diphtheriae;*
   (c) *Salmonella typhi.*
- Describe the various avenues through which infection can spread.
- List the factors that are of importance in predicting whether a particular infection will spread.
- List five examples of opportunistic infection.

In the past, infectious disease has been a leading cause of death, and its study has comprised a major component of medical practice. Gastroenteritis and acute viral infections have been leading causes of death in infancy and childhood. Tuberculosis took a heavy toll in young adults, and pneumonia was poised to strike individuals of all ages, particularly if they were weakened by starvation or disease. Severe epidemics of plague, typhus, or influenza have periodically decimated populations, but with the advent of artificial immunization, the discovery of the sulfonamides, and the introduction of the antibiotics active against a wide range of organisms, it seemed that infectious diseases were finally beaten. The battle was won, but the war is not over. Organisms have developed resistance to antibiotics, and new methods of transmission have evolved. New infective agents have been identified, e.g., the bacterial agents of Lyme disease and legionnaire's disease. The AIDS epidemic is emerging, and it seems as difficult for us to control as were the previous epidemics for our predecessors. Furthermore, the use of immunosuppressive agents has revealed that organisms previously regarded as inconsequential and almost avirulent are able to cause severe, often lethal infection. Infectious diseases are again a common event in our community and hospitals, and this has led to the formation of special infectious disease units with specifically trained health care staff. This chapter describes the general aspects of infection, its source, its spread, and the defenses that the body has against it. Individual organisms are described in the chapters that follow.

From the moment of conception, the human body is exposed to microorganisms, some of which can produce lethal effects. The developing fetus is well protected from the environment, and intrauterine development is rarely complicated by infection; the main microbial assault occurs after birth. Organisms can cause disease in two ways: either they gain access to the tissues of the host, multiply, and cause *infection*, or they manufacture powerful toxins that are subsequently introduced into the body and cause an *intoxication*.

INTOXICATION

Staphylococcal food poisoning provides an important example of an intoxication. If staphylococci of a suitable strain are allowed to grow for a few hours in a sample of food, the unfortunate victim who eats it will subsequently develop an acute attack of enteritis with accompanying diarrhea and vomiting. This reaction occurs even if the food is cooked, because even though heat kills staphylococci, it does not inactivate the toxin. It is obvious that anyone with a staphylococcal skin lesion, such as a boil, should not be allowed to handle food. Another example of intoxication is *botulism*, which fortunately is very rare. It occurs after food contaminated with *Clostridium botulinum* is eaten, when sufficient time has elapsed for the organism to grow and produce its toxin. Most outbreaks have been due to

the ingestion of home-canned food in which the sterilizing process has been inadequate to destroy the highly resistant spores of the organism. When food containing toxin is ingested, the toxin is absorbed into the blood stream and affects the nervous system—apparently by interfering with acetylcholine release at nerve endings. Paralysis results, and in many instances it is progressive and fatal.

SOURCES OF INFECTION

The most important method whereby microorganisms cause disease is by their *invasion of and multiplication in the living tissues of the host*. This is the definition of *infection*, and organisms capable of producing it are termed pathogens. An infection can be acquired from several possible sources.

Congenital Infection

Infection of the fetus via the placental circulation is uncommon. The infections that cause severe generalized infection of the fetus may be remembered by the letters TORCH for *t*oxoplasmosis, *r*ubella, *c*ytomegalovirus infection, and *h*erpes simplex infection. Herpes usually infects the infant during its passage through the birth canal. Syphilis, once common, is now a rarity.

Postnatal Infection

Endogenous Infection

If the source of infection is from within the person, the infection is termed *endogenous*. Endogenous infections usually occur when the organism leaves its normal habitat. Intestinal organisms cause wound infection and urinary tract disease, whereas nasopharyngeal organisms cause bronchopneumonia when they migrate down to the lower respiratory tract.

Exogenous Infection

Infection acquired from the external environment is termed exogenous. The organisms may be derived from the following sources.

Patients. In diseases that run an acute or self-limiting course, the source of infection is a patient. Tuberculosis, whooping cough, measles, and influenza provide examples.

Carriers. In the case of some other diseases, *carriers* play a major role. A carrier harbors the organisms but does not exhibit any clinical disease. The carrier state may follow a clinical attack of the disease *(convalescent carrier)* or a subclinical attack *(contact carrier)*. Streptococcal, staphylococcal, pneumococcal, and meningococcal infections, diphtheria, typhoid fever, bacillary dysentery, and poliomyelitis provide examples.

Infected Animals. Some pathogens are primarily a cause of animal disease but occasionally infect humans. Such an animal disease is called a *zoonosis*. Bovine tuberculosis, *Salmonella* food poisoning, rabies, and psittacosis are good examples.

Soil. A number of organisms live in the soil and contaminate wounds. Some are derived from feces (the clostridia), whereas others are soil saprophytes (see maduromycosis, Chapter 10).

Transmission of Organisms to the Body. The exogenous organisms that cause infection may be injected directly into the host by the bite of an insect or through an injury, but more often they are first deposited on the surface of the body, which is thereby contaminated. Contamination may or may not be followed by infection.

The following modes of transmission are important.

Physical Contact. The causative agents of syphilis, gonorrhea, and other venereal diseases pass from one individual to another by *direct contact*. So also do staphylococci when they are transferred from the hands of one person to the skin surface or wound of another. The transfer of organisms from one individual to another may be by *indirect contact* through fomites, *i.e.,* clothing, bedding, cups, and other articles that are contaminated by an infected person or a carrier and subsequently handled by another individual. This mode of transfer applies to hardy organisms (staphylococci and coliforms) that can withstand drying for some hours.

Inhalation. Some diseases (*e.g.,* measles and chickenpox) are transmitted by inhalation of contaminated droplets or dust particles. Droplets are formed during talking, coughing, and sneezing when air passes rapidly over a mucous membrane covered by salivary, tracheal, or nasal secretions. Droplet nuclei are formed when the droplets evaporate.

Some respiratory diseases are caused by the inhalation of dust derived from dried contaminated secretions. These secretions may be on handkerchiefs, clothing, bedding, floors, or other surfaces and on drying become converted into dust, which can easily be stirred by movement such as walking, dressing, or bedmaking. Airborne transfer of organisms is particularly important within enclosed areas. This therefore applies to hospital wards and operating rooms, where all efforts should be made to keep dust to a minimum. Avoidance of unnecessary movement and adequate ventilation within an operating room are important procedures designed to reduce wound infection.

Ingestion. Food is a common vehicle of transmission of organisms and can be contaminated in a variety of ways.

Flies can carry organisms from feces, on which they feed, to human food, on which they alight so readily. This is one way in which typhoid fever, bacillary dysentery, amebiasis, poliomyelitis, and hepatitis A are transmitted. *Food handlers* who are carriers of intestinal parasites (*e.g.,* helminths, *Entamoeba histolytica,* and salmonellae) are another source of contamination. The use of human feces as fertilizer may directly contaminate vegetables.

Milk may contain bacteria because the animal itself is diseased; for example, brucellosis in goats and bovine tuberculosis in cows can be transmitted to people via the milk of these animals. *Salmonella* infections of fowls are passed on in their eggs. Contamination of water supplies is an important means of transmission of some infections, such as cholera and typhoid fever.

Role of Arthropod Vectors. Insects (which together with spiders constitute the phylum of arthropods) play a variety of roles in the transmission of certain infective organisms to humans.

There may be direct transfer as when feces are transferred to food on the hairy legs of house flies. Of greater importance is the transfer of those organisms that are present in the blood of infected individuals; these can be spread by the bite of one of the blood-sucking arthropods such as the mosquito (malaria and yellow fever), flea (plague), louse (epidemic typhus fever), tick (Rocky Mountain spotted fever), mite (typhus), or tsetse fly (trypanosomiasis).

The actual mode of infection varies. The organism may be injected into the next victim via the insect's saliva (malaria), or it may be passed in the feces. In the latter event, the organism is inoculated by the scratching of the victim.

Hospital Infection (Nosocomial Infection)

Whenever human beings live together in confined quarters, there is always the danger that there will be carriers of pathogenic organisms. Although not suffering from clinical illness themselves, they may pass on the organisms to others who succumb to the infection because of their reduced resistance. In turn, they further transmit the disease. This process is called *cross-infection;* in the past there have been many examples of epidemics of meningococcal meningitis and dysentery occurring in nurses' homes, army camps, and other places housing large numbers of people.

In hospitals, it is not uncommon for patients to acquire severe infections from their environment; this is hardly surprising, because many patients are debilitated and their resistance to infection is lowered. Furthermore, surgical incisions provide a ready avenue for the invading bacteria. Extensive burns are particularly liable to become infected, and such patients should be isolated from possible sources of infection. This is termed *reverse isolation.*

A particularly unfortunate feature in hospitals is that the staff acquire pathogenic organisms from their patients, become carriers, and further disseminate the organism. Often, the strain is one that is resistant to the antibiotics in common use in that particular hospital. The infection is therefore all the more serious.

In the past, streptococcal infections have been serious, particularly in maternity wards. Identification of the strain of organism involved and a subsequent search for the source of infection has usually incriminated microbes in the throats of a few members of staff. The exclusion and treatment of such carriers and general measures designed to improve aseptic techniques have usually brought such epidemics to a halt. Penicillin therapy is very effective in streptococcal infections because resistant organisms do not occur. It follows that outbreaks of streptococcal hospital infection are not a problem at the present time.

The staphylococcus has, on the other hand, attained a much more prominent position. Outbreaks of postoperative wound infection are not uncommon, and the methods of control that proved effective with streptococcal outbreaks are quite inadequate. Often the majority of the staff are found to be carriers; in addition, the hospital itself—the floors, air-conditioning system, and patients' bedclothes—is also contaminated with a virulent strain of staphylococcus. Although human carriers provide the reservoir, the hardy staphylococcus often infects patients by indirect means: for instance, in airborne dust particles. The problem of control is not easy; indeed, there is no simple answer to an outbreak of staphylococcal wound infection.

Other organisms that sometimes cause hospital infection are the coliform groups, particularly the *Proteus* species, and *Pseudomonas aeruginosa.* As with the staphylococcus, the transfer of these organisms is usually indirect—via dust, contaminated articles, and fomites. The source of organisms is often a patient with urinary tract infection who contaminates the immediate environment—bedclothes, urine bottle, and other articles with which the patient has contact.

THE BODY'S DEFENSES AGAINST INFECTION

It is evident that the body surfaces are commonly contaminated by pathogenic organisms. Whether infection follows depends on two factors: (1) the mechanical integrity of the body surface; and (2) its powers of removing organisms, *i.e.,* its powers of *decontamination.*

The protective mechanisms vary greatly from one tissue to another. Some examples are considered in the following; others are described under individual organs.

Mechanical Integrity of Body Surfaces

The mechanical strength of the epidermis with its tough outer layer of keratin is an important defense mechanism. Intact skin appears to be completely impervious to invasion by organisms, and it is only after injury that infection is established. Excessive sweating may macerate the keratin layer and render it incapable of repelling organisms. For this reason, skin infections are very common in the tropics, and boils are frequently seen in moist areas like the axillae (armpits). Likewise, yeast infections (ringworm and candidiasis) are generally encountered between the toes, in the groin, in the axillae, or under pendulous breasts. Boils are also common on the buttocks, a condition presumably related to the trauma of continual pressure in the sitting posture.

In other areas, the integrity of the covering epithelium is of less importance in repelling infection. In the mouth, esophagus, and stomach, minor trauma causing superficial ulceration is common, and yet infection rarely occurs. In these situations, the underlying connective tissue seems to have some special ability to prevent infection. The nature of this local immunity is not understood, but without it, every dental extraction would present a severe hazard, for not only is the underlying fibrous tissue exposed, but also the socket penetrates deeply into the bone of the jaw. In other situations, exposed bone is readily infected, and yet osteomyelitis in the jaw is very uncommon following dental extraction.

Decontamination

Pathogenic organisms that are deposited on a body surface are generally removed expeditiously. Contamination is followed by decontamination. In the case of the skin, this can be readily demonstrated by deliberately contaminating the hands with a marker organism and subsequently estimating its rate of disappearance by taking swabs at regular intervals. The organisms often disappear within 2 or 3 hours.

The mechanisms of decontamination vary with each individual surface and can be considered under three headings: *mechanical, biologic,* and *chemical.*

Mechanical. The surface keratin flakes of the skin are continually being rubbed off. This shedding carries away any surface organisms. Mucous membranes have a covering of fluid, and its washing effect tends to remove organisms. The flow of tears over the conjunctiva, the upward moving sheet of mucus of the respiratory tract, the flow of saliva in the salivary ducts, and the flow of urine in the urinary tract are all mechanical methods that serve to wash away any organisms that have contaminated the surface. If this flow of fluid is diminished or impeded, then infection soon follows.

Biologic. Most body surfaces are not sterile but are contaminated by organisms constituting the *resident flora.* This flora is characteristic of each particular surface. In the skin, it includes *Staphylococcus epidermidis* and diphtheroids. In the mouth, alpha-hemolytic streptococci (*Streptococcus viridans*) predominate. In the large intestine, on the other hand, bacteroides, coliforms, and enterococci abound. These organisms, constituting the resident flora, are so adapted to their environment that they do not normally cause infection. In fact, they provide protection to the host by producing antibiotic substances, by competing with other organisms for essential foodstuffs, and by adhesion to epithelial cells thereby blocking the adhesion of pathogens. If the resident flora is upset by antibiotic therapy, subsequent contamination by pathogenic organisms can lead to infection. This is sometimes seen when potent broad-spectrum antibiotics are administered by mouth. The flora of the intestine is so altered that an acute, fulminating—sometimes lethal—pseudomembranous colitis can result from infection with *Clostridum difficile. Candida albicans* can likewise cause a troublesome stomatitis or vaginitis after oral antibiotic therapy, *e.g.,* tetracycline given for acne vulgaris.

Chemical. The various secretions found on each body surface contain chemicals that destroy unwanted pathogens. The chemicals vary from one tissue to another. In the stomach, the hydrochloric acid is of great importance and destroys many pathogens such as pneumococci and streptococci. The stomach also forms an important defense mechanism for the respiratory tract, because pathogens present in the expectorated mucus are destroyed when this is swallowed.

Two other antibacterial substances are noteworthy in body secretions. *Lysozyme* is an enzyme present in many secretions and is capable of removing the cell wall of some bacteria. This was first described by Fleming, who is better known for his discovery of penicillin. The other important chemical agent is immunoglobulin (see IgA, Chapter 6).

HOST-PARASITE RELATIONSHIP

The relationship between the host and organisms is complex. In part it is related to the presence of an immune response (Chapter 6), but in addition there is a type of immunity not dependent on an immune response to the organism or its products. Cellular, humoral, and genetic factors are involved.

Nonpathogenic organisms are unable to multiply in body tissues and are soon phagocytosed and destroyed in the cytoplasm of polymorphs and macrophages. Humoral factors are also involved. Complement is considered in Chapter 6. Natural opsonin is a protein in serum that can coat relatively avirulent organisms, rendering them more easily phagocytosed by polymorphs. This resistance to infection is called *innate immunity* and is closely related to genetic factors. Examples of innate immunity may be considered under three headings—species, racial, and individual.

An example of *species immunity* is the almost complete immunity that humans have to many animal diseases, such as distemper; they almost never affect humans. Likewise, it is extremely difficult to infect animals with the agents of syphilis and leprosy. The selective breeding of disease-resistant plants and animals is well known, but it is very difficult to prove that *racial* differences exist in humans. Certainly some *individual* examples of immunity exist. For instance,

individuals with the sickle cell trait are resistant to *Plasmodium falciparum* malaria. The fact that certain diseases are associated with particular HLA types lends support to the concept that an individual's genetic make-up determines his or her immune response to particular antigens and hence immunity to infection. Thus, susceptibility to *Haemophilus influenzae* epiglottis and meningitis has been shown to be related to a major histocompatibility gene in the human.

One aspect of innate immunity is the lack of appropriate receptors on the host cell to which the organisms (*e.g.,* bacteria or viruses) can adhere. For example, the specific adhesion of *Escherichia coli* to epithelial cell receptors of urinary tract epithelium is believed to be an important first step in some urinary tract infections. Therefore, absence of receptors would render a person immune.

PATTERNS OF INFECTION

The manner in which organisms produce damage must now be examined. Three main patterns of infection are described:

1. Invasive organisms producing local damage.
2. Toxic organisms.
3. Invasive organisms producing little local damage but showing widespread dissemination.

Invasive Organisms Producing Local Damage. Some infecting organisms produce toxins that, by causing local tissue destruction, excite an acute inflammatory reaction. *Staphylococcus aureus* is an example of an organism that produces such an infection; in the skin, this response can vary from a mild *folliculitis* involving the superficial part of a pilosebaceous follicle to a *boil* involving the whole hair follicle apparatus and leading to abscess formation. Local spread of infection leads to involvement of the subcutaneous tissues so that a *carbuncle* is formed (see Fig. 8–1). Spread into the lymphatic vessels leads to inflammation of the tissues around these vessels (*lymphangitis*). When these vessels are superficial, the inflammation appears as red streaks under the skin. When organisms reach the regional lymphatic nodes, there is swelling and tenderness of the nodes as evidence of *lymphadenitis*. Finally, the organisms may penetrate the barrier of the lymph nodes and enter the blood stream via the thoracic duct. The local tissues and the inflammatory reaction form the *first defense against infection,* and the *lymph nodes form the second,* but it is in the blood stream that the third and most effective defense mechanism is encountered. This is the mononuclear phagocyte system. The cells of this system have the property of being able to phago- cytose circulating organisms, and frequently they destroy them. If the cells of the mononuclear phagocyte system are capable of destroying such organisms, the presence of organisms in the blood is of both short duration and little conse- quence. It sometimes happens that during the course of an infection, blood is taken for culture and organisms are grown. The presence of these organisms in the blood is termed *bacteremia,* and it signifies the presence of a positive blood cul- ture in the absence of any marked symptoms.

Sometimes organisms engulfed by the mono- nuclear phagocyte system are not destroyed but are allowed to proliferate in the cytoplasm of the cells. This situation occurs when immunity is low and results in vast numbers of organisms being produced in the cytoplasm of the cells. When these cells undergo necrosis, the organisms and their toxic products are released into the blood stream. The blood culture is again positive, but on this occasion the patient is gravely ill. Such a condition is known as *septicemia*. It indicates a positive blood culture and a complete over- whelming of the defenses of the body. It is therefore a grave condition that frequently proves fatal.

Toxic Organisms. Some organisms manufac- ture extremely potent exotoxins that produce local tissue damage. In addition, these toxins can enter the blood stream and cause damage at distant sites. An excellent example of this type of infection is diphtheria. When the causative organism, *Corynebacterium diphtheriae,* contami- nates the surface of a tonsil, it proliferates and produces diphtheria toxin. This leads to local tissue necrosis and a local acute inflammation, recognized clinically as a sore throat. The tonsils are covered by a layer of necrotic epithelium and exudate, which is called a *pseudomembrane*. Sur- rounding edema can be so severe that life is threatened by involvement of the larynx. How- ever, the more frequently dangerous effects of diphtheria are related to the effects of dissemi- nated toxin. Damage to nerves can cause paral- ysis, *e.g.,* of the palate, and damage to the heart leads to a toxic myocarditis and heart failure. It should be noted that the manifestations of diph- theria are entirely due to the exotoxin. The or- ganisms themselves are not invasive but remain on the surface of the tonsils or on the pharyngeal wall.

In tetanus, there is a similar pattern of disease. Spores of the organism are introduced into a wound, germinate if circumstances are favorable, and produce tetanus exotoxin. This agent is ab- sorbed both via perineural spaces and directly into the blood stream. When the toxin reaches the central nervous system, its actions lead to violent spasms of skeletal muscles and ultimately to paralysis and death. Once again the organisms remain localized, but the disease is attributable to the effects of exotoxin. Gas gangrene is an- other example of an infection with a toxic organ- ism.

Invasive Organisms Producing Little Local Damage but Showing Widespread Dissemina- tion. Some organisms produce little or no local tissue damage and therefore no inflammatory response at the site of entry. Such organisms can proliferate rapidly and spread throughout the body via the lymphatics and ultimately via the blood stream. Infection with this type of organ- ism is common, and the manner by which lesions are produced can be understood by a study of the disease typhoid fever.

Pathogenesis of Typhoid Fever. The pathogen- esis of mouse typhoid (infection with *Salmonella typhimurium*) has been studied in considerable detail. By analogy, the sequence of events in humans is as follows.

Typhoid fever is contracted by the ingestion of food or water contaminated with *Salmonella typhi.* The organisms reach the lumen of the intestine and are taken up by phagocytes on its mucosal surface. In the cytoplasm of these cells, the organisms are carried into the mucosa itself and then to the local lymphoid tissue (Peyer's patches). Scarcely any local tissue damage oc- curs, and little or no inflammation ensues. The organisms multiply, and some pass on through lymph vessels to the mesenteric nodes and finally the blood stream via the thoracic duct. In this way a bacteremia develops and the phagocytic cells of the mononuclear phagocyte system engulf them. However, since the bacteria are pathogens, they are able to live and multiply in the cells; by about the tenth day, the parasitized cells undergo necrosis and cause the blood stream to be flooded with large numbers of bacilli. This is the end of the *incubation period* (usually 10 to 14 days), and the patient becomes seriously ill with septicemia (Fig. 7–1).

The *septicemic phase* lasts about a week and is characterized clinically by a progressive stepladder rise in temperature, by constipation, and by severe constitutional symptoms. The mind becomes clouded, coma ensues, and death may occur. Diagnosis rests on obtaining a positive blood culture.

The next phase of the disease is marked by the onset of diarrhea associated with ulceration of the small intestine and by the appearance of organisms in the feces. The bacilli reach the gut via the bile, which is heavily contaminated as a result of passage of bacteria from the Kupffer cells of the liver. The ulceration occurs over the inflamed Peyer's patches and is accompanied by enlarged mesenteric lymph nodes. In both the ulcers and the lymph nodes, there is an accu-

mulation of macrophages; polymorphs are conspicuously absent. At this stage, the two most dreaded complications are intestinal hemorrhage and intestinal perforation leading to peritonitis. The most likely explanation of these events is that after the initial infection, the local lymphoid tissue of the gut becomes sensitized to the organisms or their products, and subsequent contact with the organisms produces damage. The sensitizing antibodies are presumably produced locally, because the blood level of antibodies detectable as agglutinins does not rise until later in the course of the disease. During the second week of typhoid fever, diagnosis depends on finding the organism in the feces. The characteristic *rose spots* appear in crops between the seventh and twelfth days. They are small red papules seen on the skin of the trunk and are due to bleeding secondary to an acute vasculitis comparable to the lesions of gonococcal bacteremia.

Typhoid fever therefore represents an infection by a highly invasive organism in which tissue damage appears to be produced by some type of immune reaction. Since antibody production takes 10 to 14 days to begin, it follows that symptoms do not occur until after the organism has spread widely. The incubation period is therefore long and contrasts with the short incubation period of diseases caused by invasive

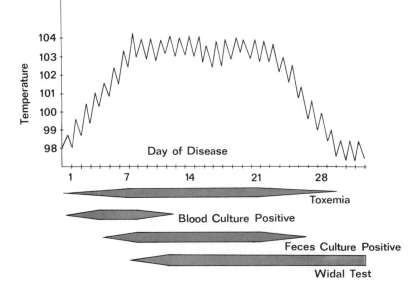

Figure 7–1 Chart correlating the clinical course of a typical case of untreated typhoid fever with the principal methods of bacteriologic diagnosis. Note the stepladder rise in temperature during the first week.

organisms that produce direct local tissue damage, *e.g.,* staphylococci and streptococci.

Toward the end of the second week of typhoid fever, antityphoid antibodies appear in the blood, and their titer subsequently rises. These antibodies are usually detected as agglutinins; the test employed is referred to as the *Widal reaction* (see Fig. 6–9). A rising titer of agglutinins is particularly significant in the diagnosis, and a specimen of blood should be taken early in the course of a suspected case of typhoid fever so that its titer of antibodies can be compared with that of later samples. This method of confirming the diagnosis of an infective illness is particularly useful in viral disease, because the infective agent is often difficult to isolate once the disease is clinically apparent. The method is also of use if the virus laboratory is not immediately at hand.

During the third week of typhoid fever, the patient gradually recovers, the diarrhea abates, and the temperature returns to normal. Nevertheless, even with chloramphenicol therapy, there is a relapse rate of 10 to 20 per cent; the blood culture again becomes positive, and symptoms, including the rose spots, return.

Other invasive organisms produce a disease similar in overall pattern to that of typhoid fever. In syphilis, there is widespread dissemination of organisms, and a local ulcer does not appear for 3 to 4 weeks (Chapter 8). In many viral infections (*e.g.,* chickenpox and measles), widespread dissemination of the organisms occurs before the onset of the characteristic disease. Once again, the incubation period tends to be about 2 weeks. It is interesting that in many instances, the ability of the organisms to spread is inversely proportional to their ability to produce immediate local tissue damage. Staphylococci produce local inflammatory lesions but tend to remain localized, whereas the organism of syphilis produces no immediate damage yet is highly invasive.

Other Patterns of Infection. Many other patterns of infection can be recognized. Some organisms can produce a local lesion with minimal inflammation such that the incident goes unnoted. This is a *subclinical* infection. Some organisms can enter into a symbiotic state with their hosts—either permanently or between phases—when they cause damage. An example of the type of infection that has phases of damage is the common coldsore due to the herpes simplex virus. The virus causes the characteristic blisters of the skin; between attacks, however, it resides in the ganglion of a sensory nerve supplying the part. A special group of virus infections (oncogenic viruses) is known that will produce tumors; these are described in Chapter 12. It is evident that infection proceeds according to many different patterns, and the situation is further complicated by the fact that one particular strain of organism can, under different circumstances, produce different types of infective illness. Thus, *Streptococcus pyogenes* can, on the one hand, produce a relatively minor local infection in the form of a sore throat but, under other circumstances (*e.g.,* when it is introduced into a cut sustained while a necropsy examination is performed), can lead to a fulminating septicemia. Likewise, the herpes simplex virus can remain as a latent infection in some individuals, whereas in others it causes coldsores, pneumonitis, or encephalitis.

SPREAD OF INFECTION

Following is a summary of the ways in which infection can spread (Fig. 7–2).

Spread by Continuity: Direct Spread

The natural cohesion of tissues tends to prevent the spread of organisms. Nevertheless, the tissue fluids are in constant motion because of movement of the part, and organisms are carried in any stream of fluid that may be present. Because muscular activity causes considerable fluid movement, the time-honored treatment of inflammation is to rest the part. Two features should be noted. First, the actual motility of the organism appears to play no part in the spread of infection. *Clostridium tetani* is a motile organism, but the infection (tetanus) is a localized affair. Second, the degree of local spread is inversely proportional to the amount of damage produced by the organism. Damage leads to an inflammatory reaction, and this is often an efficient local defense mechanism. The deposition of fibrin is important in walling off an infection; for example, fibrinous adhesions prevent the

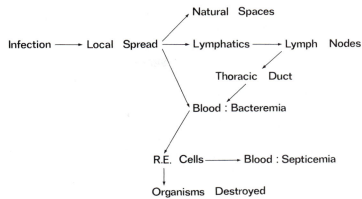

Figure 7–2 Diagram illustrating the sequence of events that can follow the spread of infection.

spread of infection from an acutely inflamed appendix (Chapter 23).

Local spread can occur in an entirely different way. Some organisms are ingested by phagocytes and are transported by these cells. This is an important means of spread in tuberculosis and almost certainly occurs in other infections.

Spread by Natural Channels

If local spread implicates a natural passage, infection may extend by this route. The following examples are important.

Peritoneum. Infection may spread rapidly throughout the peritoneal space from a localized lesion. In this way, the entire peritoneal cavity can become infected as a complication of acute appendicitis. A large surface is involved, and there is rapid absorption of toxic substances, causing the patient to become severely ill. Likewise, infection can spread throughout the pleural cavity, the subarachnoid space, the pericardium, or a joint space.

Infection can also spread along tubes, such as the bronchi (with bronchopneumonia and tuberculosis), the ureter, and the gut.

Lymphatics. In acute inflammation, the lymphatic vessels are held wide open by the increased tissue tension. The permeability of the vessel walls is increased, and so also is the flow of lymph. Invading organisms that gain access to the lymphatics are carried to the nearest lymph node, where, for a time at least, they are held up by the local mononuclear phagocytes. Lym-

phangitis and lymphadenitis are characteristic of certain types of infection, *e.g.*, streptococcal and tubercular infections.

Blood Stream. A few organisms may invade the blood vessels during the course of any local infection. The infection may itself be quite trivial, but the adjacent blood vessels can be ruptured by trauma, thereby allowing organisms to enter. Gingival infection or abscesses related to the apices of the roots of teeth are common lesions in which this invasion occurs. Such spread of infection often follows dental extraction, scaling of teeth, or even chewing hard food. When small numbers of organisms enter the blood stream in this way, they are rapidly removed by the reticuloendothelial system, and the bacteremia that occurs causes no symptoms. An exception to this is bacteremia caused by one of the gram-negative bacilli of the coliform group. In this instance, the patient sometimes has rigors and develops a fever. This is occasionally seen in the bacteremia that follows passage of a catheter up the urethra.

Bacteremia cannot be dismissed as a completely inconsequential event. Under certain circumstances, it can lead to serious sequelae.

Metastatic Lesions. Experimentally it can be shown that when an animal has a bacteremia, histamine injected at any site will precipitate a local infection by the organism concerned. Trauma has a similar effect. It is believed that this is the pathogenesis of acute osteomyelitis. A child who happens to have a staphylococcal bacteremia and traumatizes a limb then develops an acute infection of the bone (Chapter 30). Another danger of a bacteremia is that the organisms can be filtered off by the kidneys, and if there is a simultaneous obstruction of the outflow of urine, a kidney infection *(pyelonephritis)* results. A further hazard of bacteremia is that the organisms may colonize a damaged heart valve and cause endocarditis (Chapter 20).

Septic Thrombophlebitis. When infection spreads to a vein, its walls become inflamed and thrombosis occurs. The condition is called *thrombophlebitis.* If the thrombus is invaded by a pyogenic organism, it may soften and parts of it become detached, leading to pyemia (Chapter 19).

Organisms not held up in the tissues at the site of entry or in the lymph nodes reach the venous circulation via lymphatic ducts. This has already been described in the instance of typhoid fever.

Along Nerves. This route of infection is restricted to some viruses, such as the virus of rabies.

The following sections include a summary of the factors that determine whether a particular organism is likely to spread from the site of infection or to remain localized.

Factors Influencing the Spread of Infection

Whether a particular infection spreads depends on many factors. The dose of the infecting organism, its virulence, and the site of infection all play a part. Sometimes two organisms acting together exhibit a synergistic effect as when a pyogenic organism aides the establishment of an anaerobic clostridial infection.

The ability of the host to repel an infection also depends on many factors. The general health of the host is important. Patients who are starved or who suffer from chronic debilitating diseases such as renal failure or diabetes mellitus are less capable of resisting infection. The mechanism is complex and probably involves both humoral factors (*e.g.,* a low serum complement level) and an impaired activity of phagocytes. Defective B- or T-cell function can render an individual highly susceptible to infection, as has been highlighted in AIDS. Infections tend to be more severe and spread more easily if the neutrophil polymorpho-

nuclear count is low. Likewise, abnormal function of the white cells can be a factor. Occasional patients are encountered who suffer from repeated bacterial infections that commence in childhood and whose white cells are abnormal. Various syndromes are recognized in which the polymorphs show poor chemotaxis, poor phagocytosis, or inability to kill certain ingested organisms. Specialized tests are available for investigating the phagocytic and bactericidal activity of polymorphs *in vitro*.

Local factors are also important. The presence of necrotic tissue is an important predisposing cause of local infection. Foreign bodies and chemicals that cause necrosis are therefore harmful. Another important factor is the local blood supply. Ischemia of any origin, by impairing the local inflammatory reaction, is detrimental to the body's efforts at repelling infection. Infection and ulceration can follow quite trivial injuries to the legs of patients who have varicose veins or suffer from arteriosclerosis. Likewise, tetanus can sometimes follow the local injection of epinephrine (which causes contraction of the blood vessels) if a dirty needle is used.

OPPORTUNISTIC INFECTIONS

It is now apparent that some organisms that in the past have been considered to be avirulent can cause infection under certain circumstances. This is called *opportunistic infection* and may occur when either local or general factors operate in favor of the organism.

Abnormal Local Conditions. Prosthetic heart valves provide an admirable site for infection with a wide range of organisms, including rickettsiae and fungi, which normally do not produce endocarditis. Another example is related to the use of broad-spectrum antibiotics. As noted previously, these drugs can so alter the flora of the gut that pseudomembranous colitis can be caused by *Clostridium difficile.* Secondary infections stemming from alteration of the microbial flora by antibiotic therapy are usually called *superinfections.*

Immunologically Suppressed Patient. The administration of glucocorticoids and anticancer drugs, particularly to patients with malignant disease of the lymphoreticular system (*e.g.,* Hodgkin's disease), can create conditions favorable to opportunistic infections. It is not uncommon for such patients to die of infections by fungi that in normal people rarely cause infection. Furthermore, organisms (*e.g., Candida)* that commonly produce a local infection can become widely disseminated in the immunologically suppressed patient, such as one with AIDS (Chapter 6).

The traditional division of organisms into pathogens and nonpathogens, although serving a useful purpose under most circumstances, is an artificial separation. Before deciding whether an organism is causing a particular infection, one must consider the organism in relation to the circumstances of a particular patient. In the ongoing battle between man and microbe, there are no simple rules for distinguishing friend from foe.

Summary

- Intoxication, *e.g.,* botulism, occurs when a preformed bacterial toxin is absorbed.
- Infection occurs when pathogens invade and multiply in the tissues. It may be congenital when acquired *in utero,* or it may be acquired postnatally from either an endogenous source (*e.g.,* the gut) or an exogenous source by physical contact, by inhalation or ingestion, or from the environment—commonly patients, carriers, animals, or soil. Insect vectors are sometimes important.
- Nosocomial or hospital infection is commonly caused by streptococci, staphylococci, and gram-negative coliforms.
- The body's defenses against infection include the mechanical integrity of the body surfaces and the mechanisms of decontamination—mechanical, biologic, and chemical—depending on the surface considered.
- Immunity may be innate (individual, racial, or species) or related to an immune response.
- Bacteria can produce damage by toxin production or by invading tissues. Damage may follow widespread dissemination as in typhoid fever and syphilis.
- Infection can spread locally or along preformed channels such as lymphatics and blood vessels. The tendency to spread depends on the nature of the organism itself, local conditions such as blood supply, and general factors such as the function of white cells and the immune response.

Selected Readings

Braude, A. I.: Infectious Diseases and Medical Microbiology. 2nd ed. Philadelphia, W. B. Saunders Co., 1986.

Eikoff, T. C.: Nosocomial infections. N. Engl. J. Med. *306*:1514, 1982.

Källenius, G., et al.: Structure of carbohydrate part of receptor on human uroepithelial cells for pyelonephritogenic *Escherichia coli.* Lancet 2:604, 1981.

Mackowiak, P. A.: The normal microbial flora. N. Engl. J. Med. *307*:83, 1982.

Osserman, E. F.: Lysozyme. N. Engl. J. Med. *292*:424, 1975.

Quie, P. G., and Hetherington, S. V.: Patients with disorders of phagocytic cell function. Pediatr. Infect. Dis. 3:272, 1984.

Youmans, G. P., Paterson, P. Y., and Sommers, H. M.: The Biologic and Clinical Basis of Infectious Diseases. 3rd ed. Philadelphia, W. B. Saunders Co., 1985.

Bacterial Infections

After studying this chapter, the student should be able to:

- Describe the characteristics of the following organisms and the common diseases caused by them: staphylococci, streptococci, pneumococci, gonococci, meningococci, and the gram-negative intestinal coliforms.

- Describe the main features of diphtheria and compare them with a disease caused by an invasive organism.
- Discuss the prophylaxis of tetanus in relation to the immune state of the patient.
- List the mycobacteria that are pathogenic to humans.
- Describe the properties of *Mycobacterium tuberculosis* and the tissue reaction to the organism.
- Describe the Koch phenomenon and relate it to the differences between human childhood and adult types of tuberculous infection.
- List the factors that predispose to tuberculosis.
- Differentiate between lepromatous and tuberculoid leprosy with respect to
  (a) tissue reaction;
  (b) the immune state;
  (c) the number of bacilli present in the lesions;
  (d) clinical features.
- Describe three diseases caused by organisms of the genus *Borrelia*.
- Outline the sources of infection and the clinical features of human leptospirosis.
- Describe the three stages of syphilis and relate the gross findings to
  (a) the pathogenesis of the disease;
  (b) the number of organisms present in the lesions;
  (c) the diagnosis of the disease.

Bacteria are responsible for a wide range of common infections. One group, termed the pyogenic organisms, includes staphylococci, streptococci, pneumococci, gonococci, meningococci, and the coliform organisms. Infection with these organisms causes an acute inflammatory response culminating in a massive infiltration by polymorphs. If the inflammation succeeds in destroying the organisms, the lesion abates. If the organisms gain the upper hand, the condition proceeds to tissue destruction and suppuration.

The anaerobic clostridia form a separate group, causing tetanus and various forms of gangrene, whereas another group of organisms, typified by the tubercle bacillus, usually causes a chronic granulomatous inflammatory response. Nevertheless, a similar granulomatous response can be caused by the staphylococcus (see chronic granulomatous disease in Chapter 5), and likewise the tubercle bacillus can cause an inflammatory response with many polymorphs. There are no rules that enable one to predict the response to a particular organism, and each must be considered separately.

STAPHYLOCOCCAL INFECTIONS

Staphylococci are hardy gram-positive cocci that tend to grow in clusters. They are common inhabitants of the skin and can be divided into two groups based partly on the color of their colonies but mainly on their ability to produce coagulase, an enzyme that causes coagulation of citrated plasma. Coagulase-negative organisms are infrequently pathogenic, whereas the coagulase-positive ones are pathogens.

Staphylococcus aureus

This organism is coagulase-positive and is found on the skin of some normal people, particularly those who live in crowded communities such as those of hospitals. The reservoir of pathogenic staphylococci is in the anterior part of the nose. About 40 per cent of healthy adults are nasal carriers, but the figure may rise to over 70 per cent in a hospital population. From the nose, the organisms are readily transferred to the skin, particularly the hands. Here the organisms can multiply and spread to other objects and to other people.

The typical staphylococcal lesion is a circumscribed area of inflammation with suppuration.

Skin lesions are frequent and include stitch abscesses, boils, carbuncles, paronychia (inflammation of the nail fold), and impetigo (Fig. 8–1).

In *impetigo,* the organisms invade the superficial layers of the skin and produce characteristic subcorneal bullae and pustules. This is common on the face in children. The blisters soon rupture and become covered by a honey-colored crust. Local action of the exotoxin exfoliatin produces the blisters.

Infection of the hair follicles is common; the type of lesion produced depends on how deeply the organisms penetrate. Since pus is produced, the term *pyoderma* is employed to describe this whole group of skin diseases. In *superficial folliculitis,* numerous small pustules are seen at the openings of adjacent hair follicles. The face is a common site for this eruption to occur.

A more destructive and severe infection of the hair follicle is the *boil,* or *furuncle;* when pus is produced, it is discharged from a single opening. A *stye* is a particular type of boil in which an eyelash is implicated. Boils are particularly common in the axillae and on the back of the neck.

In a *carbuncle,* the staphylococcal infection extends to the underlying fatty subcutaneous tissue and spreads laterally. The subcutaneous tissue is divided into compartments by fibrous septa, which extend from the deep fascia to the dermis. It therefore follows that subcutaneous infections tend to be loculated, with each individual abscess bursting to the surface through its own hair follicle orifice. Thus, a carbuncle has multiple heads, and extensive areas of skin become undermined and are eventually sloughed off.

Staphylococci are a common cause of postoperative wound infection and other nosocomial infections. Other important staphylococcal infections are bronchopneumonia, enterocolitis, and osteomyelitis, all of which are discussed elsewhere in this text. Staphylococcal infections sometimes involve veins (a condition called *phlebitis*), and this leads to thrombosis. If the thrombus is invaded by the organisms, it tends to soften and break off, forming septic emboli. This condition is called *pyemia* and is characterized by multiple pyemic abscesses and septic infarcts (Chapter 19).

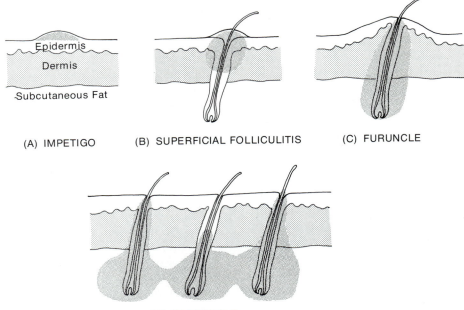

Epidermis
Dermis
Subcutaneous Fat

(A) IMPETIGO   (B) SUPERFICIAL FOLLICULITIS   (C) FURUNCLE

(D) CARBUNCLE

Figure 8–1 Diagram illustrating some staphylococcal infections of the skin. *A,* Impetigo. The infection is very superficial, and a pustule forms beneath the stratum corneum of the epidermis. *B,* Superficial folliculitis. The suppurative inflammation involves the superficial part of a hair follicle. Clinically this appears as a small pustule, and the condition is also known as impetigo of Bockhart. *C,* Furuncle or boil. The infection involves the entire hair follicle, and the inflammatory edema produces a considerable swelling, 1 cm or more in diameter. Nevertheless, a boil has one head only. *D,* Carbuncle. The infection involves the subcutaneous tissues, and loculated pockets of pus are present. These pockets are formed between fibrous septa, which are not shown in the diagram. Note the multiple heads through which pus can be discharged. (Drawing by Margot Mackay, University of Toronto Faculty of Medicine, Department of Surgery, Division of Biomedical Communications, Toronto.)

Staphylococcal Toxins

Although staphylococci are typically invasive organisms, some strains produce particular toxins that have important effects. Four conditions should be noted (Fig. 8–2).

Staphylococcal Food Poisoning. This is due to ingestion of preformed heat-stable enterotoxin formed by organisms growing in food products.

The Scalded Skin Syndrome. Certain strains of staphylococci produce an epidermolytic toxin (exfoliatin); when this organism affects young babies, there is extensive shedding of the superficial layers of the skin so that the child appears to have been extensively scalded.

Scarlatiniform Eruption. An eruption resembling scarlet fever produced by streptococcal infection is occasionally seen with staphylococcal infections by organisms producing the exotoxin exfoliatin.

Toxic Shock Syndrome. Another epidermal toxin is produced by certain staphylococci. Infec-

tions by these organisms may be accompanied by a severe illness—high fever, generalized reddening of the skin, conjunctival hyperemia, watery diarrhea, hypovolemia, and renal failure. The syndrome was first described in children; in those who recover, there is extensive desquamation of the affected skin and peeling of the palms and soles during convalescence. This toxic shock syndrome has also been described in previously healthy young women who use particular types of tampons during menstruation. Characteristically there is a sudden onset of high fever, diarrhea, and the other symptoms noted. The pathogenesis is thought to be that the staphylococci multiply in the tampon and produce toxin, which after absorption causes the syndrome.

Coagulase-Negative Staphylococci

This group of staphylococci, of which *Staphylococcus epidermidis* is one, are normal members

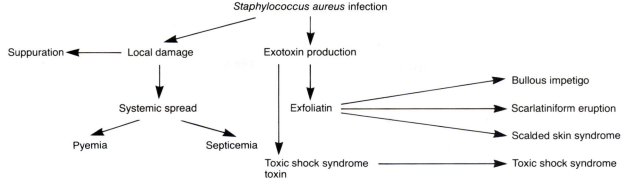

Figure 8–2 The effects of staphylococcal infection.

of the skin's flora. They are almost nonpathogenic but occasionally cause urinary tract infection. Also they can cause endocarditis in mainline drug abusers and after open heart surgery. Contamination of intravenous catheters may lead to bacteremia.

STREPTOCOCCAL INFECTIONS

Streptococci are gram-positive organisms that tend to grow in chains, particularly in a fluid culture; four major groups are recognized by the type of colony produced on blood agar.

1. *Alpha-hemolytic streptococci,* also called *Streptococcus viridans,* grow on a blood-agar plate as small colonies that produce a greenish pigmentation with an ill-defined surrounding narrow zone of partial hemolysis. Two important infections produced by this group of organisms are on the one hand the relatively trivial apical infections of teeth and on the other its lethal complication, subacute bacterial endocarditis (Chapter 20).

2. *Beta-hemolytic streptococci* produce a sharply demarcated zone of complete hemolysis on the agar plate. Many groups have been defined. Group A beta-hemolytic streptococcus is termed *Streptococcus pyogenes* and is the common human pathogen; it causes over 90 per cent of human streptococcal infections. Other groups produce disease in animals, such as bovine mastitis, in which the udder is infected. These organisms may be present in milk but are harmless to humans. Group B streptococcus, *S. agalactiae,* is a common commensal in the female genitourinary tract and can cause *severe perinatal infections.* The manifestations are those of respiratory distress with shock, septicemia, and meningitis. Group C and group G streptococci are occasional causes of *wound infection* and *puerperal sepsis.*

3. *Nonhemolytic streptococci,* also called *enterococci,* are included in the group D streptococci; they form part of the normal flora of the gut and are a cause of peritonitis, wound infection, urinary tract infection, and bacterial endocarditis.

4. *Anaerobic streptococci* are normal inhabitants of the bowel and vagina. They were important causes of puerperal infection in the past and occasionally are associated with wound infection and gangrenous lesions.

Lesions Produced by Streptococcus pyogenes

The typical streptococcal lesion is a spreading infection of the connective tissues, a condition called *cellulitis.* Abscesses occur later than in staphylococcal infections, and the pus tends to be watery and often blood-stained. Streptococci are occasional causes of wound infection and are also responsible for a number of cases of *impetigo. Erysipelas* is a classic streptococcal lesion and consists of a spreading infection in the dermis. It affects the face and is seen as a raised, bright red plaque with a sharply defined edge that steadily advances.

Streptococci are important causes of *tonsillitis* and *pharyngitis.* Infection can spread to the middle ear to produce *otitis media* and down the tracheobronchial tree to lead to *bronchopneumonia.*

In days gone by, streptococcal infections of the uterus after labor were common *(puerperal sepsis).* Before the introduction of aseptic techniques and chemotherapy, this was one of the major causes of death after childbirth.

Some streptococci produce an *erythrogenic toxin,* which is absorbed into the blood and produces a punctate erythematous rash termed *scarlet fever.* The skin lesions are sterile, since they are produced entirely by this exotoxin. The usual streptococcal infection leading to scarlet fever is a sore throat.

Two other important diseases associated with streptococcal infections are *acute rheumatic fever* and *acute glomerulonephritis.* Both are thought to be related to the development of hypersensitivity and to be manifestations of immune-complex reactions (Chapter 6).

PNEUMOCOCCAL INFECTIONS

Pneumococci closely resemble streptococci but have a well-defined capsule and tend to occur in pairs. The organism, now called *Streptococcus pneumoniae,* is a common commensal of the throat; about 80 different serotypes are known. A few of these types are highly virulent and can cause infection in healthy individuals. The organisms penetrate the defenses of the respiratory tract, invade the lung, and cause *lobar pneumonia.* This is accompanied by a septicemia that at times is complicated by metastatic lesions such as meningitis. The other category of pneumococci tends to be relatively avirulent, but they can act as secondary invaders causing *bronchopneumonia* either in elderly debilitated patients or in persons who have had a previous virus infection (Chapter 22).

GONOCOCCAL INFECTIONS

Neisseria gonorrhoeae, the gonococcus, is a gram-negative diplococcus whose only known host is humans. The organism is generally transmitted by sexual intercourse and causes the important venereal disease *gonorrhea.* In the male, an *acute urethritis* appears 2 to 8 days after infection. A purulent penile discharge is the main symptom and is combined with difficulty and pain on passing urine. A smear of the pus on a glass slide when stained by Gram's method reveals typical *intracellular diplococci.* Diagnosis is confirmed by culture of the organism on special media. If treated, usually with tetracycline or spectinomycin, the disease usually clears up rapidly. Untreated, the infection can spread to involve the seminal vesicles and epididymis. Chronic infection and its attendant fibrosis is a well-known cause of *urethral stricture.*

In the female, gonorrhea causes acute urethritis and cervicitis, but symptoms are frequently ignored or absent, and the infection goes unnoticed. These asymptomatic females are the main reservoir of gonorrhea in our society. Spread to involve the fallopian tubes leads to *acute salpingitis* and associated peritonitis. This event can present as an acute surgical abdominal emergency; the patient presents with abdominal pain and fever. Chronic gonococcal infection is a very common cause of *pelvic inflammatory disease* and may follow an acute attack or appear *de novo.* Salpingitis leads to fibrosis of the fallopian tube, which is an important cause of *sterility* in the female.

When the sulfonamides, and later the antibiotics, were introduced, it was hoped that gonorrhea could be eliminated from our society because the organism was very sensitive to these agents. Unfortunately, these hopes have not been fulfilled. Some cases are missed and continue to provide a source of infection. At the same time, drug-resistant strains of the gonococcus have evolved. The control of gonorrhea is an important public health function, and a vital aspect of this is the tracing of patient contacts. As with syphilis, the source of infection is another human being. There can never be an isolated case of either of these venereal diseases!

Two nonvenereal infections with the gonococcus are worthy of note.

Acute Vulvovaginitis. This can occur in epidemic form in girls' schools and is transmitted by towels and communally used clothing. This infection does not occur after puberty, because the hormonal activity associated with sexual maturity leads to an acid pH in the vagina, and this acts as an efficient bactericidal chemical barrier.

Gonococcal Conjunctivitis and Ophthalmitis. Infection of the baby's conjunctiva during delivery results in an acute purulent conjunctivitis. Corneal involvement with ulceration and even perforation is a dreaded complication, since it leads to blindness. This disease was said to be responsible for about 50 per cent of blindness in children before effective prophylaxis abolished it. As a routine, a drop of 1 per cent silver nitrate or an antibiotic, such as erythromycin, is placed in each conjunctival sac of a newborn child.

Gonococcal conjunctivitis is occasionally seen in adults when pus from a urethral discharge is transmitted to the eyes, generally by the patient's own hands.

The introduction of the gonococci usually leads to a local infection, but the invasive potential of the organisms should not be forgotten. Bacteremia can result in metastatic lesions, of which acute septic arthritis is the most common. Gonococcal septicemia has recently become an important complication. It usually affects young women, and its onset is triggered by a menstrual period. The fever, arthralgia (pain in the joints), and development of skin lesions due to vasculitis are the outstanding symptoms of the condition (Fig. 8–3).

Case History I

The patient was a 24-year-old woman who gave a 5-day history of pain flitting from one joint to another (polyarthralgia). The onset of the pain dated from the onset of her last menstrual period. Pain and discomfort were particularly marked in the right knee. On examination, this joint was swollen and somewhat tender. A day or two after the onset of the arthralgia, she noted a rash that consisted of scattered lesions on the distal part of the arms and legs. Some of these lesions were small erythematous papules, but others were petechial and palpable. Some of these developed hemorrhagic necrotic centers (Fig. 8–3), and biopsy showed an acute leukocytoclastic vasculitis (Fig. 21–8). During the course of the disease, the patient felt unwell, lost her appetite, and developed a mild fever every evening. The history, together with the clinical and pathologic findings, suggested a diagnosis of gonococcal septicemia. A slight vaginal discharge was noted, and a swab from the cervix subsequently grew gonococci. Penicillin therapy was started, and an uneventful recovery ensued. The patient had been on vacation 2 weeks before the onset of the illness. During that time she had unprotected intercourse with a casual acquaintance.

MENINGOCOCCAL INFECTIONS

The meningococcus closely resembles the gonococcus morphologically and is a normal commensal of the nasopharynx. The first encounter with the organism causes an inconsequential infection in most individuals, but occasionally the organism spreads to produce a septicemia; finally, it settles in the subarachnoid space to cause *meningitis*. Septicemia is usually accompanied by a petechial skin rash, which gives the disease its alternative name of "spotted fever." Meningitis usually occurs in those individuals who lack immunity (usually children), but it also may appear in susceptible adults. The disease occasionally becomes epidemic when large numbers of adults are crowded together in confined quarters, such as in army barracks.

INFECTIONS WITH GRAM-NEGATIVE INTESTINAL BACILLI

This is a large group of rod-shaped bacteria; the pus-producing members include *Escherichia coli*, *Proteus* species, and *Pseudomonas aeruginosa*. The organisms, commonly grouped as the "coliforms" or "gram-negative rods," are normal commensals of the lower small intestine and the colon, where, with the exception of certain enteropathic strains considered in Chapter 23, they cause no damage; indeed, their presence is beneficial. Once outside the confines of the gut, they cause infection with suppuration. They are always predominant in infective lesions derived from the bowel contents, *e.g.*, appendicitis and generalized peritonitis following perforation of the gut. Furthermore, the coliforms are the commonest agent in *urinary tract infections*, reaching the kidney as part of a normal bacteremia from the colon, or else ascending to the bladder from the perineum. The coliform organisms are sometimes troublesome causes of *wound infection* in hospitals. Not infrequently they cause *bronchopneumonia* and *middle ear infection*. Septicemia may complicate any of these infections and is a potent

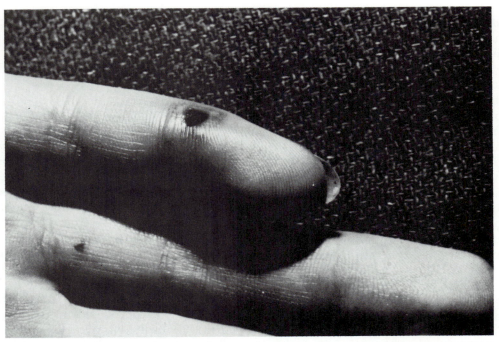

Figure 8–3 Gonococcal vasculitis. Two vasculitic lesions are shown. Both show hemorrhagic papules that have developed a central area of necrosis. The lesion on the fifth finger is the more advanced. See Case History I for details.

factor in inducing shock (Chapter 19). The common pyogenic infections are summarized in Table 8–1.

Salmonella and *Shigella* are important members of the gram-negative intestinal bacilli, and their pathogenic activity is largely confined to the intestinal tract. *Food poisoning* and *bacillary dysentery* are described in Chapter 23.

Table 8–1 COMMON PYOGENIC INFECTIONS

Organism	Source of Infection	Common Infections
Staphylococcus		
S. aureus	Skin of carrier or patient	Wound and skin infections; pyemia; pneumonia; osteomyelitis
Coagulase-negative staphylococci	Normal flora of skin	Mild wound infections; endocarditis
Streptococcus		
S. pyogenes	Throat of carrier or patient	Throat infections; wound infections; pneumonia
S. viridans	Normal flora of mouth	Apical tooth infection; endocarditis
Nonhemolytic streptococci (enterococci)	Normal flora of intestine	Wound infections; urinary tract infections; peritonitis
Pneumococcus	Normal flora of nose and throat; carriers	Pneumonia; meningitis
Gonococcus	Patients with chronic genital infection	Genital tract infections; gonococcal conjunctivitis and ophthalmitis
Meningococcus	Normal flora of nose and throat carriers	Meningitis
Gram-negative intestinal bacillus		
Escherichia coli	Normal flora of intestine; fomites	Wound infections; urinary tract infections; peritonitis; pneumonia
Proteus species		
Pseudomonas aeruginosa		

DIPHTHERIA

Diphtheria is an acute infectious disease caused by *Corynebacterium diphtheriae*. This organism is a gram-positive curved bacillus that produces characteristic colonies on special growth media. Spread is by inhalation of droplets or airborne particles from an active case or a carrier. Generally the organism settles on the tonsils, adjacent soft palate, or nasopharynx; less commonly affected are the nose and larynx. The bacteria multiply on the surface, and after an incubation period of 1 to 7 days, there are sufficient organisms present to produce enough of their powerful exotoxin to cause the epithelium to undergo necrosis. There is a severe underlying inflammatory reaction so that fibrin and neutrophils are added to the necrotic tissues to form the characteristic gray, tough, adherent *pseudomembrane*. Forcible attempts to remove this membrane lead to bleeding. This is in contradistinction to the exudate of acute streptococcal sore throat or of a *Candida* infection, which can easily be removed. Of interest is the origin of the term diphtheria—it is derived from a Greek word meaning skin or hide.

Clinically, the patient with diphtheria complains of a sore throat, and tender enlarged regional lymph nodes may be felt. If the larynx is involved, there may be sufficient edema to cause respiratory difficulty; partial detachment of the diphtheritic membrane can add to this serious complication. Fever, malaise, and a neutrophil leukocytosis are present.

It must be stressed that the diphtheria bacilli do not invade the tissues, but their exotoxin produces damage not only locally but also to other tissues, such as myocardium and nervous tissue, which it reaches via the blood stream.

After recovery from diphtheria, the subject has sufficient antitoxic immunity to prevent reinfection (Chapter 6). Nevertheless, the throat (or other site) may still harbor *C. diphtheriae*. Such a person is immune to diphtheria but is a carrier of the organism and can infect other people.

Immunity to diphtheria can be assessed by performing the *Schick test,* in which a minute amount of diphtheria toxin is injected into the skin and the effect observed over the next week. If an acute inflammatory reaction ensues, it means that the subject has no antitoxins and is therefore susceptible to diphtheria. A negative reaction implies immunity.

Diphtheria was at one time common in Europe and North America, particularly in children; but since the introduction of mass immunization with toxoid, it is now rare. However, the disease is not uncommon in the developing countries, and even in North America small outbreaks still occur. This emphasizes the necessity for continuing the immunization program.

PLAGUE

Plague is caused by *Yersinia pestis,* an organism that normally infects rodents such as the rat, but infection can spread to humans by the bite of the rat flea. Plague is generally a problem in times of war when large numbers of people are herded together under poor conditions. Nevertheless, the disease is still endemic in certain parts of North America (New Mexico and California), and small outbreaks are to be expected. After the bite of an infected flea, the regional lymph nodes (called buboes) enlarge, suppurate, and discharge pus through the overlying skin. The bite is generally on the leg, and it is the inguinal nodes that are affected. This form of the disease is called bubonic plague. Occasionally there is widespread dissemination of the infection and pneumonia occurs. Direct spread to other humans then occurs in this pneumonic form of the disease.

CLOSTRIDIAL INFECTIONS

The clostridia comprise a group of organisms that are normal commensals of the intestine, form spores that are extremely resistant to destruction, and grow only in the absence of oxygen. The strict anaerobic requirement for growth makes laboratory isolation difficult and explains the curious circumstances under which these bacilli cause human disease. *Clostridium botulinum* is described in Chapter 7. This section deals with the clostridia that cause gas gangrene as well as *Clostridium tetani,* which causes tetanus, and *Clos-*

tridium difficile, which causes a severe form of colitis.

Clostridial Wound Infections

Clostridia can be isolated from many cases of intra-abdominal and wound infections, but they probably have little pathogenic action. Sometimes there is crepitation due to gas production, but the lesions lack the diffuse spreading cellulitis that characterizes gas gangrene.

Gas Gangrene (Clostridial Myonecrosis)

Gas gangrene follows the contamination of a wound with spores of the pathogenic clostridia. Considering the ubiquitous presence of these spores and the rarity of gas gangrene, it is evident that a healthy wound that is contaminated does not develop infection. The essential factor necessary for spore germination is a reduced oxygen tension. This is present in a severely lacerated wound that contains dead tissue, particularly dead muscle that has lost its blood supply. The presence of soil in a wound is particularly dangerous, because the calcium salts in it may lead to considerable tissue necrosis. Any coincidental infection by one of the aerobic pyogenic organisms, such as staphylococci or streptococci, serves to augment the anaerobic conditions. Most examples of gas gangrene are exogenous in origin and are due to the gross contamination of a severely lacerated dirty wound. Gas gangrene is frequent in battle casualties and in agricultural accidents. Indeed, it was during World War I that this group of organisms was studied intensively and finally classified—so important was this type of infection in causing deaths. Occasionally, gas gangrene is endogenous and occurs when a wound is contaminated with the patient's own feces.

Pathogenesis and Lesions. Gas gangrene is never due to infection by a single type of clostridium; it is the result of a combined assault by several organisms working together. The true pathogens, best known of which is *Clostridium perfringens,* produce powerful exotoxins that are liberated locally and produce tissue necrosis.

Since muscle is usually involved, an extensive and progressive local muscle necrosis around the area of the original wound follows. At this stage, the muscle appears red and is obviously dead and does not contract. There is an acute inflammatory response characterized by a tremendous outpouring of fluid with remarkably few polymorphs. The extensive inflammatory edema impairs the blood supply of the muscle, so that further growth of and invasion by the organism are favored. As noted, many organisms are involved in the clinical condition of gas gangrene. The saprophytic group of clostridia, typified by *Clostridium sporogenes,* produce no potent toxins but have the property of splitting protein. They attack the dead muscle and liberate hydrogen sulfide and other foul-smelling gases. The hydrogen sulfide combines with iron from hemoglobin, and the iron sulfide so formed gives the whole area a black color. The wound that is complicated by gas gangrene rapidly becomes black and discharges foul-smelling fluid in which there are bubbles of gas. Absorption of toxic substances, particularly the exotoxins of the pathogenic clostridia, leads to shock, and the patient dies unless the limb is expeditiously amputated.

Treatment. In the treatment of gas gangrene, it is usual to give an antiserum prepared against the exotoxins of the main pathogens. Penicillin or other antibiotics are also useful because they destroy the growing bacteria. For prophylaxis, it is important that wounds be adequately treated surgically so that all dead tissue is removed and adequate drainage assured. This is as important as the administration of appropriate antibiotic therapy.

Tetanus

The spores of *Clostridium tetani* infrequently contaminate wounds, but as with gas gangrene organisms, a reduced oxygen tension is essential for their germination. The conditions conducive to tetanus infection are therefore similar to those described for gas gangrene. Nevertheless, quite often the degree of trauma may be mild, and an insignificant puncture wound, such as the prick of a thorn contaminated with manure, has quite commonly been the site of origin of a fatal tetanus infection.

Clinical Features. The incubation period varies from a few days to several weeks; the shorter it is, the worse is the prognosis. Tetanus is clinically a disease of the central nervous system. The local lesion may be so mild that only a very careful search will reveal it, yet the exotoxin produced by the local infection may be sufficient to cause death.

After peripheral absorption, the toxin reaches the central nervous system—probably by passing along the motor nerve trunks to the spinal cord or medulla oblongata. At first, the toxin acts locally, which explains the early phenomenon known as local tetanus. This consists of spasm of those muscles controlled by the same spinal segment as that supplying the area infected. Stiffness of the muscles appears, and this is soon followed by an increase in muscular tone and painful spasms. After a while, the spasms become generalized; particularly striking is contraction of the jaw muscles, resulting in closure of the lower jaw or *trismus* (inability to open the mouth, or "lockjaw"). Finally, generalized convulsions occur, and death from asphyxia follows involvement of the respiratory muscles.

Prophylaxis. Tetanus may complicate quite trivial wounds, and by far the best method of prophylaxis is active immunization. This is carried out by giving a course of three injections of tetanus toxoid, thereby inducing a high blood level of specific antitoxin immunoglobulin.

In a patient who has sustained a deep wound—particularly if there is much ragged laceration of tissue, or if it has been contaminated with animal fecal material—the procedure used depends on whether the patient has had previous active immunization. If previous injections of tetanus toxoid have been given, all that needs to be done is to give a further dose of toxoid. A rapid secondary immune response leads to a high level of antitoxin within 1 or 2 days. If, on the other hand, there has been no previous immunization, passive immunization with antitoxin must be considered. In the past, the administration of horse antitetanic serum has been advised, but the danger of inducing anaphylactic shock or serum sickness is considerable. Furthermore, the duration of passive immunity is short, particularly if the subject has had previous injections of horse serum (see Fig. 6–15). The use of human antitetanic serum obviates these difficulties, and it should be given whenever it is available. At the same time, it is also advisable to give the first injection of tetanus toxoid. The patient should be instructed to return for further toxoid administrations. Tetanus is now an uncommon disease in the Western world, but the situation in the poorer countries is quite different. It has been estimated that over one million people die of tetanus each year, and that it is the leading cause of death in hospitals in many developing countries. Injecting quinine (for malaria), ear piercing, circumcising, and applying soil or even dung to the umbilicus of the newborn are all common modes of contamination that lead to infection in the unprotected population.

Other Clostridial Infections

Clostridium difficile is a minor normal inhabitant of the human bowel, but during the course of oral antibiotic therapy, particularly with clindamycin or lincomycin, bacterial overgrowth and accompanying toxin production can lead to a severe, sometimes fatal, pseudomembranous colitis (Chapter 23).

Ingestion of food (generally a meat or poultry stew) heavily contaminated with certain strains of *Clostridium perfringens* leads to acute food poisoning. Approximately one third of all outbreaks of food poisoning are due to this cause.

BACTEROIDES INFECTIONS

The gram-negative intestinal bacilli of the genus *Bacteroides* form the bulk of organisms in the feces, and they are present also as part of the normal flora of the mouth and vagina. These organisms do not produce spores and are strictly anaerobic. They cause wound infection, pelvic abscesses, puerperal sepsis, and occasionally oral infection. In these instances, however, their role is probably secondary to infection with more pathogenic organisms. Their presence should be suspected in any infection associated with a foul odor. The organisms may on occasion invade the blood stream and cause septicemia with shock.

The important anaerobic infections of wounds are summarized in Table 8–2.

MYCOBACTERIAL INFECTIONS

The mycobacteria are acid-fast bacilli and have features that distinguish them from other bacteria. They are difficult to stain (see Ziehl-Neelsen strain in the following), and the two important human pathogens, *Mycobacterium tuberculosis* and *Mycobacterium leprae*, grow slowly *in vivo*. They have some affinity with fungi and were so named on this account (*mykes* is Greek for "fungus"). *Atypical mycobacteria* may also cause disease and are described later.

Tuberculosis

The importance of tuberculosis cannot be judged by its present incidence in the Western world. In the past it was a common and dreaded disease, but the sanitoria and hospitals for "consumption" (as the disease was once called) either have shut down or have changed their names and directed their attention to other diseases. In part, this has been effected by early diagnosis and better treatment; in the main, however, improvement in social conditions, removal of slums, and the pasteurization of milk have played the major role. In areas of the world where poverty and overcrowding are rife, so also is tuberculosis.

The Causative Organism. Tuberculosis is caused by *Mycobacterium tuberculosis*, of which there are several strains, the most important being the *human* and the *bovine* varieties. The organisms contain a waxy material in their cell walls that is responsible for their special properties. Since stains cannot easily penetrate the organism, a smear receiving the ordinary Gram stain will show no bacteria. A special stain must be employed: heating a smear with strong carbolfuchsin. Once this stain has penetrated the organism, it cannot easily be removed by acid or alcohol. This forms the basis of the *Ziehl-Neelsen (ZN) stain*. *Mycobacterium tuberculosis* is therefore spoken of as being "acid-alcohol-fast." The organism is demanding in its cultural requirements and takes several weeks to produce visible colonies. It follows that tuberculous specimens treated in a routine way will be reported as sterile. Special methods must be employed, and the laboratory technologists must be aware of the necessity for this. The organisms also grow slowly *in vivo*, and tuberculous infections tend to develop slowly and to be chronic.

Tissue Reaction to Tuberculous Infection. When tubercle bacilli are introduced into a tissue, there is a fleeting acute inflammatory response with a polymorph infiltration. It is soon followed by massive accumulation of macrophages, which ingest the bacilli and then become modified to form *epithelioid cells*. These have more cytoplasm than does the typical macrophage and lose their ability to ingest material. The accumulation of epithelioid cells tends to be focal, and small nodules or *tubercles* are formed (Fig. 8–4). These are about 0.5 to 1.0 mm in diameter and are just

Table 8–2 COMMON ANAEROBIC WOUND INFECTIONS

Organism	Source of Infection	Common Infections
Clostridium perfringens and others	Animal feces; normal flora of human intestine	Wound infection; myositis (gas gangrene); gangrenous lesion of intestinal tract
Clostridium tetani	Animal feces; occasional member of flora of human intestine	Mild wound infection with severe toxic effects (tetanus)
Anaerobic streptococci *Bacteroides* species	Normal flora of intestine, vagina, and the mouth to a lesser extent	Wound infections; gangrenous lesions of intestinal tract; peritonitis; postpartum uterine infection (puerperal sepsis)

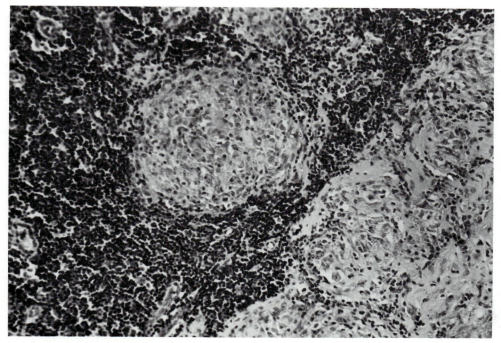

Figure 8–4 Tuberculosis of lymph node: early lesion. In the center of the picture, there is a circumscribed collection of epithelioid cells forming a follicle that stands out clearly against the dark background provided by the closely packed lymphocytes of the node. On the right-hand side, several follicles have fused together.

visible to the naked eye. Some macrophages, instead of becoming epithelioid cells, form giant cells that are of the Langhans type. Surrounding the mass of epithelioid cells, there is a diffuse zone of lymphocytes with a few plasma cells and fibrocytes. Within 2 weeks, necrosis begins in the mass of tissue containing not only the epithelioid cells but also those cells peculiar to the part involved. The necrosis is called *caseation,* and the dead tissue forms a dry, firm, coagulated mass, which has fancifully been likened to cheese. Caseation is probably caused by the development of hypersensitivity to the products of the bacilli, as explained in Chapter 6.

The end result is a fully formed tubercle follicle (Fig. 8–5). It consists of a central mass of caseation surrounded by epithelioid cells and occasional giant cells. This, in turn, is surrounded by a wide zone of small round cells. The appearance is highly characteristic of tuberculosis, but a similar reaction can be seen in other infections, particularly those caused by fungi. Adjacent tubercles tend to fuse, and as the caseous process extends, wide areas of tissue are destroyed. The

lesion can now be seen with the naked eye, and the caseation can extend for many centimeters. Progressive caseation is the hallmark of spread of tuberculosis. In some instances, the firm caseous tissue undergoes liquefaction. The precise reason for this is not known, but the development of a high degree of delayed type hypersensitivity is generally incriminated. A cavity is then formed containing liquefied caseous material that is teeming with bacilli. Conventionally, this is called pus, although technically this term is inaccurate because few polymorphs are present. The tuberculous pus tends to track in the line of least resistance, providing one means by which a tuberculous lesion can extend.

Tubercle bacilli are typically intracellular parasites and can be spread locally in the tissues by the migration of macrophages. Satellite lesions are formed, and their eventual fusion with the original focus is the means by which the lesion enlarges. Tubercle bacilli also spread via the lymphatic vessels, causing the regional lymph nodes to contain typical tubercles. In susceptible individuals, this spread continues to the blood

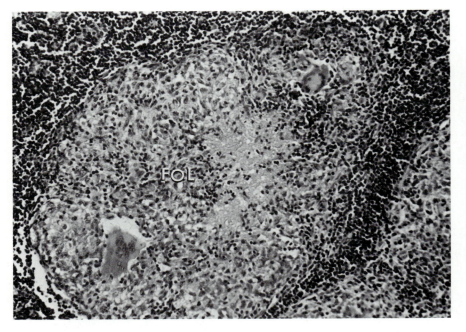

FOL

Figure 8–5 Tuberculosis of lymph node: follicles with caseation. Compared with the lesion shown in Figure 8–4, this tuberculous follicle (Fol) has enlarged, and its center has become caseous. Two giant cells are shown. The one with many nuclei arranged around its periphery has the characteristic features of a Langhans giant cell. Although this is an active tuberculous lesion, bacilli are scanty and would be very difficult to find in a section stained with Ziehl-Neelsen's carbolfuchsin. Culture in a suitable medium or guinea pig inoculation is used to isolate the organism.

stream, and widespread dissemination occurs. The subject becomes severely ill, having numerous tubercles, particularly in those organs with a high content of mononuclear phagocytes such as the spleen, bone marrow, and liver. The meninges are also affected, and *meningitis* frequently accompanies this condition, which is called *generalized miliary tuberculosis.* The name is derived from the numerous small tubercles that at one time were likened to millet seeds.

Tuberculosis Due to the Bovine Strain

Tuberculosis causes mastitis in cows, and the organism is therefore present in their milk. On ingestion of the milk by humans, a local infection occurs either in the tonsils or in the small intestine. This local lesion is small and clinically silent, but the organism spreads to involve regional lymph nodes in a massive way. The situation is similar to that of tuberculosis in the guinea pig. Bovine tuberculosis was once common in children, in whom large masses of caseous cervical or mesenteric lymph nodes were characteristic. Human beings have considerable innate immunity to tuberculosis, and the disease usually stopped its spread at this point. Occasionally,

continued spread resulted in miliary tuberculosis and death.

The eradication of tuberculosis from our herds and the almost universal pasteurization of milk have made bovine tuberculosis so rare that this form of the disease has virtually ceased to exist in the Western world.

Tuberculosis Due to the Human Strain

The mode of infection is by the inhalation of organisms present in fresh droplets or in the dust of dried sputum expectorated by a person having an open case of pulmonary tuberculosis.

It has been recognized for a long time that tuberculous infection manifests itself differently in children and adults. At all ages, the lung is the principal organ involved.

Childhood Tuberculosis. In childhood, the primary focus (the Ghon focus) is a small lesion situated at the periphery of the lung field. This subpleural focus may heal and produce no clinical illness, whereas the infection may spread to the hilar lymph nodes, which become greatly enlarged and caseous and eventually form a conspicuous primary complex (Fig. 8–6A). Either it heals and calcifies (Fig. 8–7), or the infection

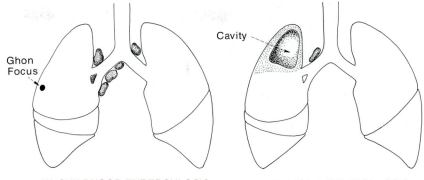

Figure 8–6 Pulmonary tuberculosis. In childhood tuberculosis, the lung lesion is small but the spread to hilar and mediastinal nodes is extensive. In adult tuberculosis, there is a destructive lung lesion (often apical and with cavitation), and the lymphatic spread to the hilum is minimal. (Drawing by Margot Mackay, University of Toronto Faculty of Medicine, Department of Surgery, Division of Biomedical Communications, Toronto.)

Ghon Focus

Cavity

(A) CHILDHOOD TUBERCULOSIS

(B) ADULT TUBERCULOSIS

spreads and the child dies of miliary tuberculosis with meningitis.

Adult Tuberculosis. In adult life, a pulmonary focus is almost always either atypical or subapical. The lesion either heals or progresses slowly with softening and liquefaction. In this way a cavity is formed (Figs. 8–6B and 8–8). The destruction of lung tissue causes bleeding, which often leads to hemoptysis. This is accompanied by a chronic cough, low-grade fever, weight loss, and a raised erythrocyte sedimentation rate. The patient feels unwell and lacks energy. Depending on the resistance of the patient, there is a tendency for either healing with fibrosis or extension of the cavitating process. In severe cases, there can be great destruction of lung tissue. At any time, caseous debris may be inhaled into other bronchi to produce areas of tuberculous bronchopneumonia. This may occur on a small scale and result in extension of the disease, but if it is widespread in a highly sensitized person, it can lead to massive consolidation of lung tissue. This is quite uncommon nowadays.

In summary, adult tuberculosis is a chronic disease in which phases of spread alternate with phases of healing and fibrosis.

Precisely why the morphology of adult tuberculosis of the lung is so different from that seen in childhood is not known. One explanation is that the adult type is a reinfection or reactivation of a previous infection. The previous infection induces immunity; with a reinfection, the disease does not spread but remains localized to the lung. Unfortunately, delayed type hypersensitivity leads to extensive destruction of lung tissue. Undoubtedly, there is some truth in this expla-

nation, but although the situation is similar to that seen in the Koch phenomenon, it is not exactly the same. In the Koch phenomenon, the lesion of reinfection heals because immunity develops (Chapter 6), whereas in human pulmonary adult tuberculosis, the lesion tends to heal slowly, and the disease remains chronic and progressive.

Metastatic Tuberculosis. At any stage in the development of a tuberculous lesion, a transient bacteremia can occur. This can result in small metastatic tuberculous lesions being produced in virtually any organ of the body. These usually remain quiescent, but years later they may become active and produce active tuberculous lesions at that site. Bone, kidney, brain, epididymis, fallopian tube, and joints are areas where this response is particularly frequent. The lesions are typically those of a chronic inflammation with progressive destruction of parenchyma and its replacement by fibrous tissue. Caseation is usually an obvious feature; if there is liquefaction, the tuberculous ''pus'' can spread in the line of least resistance. With renal tuberculosis, the pus ruptures into the pelvis of the kidney and is passed in the urine. Large cavitated areas extend from the pelvis of such a kidney. When tuberculous pus is formed adjacent to tuberculosis of the spinal column, the pus enters the psoas sheath, tracks down to below the inguinal ligament, and finally opens onto the skin surface.

Factors Determining the Response of Tissues to Tuberculous Infection

It is evident that a tuberculous infection may be followed by a minimal reaction that heals

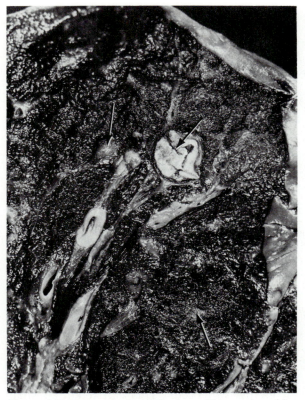

Figure 8–7 Tuberculosis of the lung. This section of lung shows a circumscribed, partly calcified lesion called a Ghon focus (see also Fig. 8–6A), which is indicated by the upper right arrow. This is thought to be the primary focus of a previous tuberculous infection. The adjacent pleura is thickened, and the overlying pleural space is obliterated by fibrous adhesions. In Europe, this type of lesion is usually due to a previous tuberculous infection; however, it is often difficult to prove this by finding organisms in the focus itself. In North America, histoplasmosis can produce a lesion with an identical appearance.

The specimen was from a patient who had died of miliary tuberculosis. The Ghon focus had evidently become reactivated; the bacilli had spread throughout the body via the blood stream. Two miliary tubercles are identified by arrows. (Specimen courtesy of the Body Museum, University of Toronto.)

rapidly or may lead to a progressive disease with rapid spread culminating in death. Many factors determine the response to tuberculous infection. These include the dose and virulence of the organism on the one hand, and the age, sex, and general health of the individual on the other. Silicosis renders the lung particularly liable to infection. Even more important is the immune state of the individual. Treatment with immunosuppressive drugs and diseases of the lymphoreticular system (*e.g.*, Hodgkin's disease), particularly when T-cell function is depressed, render the patient susceptible to a severe fulminating tuberculous infection. For example, an attack of measles can activate a previously quiescent tuberculous focus. Of greater current interest is AIDS, because tuberculosis is one of the many infections that are common in this disease.

Atypical Mycobacteria

Sometimes cases of human tuberculosis are encountered in which atypical bacteria are isolated. The organisms differ from *M. tuberculosis* in their resistance to antituberculous drugs and in their pathogenicity to the guinea pig. The disease that they cause is generally milder than is classic tuberculosis. The atypical bacteria or "mycobacteria other than tubercle bacilli" (MOTTS) have been subdivided into groups based on their cultural characteristics and pathogenicity. *M. fortuitum, M. cheloni,* and others occasionally cause wound infection, particularly after heart surgery. *Mycobacterium avium intracellulare* is now recognized as an important opportunistic pathogen in patients with AIDS. It causes a disseminated infection, and organisms are frequently present in vast numbers in the lungs, spleen, and lymph nodes. The organisms can be isolated from many specimens, including blood and stool. They are characteristically highly resistant to most antituberculous drugs; the response to treatment is usually poor.

Mycobacteria Causing Skin Infections

In addition to the cutaneous infections with *M. tuberculosis,* such as lupus vulgaris, two other organisms have been implicated in chronic ulcerations of the skin. Both organisms are characterized by growing best at 31° to 33°C, a property that resulted in their being overlooked until 1948.

Mycobacterium ulcerans. This organism causes chronic undermined ulcers of the skin, most commonly of the limbs. The disease is remarkable for the lack of inflammation, considering the extent of the necrosis. It bears little resemblance histologically to tuberculosis. The

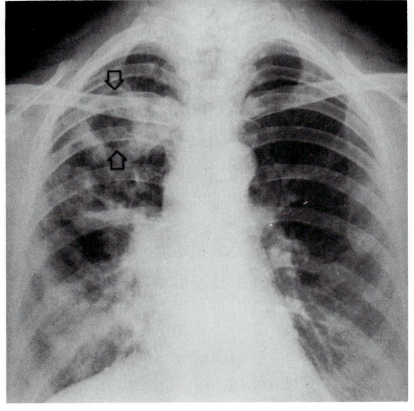

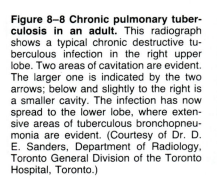

Figure 8–8 Chronic pulmonary tuberculosis in an adult. This radiograph shows a typical chronic destructive tuberculous infection in the right upper lobe. Two areas of cavitation are evident. The larger one is indicated by the two arrows; below and slightly to the right is a smaller cavity. The infection has now spread to the lower lobe, where extensive areas of tuberculous bronchopneumonia are evident. (Courtesy of Dr. D. E. Sanders, Department of Radiology, Toronto General Division of the Toronto Hospital, Toronto.)

disease is common in Uganda, where it is known as Buruli ulcer.

Mycobacterium marinum. This organism, formerly called *M. balnei,* causes infections of abrasions and may be acquired in swimming pools (hence its former name) or sometimes from tropical fish tanks. The ulcers are usually solitary, and the elbow or knee is the common location. The lesions tend to heal spontaneously.

Leprosy (Hansen's Disease)

Leprosy is caused by *Mycobacterium leprae,* which was one of the first bacteria to be incriminated as a cause of human disease and will probably be the last to be cultured in an artificial medium. Investigation of the disease, in particular the sensitivity of the organism to antibiotics, has been greatly hindered by our inability to grow the organism and the great difficulty encountered in infecting laboratory animals. So far, the organism has been grown only in the foot pads of mice and in the nine-banded armadillo. In practice, pathologic diagnosis depends on demonstrating the organism by staining of smears or sections. A modified Ziehl-Neelsen stain is used (the Fite stain).

Although the disease is very old, its precise origin is shrouded in mystery and superstition. The Old Testament accounts of leprosy almost certainly described conditions (possibly lupus erythematosus, lupus vulgaris, and skin cancers) other than the disease as we understand it today. Leprosy is generally believed to have had its origin in India, for there is evidence that it existed there in the sixth century B.C., at a time when its presence elsewhere cannot be substantiated. The disease was unknown to Hippocrates (c. 400–370 B.C.), but its appearance in Greece coincided with the return of the armies of Alexander the Great from the Indian campaign in 327 to 326 B.C. The return of the armies of Pompey in 62 B.C. helped to spread the disease to Italy, and the legions of Rome further disseminated it to the then civilized world. The returning Crusaders are also credited with spreading leprosy throughout Europe. The disease was common in Europe during the Middle Ages, but by the fifteenth century its incidence was declining, possibly because of improved living standards or possibly as a result of various great plagues that killed millions of people, particularly those who were already ill. The disease has now retreated from Europe but is endemic in the Far East, India, the Middle East, Africa, and Central and South America. It is estimated that there are over 12 million cases of leprosy in the world today; its incidence is related not to climate, but rather to the presence of overcrowding and poverty. The disease is believed to have been introduced into the continental United States by the black slaves from Africa, and it is still endemic in some southern states and in Hawaii.

Mode of Infection

The mode of infection is probably by inhalation of material from contaminated nasal secretions. It has been estimated that over 90 per cent of humans have such high innate immunity to the lepra bacillus that they are very unlikely to develop infection even if exposed to the disease. The remaining 5 to 10 per cent are susceptible. The disease is generally acquired in childhood, and the first lesion is an insignificant scaly skin patch. This *indeterminate lesion* may heal spontaneously or progress to one of the two major forms of the disease (Fig. 8–9).

Types of Leprosy

Tuberculoid Leprosy. This type of leprosy occurs in individuals with a relatively high state of natural immunity. The skin lesions consist of one or several *well-demarcated* papules or plaques, which are associated with local nerve involvement, causing the skin of the area to become hypoesthetic. On microscopic examination, the skin and involved nerves show a noncaseating tuberculoid reaction similar to that seen in early tuberculosis. Lepra bacilli are extremely sparse. The lepromin reaction (Fernandez reaction),* which is similar to the Mantoux, is positive and indicates a high state of cell-mediated immunity.

Lepromatous Leprosy. In lepromatous leprosy, the lesions consist of multiple macules, papules, and plaques, which are of *widespread distribution* and tend to be *symmetric*. The lesions are *poorly delineated*, and often there is a diffuse infiltration of the skin. On microscopic examination, the dermis is diffusely packed with macrophages, which are themselves stuffed with lepra bacilli. Since the lesions tend to occur in the cold parts of the body, the hands and face are particularly affected. The diffuse thickening of the skin of the face leads to a lionlike appearance (leonine facies). There is diffuse involvement of nerves, so that a symmetric peripheral neuritis is characteristic.

In lepromatous leprosy, the nasal mucosa is also infiltrated by bacteria-laden macrophages, and the destruction of the nasal bones leads to the characteristic appearance (Fig. 8–10). Because the nasal secretions contain a large number of bacilli, it is probable that this is the manner by which the disease is disseminated.

There is defective T-cell immunity in lepromatous leprosy, which causes the lepromin reaction to be negative. As if to compensate for this, there is an overproduction of immunoglobulins, and the hyperimmunoglobulinemia is associated with *acute reactional phases* that are a great hazard in leprosy. Exacerbation of the skin lesions, iridocyclitis, orchitis, nerve damage, fever, prostration, and death can occur during these acute phases, which may either develop spontaneously or be precipitated by treatment. The damage in some types of reaction is me-

---

*The lepromin test is performed by injecting a preparation of human or armadillo lepromatous tissue into the skin. An inflammatory reaction at 48 to 72 hours is comparable to a positive Mantoux test. It is termed the *Fernandez reaction* and is positive in tuberculoid leprosy. A reaction that develops at 3 weeks or more *(Mitsuda reaction)* indicates that the individual can react to the lepra bacillus with a granulomatous reaction. *The test is positive in many uninfected normal people* and indicates that their innate immunity is very high and that they are unlikely to develop leprosy. A negative Mitsuda reaction, on the other hand, indicates a low resistance to infection; should such an individual become infected, the lepromatous form of the disease will probably ensue.

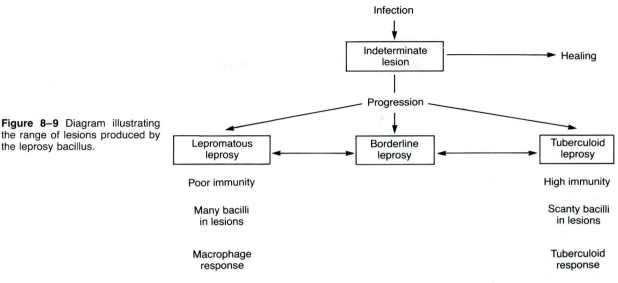

Figure 8–9 Diagram illustrating the range of lesions produced by the leprosy bacillus.

diated by the deposition of immune complexes with antigen excess. The large number of bacilli present in the lesions provides the antigen for the formation of these complexes. These lesions resemble erythema nodosum (erythoma nodosum leprosum).

Leprosy provides a fascinating example of the effects that an immune response has on the pattern of an infection. In the tuberculoid type, T-cell immunity is well developed, the lepromin test is positive, few bacilli are present in the lesions, and the inflammatory response is characterized by a tuberculoid reaction with plentiful Langhans giant cells. The pattern of reaction is similar to that encountered in the common type of tuberculous infection. In lepromatous leprosy, on the other hand, T-cell function is in abeyance and vast numbers of bacilli are present in the lesions, which are characterized by a diffuse infiltration by macrophages ("lepra cells"). Occasionally, an analogous situation is encountered in tuberculosis. In the terminal stages of miliary tuberculosis, the tuberculin test becomes negative, and the lesions teem with bacilli.

Borderline or Dimorphous Leprosy. Cases occur in which the clinical and pathologic features are between the two polar types of tuberculoid and lepromatous leprosy. In these borderline cases, acute reactional states are particularly common, and the disease tends to terminate in one of the two major forms, often the lepromatous type.

Leprosy is a chronic disease that is now amenable to treatment with a number of chemotherapeutic drugs. The sulfones are the mainstay of these drugs, because they are not only effective but also readily available and cheap. Multiple-drug treatment regimens are currently recommended in North America owing to the emergence of drug-resistant strains of the organism. When treated, the disease soon becomes noninfectious, so that there is no need for patients with Hansen's disease to be isolated.

SPIROCHETAL DISEASES

Spirochetes are long, slender, spiral filamentous organisms. The human pathogens are classified according to three genera: *Borrelia, Leptospira,* and *Treponema* (Table 8–3).

Borreliosis

Two species of *Borrelia* cause *relapsing fever.* The European type is spread by lice, whereas the African variety is tick-borne. Relapsing fever has an incubation period of 3 to 4 days and is characterized by an abrupt onset, a high fever,

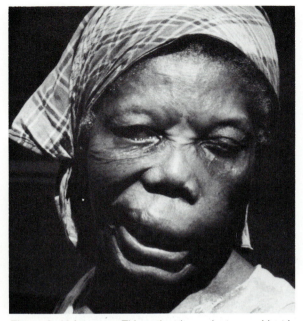

Figure 8–10 Leprosy. This patient is a voluntary resident in a leper colony in the Caribbean. Years before this picture was taken, she was found to be suffering from lepromatous leprosy and had been taking a sulfone or other antileprous drug ever since. Her disease is not now infectious; indeed, she may be completely free of the lepra bacillus, although this is difficult to prove. Nevertheless, she exhibits some of the devastating effects of the disease. Inflammation of the nasal mucosa (rhinitis) accompanied by destruction of the nasal bones has resulted in collapse of the bridge of the nose. Repeated attacks of iritis have led to glaucoma and cataract so that the sight of both eyes has been gravely affected. The left eye is completely blind, but the right eye is able to detect movement and the difference between light and dark. Because the patient has a left-sided facial nerve paralysis, the muscles of the left side of the face do not move. This can be detected by the drooping of the left eyelid and the failure of the left side of the mouth to move backward when the patient smiles or talks.

and the appearance of spirochetes in the blood stream. After 3 to 5 days, circulating immunoglobulin antibodies appear, the blood is cleared of organisms, and the fever abates. Some days later, organisms return to the blood, and another attack of fever ensues. Up to ten similar attacks may occur, thereby giving the disease its descriptive name.

The pathogenesis of this remarkable relapsing disease is that the organisms are able to mutate with extreme rapidity. No sooner does the immune response develop and kill off the organism than a new immunologic variant emerges, followed by a relapse of fever until the host has had time to develop new specific antibodies. A similar type of relapsing fever is also seen in trypanosomiasis; this, too, is due to the high mutability of the organism.

Borrelia vincentii is another large spirochete; it is a naturally occurring contaminant of the mouth. When local resistance is impaired, *e.g.,* in agranulocytosis and leukemia, the organism in association with *Bacteroides* causes ulcerative oral lesions. It is also an important member of the bacteria that are incriminated in gingivitis. During World War I, the condition of acute ulcerative gingivitis was so common in soldiers that it was known as "trench mouth." This was due to poor nutrition and poor dental hygiene.

Lyme Disease

Lyme disease first came to medical attention as a result of the observation of two mothers in Lyme, Connecticut, whose children were diagnosed as having the rare disease juvenile rheumatoid arthritis. They notified the health department, and it became apparent that the patients were not isolated cases; indeed, in the townships of Lyme, New Lyme, and East Haddam, the incidence of this form of arthritis was much higher than could be expected. In one small area, the incidence was 100,000 times greater than could be expected. Research by Dr. Allen C. Steere suggested that the disease was due to an infection, and he concluded that a tick was the likely vector. This vector was later identified as the deer tick *(Ixodes dammini),* and the causative organism is a spirochete now called *Borrelia burgdorferi.* The organism is transmitted by the bite of the tick; in most cases, a red papule appears at the site of the bite and is followed by the development of an zone of erythema that expands to reach a size of 50 cm or more over a period of 2 to 3 weeks *(erythema chronicum migrans).* Fever, headache, and backache may be present. Even without treatment, patients often recover completely from this first stage of the illness. Other patients, however, develop the second stage that is characterized by neurologic complications and, in a few cases, cardiac abnormalities. The third stage commences within 2 years of infection and affects about 60 percent of

Table 8–3 COMMON SPIROCHETAL INFECTIONS

Organism	Source of Infection	Disease Produced
Borrelia		
B. recurrentis	Body louse	European relapsing fever
B. duttonii	Ticks	African relapsing fever
B. vincentii	Normal flora of mouth	Gingivitis, gangrenous lesions of mouth
B. burgdorferi	Tick	Lyme disease
Leptospira		
L. icterohaemorrhagiae and others	Urine of rodents, dogs, and many other species	Leptospirosis (Weil's disease)
Treponema		
T. pallidum	Human case of syphilis	Syphilis
T. pertenue	Human case of yaws	Yaws

untreated patients. It is characterized by an arthritis that closely resembles rheumatoid arthritis; it may occur without any preceding skin manifestations.

Leptospirosis

Many strains of leptospira are known and are normally carried in the kidneys of many species of animals such as rodents, dogs, cattle, birds, and amphibians. The organisms rarely cause harm in their usual host, but if transmitted accidentally to another animal species or to human beings, they give rise to a clinical infection called leptospirosis. Leptospirosis is transmitted to humans in water contaminated by the urine of carrier animals, usually rats or dogs. It is therefore an occupational hazard of such persons as sewer workers, military personnel, and veterinarians. The disease is now more often encountered in children and young adults who acquire the infection during swimming or wading in contaminated water.

Leptospirosis can vary from a mild influenza-like disease to a severe illness with renal and hepatic damage. The latter type is known as Weil's disease. Occasionally meningitis is a dominant feature of the clinical presentation.

Treponemal Diseases

The most important member of the treponematoses is venereal syphilis. An epidemic of this disease erupted in Europe at the end of the fifteenth century. One theory maintains that the infection was introduced by the sailors of Christopher Columbus in 1493 when they returned from the New World. However, the situation is confusing because various forms of *nonvenereal treponemal diseases*, such as yaws, pinta, bejel, and others, are found in various underprivileged, overcrowded parts of the world. These diseases resemble venereal syphilis closely, with primary, secondary, and tertiary lesions, but are transmitted by contact often during early childhood. Also, the severe cardiovascular and nervous system lesions that characterize tertiary venereal syphilis do not occur. The causative organisms of nonvenereal syphilis cannot be distinguished morphologically or serologically from the organism that causes venereal syphilis. Presumably venereal syphilis developed as a mutation from one of these nonvenereal forms.

Nonvenereal Treponemal Diseases

This group includes a number of diseases that occur in various parts of the world, *e.g.*, pinta (Central and South America), endemic syphilis (known as bejel in the Middle East), and yaws. Yaws is the best known and is common in many tropical countries; its greatest incidence is in central Africa. The primary lesion is extragenital; secondary and tertiary stages follow but affect skin and bones.

Venereal Syphilis

The causative organism of venereal syphilis is *Treponema pallidum,* a delicate spiral filament or spirochete 6 to 15 μm long. It cannot be stained by the usual techniques, but a special silver impregnation method is available. The organism has never been cultivated artificially, nor does animal inoculation play any part in its diagnosis. Rabbits develop an acute orchitis after intratesticular inoculation of the organism. This method is used to obtain a supply of organisms for such procedures as the TPI and FTA tests.

During the course of infection, the patient develops immunoglobulins that are of great diagnostic importance. The best known is the Wassermann antibody, which fixes complement in the presence of a phosphatide extract of heart muscle (cardiolipin) or produces a precipitate in the presence of a similar type of antigen (Kahn reaction, the Venereal Disease Research Laboratory [VDRL] test, and other modifications). Since the antigen used is not a specific component of the spirochete, it is not surprising that these *standard tests for syphilis (STS)* are also sometimes positive in nonspirochetal diseases—for example, leprosy, malaria, and systemic lupus erythematosus. Pregnancy, too, is occasionally associated with a false-positive reaction.

In recent years, it has been found that syphilitics also develop a specific treponemal antibody in their sera. When mixed with a suspension of live organisms, the antibody leads to immobilization of the organisms, and this forms the basis for the *treponemal immobilization (TPI) test.* Specific treponemal antibody will adhere to the organism, and this can be detected by a fluorescent technique *(fluorescent treponemal antibody test [FTA]).* Dead organisms adherent to a slide are used in this test, in contrast to the living, and therefore infectious, organisms required for the TPI test. If nonspecific antibodies are first absorbed by mixing the patient's serum with a nonpathogenic strain of treponema (the Reiter strain), the test is made more specific for syphilis. This is the *FTA-ABS* test and is the one most commonly performed. These *treponemal tests* are not performed routinely but are of great value in verifying ambiguous results and eliminating false-positive reactions. It is unfortunate that even the specific tests cannot distinguish syphilis, yaws, and other types of nonvenereal syphilis.

Apart from congenital syphilis, the infection is nearly always acquired venereally. Unlike the tubercle bacillus, *T. pallidum* is very rapidly destroyed both in water and by drying. Intimate direct contact is therefore necessary for infection to occur. The spirochete is one of the most invasive organisms known, for once having penetrated the surface, it spreads along the lymphatics to the regional nodes and reaches the blood stream in a matter of hours. Therefore, systemic dissemination occurs long before any local manifestations appear.

The disease is divisible into three active stages.

Primary Syphilis. The primary lesion of syphilis is the *chancre,* which usually appears on the genital area 3 to 4 weeks after infection. It commences as an indurated nodule, which breaks down to form an ulcer that characteristically is painless and is accompanied by enlargement of the regional lymph nodes (Fig. 8–11). Extragenital chancres are not uncommon (*e.g.,* around the anus, and on the lips, tip of tongue, tonsil, or other part of the oral cavity). The chancre heals even without treatment and leaves an inconspicuous atrophic scar. Its occurrence can easily be missed, particularly in women, in whom the lesion can be on the cervix or vaginal vault. Likewise, anal lesions in either sex can easily evade detection.

Case History II

The patient (see Fig. 8–11), who had been consorting with a number of sexual partners, had noticed a small ulcer on the penis about a week before this picture was taken. This ulcer had steadily enlarged. Although it was not painful, he was persuaded to seek medical advice when he noticed swelling of his left inguinal region. On examination, an oval ulcer with a firm base on the penis was noted, and this was associated with large inguinal lymph nodes on the left side. Characteristically, the ulcer was not painful. The ulcer was firmly squeezed, and its base gently rubbed with a bacteriologic loop. The drop of fluid that was obtained was examined by dark-field illumination and showed numerous active spirochetes. A blood sample taken at this time showed a negative VDRL. After the administration of penicillin, the ulcer healed and the lymphadenopathy subsided. The patient's sexual partners were traced, and only two were found to have had intercourse with him during the last 3 months. Both were found to have a positive VDRL and were treated

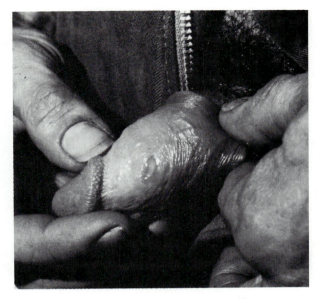

Figure 8–11 Primary chancre of syphilis. For a more complete description, see Case History II.

for syphilis. This cases illustrates three important points: (1) A VDRL can be negative during the early stages of primary syphilis. (2) The response to penicillin is dramatic. (3) Contacts must be traced in an effort to prevent the further spread of the disease. Tracing the contacts is an important public health function.

The fact that the spirochetes become disseminated long before there is any local lesion suggests that hypersensitivity plays an important part in the pathogenesis of the lesion. The chancre is not comparable to a boil, for it is not a local inflammatory reaction tending to limit the infection. A possible explanation is that sensitizing antibodies are first formed at the site of infection and in the regional lymph nodes. During the incubation period, the organisms multiply; as sensitizing antibodies are produced, a damaging antigen-antibody reaction occurs to produce the primary lesion and its associated lymphadenitis.

A definite diagnosis of primary syphilis rests entirely on finding the organisms in the lesion by direct microscopic examination with use of the dark-field method (Chapter 1). Soon after the appearance of the chancre, antibodies appear in the blood, and the serologic tests for syphilis become positive.

Secondary Syphilis. Within 2 to 3 months of exposure, the disease becomes clinically generalized. When the virulent form of syphilis was introduced into Europe, the disease was sometimes fatal and indeed sufficiently severe to warrant naming it the Great Pox. The disease spread rapidly like a plague throughout Europe, reaching as far as Scotland by 1497. Even to this day, *lues* (from the Latin for pestilence) is used as an alternative name for the disease. Nowadays, secondary syphilis is much milder and is characterized by the appearance of a generalized macular or papulosquamous erythematous rash. Characteristically, this does not itch and affects the whole body, including the palms and soles (Fig. 8–12).

Papules affecting moist areas such as the genital, axillary, and submammary regions can enlarge to produce flat, warty lesions (*condylomata lata*). The primary chancre may still be present or may have healed by the time the secondary lesions appear.

Case History III

The patient (see Fig. 8–12) had developed a generalized nonitching rash composed of red palpable lesions (0.2 to 1.0 cm in diameter) covered by loose, keratin scales (this constitutes a generalized, nonpruritic, erythematous, papulosquamous eruption; see Chapter 31). Lesions were most obvious on the trunk, but they were also present on the limbs, including the palms and soles. Because the patient was in the habit of taking a barbiturate sleeping pill each night, the

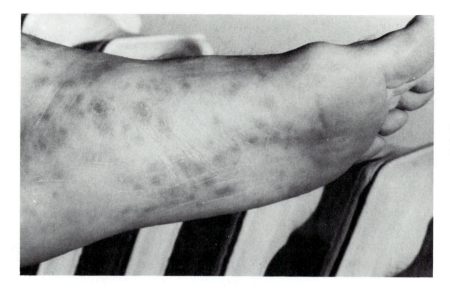

Figure 8–12 Lesions of secondary syphilis. For a more complete description, see Case History III.

possibility of the rash being due to an adverse drug reaction was also considered. However, drug rashes generally itch, and the presence of a nonitching rash, particularly if it affects the palms and soles, is very suggestive of secondary syphilis. The patient denied ever having had an ulcer on his penis but admitted to having had homosexual encounters. Blood was taken for a VDRL test. The patient was treated with penicillin. Within 8 hours he had developed a fever, and the rash had become more obvious before it faded. The VDRL was subsequently reported as being strongly positive.

This case illustrates the following points:

1. Any generalized nonpruritic papulosquamous rash, particularly one affecting the palms and soles, should be diagnosed as syphilis until proved otherwise.

2. The VDRL test is always positive in secondary syphilis.

3. No history of a primary lesion is obtainable in some patients, particularly in females and in male homosexuals.

4. Successful treatment with penicillin often causes an immediate accentuation of the lesions. This response is known as the Herxheimer reaction and is presumed to be due to the massive release of bacterial antigen as the organisms are killed.

5. The patients should be treated before laboratory confirmation is obtained. This helps prevent the spread of the infection.

A low-grade fever, headaches, joint pain, anemia, generalized lymph node enlargement, iritis, and many other symptoms may be noted at this stage. Shallow ulcers may occur on the mucous membranes; these, like other secondary lesions, particularly the condylomata, are teeming with organisms and are highly infectious. Diagnosis at this stage depends either on identification of the organism by microscopy or on confirmation by serologic means. The serologic tests are always positive in secondary syphilis. If a negative result is reported, the prozone phenomenon should be suspected (Chapter 6).

Even without treatment, the lesions of secondary syphilis heal, and the patient enters into a latent phase.

Latent Syphilis. This is an asymptomatic state that can be diagnosed only on history and by obtaining a positive serologic test for syphilis. It is divided into two phases.

Early Latent Syphilis. This is usually defined as the period under 2 years after infection. Some authorities extend it to 4 years. The patient is still infectious during this phase and can at any time develop lesions of secondary syphilis.

Late Latent Syphilis. This period extends from 2 years after infection. There is virtually no tendency to develop secondary type lesions, and the patient may be considered almost noninfectious. Nevertheless, a woman can still bear a syphilitic child. The patient may remain in this stage of latent syphilis for life, but approximately one third of the patients with untreated syphilis develop one of the tertiary lesions. The remaining two thirds remain asymptomatic for life, although about half of them are seropositive for life.

Tertiary Syphilis. Local destructive lesions may appear 2 to 3 years after infection and continue to erupt sporadically for many years. The lesions are presumably due to marked hypersensitivity, because spirochetes are few and the reaction to them is excessive. Two types of lesions can be recognized: localized gummas and diffuse inflammatory lesions characterized by parenchymatous destruction.

Gummas. The gumma is the classic lesion of tertiary syphilis. It is usually a solitary tumorlike mass and consists of a central large area of coagulative necrosis that has a slimy, stringy, gumlike mass from which the name gumma is derived. The necrotic tissue is surrounded by a granulomatous inflammatory reaction. Gummas are described as being most frequent in the liver, testes, subcutaneous tissues, and bones—including the nasal and palatal bones. In the palatal bones, the destruction produced by the gummas leads to perforation of the hard palate. With the introduction of penicillin and other antibiotic treatment of syphilis, *gummas are now extremely uncommon.*

Diffuse Lesions. The really severe effects of tertiary syphilis fall on the cardiovascular and the nervous systems.

In *syphilitic aortitis,* the elastic aortic wall is steadily destroyed by a chronic inflammatory reaction and is replaced by fibrous tissue. The weakening of the aorta results in aneurysmal dilation; ultimately, the vessel may rupture. The disease tends to affect the thoracic aorta, causing widening of the aortic ring, which can lead to aortic regurgitation.

Neurosyphilis may be meningovascular or parenchymatous. In the meningovascular type, there is focal meningitis and vascular occlusion of small vessels. Isolated cranial nerve paralyses are produced.

Parenchymatous neurosyphilis includes the two well-known conditions of general paralysis of the insane and tabes dorsalis. *General paralysis of the insane* is a chronic syphilitic meningoencephalitis in which the frontal lobes are particularly affected. This results in progressive dementia and paralysis. *Tabes dorsalis* is a degenerative condition of the posterior columns of the spinal cord and the posterior roots of the spinal nerves. The loss in sensation leads to loss of postural sense and a typical staggering gait.

The diagnosis of tertiary syphilis is primarily clinical, but it may often be substantiated by serologic examination of the blood and cerebrospinal fluid. In most cases of overt syphilis, the serologic reactions are positive. Gummas are usually diagnosed by biopsy or following excision. It has frequently been stressed that syphilis is the great mimic in medicine and that virtually any lesion or disease can be faithfully copied by syphilis. Hence, a routine VDRL test is a common clinical procedure. Note, however, that the serologic tests for syphilis frequently remain positive during the latent periods and that a syphilitic patient can suffer from other diseases. Thus, a mass present in the lung in a patient with a positive VDRL is more likely to be a carcinoma, which is common, than a gumma, which is rare.

Congenital Syphilis. During the first 2 years of infection, an untreated syphilitic mother is very liable to transmit the disease to her fetus, particularly in the later months of pregnancy. Abortion may result, or a severely affected infant may be born alive but die soon after birth.

More frequently, the child survives and may then exhibit early stigmata of the infection: skin eruptions, nasal infection (snuffles), and involvement of bones. Destruction of the nasal bones leads to a saddle-shaped deformity of the nose. Sometimes stigmata appear only in later childhood. The notched, deformed upper incisor teeth, inflammation of the cornea (interstitial keratitis), periostitis, and nerve deafness are all well-known features. In effect, the early lesions of congenital syphilis are comparable to those of the secondary stage, whereas the later manifestations have the destructive features of tertiary syphilis as encountered in the adult.

NOCARDIOSIS

The causative nocardia are soil saprophytes and occasionally cause infection of the lungs or skin.

ACTINOMYCOSIS

The causative organism, *Actinomyces israelii*, is a normal inhabitant of the mouth and occasionally causes a chronic suppurative infection of the jaw. The organism resembles the nocardia in growing as long branching threads the same width as bacteria. In pus, the masses of organisms are visible as clusters called grains. This group of higher bacteria bear considerable resemblance to fungi but are now classified as bacteria.

Summary

- The pyogenic organisms cause inflammation with numerous neutrophils and often the formation of pus. Staphylococci, streptococci, and gram-negative coliforms affect many sites; pneumococci, gonococci, and meningococci tend to affect lung, genitalia, and meninges, respectively.
- *Staphylococcus pyogenes* also elaborates exotoxins that cause food poisoning, the toxic shock syndrome, and skin eruptions.
- *Streptococcus pyogenes* also causes scarlet fever, glomerulonephritis, and rheumatic fever.
- *Corynebacterium diphtheriae* elaborates a powerful exotoxin that leads to the manifestations of the disease.
- Anaerobes include the clostridia and *Bacteroides* species. *Clostridium tetani* contaminates wounds and causes tetanus, a disease that can be prevented by prior immunization with toxoid. Clostridial myositis or gas gangrene complicates deep wounds in which muscle is damaged or rendered ischemic; toxemia and shock are characteristic. *C. difficile* causes pseudomembranous colitis. *Bacteroides* infection complicates wounds contaminated by feces.
- *Mycobacterium tuberculosis* is acid-alcohol-fast, grows slowly *in vitro*, and causes an infection characterized by a caseating tuberculoid granulomatous reaction. The lung is the primary site of infection, but later any organ may be affected. In infants, rapid spread may occur (miliary tuberculosis), but in adults the disease is usually chronic.
- Atypical mycobacteria cause a variety of skin and lung infections. They may cause an opportunistic infection in patients with AIDS.

- *Mycobacterium leprae* causes leprosy. Infection mainly affects nerves and skin and is probably acquired by inhalation. The disease ranges from an indolent and localized form if immunity is high (tuberculoid leprosy) to a generalized and disfiguring form if immunity is low (lepromatous leprosy). Immunologic reactions are common and result in much damage.
- Borrelia are spirochetes; two species cause relapsing fever. *Borellia vincentii* is associated with gangrenous lesions; *B. burgdorferi* causes Lyme disease. This is a tick-borne infection characterized by erythema chronicum migrans sometimes complicated by arthritis and cardiac and nervous manifestations.
- Leptospirosis is a generalized infection usually acquired by swimming in contaminated water.
- Treponemal infection causes a nonvenereal disease that includes yaws and the more important venereal syphilis. Syphilis commences as a localized primary chancre followed by a generalized secondary stage with skin lesions. A latent phase may later be followed by gummas or diffuse lesions affecting the aorta or nervous system. A variety of antibodies are produced after infection and are useful aids to diagnosis. The VDRL is the best known but is not specific.

Selected Readings

Binford, C. H., and Connor, D. H. (eds.): Pathology of Tropical and Extraordinary Diseases. Washington, D. C., Armed Forces Institute of Pathology, 1976.

Davidson, P. T.: Tuberculosis. New views of an old disease. N. Engl. J. Med. 312:1514, 1985.

Holmes, K. K., et al. (eds.): Sexually Transmitted Diseases. 2nd ed. New York, McGraw-Hill, 1990.

Leading article: Infant botulism. Lancet 2:1256, 1986.

Leading article: Neonatal infection with group B streptococci. Lancet 2:181, 1981.

Leading article: Tick-borne *Borrelia*. Lancet 2:1134, 1984.

Lennette, E. H., et al. (eds.): Manual of Clinical Microbiology. 4th ed. Washington, D. C., American Society for Microbiology, 1985.

Sheagren, J. N.: *Staphylococcus aureus*. The persistent pathogen. N. Engl. J. Med. 310:1368 and 1437, 1984.

Shepard, C. C.: Leprosy today. N. Engl. J. Med. 307:1640, 1982.

Stead, W. W., and Dutt, A. K.: What's new in tuberculosis? Am. J. Med. 71:1, 1981.

Stead, W. W., et al.: Tuberculosis as an endemic and nosocomial infection among the elderly in nursing homes. N. Engl. J. Med. 312:1483, 1985.

Mycoplasmal, Chlamydial, Rickettsial, and Viral Infections

After studying this chapter, the student should be able to:

- Outline the main features of mycoplasmal pneumonia and the organism that causes it.
- Compare chlamydia with mycoplasma and describe the important human diseases caused by members of the chlamydial group of organisms.
- List the four types of typhus fever and describe the main features of one of them.
- Describe the main features of Q fever.
- Compare and contrast viruses with higher organisms with respect to the following:
  (a) size;
  (b) structure;
  (c) chemical composition.
- Describe how viruses enter a cell, how new viral material is produced, and how new particles are released.
- Describe the range of effects that a viral infection can have on a cell.
- Describe the immunity that a viral infection can evoke, particularly in relation to the following:
  (a) immunoglobulin formation;
  (b) T-cell immunity;
  (c) interferon production.
- Distinguish among the following: the incubation period, the prodromal stage, enanthem, and exanthem. Use measles and smallpox as examples.
- Describe the pathogenesis of poliomyelitis as well as the means available for preventing this disease.
- Describe the methods of treating viral infections.
- Outline the laboratory investigations available for the diagnosis of a viral infection.
- List the nine families of viruses described in this

chapter and give examples of the common members within each group.
- Describe the types of infection caused by herpes simplex virus.
- Indicate how humans become victims of rabies and how this may be averted.
- Discuss the relationship between varicella and zoster. Outline the clinical features of each.

MYCOPLASMAL INFECTIONS

Mycoplasmas are the smallest organisms (150 to 250 nm) that are capable of growth in a cell-free medium. They lack a cell wall and therefore tend to be very pleomorphic; coccobacillary, filamentous, and branching forms are common. The only definite human pathogen is *Mycoplasma pneumoniae,* an organism causing a type of pneumonia that tends to occur in small epidemics. The onset is insidious, and the x-ray changes of patchy consolidation are often more extensive than the clinical picture would suggest (Fig. 9–1). Recovery is invariable and can be hastened by tetracycline therapy. Before the nature of the causative organism was understood, the disease was labeled "primary atypical pneumonia" or "viral pneumonia" (see Case History I). Two

curious features of the disease are the development of cold autohemagglutinins (Chapter 18) and a positive standard test for syphilis. A complement fixation test is available and is the most widely used method of diagnosis.

Case History I

The patient (see Fig. 9–1) was a 36-year-old female who had developed an upper respiratory infection that persisted for 2 weeks and was accompanied by a dry, hacking cough. Although she was treated with penicillin, she showed no improvement. At the end of the third week, the patient still felt ill and was troubled by a persistent cough, shortness of breath, and an evening fever. A diagnosis of mycoplasmal pneumonia was confirmed by the finding of specific antibodies to a titer of 1 in 3000.

Since the patient was found to be 3 months pregnant, she was not administered tetracycline, the usual drug of choice. Tetracycline is contraindicated in pregnancy, particularly during the last 3 months, because it impairs fetal tooth development. The patient was given erythromycin and made a slow recovery.

Some species of *Mycoplasma* have been implicated as a cause of nongonococcal urethritis.

CHLAMYDIAL INFECTIONS

The chlamydiae are small, obligatory intracellular parasites about 300 nm in diameter. Several

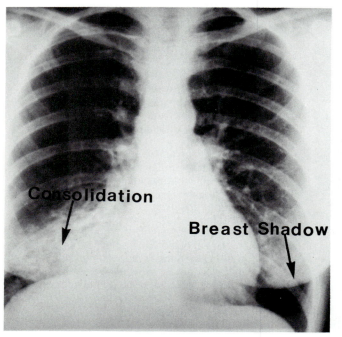

Figure 9–1 Chest radiograph of patient with mycoplasmal pneumonia. There is patchy, bilateral consolidation most marked in the lower lung fields, particularly on the right side. For clinical details, see Case History I. (Courtesy of Dr. D.E. Sanders, Department of Radiology, Toronto General Division of the Toronto Hospital, Toronto.)

are pathogenic to human beings. Since growth in tissue cultures is difficult, the organisms are generally isolated by injecting the yolk sac of the chick embryo. Chlamydiae contain both DNA and RNA and have been divided into two species, *Chlamydia trachomatis* and *Chlamydia psittaci*. Various serotypes of *C. trachomatis* cause trachoma, inclusion conjunctivitis, lymphogranuloma, and the other sexually transmitted infections. *C. psittaci* strains cause psittacosis and ornithosis.

Trachoma

Trachoma is an infection of the conjunctiva that becomes chronic, tends to spread to the cornea, and causes scarring. The disease is uncommon in the Western world but is a very important cause of *blindness* in the Middle East and other areas of poverty and overcrowding. Diagnosis is confirmed by isolating the organism or demonstrating the inclusion bodies in a smear from the conjunctiva.

Inclusion Conjunctivitis

This disease is so named because inclusion bodies can be seen in infected cells. It affects newborn babies (in whom it forms a type of ophthalmia neonatorum) as well as adults (causing "swimming pool conjunctivitis"). The organism is transmitted venereally and causes urethritis in the male.

Chlamydial Urethritis and Cervicitis

Chlamydial urethritis accounts for about 50 per cent of nongonococcal urethritis in the male. Double infections are common; because the incubation period of chlamydial urethritis is longer than that of gonorrhea, treatment with penicillin cures the obvious gonorrhea but does not affect the resistant chlamydial infection. About 70 per cent of postgonococcal urethritis is due to chlamydiae.

Chlamydiae cause cervicitis in the female, but the infection can be clinically inapparent and therefore remains untreated; indeed, the female genital area is an important reservoir of infection. Transfer to the eyes of babies occurs during labor; transfer in adults occurs via the hands or imperfectly chlorinated pool water.

Lymphogranuloma Venereum

This is an uncommon venereal disease characterized by the appearance of a local genital ulcer and regional lymph node enlargement.

Psittacosis (Ornithosis)

Psittacosis is a disease of birds of the parrot family (psittacine birds). Ducks, chickens, turkeys, pigeons, gulls, and other birds may also have the disease, in which case it is termed ornithosis. Diagnosis is confirmed by a complement fixation test. Infection in humans is caused by inhalation of dust containing contaminated bird excreta, and it usually presents as a type of pneumonia. The regulations relating to the importation of psittacine birds have made this an uncommon disease. Occasional outbreaks still occur, however, because native birds, such as poultry and pigeons, can harbor the organism.

RICKETTSIAL INFECTIONS

The rickettsial organisms are obligatory intracellular parasites that are widely distributed in nature, infecting many species of mammals that form their natural reservoir. Infection is transferred by lice, fleas, ticks, and mites. Humans are infected when they accidentally intercept the life cycle of infection from insect vector to animal reservoir. The only exception to this mode of transfer is with epidemic typhus, in which humans, themselves, are the only known reservoir.

The organisms are named after Dr. Howard T. Ricketts, an American pathologist who first identified the causative agent of Rocky Mountain spotted fever in a patient and in the tick that transmits the disease. His subsequent work with typhus led to his own death from rickettsial infection.

Rickettsial organisms are responsible for the typhus group of infections, rickettsialpox, and Q fever.

Typhus

The typhus group of fevers is currently of little day-to-day importance; in the past, however, it has been responsible for epidemics of ferocious intensity. These have occurred in time of war when humans, rats, fleas, and lice have shared a common habitation. No doubt, future catastrophes will once again highlight the virulence of the rickettsiae, and it is for this reason that some knowledge of this group of diseases is important.

Mode of Infection. Some rickettsiae are injected by the bite of an infected tick or mite. On the other hand, lice and fleas pass contaminated feces as they feed on their animal host, causing rickettsial organisms to be introduced when the site of the bite is scratched.

The typhus fevers have an incubation period of 7 to 10 days, and their onset is of dramatic suddenness with rigors, fever, and severe headaches accompanied by prostration. The organisms multiply in the endothelial cells of blood vessels; the far-reaching vascular damage accounts for the widespread nature of the lesions seen in the disease. A skin rash appears in most cases about the fourth day of clinical illness.

Types. The following types of typhus are important.

*Epidemic, Louse-borne Typhus.** Caused by *Rickettsia prowazekii*, this disease is associated with a high mortality and was responsible for the typhus epidemics of the two World Wars. DDT, with its lousicidal activity, proved to be an effective weapon in controlling this disease. Unlike the case in all other forms of typhus, with this disease humans are the only mammal host. Since infected lice soon die, one would expect the disease to die out. A parasite that often kills

---

*In addition to rickettsiae, the body louse also transmits the European type of relapsing fever due to *Borrelia recurrentis*. Infestation can generally be recognized by the presence of itchy papules and numerous scratch marks ("vagabond's disease"). It is important to note that the parasite lives in clothing and not on the skin. Hence, when infestation is suspected, the underclothing—particularly its seams—should be carefully examined.

its only hosts should not be successful. The explanation of the paradox is that after an attack of the disease, humans can harbor the organism for many years. A recrudescence of the disease (Brill-Zinsser disease) can occur; the illness is mild but of great importance, because the victim constitutes a potential source of infection. If the individual happens to harbor lice and lives in overcrowded squalor, the next epidemic can be initiated.

Endemic, Flea-borne Typhus. This disease is endemic in many parts of the world, including the United States. It is caused by *Rickettsia typhi (mooseri)* and is transmitted by the *rat flea.*

Rocky Mountain Spotted Fever. This disease, endemic throughout North America, is caused by *Rickettsia rickettsii* and is a severe form of typhus transmitted by the bite of a tick. The disease is characterized by a sudden onset, fever, and a severe headache. The characteristic rash appears about the fourth day of illness, is initially maculopapular, but subsequently becomes petechial and hemorrhagic—features that give the disease its name. Similar types of tick-borne diseases occur in other parts of the world.

Scrub Typhus. This was the mite-borne type of typhus that constituted a problem in the Pacific area in World War II.

Laboratory Diagnosis. Patients with typhus develop antibodies that by chance agglutinate certain strains of *Proteus* organisms. This reaction has been utilized in a diagnostic test, the *Weil-Felix reaction,* that is analogous to the Widal reaction for typhoid. A rising titer during the course of a febrile illness helps confirm the diagnosis. Specific antirickettsial complement-fixing antibodies can also be demonstrated. Isolation of the organism is performed by inoculating a suitable laboratory animal.

Treatment. Treatment of typhus has been revolutionized by the introduction of chloramphenicol and tetracycline. Typhus now has a low mortality, unless the patient is already the victim of other disease or starvation.

Rickettsialpox

This mild febrile illness is accompanied by a widespread skin rash. The disease was first noted in New York City and is due to infection by *Rickettsia akari* transmitted from mouse to human by the bite of a mite.

Q Fever

Q (for *query*) fever, caused by *Rochalimaea* (formerly *Coxiella) burnetii,* is transmitted from animal to animal by the bite of a tick. Sheep, goats, and cows are naturally infected, and human disease is caused either by drinking contaminated milk or by inhaling dust contaminated by animal material. Q fever in humans is characterized by a long incubation period (about 19 days). The disease resembles other forms of typhus, except that although a rash is very uncommon, evidence of pneumonia or hepatitis is frequently found.

VIRAL INFECTIONS

Viral infections are common and are of many types. At times, some have reached epidemic proportions and have been so severe that through the ages strenuous attempts have been made to prevent them; by chance, some attempts have been successful. Thus, Jenner, who knew nothing of virology, found a way to prevent smallpox. Pasteur postulated that the cause of rabies was an infinitesimally small microorganism, and without ever isolating it, he devised a means of protecting against rabies. The theory that disease could be caused by organisms smaller than bacteria was finally confirmed by Iwanowsky in 1892, when he showed that tobacco mosaic disease was due to an agent so small that it could pass through the pores of a filter that would retain all known bacteria. It was at the turn of the century that the first human disease, yellow fever, was proved to be caused by a similar ultramicroscopic, filterable virus. The properties of viruses and their mode of action can best be understood by comparing them with bacteria.

General Properties of Viruses

Bacteria are all within the range of the light microscope and are complete cells surrounded by a cell membrane and often by a cell wall.* They contain both DNA and RNA together with many chemicals, such as enzymes, for their own maintenance and reproduction. They multiply by simple division. Since bacteria are complete cells, the majority of them can be grown by the bacteriologist on an artificial medium; the causative organisms of leprosy and syphilis are the two notable exceptions. Viruses, on the other hand, are much smaller, although the large poxviruses are just within the range of the conventional light microscope.

The only feature that distinguishes viruses from all other organisms is that during the process of multiplication, viruses enter a noninfective, or "eclipse," phase. Their nucleic acid is either RNA or DNA, but never both. They contain neither ribosomes nor mitochondria and cannot produce high-energy adenosine triphosphate (ATP). They do not possess the necessary enzyme systems for the synthesis of viral material and are therefore dependent on those of the parasitized cell for survival and multiplication. Indeed, the essential difference between viruses and other organisms is that the synthetic processes that attend multiplication take place within the protoplasm of the infected cells in the case of viruses, but in the body of the organism itself in other infective agents.

Structure of Viruses

A complete infective virus particle that can exist outside a cell is called a *virion,* and it consists of a core of either DNA or RNA, which is surrounded by a protein coat, or *capsid.* Some viruses, *e.g.,* herpes simplex virus, have an outer *envelope* derived from the nuclear membrane or the plasma membrane of the cell from which the virus was released.

Electron microscopy has shown the coat to consist of subunits, or *capsomeres,* each of which is made of protein and consists of a hollow tube pointing outward. The capsomeres are closely packed and so arranged with their neighbors that

---

*Animal cells do not possess a cell wall. Penicillin acts by inhibiting the formation of cell wall material. After division, penicillin-treated bacteria have a defective cell wall, are fragile, and are easily killed.

the virion has a definite geometric shape. Three major types of viruses can be recognized: *viruses with cubic symmetry*, which have the form of an icosahedron, a solid, roughly spherical structure with 20 facets, each consisting of an equilateral triangle and meeting at 12 corners (Fig. 9–2); *viruses with helical symmetry*, which consist of a filament with capsomeres arranged around the nucleic acid as a *helix* (Fig. 9–3); and *complex viruses*, in which the virus particle does not conform to either cubic or helical symmetry, *e.g.*, bacteriophages and poxviruses (Figs. 9–4 and 9–11). Bacteriophage is a virus that infects bacteria and is commonly called "phage" for short; it has a head attached to a central core from which arise six tail filaments.

Growth of Viruses

Viruses will grow only in living cells. In the early days of virology, whole live animals were used for growth of these structures, but the animal's immune response was a complicating factor and the method was ethically undesirable

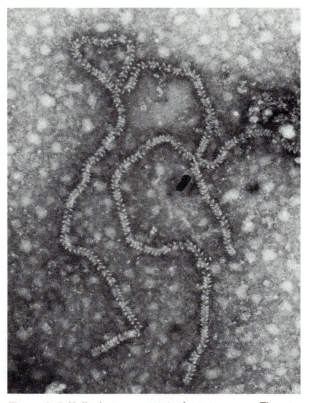

Figure 9–3 Helical arrangement of capsomeres. The covering envelope of a paramyxovirus has been ruptured to release its RNA content. The photograph shows the long thread of nucleoprotein surrounded by the capsomeres arranged in a helical manner ($\times$117,450). (Courtesy of Micheline Fauvel, Laboratoire Santé Publique du Québec.)

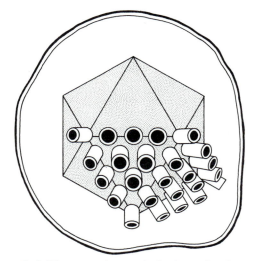

Figure 9–2 Diagram of a typical virus showing cubic symmetry. The core of the virus has the form of an icosahedron with 20 facets. It is covered by symmetrically arranged capsomeres, each consisting of a hollow tube. The covering of capsomeres constitutes the viral capsid. The virion (consisting of the genetic material and the capsid) has an outer membrane derived from the altered host plasma or nuclear membrane. (Drawing by Frederick Lammerich, Department of Art as Applied to Medicine, University of Toronto.)

as well as expensive. Also, the animals often harbored their own viruses, and these sometimes served as contaminants. Embryonated hen's eggs were next used, but apart from the absence of an immune response, they had similar disadvantages. Cell culture has now largely replaced these methods.

Animal cells (*e.g.*, kidney cells or fibroblasts) will grow as a single monolayer on a glass surface if this is covered by a suitable culture medium. Subcultures can be obtained from such a growth, but after repeated subculture, the cells cease to multiply and die off. Apparently, normal animal cells cannot live forever. Occasionally, the cells undergo an alteration and continued subculture is possible. The process is called *transformation*, and the cells are malignant (Chapter 12). Established cell lines of this type can be kept growing

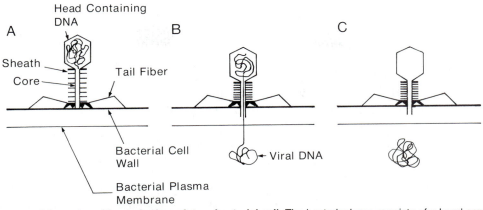

Figure 9–4 Diagram of the entry of bacteriophage into a bacterial cell. The bacteriophage consists of a head containing DNA, a rigid core surrounded by a sheath to which is attached a tail piece and tail fibers. *A*, The first event in the entry of the phage is the attachment of the tail fibers to the receptors of the bacterial cell wall. *B*, Contraction of the sheath results in the injection of viral DNA into the bacterial cell substance. *C*, The protein component of the phage shown attached to the cell wall is subsequently lost, leaving the viral DNA within the substance of the bacterium. Here, it can replicate and lead to lysis of the bacterial cell, or it can remain latent as prophage.

indefinitely and are used for virus culture. The best known of these is the HeLa cell.

The first stage of virus-cell interaction is *attachment* of the virion to the cell surface. This is believed to be the result of an affinity of the virus for some specific cell receptors. With the relatively simple bacteriophage, the protein capsid of the organism remains on the outside of the cell, but the phage acts as a type of microsyringe, its DNA content being squirted into the cell substance (Fig. 9–4). With animal viruses, the process is less simple, because the stage following attachment is *penetration* of the virus particle into the cell by a process of *endocytosis*. Initially, the virus is contained within a phagosome; then, by means that are not clearly understood, it escapes from the phagosome and enters the cytoplasm proper. The next stage is one of *uncoating* of the virus so that the free nucleic acid is released. The virus now ceases to exist as a particle and may not even be infective. Nevertheless, its component parts can still be detected. This stage in viral multiplication is known as the *eclipse phase* and is a feature of the reproductive cycle of all true viruses.

The information in the viral nucleic acid is transcribed and diverts the host's cell activity into synthesizing viral coded enzymes, regulating protein synthesis and ultimately leading to the production of more viral nucleic acid and viral structural proteins. The precise way in which this occurs varies considerably from one virus to another.

DNA Viruses. The viral DNA encodes for specific mRNA, and this is translated on host ribosomes. This leads to the formation of enzymes that are needed later for the subsequent synthesis of new viral DNA and structural proteins that form the viral coat.

RNA Viruses. Viruses in this group vary considerably in how they replicate within cells. With some viruses (*e.g.*, poliovirus), the viral RNA acts as messenger RNA that encodes for enzymes and viral proteins and as a complementary RNA that is used as a template for the formation of new viral RNA. With other viruses, especially those that are enveloped, such as the myxoviruses, the viral RNA leads to the formation first of a complementary strand of RNA, which then acts as mRNA for the production of new enzymes, viral protein, and new viral RNA. The replication of RNA retroviruses is quite different from either of the two previous methods. Virus-specific DNA is formed by reverse transcriptase and becomes incorporated in the host cell's genome. Virus RNA is transcribed from this virus-specific DNA.

It is evident that the replication of viruses is a complex affair. The result is that the specific nucleic acid, either RNA or DNA, is manufactured together with the protein component of the capsomeres. The final result is assembly of mature virus particles, and this may occur either in the cytoplasm or in the nucleus. Finally, the particles are released from the cell.

Release of Virus Particles. The virus-infected cell may be so damaged that it disintegrates, and mature virus particles are released in a burstlike fashion. Under other circumstances, the cell is not destroyed, and virus particles are released slowly. In the latter type of infection, the virus frequently receives an additional coat, termed an *envelope*, from a cell membrane. Thus, the ortho-myxoviruses receive an envelope of cell membrane (Fig. 9–5). This membrane is not a completely normal cell membrane, but one that has been modified by the effect of virus and contains viral type antigens. Herpesvirus, a DNA virus that is assembled in the nucleus, acquires an envelope of modified nuclear membrane from the host cell (Fig. 9–6C).

Cell and Tissue Reactions to Viruses

Viruses are obligatory intracellular parasites, and the initial cellular damage they produce is

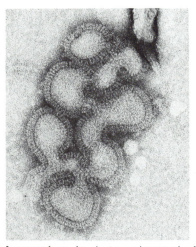

Figure 9–5 A myxovirus. An electron micrograph of influenza A/2, England 4272, which is demonstrated by negative staining. The irregular shape of the virus is clearly seen, and the well-marked covering membrane from which numerous prickles project is also observable. These projections contain hemagglutinin; it is to these structures that red blood cells become adherent. The RNA within the virion is not apparent in this photograph (×120,000). (Courtesy of Micheline Fauvel, Laboratoire du Santé Publique du Québec.)

followed by a local inflammatory reaction. In infected animals, the effect of a viral infection may be to cause cell necrosis as illustrated by the epidermal necrosis encountered in herpes simplex infection or the nerve cell necrosis in poliomyelitis. Indeed, in most human viral diseases, cellular destruction is the predominant lesion. The respiratory viruses, such as the influenza viruses, destroy the tracheal and bronchial surface epithelia. The viruses of hepatitis and yellow fever cause liver cell necrosis. On the other hand, a cell infected with a virus can undergo proliferation; the common wart provides a good example. Whether a cell degenerates or proliferates depends on the type of cell involved as well as on the particular infecting virus. With labile cells like those of surface epithelia, viral infection may produce proliferative or degenerative lesions. With permanent cells, *e.g.,* neurons that cannot divide after birth, viral infections are necessarily always destructive in tendency.

As noted, viruses sometimes kill the cells that they infect. In tissue culture, this is termed a *cytopathic effect* and is useful in diagnostic virology. If known specific antiserum is added to a culture, inhibition of the cytopathic effect helps identify an unknown virus (Figs. 9–7 and 9–8).

Sometimes an infecting virus alters the cell, but it does not kill it. A common effect is the formation of a mass of homogeneous material, called an *inclusion body,* either in the nucleus or in the cytoplasm of the infected cell. Inclusion bodies consist of maturing viral material and can be used as markers in the identification of a viral disease. Thus, the finding of characteristic inclusion bodies (Negri bodies) in the neurons of a dog is diagnostic of rabies.

Viral nucleic acid can sometimes enter the nucleic acid pool (genome) of the host cell and become incorporated into the host's genetic material. The viral nucleic acid then replicates when the cell divides; in fact, it behaves like a gene. This symbiotic relationship can result in the cell's showing no evidence of infection. The virus is *latent.*

Under certain circumstances, the nucleic acid of a latent virus can replicate and behave once more as an infective agent. The cell may then be damaged. Some examples illustrating the impli-

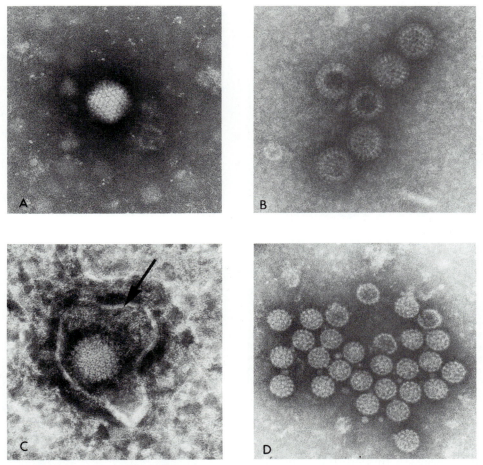

Figure 9–6. *A,* Adenovirus. This virus, which is demonstrated by negative staining, has the typical icosahedral form and has no outer envelope (×167,760). *B,* Rotavirus. This virus has not yet been grown in tissue cultures. It can be found by electron microscopy in the stools of some infants with acute gastroenteritis. This disease is a major cause of illness during childhood and is particularly common in infants under the age of 2 years; it often occurs in winter. Some cases are due to bacterial infection *(e.g., Salmonella, Escherichia coli),* but most cases appear to be due to viruses (×136,300). *C,* Herpes simplex virus. The envelope, which is clearly shown (arrow), is derived from the modified nuclear membrane of an infected cell. The hollow capsomeres of the virion are clearly visible (×139,800). (Compare this with Fig. 9–2.) *D,* Papovavirus, S.V. 40. This organism was found as a contaminant in a culture of African green monkey kidney cells. Another important member of this group of viruses is the polyoma virus. In tissue culture, the cells show characteristic vacuolation. The name papova is derived from *pa*pilloma, *po*lyoma, *va*cuolating agent (×136,300). (Courtesy of Micheline Fauvel, Laboratoire de Santé Publique du Québec.)

cations of this remarkable relationship are as follows.

Some bacteria contain a latent bacteriophage. Such a cell may show altered function. For example, production of toxin by the diphtheria bacillus is determined by the presence of a phage. A latent virus may suddenly lead to lysis of a whole culture. Such a strain of bacteria is termed lysogenic. A similar phenomenon occurs in varicella (chickenpox) infection. The virus can re-

main latent for many months or years in human beings. At any time, it can be reactivated and cause herpes zoster (shingles).

Secondary to the cellular damage produced by viral infection there is an acute inflammatory reaction with vascular dilation and an exudate containing lymphocytes and macrophages. Polymorphs are usually few in number. Most viral diseases are acute and of short duration, terminating in either rapid death of the patient or

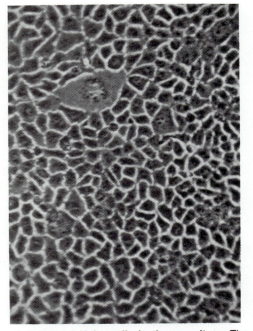

Figure 9–7 Normal HeLa cells in tissue culture. The confluent sheet is composed of plump polygonal cells derived from a malignant epithelial cell line that originated from a carcinoma in a patient named Helen Lane, hence the name "HeLa." A giant cell form is conspicuous in this field. This photograph was obtained by use of phase contrast microscopy (×200). (From Walter, J.B., and Israel, M.S.: General Pathology. 6th ed. Edinburgh, Churchill Livingstone, 1987.)

recovery. Exceptions to this are the tumor-producing viruses including the papilloma or wart virus, the slow viruses, hepatitis B virus, and those viruses producing latent infections, *e.g.,* measles, varicella-zoster viruses, and herpes simplex.

The General Body Reaction to Viral Infection

Viruses first contaminate and then infect a surface integument by inhalation (*e.g.,* influenza), by ingestion (*e.g.,* poliomyelitis), or by the bite of an arthropod vector (*e.g.,* yellow fever). If infection is established, some viruses produce a localized infection (*e.g.,* human papilloma virus causing warts), whereas others spread via the blood stream and produce infection in an organ remote from the site of primary infection (*e.g.,* the nervous system in poliomyelitis). Some viruses spread widely to many organs. During this early viremic phase, there is often fever. This may be followed by a short remission, but fever returns when the virus becomes clinically evident at its organ of destination. Sometimes the infection involves many organs, and this systemic type of infection is associated with constitutional symptoms that are much more pronounced than the localized one.

When a vital organ, such as the liver in hepatitis, is severely damaged, the cause of death is obvious—the patient dies of liver failure. In other diseases, the mode of death is less obvious. A state of "shock" develops; it is suggested that this is due to virus invasion of endothelial cells and vascular damage.

Immune Response

With most viral infections, there is a brisk immune response; a high titer of immunoglobu-

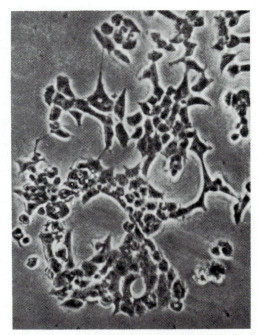

Figure 9–8 HeLa cells in culture infected with adenovirus. The sheet of cells is broken up, and the swollen, refractile cells have fused to form irregular masses. This response is called the cytopathic effect of the virus. Specific antisera will inhibit this effect. Using known antisera, one can identify a particular virus. Likewise, if cultures of a known virus are used, the ability of a serum to inhibit the cytopathic effect can be used to estimate the titer and specificity of antibody (×200). (From Walter, J.B., and Israel, M.S.: General Pathology. 6th ed. Edinburgh, Churchill Livingstone, 1987.)

lins is present during convalescence, and their detection is useful in retrospective diagnosis. With some generalized viral infections, such as chickenpox, measles, and mumps, the immune response is marked, and a second attack of these diseases is very uncommon. In the case of the common cold, a localized infection, there is some antibody formation, but the degree of immunity produced is slight, and repeated infections are common. An additional reason for recurrent attacks of this particular infection is that there are over 100 different antigenic strains of rhinoviruses. The element of *hypersensitivity* in viral infections is evident in the pathogenesis of the skin eruption that occurs in the course of generalized infections such as chickenpox and measles. These diseases have an incubation period of about 2 weeks, during which interval the skin is sensitized to viral products. When a secondary viremia occurs, the skin reacts with the characteristic exanthem of the disease. The pathogenesis resembles that of typhoid fever.

Immunity to viral infection may be related to the presence of antibodies or it may be cell mediated.

Cell-Mediated Immunity. If T-lymphocyte function is deficient, simple viral infections, such as chickenpox and herpes simplex, can be severe and lead to death. This indicates the key role that T cells play in defense against viral infection. In contrast, subjects with agammaglobulinemia can resist most viral infections but are susceptible to some bacterial infections. The T-cell response to viral infection is directed against the products of viral genes in combination with products of the major histocompatibility complex of the host cell. *Specific cytotoxic T cells* directly kill the virus-infected cell. *Delayed type hypersensitivity* is another consequence of T-cell immunity. The tissue necrosis and inflammatory reaction that occur also result in viral destruction. Finally, T cells release interferon-gamma.

Interferon. The infection of a cell with one type of virus can prevent an infection by another type virus, a phenomenon termed viral interference. The mechanism is the production of a protein of low molecular weight called interferon that enables the cell to prevent a second infection. Furthermore, interferon can diffuse to adjacent cells and render them resistant to infec-

tion. Interferon causes a cell to produce agents called translation-inhibiting proteins, which are thought to prevent translation of viral mRNA without impairing the cell's own protein synthesis. The production of interferon does not save an infected cell but, by its effects on adjacent cells, prevents the spread of the infection within the body and is probably a major factor in recovery from an acute attack. Interferon does not produce lasting immunity to viral infection.

Various attempts have been made to use interferon as a prophylactic agent; however, it is species specific, and only human interferon is effective in the treatment or prophylaxis of human disease. Human interferon was initially manufactured from human cells in culture, but by the employment of recombinant DNA techniques, it can be produced in large quantities.

The Diagnosis of Virus Disease

Viruses survive for a number of hours or days in special transport media that are used for conveying unfrozen specimens to the laboratory, where they can be cultured by use of the living cell systems already described. The virus may then be typed by means of complement fixation and neutralization tests with use of specific antisera. Some viruses with a characteristic shape can be identified by electron microscopy; by use of negative contrast techniques, they may be detected within a few minutes of receipt of the specimen. For practical purposes, this method is used for examining specimens obtained from readily accessible sites that contain high concentrations of virus (*e.g.*, poxviruses and herpesviruses from skin lesions; rotaviruses, adenoviruses, and hepatitis A virus from the feces).

Immunofluorescence techniques using monoclonal antibodies are also valuable in the rapid diagnosis of viral disease; either secretions or sections of tissue may be used. The method is more sensitive than is electron microscopy.

Diagnostic inclusion bodies may be found in viral lesions in either smears or sections, but this method of diagnosis is of value only in a few diseases (*e.g.*, Negri bodies in rabies; skin with varicella-zoster and herpes simplex infections).

Antigen Detection in Diagnosis. Viral antigen

can be found in the blood or tissue fluids in certain viral infections, *e.g.,* carriers of hepatitis B virus.

Examination of Convalescent Serum. There is often a rise in titer of antibodies against the agent during the course of the disease and during convalescence—stages at which the virus itself cannot be easily detected. Hence, in practice, viral diseases are often diagnosed retrospectively from serologic analysis. It is important to obtain a sample of serum early in the disease; this furnishes a baseline against which to judge any subsequent rise.

Viral Chemotherapy

The fact that the infected cell's own metabolic pathways and ribosomes are used for virus reproduction made it seem unlikely that a specific blocking chemotherapeutic agent could be found. This initial pessimism was not justified, and it is evident that viruses have very specific actions: attachment to the cell membrane, penetration, uncoating, production of new viral material, and finally the assembly and release of mature viral particles. These are highly specific events, each of which is a point of attack. Already a number of compounds are known that will act as chemotherapeutic agents, but unfortunately most of them are too toxic to be of clinical use. Amantadine specifically blocks the penetration of influenza A virus into cells and can be used as a prophylactic drug in the event of a widespread epidemic. 5-Iodo-2′-deoxyuridine (idoxuridine or 5-IDU) inhibits the growth of vaccinia and herpes simplex viruses; but in practice, its use for the common herpes infection (coldsores) of the skin is very disappointing. Cytosine arabinoside and adenine arabinoside (ARA-A) have been used in the treatment of herpetic encephalitis and severe varicella-zoster infections. Like 5-IDU, they are too toxic to be useful agents except in desperate situations. *Acyclovir* is an acyclic purine thymidine analogue. Before affecting a virus, it must first be activated by enzyme thymidine kinase produced by the virus itself. Hence, it is active only in virus-infected cells. Acyclovir is used topically and systemically against herpes simplex and varicella-zoster infections. *Ribavirin* is a

guanosine analogue that is effective in the treatment of respiratory syncytial virus infections. *Zidovidine (AZT)* and other drugs have been developed for the treatment of AIDS. Some palliation is to be expected, but a cure is not in sight. This applies also to our current treatment of many viral infections; it is hoped that in the future more effective and less toxic drugs will be developed.

Classification of Viruses

The classification of viruses is based on size; morphologic features, including the presence or absence of an envelope; antigenic structure; and the disease caused by the organism. Of equal importance is the type of nucleic acid present, its relationship to viral mRNA, and the mode of replication of the virus. A complex classification has evolved and is under constant review. Some viruses are not easy to place in this classification, *e.g.,* the virus of hepatitis B that is described in Chapter 24.

Table 9–1 shows the main viruses described in this chapter.

Some Common Viral Infections

Adenoviruses

The adenoviruses are DNA-containing viruses that are common commensals of the upper respiratory tract. They cause a variety of mild upper respiratory tract infections and conjunctivitis (Fig. 9–6A).

Herpesviruses

The herpesviruses are medium-sized, spherical, double-stranded, enveloped, DNA-containing viruses that produce a characteristic cytopathic effect in cells grown in tissue culture (Fig. 9–6C). After the initial primary infection, the herpesviruses have the ability to remain latent in the host tissues for long periods. The six human herpesviruses are described: herpes simplex type

Table 9–1 COMMON VIRUS INFECTIONS

Family	Individual Species
DNA Viruses	
Adenoviridae	Human serotypes of adeno-viruses
Herpetoviridae	Herpes simplex viruses
	Varicella-zoster virus
	Cytomegalovirus
	Epstein-Barr virus
Poxviridae	Smallpox virus
	Vaccinia virus
Papovaviridae	Human papillomaviruses
RNA Viruses	
Picornaviridae	Polioviruses
	Coxsackieviruses
	Echoviruses
	Other enteroviruses
	Common cold viruses
Togaviridae	Encephalitis viruses
	Yellow fever virus
	Dengue virus
Orthomyxoviridae	Influenza viruses
Paramyxoviridae	Parainfluenza viruses
	Mumps virus
	Measles virus
	Respiratory syncytial virus
Rhabdoviridae	Rabies virus
Retroviridae	Animal tumor and leukemia viruses
	HTLV-1 and HTLV-2 in humans
	Human immunodeficiency viruses

Modified from Walter, J.B., and Israel, M.S.: General Pathology. 6th ed. Edinburgh, Churchill Livingstone, 1987.

1 and type 2, varicella-zoster virus, cytomegalovirus, Epstein-Barr virus, and herpes 6 virus.

Herpes Simplex Virus. Herpes simplex virus (HSV), of which there are two strains, is one of the most widely distributed viruses in human beings; by the age of 70 years, virtually all individuals have been infected as judged by the presence of antibodies. HSV-1 usually affects mucous membrane of the mouth or the surrounding skin; HSV-2 commonly affects the genital region and is transmitted venereally. It is now one of the most important sexually transmitted diseases. Herpes occurs as a primary infection and is sometimes followed by recurrent lesions.

Primary Infections. The primary infection usually passes unnoticed by the patient but in about 10 per cent or less of individuals is clinically apparent as acute gingivostomatitis, keratoconjunctivitis, vulvovaginitis, or cervicitis. Abrasions of the skin predispose to primary herpetic infection (traumatic or inoculation herpes simplex). A good example of this is the very painful *herpetic whitlow,* which is seen in individuals such as nurses, dentists, and anesthetists who come in contact with nasobronchial secretions. About one third of young adults lack antibodies to herpes simplex and are susceptible to infection. *Herpetic proctitis* occurs in the passive partner after anal intercourse. A chronic herpetic proctitis is a common feature of AIDS.

The most severe form of herpes infection is generalized visceral herpes simplex, a fatal infection in which necrotic lesions are present in many organs. It is encountered in patients with T-lymphocyte deficiency. A similar severe infection can occur in the neonatal period, the infant having been infected from genital lesions of the mother. Indeed, the presence of active genital herpes at term is an indication for cesarian section because of this grave risk to the newborn infant. Acute necrotizing encephalitis is another severe form of herpes simplex infection.

Recurrent Herpetic Infections. After the primary infection, a number of subjects develop recurrent lesions, often in the same general area of the body. The most common manifestation is recurrent "coldsores" on the lips or adjacent skin of the face; unlike a primary infection, the mucous membrane of the mouth is rarely affected. Nevertheless, involvement of the eye can occur and is a serious complication because the cornea can be scarred. Any part of the skin can be involved, and the recurrent vesicular lesions at one site should always suggest herpes.* Attacks can be precipitated by a number of events, some quite trivial, *e.g.,* a common cold, exposure to strong sunlight, or emotional stress. *Recurrent genital herpes* is an important condition because apart from the discomfort it causes, it limits sexual activity and is psychologically disturbing. There is as yet no effective cure, but acyclovir is a useful drug especially in controlling symptoms and reducing the frequency of recurrences.

The skin lesions of herpes simplex cannot always be clinically distinguished from those of shingles. Virus particles can readily be identified

_____

*A fixed drug eruption is another cause.

in vesicle fluid by electron microscopy, but distinction between herpes simplex virus and varicella-zoster virus must rely on serologic investigations or culture. Varicella-zoster virus grows slowly in tissue culture; herpes simplex virus produces a massive cytopathic effect, usually within 24 hours.

Varicella and Zoster. Although the well-known clinical features of varicella (chickenpox) and zoster are poles apart, there is good evidence that they are both caused by the same virus.

Chickenpox. This disease has a pathogenesis similar to that of smallpox. It exhibits an enanthem with vesicles on the oral mucosa followed by an exanthem of vesicles on the skin, which subsequently become pustular. The skin eruption tends to occur in crops, so that lesions at different stages of development are present at the same time, and the distribution of the rash is different. In chickenpox, the lesions are not clustered in areas of pressure and tend to be most profuse on the trunk. In smallpox, the limbs, face, and back are most severely affected.

Congenital Varicella Syndrome. If the mother develops chickenpox during the first 6 months of pregnancy, infection of the fetus can lead to severe damage including underdevelopment of the limbs, brain damage, chorioretinitis, and cataract. Transmission of the virus later in pregnancy may result in a severe systemic illness but not the development of malformations.

Zoster (Shingles). After an attack of chickenpox, the virus may lie latent in the posterior root ganglia of the spinal, trigeminal, or facial nerves. In later life, the virus can be reactivated and can spread down the nerve fibers to the skin, producing the lesions of herpes zoster (Fig. 9–9).

The onset of an attack is characterized by discomfort or pain in the area affected. Next, erythema (redness) and swelling appear, followed by crops of papules and vesicles, which often become hemorrhagic before maturing to form pustules (see Chapter 31 for definitions of these terms). These dry, and the crusts finally fall off to leave areas of scarring and irregular pigmentation. Shingles commonly involves one or more of the branches of the fifth cranial nerve; if the eye is affected, special care is needed to prevent permanent damage to the cornea (Fig. 9–10). Pain is a feature of shingles and is often

severe when the face is involved. The pain can persist for many months after the skin lesions have healed *(post-herpetic neuralgia)*. This emphasizes the fact that shingles is primarily an infection involving nerves.

Children exposed to a patient with zoster can develop chickenpox if they are susceptible.

Cytomegalovirus. Infection by this virus of the herpes group causes a variety of syndromes. Infected cells are enlarged and develop large intranuclear inclusions, a feature that has given the organism its name. Transplacental infection of the fetus can cause a fulminating disease. Children and adults can acquire the infection either in a subclinical form or as an illness that resembles infectious mononucleosis. Widespread infection can occur in the immunosuppressed patient. It is one of the infections that can kill patients with AIDS.

Epstein-Barr Virus. This herpesvirus is the cause of infectious mononucleosis. It is also associated with nasopharyngeal carcinoma and Burkitt's lymphoma (Chapter 12).

Herpes 6 Virus. Recently, herpes 6 virus (human B lymphotropic virus) has been associated with roseola infantum, sometimes called sixth disease. This infection of young children causes a brief febrile illness followed by an exanthem of rose-red macules on the trunk and face. They fade after about 2 days.

Poxviruses

The poxviruses are large, brick-shaped, DNA-containing viruses that produce vesicular and pustular lesions of the skin. Many animals have their own variety of pox disease, *e.g.,* mousepox and cowpox. The human equivalent is smallpox, or variola. The virus that causes the common skin disease molluscum contagiosum is also a poxvirus (Fig. 9–11).

Smallpox. This disease is acquired by inhalation of virus; the primary site of infection is in the nasopharynx. The virus multiplies locally, spreads via the lymphatics, and finally reaches the blood stream. There is involvement of the mononuclear phagocyte system. Viral multiplication is followed by a second phase of viremia about 10 days later, and this coincides with the

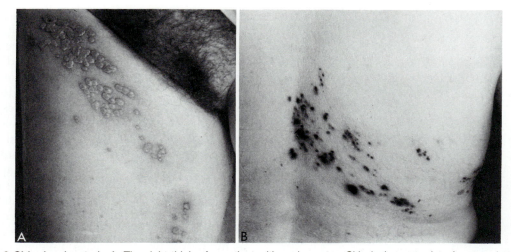

Figure 9–9 Shingles (zoster). *A,* The right thigh of a patient with early zoster. Skin lesions consist of grouped, tender water blisters (vesicles), each surrounded by a zone of redness (erythema). The lesions are distributed along the second lumbar nerve. As the disease progresses, the lesions dry up and become encrusted. *B,* A typical case of zoster at the stage of crusting. Note how the lesions follow the line of the cutaneous nerves that parallel the ribs. The lesions do not cross the midline; this is an important sign that helps distinguish zoster from other localized blistering diseases, such as a contact dermatitis. The lesions of zoster heal with scarring and are often painful, particularly in elderly patients.

onset of the prodromal stage with symptoms such as malaise, headache, and fever. About 4 days later, the skin eruption develops and the patient becomes seriously ill. Smallpox is highly infectious; in the past, there have been severe epidemics with a mortality of up to 50 per cent. In those who survive, the skin lesions heal with scarring, which leaves the typical "pockmarks" on the face.

Edward Jenner discovered that the natural pox infection of bovine animals, cowpox, could produce a localized lesion in human beings and that this provided protection against subsequent smallpox infection. The development of a live vaccine followed, but the precise origin of the vaccinia virus is not certain. It is probably a mutant of either variola or cowpox virus. Widespread and compulsory vaccination has finally eradicated smallpox. The last naturally occurring case was in Somalia in October 1977. There was one other case of smallpox in September 1978. It occurred in Birmingham, England, and was acquired accidentally in a research laboratory. Since no known carrier state exists, smallpox is now regarded as having become extinct. The only possible way of acquiring the disease is from a strain of virus kept in a reference laboratory.

Vaccination against the disease is a thing of the past.

Papillomaviruses: Infectious Warts

The human papillomavirus (HPV) that causes warts can be demonstrated electron microscopically but has yet to be cultured *in vitro*. At least 32 distinct serotypes has been identified, and each has a particular pattern of infection. Thus, HPV-1 is associated with deep plantar warts, HPV-2 and HPV-4 with common warts, and HPV-6 and HPV-11 with condylomata acuminata.

The papilloma viruses belong to a larger family of viruses termed the *papovaviruses*. This also includes polyoma virus and the JC virus. Infection with JC virus is common. It causes a trivial upper respiratory illness in childhood. However, the virus persists and can become reactivated in immunodeficiency states (*e.g.,* AIDS). A severe degenerative neurologic disease (progressive multifocal leukoencephalopathy) is the result.

Enteroviruses

The enteroviruses are small, single-stranded RNA viruses found particularly in the intestine.

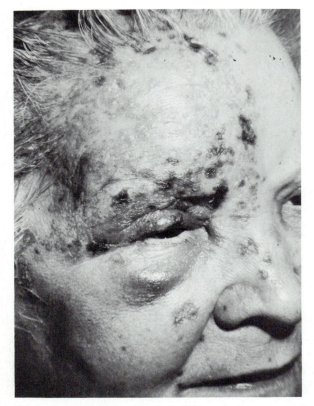

Figure 9–10 Shingles (zoster). This patient has well-advanced lesions of zoster involving the ophthalmic and maxillary divisions of the right fifth cranial nerve (trigeminal nerve). Although the eyelids are swollen and show vesicles with crusting, the conjunctiva and cornea were spared. The branch that supplies the cornea also supplies the tip of the nose, which in this patient is also uninvolved.

They cause a variety of infections and are particularly associated with neurologic involvement. Enterovirus type 72 is now recognized as the cause of hepatitis A. Polioviruses, coxsackie viruses, and echoviruses are the major species in the enterovirus genus.

Poliovirus. Poliomyelitis (infantile paralysis) is caused by the poliovirus, of which there are three strains. The disease is acquired by ingesting material contaminated by virus-containing feces. The virus proliferates in the cells of the bowel, and if the infection is not arrested at this stage, the virus enters the blood stream via the lymphatics. It multiplies in various extraneuronal sites; after 7 to 14 days (the incubation period of the disease), virus particles re-enter the blood stream and fever commences. Even at this stage

of viremia, the disease may be arrested without severe effect.

If the condition proceeds, the virus finally invades the central nervous system and localizes in the motor nerve cells of the medulla and spinal cord. Some of the infected cells are destroyed, and paralysis ensues. It should be stressed that although many people are infected with poliomyelitis, only a few develop a clinical disease, and of these, only some develop paralysis. A number of factors are known that appear to precipitate paralytic poliomyelitis. One of these is local trauma. If a patient who is already infected with poliomyelitis has his tonsils removed, paralysis of the pharynx can occur. This is known as the bulbar type of disease. Likewise, an injection at any site can precipitate paralysis. Therefore, it is important that during an epidemic of poliomyelitis, no one should be subjected to

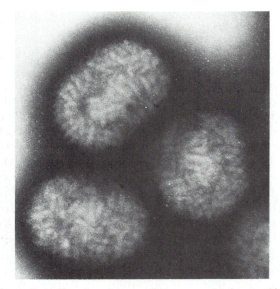

Figure 9–11 Poxvirus from molluscum contagiosum. Molluscum contagiosum is a viral disease of the skin that is characterized by the formation of small umbilicated papules. It is common in children and is a self-limiting disease. A suspension of material from a human lesion was mixed with a solution of 2 per cent phosphotungstic acid and allowed to dry on a suitably prepared copper grid coated with a film of carbon. Under the electron microscope, the electron-dense background produced by the phosphotungstic acid allows the viral particles to stand out quite clearly. This technique, which is known as negative staining, is frequently used to demonstrate viral particles. Poxviruses are large, square, and structurally complex. The outer protein layer consisting of strands is shown here (×105,850). (Courtesy of Micheline Fauvel, Laboratoire de Santé Publique du Québec.)

unnecessary surgical trauma, nor should injections for immunization against other disease, such as diphtheria, be given.

Active Immunization. The first effective vaccine was devised by Salk, who used poliovirus grown in monkey kidney cells and subsequently inactivated by formaldehyde. The Salk vaccine is administered by intramuscular injection, and three or four doses are given to ensure adequate antigenic stimulation. The vaccine stimulates the production of immunoglobulins. This does not prevent infection of the intestine with poliovirus, but it does prevent subsequent spread of the virus to involve the central nervous system. The vaccine can advantageously be combined with other vaccines and toxoids.

The vaccine developed by Sabin is a live attenuated virus and is given by mouth. The attenuated virus causes an intestinal infection that, like the Salk vaccine, stimulates the formation of immunoglobulin antibodies. However, there is one important difference between the vaccines: the Sabin vaccine also produces intestinal immunity because of the local formation of IgA. Thus, the Sabin vaccine prevents the subsequent infection with poliovirus, and if large populations are immunized with Sabin vaccine, virulent wild strains of the virus are replaced by Sabin type virus. Indeed, the few cases of poliomyelitis that still occur in the United States are due to Sabin-derived viruses.

Because the Sabin vaccine is easier to administer and more effective, it has become the more popular of the two methods of immunization. It is usual to give the three separate strains of poliovirus. As noted previously, the infection of a cell with one virus sometimes prevents infection with other viruses. To overcome this interference, three separate doses of the trivalent vaccine are administered.

The Coxsackieviruses. This group was so named because they were first isolated in the town of Coxsackie in New York State. There are a large number of viruses in this group, and they cause a variety of illnesses ranging from an upper respiratory infection resembling a cold to meningitis and myocarditis.

The Echoviruses. There are many types, causing a variety of infections, as do the coxsackieviruses.

The enteroviruses belong to a larger family termed *picornaviruses,* so named because of their size and nucleic acid content (*pico,* small + RNA). Two other genera are important, *rhinovirus* and *calicivirus.*

Rhinoviruses

These are small RNA-containing viruses that cause the common cold, by far the most frequent form of respiratory viral infection. The incubation period is 2 to 4 days; the disease is characterized by nasal discharge, sore throat, cough, and fever. There are a large number of different subtypes; repeated attacks can occur because neutralizing antibodies merely have a protective effect against reinfection with the particular serotype responsible.

Caliciviruses

These viruses cause gastrointestinal infections in animals and probably also in humans.

Togaviruses

This group of viruses contains members that cause encephalitis, yellow fever, dengue fever, and rubella (German measles). Many of these infections are spread by the bite of an arthropod and in the past have been classified as arthropod-borne viruses or *arboviruses.* This grouping is not currently used because its members differ widely in other important respects.

Togavirus Encephalitis. Many types are known and tend to be restricted to particular parts of the world. Some (*e.g.,* Western equine encephalitis of North America and Venezuelan equine encephalitis) are mild; others (*e.g.,* Eastern equine encephalitis of North America and Japanese B encephalitis) are severe.

Yellow Fever. One of the most severe diseases of the togavirus family is *yellow fever,* which is caused by a flavivirus and is spread by a mosquito. The disease is endemic in West Africa and

---

*Echo is the acronym for *e*nteric, *c*ytopathic, *h*uman, *o*rphan viruses. These viruses were first noted in children's feces and could not at first be linked with any disease.

Central America. The virus causes a severe illness characterized by hepatic necrosis resulting in jaundice, renal failure, and a high mortality.

Other Togavirus Fevers. *Dengue* is a major health problem in Southeast Asia, India, and the Pacific Islands. The disease is characterized by a severe febrile illness with a rash and severe pains in the limbs. It is rarely fatal, except in young children, in whom it may cause the *dengue hemorrhagic shock syndrome*. Clinically, this resembles a number of other distinct viral infections that are collectively known as the *hemorrhagic fevers* and have a high mortality. They are caused by viruses of different families (bunyaviruses and arenaviruses).

Orthomyxoviruses

This is a family of spherical or irregularly shaped viruses having a characteristic envelope that has the property of adhering to red blood cells (Fig. 9–5). Within the envelope, there is a strand of ribonucleoprotein having helical symmetry (Fig. 9–3). The orthomyxoviruses cause influenza, an illness characterized by an acute tracheobronchitis of abrupt onset. The severity of the illness varies from a mild upper respiratory infection with fever and chest pains (the flu) to a rapidly fatal illness with extensive pneumonia. The pneumonia may be due to the virus itself or to a coexistent bacterial infection, generally streptococcal or staphylococcal. Three types of influenza virus are known. *Influenza virus type A* is the most important and causes epidemics or pandemics of varying severity. In some, such as the pandemic of 1918, tens of millions of people died. Influenza virus type A readily mutates, so that new strains are continually appearing. Occasionally a virulent strain emerges, and an epidemic ensues because the population has no immunity to it. *Influenza virus type B* causes endemic cases and occasional epidemics, although these tend to affect a localized area. Type B virus shows less antigenic variation than does type A. *Influenza virus type C* appears to exist as one single type and causes a subclinical or very mild upper respiratory infection.

Paramyxoviruses

These viruses resemble the orthomyxoviruses in morphologic features but are larger and more pleomorphic. The group includes the viruses described in the following.

Parainfluenza Viruses. These cause respiratory infections similar to influenza. In infants, parainfluenza viruses cause *croup* or *acute laryngotracheobronchitis*. This is characterized by hoarseness and cough and may lead to severe respiratory distress. Bronchiolitis and pneumonia may occur.

Respiratory Syncytial Virus. This virus produces a cytopathic effect in tissue culture, and the virus-infected cells tend to fuse together to form giant cells or a syncytium, from which the virus acquires its name. Infection may occur at any age to produce a common cold–like illness, but the importance of this virus is that it is a common cause of *bronchiolitis and pneumonia in infants* under 1 year of age and is indeed the most common cause in those under 6 months.

Mumps Virus. Mumps is a disease that has a long incubation period (18 to 21 days) and is characterized by fever and enlargement of one or both parotid glands (acute parotitis). In adult males, this may be complicated by involvement of one or both testes (acute orchitis). Infection of the ovaries may also occur. In both sexes, meningoencephalitis and pancreatitis are well-recognized complications.

Measles (Morbilli). This is the most infectious of the common fevers. A 10-day incubation period is followed by a 4-day illness with fever, tracheobronchitis, and conjunctivitis. The characteristic enanthem appears on the buccal mucosa as grains of salt on a red background; these "Koplik's spots" are diagnostic of the disease during this early catarrhal infectious phase. On the fourteenth day after exposure, the characteristic maculopapular exanthem appears. *German measles* (rubella) resembles measles clinically, but has a longer incubation period (16 to 18 days), and the prodromal stage is mild or absent. This otherwise trivial disease is of importance because it causes malformations and other abnormalities in the unborn children of pregnant women who contract the disease (Chapter 11). The virus of German measles is not paramyxovirus and is now classified as a rubivirus. It is included here for convenience.

Rhabdoviruses

Rabies. Rabies is caused by a bullet-shaped virus that normally infects certain species of animals. The disease is rare in human beings, but it is of intense interest for two reasons. With one possible exception, there has never been recorded a human case of rabies in which the patient survived. Although many diseases are fatal, the mode of death in rabies is particularly unpleasant. An initial phase of excitement with spasms and convulsions is characteristic. Particularly common are painful contractions of the pharyngeal muscles initiated by attempts to swallow water. Hence the term *hydrophobia,* meaning that the patients fear water. The stage of excitement is followed by one of generalized paralysis, and death usually occurs within a few days of its onset. Treatment is entirely supportive; the only hope is that the diagnosis is wrong.

Rabies is endemic in the fox population in Europe, whereas in North America it affects many other species of animals, particularly the skunk and raccoon. After the bite of an infected animal, the virus spreads to the nervous system via the nerve fibers. Rabies in dogs is invariably fatal within 10 days; if a person is bitten by a dog, it is important to keep the dog under surveillance for this period. If the dog dies or is killed, examination of the brain for Negri bodies is an important investigation.

If the person is bitten by a rabid animal or by an animal that escapes, the question of immunization is of paramount importance. It has been estimated that about 30,000 persons in the United States are given treatment each year for rabies immunization.

The original method of immunization against rabies was devised by Pasteur. He injected a vaccine derived from the dried spinal cords of infected rabbits. The method was painful, and repeated injections of foreign spinal cord tissue occasionally led to autoimmune encephalomyelitis (Chapter 6). Currently, the prevention of rabies after the bite of a suspected animal involves both the administration of rabies immune globulin and commencement of rabies vaccination. The vaccine consists of an inactivated virus grown in tissue culture (the human diploid cell rabies vaccine, HDCV) administered in five doses over 28 days.

Retroviruses

The retroviruses are an important group of RNA viruses that have a unique mode of reproduction. They contain an enzyme called reverse transcriptase that is used to make a DNA molecule that is complementary to viral RNA. This DNA provirus is integrated into the host cell's genome and directs the formation of viral encoded RNA. If the virus contains an oncogene, or activates a cell oncogene, the infected cell is transformed to a malignant cell (see Chapter 12). Such oncogenic retroviruses are responsible for certain leukemias, lymphomas, and sarcomas in birds, mice, and cats. In humans, one such virus has been associated with a T-cell lymphoma (human T-cell lymphotropic virus type 1 ([HTLV-1]); another, HTLV-2, has been associated with a leukemia. The best known example, however, is a virus originally called HTLV-3 but renamed human immunodeficiency virus (HIV), which is the cause of the acquired immunodeficiency syndrome or AIDS (see Chapter 6).

The Slow Viruses

Scrapie is a disease of sheep that is characterized by itching and by degeneration of the brain. It can be transmitted to sheep, goats, and mice, but the incubation period is long, rarely less than 4 months. The infective agent has unusual properties: it can withstand boiling, x-irradiation, and treatment with formalin. It contains little, if any, nucleic acid. Its nature is not understood, but it is grouped with other similar agents as a *slow virus.*

Kuru is a slowly progressive degenerative nervous disease of the Fore people of New Guinea and was originally thought to be inherited. It usually affected women and children of either sex, but not men. A tribal ritual was for women and children to eat the brains of deceased relatives, including those who had suffered from kuru, and it is believed that the disease is caused by a slow virus acquired by this tribute to the dead.

These rare and curious diseases have been mentioned not because they are ever likely to be encountered by a medical practitioner, but because they reveal the existence of patterns of infective disease quite different from those previously recognized. The hope is that other diseases will be found to be of similar nature, and that ways will be found to combat them.

Persistent Viral Infections

In addition to the slow virus infections described, there are a number of viral diseases caused by "conventional viruses" acting in an unusual manner. Sometimes the virus remains dormant, concealed in a variety of tissues (*e.g.,* adenovirus in lymphoid tissue; herpes simplex and varicella-zoster viruses in the dorsal root ganglia). Periodically, however, the virus may become activated to produce clinical illness. Progressive multifocal leukoencephalopathy and subacute sclerosing panencephalitis are other examples. Subacute sclerosing panencephalitis is caused by the measles virus acting in an obscure manner to produce a disease quite different from ordinary measles.

The viruses causing persistent infections have found ways to evade the immune system. This may explain why some of them infect the central nervous system, a site that is somewhat isolated from the cells of the general immune system. Another mechanism involves the virus directly attacking the cells of the immune system. This applies to the human T-cell lymphotropic virus type 1 and type 2 as well as being the major effect of the human immunodeficiency virus causing AIDS.

Summary

- Mycoplasmas are small, yet can grow in a cell-free medium; one species, *M. pneumoniae,* causes pneumonia in humans.
- *Chlamydia trachomatis* causes trachoma (a leading cause of blindness) and a variety of other eye and genital infections (urethritis and cervicitis). *C. psittaci,* a pathogen in birds, may cause interstitial pneumonia in humans.
- Rickettsiae are intracellular parasites. They cause various types of typhus, infections that are spread by lice, fleas, ticks, or mites. Rickettsialpox is a mild mite-borne disease; Q fever of Australia is generally acquired by inhalation.
- Viruses are obligatory intracellular parasites that rely on the parasitized cell's metabolism for energy and reproduction. After attachment and entry into the cell, an eclipse phase is characteristic. Within the cell, a virus may lie latent, lead to inclusion body formation, kill the cell (a cytopathic effect), or lead to neoplasia.
- Immunity to viral infection is due to immunoglobulins, cell-mediated mechanisms, and interferon.
- Viruses are classified on the basis of their nucleic acid content, their mode of replication, the presence of an envelope, and their pathogenicity.
- Herpes simplex virus causes acute followed by recurrent skin and mucous membrane lesions; sometimes there is widespread dissemination. Recurrent genital herpes (due to HSV-2) is an important sexually transmitted disease.
- Varicella (chickenpox) is a common mild infection in children but can cause severe damage to the fetus *in utero.* Zoster (shingles) is a late recurrence of the virus and affects one or more dermatomes.
- The papillomaviruses cause warts and condylomata and are implicated in cancer of the vulva and cervix.
- The polioviruses cause poliomyelitis, a disease that has an intestinal phase sometimes followed by central nervous system involvement. It is largely controlled by the Salk and Sabin vaccines.
- Upper respiratory tract infections (sometimes followed by pneumonia) are caused by many types of virus: adenoviruses, coxsackieviruses, echoviruses, rhinoviruses, and myxoviruses. Respiratory syncytial virus (a paramyxovirus) is an important cause of pneumonia in infants.
- Togaviruses cause encephalitis, yellow fever, dengue, and a variety of hemorrhagic fevers. Some are arthropod-borne and have been grouped as arboviruses.
- Rabies is acquired by the bite of a rabid animal. No treatment can avert death, but prophylaxis is effective.
- Retroviruses are RNA viruses that by reverse transcriptase produce DNA provirus that may integrate with host DNA. Human T-cell lymphotropic virus type 1 and type 2 are associated with lymphoma or leukemia. Human immunodeficiency virus (HIV) causes AIDS.
- Slow viruses have a very long incubation period, may not contain nucleic acid, and cause neurologic disease. Persistent viral infections (*e.g.,* measles) somewhat resemble these illnesses.

Selected Readings

Belshe, R. B. (ed.): Textbook of Human Virology. Littleton, Mass. PSG Publishing, 1984.

Bockman, J. M., et al.: Creutzfeldt-Jacob disease prion proteins in human brains. N. Engl. J. Med. *312*:73, 1985.

Brunham, R. C., et al.: Mucopurulent cervicitis: The ignored counterpart in women of urethritis in men. N. Engl. J. Med. *311*:1, 1984.

Cassell, G. H., and Cole, B. C.: Mycoplasmas, agents of human disease. N. Engl. J. Med. *304*:80, 1981.

Corey, L., and Spear, P. G.: Infections with herpes simplex viruses. N. Engl. J. Med. *314*:686, 1986.

Haywood, A. M.: Patterns of persistent viral infections. N. Engl. J. Med. *315*:939, 1986.

Schachter, J.: Chlamydial infections. N. Engl. J. Med. *298*:428, 490, and 540, 1978.

Sharpe, A. H., and Fields, B. N.: Pathogenesis of viral infections: Basic concepts derived from the reovirus model. N. Engl. J. Med. *312*:486, 1985.

Timbury, M. C.: Notes on Medical Virology. 7th ed. Edinburgh, Churchill Livingstone, 1983.

Warrell, D. A.: Rabies. Med. Clin. North Am. *5*:569, 1980.

Weller, T. H.: Varicella and herpes zoster. N. Engl. J. Med. *309*:1362 and 1434, 1983.

Fungal, Protozoal, and Helminthic Infections

After studying this chapter, the student should be able to:

- Outline the main groups of infection caused by fungi.
- Describe the clinical features of amebiasis, including the mode of infection.
- Describe the effects of infection with *Giardia lambia*.
- Explain the life cycle of the malaria parasite and the effects of infection in humans.
- Describe the manifestations of toxoplasmosis in the adult and in the newborn.
- Discuss the mode of transmission of trypanosomiasis and the main features of the three forms of the disease in humans.
- Compare and contrast the three types of leishmaniasis.
- Describe the importance of *Trichomonas vaginalis* as a pathogen.
- Discuss the importance of *Pneumocystis carinii* as a human pathogen.
- Distinguish between the definitive and the intermediate host of a helminth.
- Describe the major differences between the tapeworms, the flukes, and the roundworms.
- Describe the life cycles of the helminths listed in Table 10–3 and outline the effects on humans of infection with these parasites.

FUNGAL INFECTIONS

The classification of fungi is complex and unsatisfactory, but for practical purposes four varieties can be recognized: *molds*, which grow as long filaments (hyphae) that branch and interlace to form a meshwork or mycelium; *yeasts*, which are unicellular and grow by budding only; *yeast-like fungi*, which grow partly as yeasts and partly as long filamentous forms called pseudohyphae; and *dimorphic fungi*, which can grow either as hyphae or as yeasts, according to the cultural conditions.

The great majority of fungi are saprophytic and play an important part in nature by breaking down organic material. They have been of great service to people in the production of bread, cheese, and alcoholic beverages. In the last several decades, they have attracted interest because antibiotic substances that they produce have been of great value as therapeutic agents.

Diseases Caused by Fungi

Fungal infections (the *mycoses*) may be divided into two groups. The superficial mycoses, described in Chapter 31, are very common and they affect skin only. The deep or systemic mycoses, on the other hand, are uncommon causes of clinical illness, but they have recently come to the fore because they complicate illnesses in which there is impairment of the T-cell component of the immune response. The primary lesion is usually in the lung, and these diseases are described in Chapter 22.

Other Fungal Infections. More than 100,000 species of fungi are known; of these, about 100 are human pathogens. Apart from those previously mentioned, there are others that occasionally produce infection under particular circumstances. For the most part they act as secondary invaders in the course of other diseases, or they are encountered as opportunistic infections when immunity is weakened. Others occur under particular local conditions. Thus, in India, injuries to the feet are sometimes infected by fungi, leading to chronic suppurative lesions involving the skin, subcutaneous tissues, and bone; pathologically it resembles actinomycosis and is called *maduromycosis* or *Madura foot*. Some cases of Madura foot are caused by infection with higher bacteria, *e.g., Nocardia* and *Streptococcus* organisms.

The widespread use of immunosuppressive drugs combined with modern technology that keeps patients alive, but in a debilitated state, has led to a considerable increase in the incidence of fungal infections. Indeed, in the modern hospital, they form one of the most important and lethal examples of opportunistic infection.

PROTOZOAL INFECTIONS

Protozoa are unicellular motile animals that have a well-defined nucleus. Some travel by ameboid movement; others are ciliated or have a single flagellum. They are widely distributed in nature, but few species are pathogenic to humans. Yet one of these causes malaria, which is currently the major human infectious disease problem. Worldwide, approximately 125 million people are believed to be infected.

Amebiasis

It has been estimated that about 10 per cent of the world's population harbor *Entamoeba histolytica;* the incidence ranges from under 5 per cent in the United States to over 40 per cent in the tropics. The majority of these people are asymptomatic and act as carriers.

Entamoeba histolytica exists in two forms: an active amebic trophozoite, which is present in active lesions of the disease; and a cyst, which develops when the organism is confronted by adverse conditions. It is by the swallowing of cysts that the disease is acquired. Cysts can withstand the acidity of the gastric juice and develop into active trophozoites, which by invading the mucosa of the large intestine cause catarrhal inflammation and ulceration. After infection, symptoms are absent (in *asymptomatic carriers*), or they consist of intermittent diarrhea with the passage of blood and mucus (*chronic amebic dysentery);* sometimes the colitis is severe and has an abrupt onset. Fever, severe abdominal pain, and the passage of profuse blood-stained stools are the features of this *acute amebic dysentery.* Cases of the acute form occur sporadically and almost always in the tropics. Why the ameba is so aggressive in some people but causes a symptomless state in the majority of patients is not known. The existence of virulent strains of *E. histolytica* has been postulated; in addition, it seems that a synergistic action exists between the ameba and the intestinal flora in certain individuals.

Entamoeba histolytica occasionally penetrates the portal venous circulation, and this leads to *amebic hepatic abscess* formation. A diagnosis of this condition is often difficult because the complication is seen more commonly in cases of asymptomatic infection of the colon than in patients with overt dysentery. The diagnosis of active amebic colitis depends on identification of the active trophozoites by microscopic examination of fresh warm stool.* Serologic tests are also available. In the absence of diarrhea, the trophozoites encyst before leaving the gut. The feces of asymptomatic carriers contain cysts only and are the chief source of infection. Food is the common vehicle of transmission, being contaminated by infected food handlers or by flies. The use of human feces as fertilizer may directly contaminate vegetables. Outbreaks of amebic dysentery are generally waterborne and are never as explosive as are those of bacillary dysentery (Chapter 23).

Giardiasis

Giardiasis is a protozoal infection of the small intestine that has come into prominence during the last decade because of an increased awareness that it can cause significant disease. The causative organism, *Giardia lamblia*, exists in two forms: a *trophozoite* that is found attached to the mucosa of the jejunum; and a *cyst* that is the infective form, since on being swallowed it can resist the acid contents of the stomach. Both forms of the parasite are present in the feces during active stages of the disease when diarrhea is present.

Giardiasis can be asymptomatic, but it may also cause acute attacks of diarrhea. The infection can also be responsible for chronic diarrhea, and this may be associated with malnutrition, steatorrhea (excess of fat in the stools), and a condition resembling celiac disease (Chapter 23). Outbreaks of giardiasis have recently been held responsible for attacks of diarrhea in infant day care centers, among male homosexuals, and in travelers with "traveler's diarrhea" (Chapter 23). In the Rocky Mountains, beaver may be the source of water contamination; hence, the infection is known as beaver fever.

---

*Both trophozoites and cysts of *Entamoeba histolytica* must be distinguished from those of *Entamoeba coli*, which are part of the normal flora of the colon.

Malaria

Malaria is a protozoal disease caused by infection by a member of the genus *Plasmodium*. It is characterized by paroxysms of fever, each lasting 2 to 4 hours and initiated by a severe rigor. The paroxysm passes through the classic cold, hot, and sweating stages (Chapter 14). The infection is acquired from the bite of a female anopheline mosquito whose injected saliva contains sporozoites that travel via the blood stream to reach the liver cells, where they multiply (Fig. 10–1). This *exoerythrocytic stage* occurs during the incubation period of the disease. Finally, infective forms return to the blood stream, invade the red blood cells, and divide asexually to produce sporozoites, each of which breaks up into numerous merozoites. These are liberated as the red blood cell ruptures, and each merozoite invades another red blood cell. This asexual cycle (schizogony) takes 48 hours with *Plasmodium falciparum*. It is a remarkable fact that the maturation cycle of each parasite soon becomes synchronized. The release of merozoites is accompanied by the onset of a paroxysm—each third day with tertian malaria (due to *Plasmodium vivax* and *Plasmodium ovale*) and each fourth day with quartan malaria (*Plasmodium malariae*). Paroxysms are more erratic with malignant malaria (due to *P. falciparum*), which is so named because it is the most severe and is accompanied by two serious complications.

Cerebral Malaria. A complication of malignant malaria, cerebral malaria is characterized by the rapid development of a high fever (hyperpyrexia), coma, and death (see Fig. 14–2).

Blackwater Fever. In blackwater fever, a malarial paroxysm is followed by massive intravascular hemolysis, hemoglobinuria (which causes the urine to turn dark), cessation of urine formation (anuria), and frequently death. The pathogenesis is not understood, but this complication is usually seen in chronic falciparum malignant malaria treated episodically with quinine. An autoimmune type of anemia probably plays an important part.

Course of Malaria. The first attacks of malaria are often severe, but as time goes by, the episodes become milder. Persistence of infection is due to the persistence of the exoerythrocytic

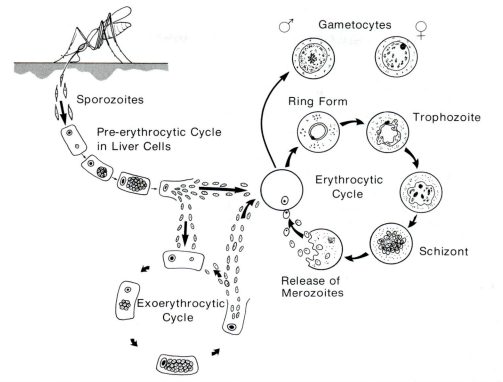

Figure 10–1 Development of malarial parasites in humans. Infection begins with the bite of an infected mosquito. The injected sporozoites travel in the blood stream and enter the liver cells, where they develop. Infective forms are released into the blood, and the majority of these enter red cells, develop into ring forms, and mature to form trophozoites. The erythrocytic cycle is completed by the development of a schizont; with the subsequent destruction of the red cell, infective merozoites are released. Except in the case of *Plasmodium falciparum,* some malaria parasites continue to multiply within liver cells and constitute the exoerythrocytic circle that is responsible for the persistence of the malarial infection. The male and female gametocytes, which are formed by some parasites, do not develop further in the human host but must await the bite of another mosquito. The precise shape and form of malarial parasites vary according to the species. In the diagram, the forms approximate those of *Plasmodium vivax.* (After Jeffrey, H.C., and Leach, R.M.: Atlas of Medical Helminthology and Protozoology. 2nd ed. Edinburgh, Churchill Livingstone, 1975. Drawing by Margot Mackay, University of Toronto, Faculty of Medicine, Department of Surgery, Division of Biomedical Communications, Toronto.)

forms in the liver. In endemic areas, reinfection constantly occurs, and a state of chronic infection ensues. This state is characterized by anemia, enlargement of the spleen (splenomegaly), debility, and cachexia, leaving the patient open to other infections. Tuberculosis, cholera, bacillary dysentery, and bronchopneumonia all take their toll in patients with chronic malaria.

Control of Malaria. The malarial parasites divide asexually in the human being, who is therefore the *intermediate host.* Gametocytes are formed in some infected red blood cells, but their maturation to form gametes and subsequent union to form zygotes occurs only in the female mosquito

(Fig. 10–2). The anopheline mosquito is therefore the *definitive host.* The control of malaria involves mosquito control and the treatment of patients, who serve as the reservoir for the disease. Neither of these has proved to be easy, and eradication of the disease has not proved to be possible. Mosquitoes have developed immunity to insecticides, and drug-resistant strains of plasmodia have emerged. Evolution, which designed the complex life cycle of the plasmodia, is not easily relinquishing such a prize.

Diagnosis of Malaria. The diagnosis of malaria rests on finding the parasite in a suitably stained blood film (see Figs. 10–2 and 14–2).

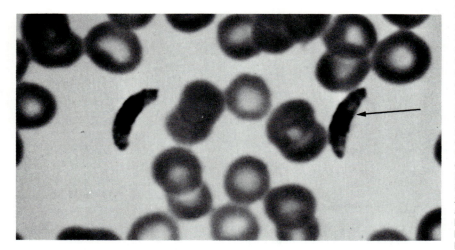

Figure 10–2 Gametocytes of *Plasmodium falciparum*. The two gametocytes shown were found in a routine blood film of a Malayan soldier. He was asymptomatic at the time. The crescentic shape of the organism is characteristic of this species of malarial parasite. One gametocyte (arrow), which has a more pointed end, is male; the other is female. The patient had a history of previous attacks of malaria, but he evidently had developed sufficient immunity to remain as an asymptomatic carrier. After a host has been bitten by a mosquito, gametocytes develop into gametes, which fuse to form a zygote. This zygote develops further and ultimately produces vast numbers of sporozoites that are ready to be injected when the mosquito bites her next victim.

Toxoplasmosis

Toxoplasmosis is caused by an infection with *Toxoplasma gondii*. The parasite primarily affects members of the cat family, which are the definitive hosts, being the hosts in which the organism reaches maturity and produces gametes. The organisms multiply in the cells of the small intestine and develop into oocysts that are passed in the feces and subsequently mature into infective forms that remain viable for months. Humans and other animals acquire the disease by eating these mature oocysts. In the intestine, the cysts develop into trophozoites that penetrate the bowel wall and migrate to lymph nodes, brain, and other tissues, where they encyst. When such cysts (*e.g.*, in a mouse) are eaten by a cat, the life cycle is completed (Fig. 10–3).

It has been estimated (as judged by the presence of antibodies) that up to 70 per cent of humans are infected by *T. gondii* but that the infection is subclinical in the vast majority of people. A very few individuals develop a severe illness with brain involvement, whereas others have a mild febrile illness that resembles infectious mononucleosis because its symptoms include lymphadenopathy and a skin rash.

Once the individual has been infected, a breakdown of immunity may be followed by overt disease. This may be evident as pneumonia, myocarditis, hepatitis, or encephalitis. Other organs may also be affected, and chorioretinitis is particularly characteristic although it is less common under these circumstances than in the congenital form of the disease. Recrudescence of toxoplasmosis is particularly common in immunocompromised patients, such as in patients with the acquired immunodeficiency syndrome (AIDS) and in those being treated for malignancy or for the prevention of graft rejection. Under these circumstances, the infection is severe and rapidly fatal, with central nervous system involvement being the outstanding feature.

The tragedy of toxoplasmosis lies in its tendency to be transmitted transplacentally to the fetus. The mother, although infected, is symptomless. The effects on the fetus vary. A very severe infection may precipitate abortion. More often, the child survives but develops a severe generalized disease a few weeks after birth. In other cases, the disease appears later, and there is severe involvement of the central nervous system and the eye.

Cryptosporidiosis

Cryptosporidium is an intestinal protozoan parasite belonging to the same family as *Toxoplasma*; it causes diarrhea in the young of many species and is an occasional cause of diarrhea in humans, particularly in those handling animals and in

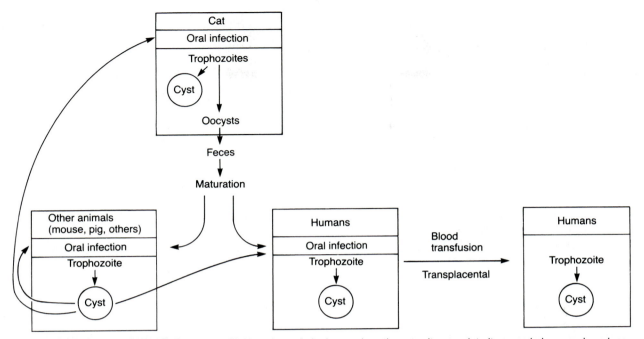

Figure 10–3 Life cycle of *Toxoplasma gondii*. Note that only in the cat does the parasite complete its sexual phase and produce oocysts. These are passed in the feces. When mature and ingested, these oocysts infect cats and other animals, including humans.

children in day care centers. The diagnosis is made by identifying the oocysts in feces by an acid-fast staining method. Severe infections can occur in patients with AIDS; in them, it causes a choleraic syndrome that results in the loss of many liters of fluid daily.

Trypanosomiasis

The trypanosomes are protozoa with a terminal flagellum and an undulating membrane. They cause infections of many animal species and pose a great economic problem in many parts of the world. Millions of acres in Africa are sparsely populated because of the impossibility of keeping domestic animals free of trypanosomiasis. Two types of infection occur in humans (Table 10–1).

African Trypanosomiasis

African trypanosomiasis is caused by infection with *Trypanosoma brucei,* of which there are two

strains. Humans are the only known victims of the Gambian strain *(T. brucei gambiense);* the Rhodesian strain *(T. brucei rhodesienses)* is primarily a parasite of wild game, with humans acting as an occasional and accidental host. Humans are infected by the bite of a fly of the genus *Glossina* (the tsetse fly), which injects infective forms with its saliva. A local skin lesion, which may pass unnoticed, is followed by a generalized infection that is characterized by fever, skin rashes, lymphadenopathy, and splenomegaly. After about 1 year, infection can involve the central nervous system, and the patient becomes lethargic and lapses into a coma. It is this latter feature that has given the disease its other name, *sleeping sickness.*

Chagas' Disease, or South American Trypanosomiasis

Trypanosoma cruzi is transmitted by a reduviid (kissing) bug, which tends to bite the face of the victim around the mouth, a habit that has earned

Table 10–1 TYPES OF TRYPANOSOMIASIS

Type	Organism	Vector	Lesions
African	*T. brucei*	Tsetse fly	Localized skin ulcer Generalized infection Brain
South American	*T. cruzi*	Reduviid (kissing) bug	Skin nodule Generalized infection Encephalitis Myocarditis

it its name. After feeding, the bug defecates and passes infective forms of the trypanosome that enter the bite wound. A local nodule appears and is followed by evidence of generalized parasitemia, with fever and involvement of many organs—skin, mucous membrane, lymph nodes, and the central nervous system.

Chronic Chagas' disease is characterized by parasitization of the heart muscle. This accounts for many cases of heart failure in some parts of South America. There is no treatment for it.

Leishmaniasis

The leishmania are protozoa that are transmitted by species of sandflies (genus *Phlebotomus*). In the fly, the organism has a flagellum; in the lesions of humans and other animal hosts, the organism is nonmotile (forming Leishman-Donovan bodies) and parasitizes macrophages (Fig. 10–4). Dogs, jackals, rodents, and other animals form the natural reservoir of infection of most of the leishmania that cause human disease. In some areas, humans are the only known host.

Three main types of leishmaniasis are known (Table 10–2).

Kala-Azar, or Visceral Leishmaniasis

Kala-azar is widely distributed, affecting the Far and Middle East; the area around the Mediterranean, particularly Malta and Greece; Africa; and, to a lesser extent, Central and South America.

Kala-azar is caused by *Leishmania donovani*, of which there are probably several types, since the disease shows considerable geographic variations. Generally there is no local lesion at the site of the sandfly bite, and the organism proliferates in the cells of the mononuclear phagocyte system of the spleen, lymph nodes, liver, and bone marrow. Compensatory hyperplasia of the mononuclear phagocyte system leads to enormous splenomegaly and hepatomegaly. Involvement of the marrow leads to anemia and a low granulocyte count.

The mortality rate in untreated kala-azar is

Table 10–2 TYPES OF LEISHMANIASIS

Type	Organism	Vector	Lesions
Kala-azar (visceral leishmaniasis)	*L. donovani*	Sandfly (*Phlebotomus*)	Local skin ulcer in some types only Generalized infection of mononuclear phagocyte system
Cutaneous leishmaniasis of the Old World (oriental sore, Aleppo button, Baghdad boil, Delhi boil, and others)	*L. tropica*	Sandfly	Skin only
Cutaneous leishmaniasis of the New World	*L. braziliensis, L. mexicana,* and others	Sandfly	Skin and sometimes mucous membranes of mouth and nose

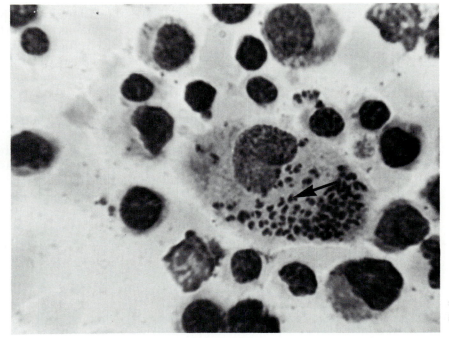

Figure 10–4 Photomicrograph of stained bone marrow of patient with leishmaniasis. The specimen illustrated here was taken from a sternal puncture. In the center is a large macrophage stuffed with parasites. Each organism has one large nucleus and a smaller rod-shaped structure called a *kinetoplast*. The arrow points to a typical organism showing these two structures. The membrane surrounding each individual organism is not clearly seen in this photograph.

about 90 per cent, but the disease responds to treatment with antimony compounds.

Cutaneous Leishmaniasis of the Old World, or Oriental Sore

Oriental sore, which is the least serious form of leishmaniasis, occurs in countries bordering the eastern Mediterranean, in Asia Minor, and in India. The causative organism, *Leishmania tropica*, produces a local infection of the skin at the site of the sandfly bite. A chronic ulcer is formed, and this heals spontaneously after a protracted course.

Cutaneous Leishmaniasis of the New World

The best-known variant of this type of leishmaniasis is American mucocutaneous leishmaniasis, or espundia, due to *Leishmania braziliensis*. One of more cutaneous lesions first appear and resemble oriental sore. However, the organisms spread to involve the mucosa of the mouth and

nose. Here, even after the skin lesions have been treated, the disease progresses and leads to great tissue destruction, secondary bacterial infection, and death. Infections with other organisms (*e.g., Leishmania mexicana*) tend to be less severe than espundia and often involve the skin only.

Trichomoniasis

Trichomonas vaginalis is the cause of a common vaginal infection that produces itching and a profuse, watery, yellow, frothy vaginal discharge. The diagnosis is made by examining a fresh specimen of the discharge under the microscope and identifying the motile trichomonads. On the fixed smear stained by the Papanicolaou method, the organisms can be seen, but often with difficulty.

In the male, a mild urethritis is the only evidence of infection. Usually the male carrier is symptomless. Transmission is by sexual contact, and both patient and sexual partners should be treated simultaneously.

Pneumocystosis

Until recently, infection with *Pneumocystis carinii* was an uncommon cause of pneumonia in malnourished or premature infants. However, it also infects immunologically deficient subjects of any age and is being recognized with increasing frequency as a cause of terminal pneumonia in patients who have an immunologic defect, either of congenital origin or due to malignant disease, administration of glucocorticoids, or therapy with antimetabolites. Patients with acute lymphocytic leukemia and AIDS are particularly susceptible (Chapter 6).

Pneumocystis carinii is probably a widely distributed organism and present in many apparently healthy people. It is thought to be a protozoan, but its life cycle has not yet been determined. The pneumonia it causes is an example of an opportunistic infection (Chapter 7).

Diagnosis of *Pneumocystis* pneumonia often presents difficulty. The organism is best demonstrated by a special silver stain (methenamine silver nitrate stain). It may be found in the sputum, but often recourse has to be made to lung biopsy. This may be transbronchial, although an open lung biopsy is often performed.

Open lung biopsy has the advantage that tissue is obtained for histopathologic examination as well as for culture for other possible opportunistic infecting organisms, such as cytomegalovirus and *Aspergillus* species.

HELMINTH INFECTIONS

The worms, or helminths, that plague mankind are classified as belonging within two phyla of the animal kingdom (Table 10–3).

The phylum *Platyhelminthes*, or flatworms, is further subdivided into two classes, *Trematoda* and *Cestoda*. The *Trematoda*, or *flukes*, are flat, leaflike creatures that live in the *intestine, liver,* or *lung* (the distomes) or in the *blood stream* (the schistosomes). The *Cestoda*, or *tapeworms*, are segmented and possess a head or scolex, a neck, and a varying number (often hundreds) of proglottides. Both cestodes and trematodes are hermaphroditic.

The phylum *Nemathelminthes* contains the roundworms, which are never segmented, possess an alimentary canal, and in general have separate sexes.

The helminths of medical importance form a

Table 10–3 CLASSIFICATION OF WORMS

Phylum	Class	Examples

Platyhelminthes (flatworms)	Trematoda (flukes)	Distomes
		  Fasciola hepatica
		  Clonorchis sinensis
		  Paragonimus westermani
		Schistosomes
		  Schistosoma hematobium
		  Schistosoma mansoni
		  Schistosoma japonicum

	Cestoda (tapeworms)	*Taenia saginata* *Taenia solium* *Diphyllobothrium latum* *Echinococcus granulosus*

Nemathelminthes (roundworms)	Nematoda (roundworms)	*Ascaris lumbricoides*
		Ancylostomes
		  Ancylostoma duodenale
		  Necator americanus
		Enterobius vermicularis (pinworm or threadworm)
		Trichuris trichiura (whipworm)
		Trichinella spiralis
		Strongyloides stercoralis
		Filariae
		  Wuchereria bancrofti
		  Onchocerca volvulus
		  Dracunculus medinensis

very small fraction of the total number known, and their study and recognition is a very specialized field. Only some common examples are described in this chapter.

The life cycle of many worms is complex. The *definitive host* is the one in which the parasite reaches maturity and produces gametes. The *intermediate host* is one in which the parasite passes through its larval stage or stages; in some instances, several intermediate hosts are required. Most parasites are extremely exacting in their demands, and knowledge of their host requirements is a valuable weapon in designing methods of eliminating them.

In general, the spread of parasites is encouraged by unsanitary conditions, overcrowding, and a warm climate. The Arctic is less hospitable for harboring these organisms than is the Nile region. It follows that helminthic infections are much more common in the tropics. Nevertheless, a worm can travel by air as easily as can its host; even in temperate climates, therefore, it is important to be aware of common "tropical diseases."

Trematodes or Flukes

The life cycle of the flukes involves one or two intermediate hosts (Fig. 10–5). Humans are the definitive host and acquire the infection by ingestion of infected fish, crayfish, or vegetation (causing *clonorchiasis, paragonimiasis,* or *fascioliasis,* respectively) or by penetration of the skin by the parasite *(schistosomiasis).* The first intermediate host is always a snail.

The Distomes

Members of this group of flukes live in the liver, the intestine, or the lung.

Liver Flukes. *Fasciola hepatica* is a common parasite of sheep and is occasionally acquired by human beings after the ingestion of watercress containing metacercariae (the resting stage of the trematode parasite). The ingested parasite enters the intestine, penetrates its wall, crosses the peritoneum, and reaches the liver, which is entered by piercing of its capsule. Parasites reach the bile ducts and mature in them. The adult flukes are 2 to 3 cm long and can obstruct the

bile ducts. They cause cholangitis, hyperplasia of the bile duct epithelium, and later portal fibrosis. Occasionally an adult fluke is found in some ectopic site—brain or subcutaneous tissues.

Clonorchis sinensis, or Chinese liver fluke, has a similar life cycle, but the metacercariae are found beneath the scales of a freshwater fish. Eating raw fish is the mode of infection. Cholangitis, bile duct obstruction, and cholangiocarcinoma are late sequelae.

Lung Flukes. Various species of the genus *Paragonimus* infect the lung. The adult flukes reside in cavities in the lung, and there is usually much surrounding inflammation and later fibrosis.

Blood Flukes or Schistosomes

Schistosomiasis (also called bilharziasis after Bilharz, who discovered the worm) is the most important disease caused by flukes because of its worldwide distribution and the severity of its lesions. It is caused by three closely related flukes. *Schistosoma mansoni* occurs in the Middle East and Africa and is the only schistosome that inhabits the New World. *Schistosoma haematobium* is found in Africa and the Middle East. *Schistosoma japonicum* is found in China, Japan, and Southeast Asia.

Life Cycle. Ova are passed in the stools or urine and, on contact with fresh water, hatch into ciliated forms, the *miracidia.* These have about 8 hours in which to search for the intermediate host, a specific snail. If the search is successful, the parasite proliferates in the snail; 1 to 2 months later, thousands of infective larvae, called *cercariae,* are liberated into the water. Cercariae are able to penetrate the skin of an unsuspecting bather, then enter venules, and finally pass through the lungs and liver, reaching the portal vein. The flukes mature in the portal venous system and after copulation migrate against the blood flow in the superior or inferior mesenteric veins to reach the vessels in the mucosa of the small intestine (*S. japonicum*), descending colon and rectum (*S. mansoni*), or bladder and other pelvic organs (*S. haematobium*). Some ova penetrate the mucosa and are passed in the stools or urine to start their remarkable life cycle once again.

Effects of Schistosomiasis. Schistosomiasis

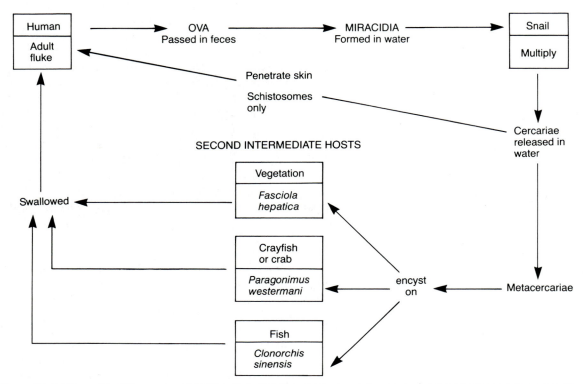

Figure 10–5 Life cycle of the common flukes. Note that the schistosomes have only one intermediate host: a *snail*. The other parasites shown have a second intermediate host: freshwater *vegetation*, a *crab* or other *crustacean*, or a *fish*.

may be divided into three stages. The penetration of the skin by cercariae leads to a local inflammatory reaction *(schistosome dermatitis or "swimmer's itch")*. Twenty to 60 days after exposure, the patient may develop a type of immune complex disease termed *katayama fever*. This is characterized by fever, diarrhea, cough, hepatosplenomegaly, generalized lymphadenopathy, urticaria, and blood eosinophilia. The phase may last for several weeks and corresponds to the time the females commence egg-laying. Katayama fever is most frequent and severe with infections of *S. japonicum*, the fluke that produces the largest number of ova. The syndrome is less common and severe with *S. mansoni* and uncommon with *S. haematobium*.

Chronic Schistosomiasis. It should be emphasized that many patients with schistosomiasis are asymptomatic. However, with heavy infections,

there is a considerable accumulation of ova in the tissues, where they cause a chronic granulomatous inflammatory reaction with many eosinophils and later fibrosis (Fig. 10–6). Delayed type hypersensitivity is believed to be responsible for much of this reaction. The effects of chronic schistosomiasis depend on the organ involved. With *S. haematobium*, involvement of the bladder causes severe fibrosis and mucosal overgrowths. In Egypt, carcinoma of the bladder appears to be an important complication, but the precise relationship between this and the infection is not clear.

S. mansoni involvement of the intestine leads to ulceration with bleeding, diarrhea, and fibrosis. Similarly, *S. japonicum* affects the small intestine. In both types, involvement of the liver is of great importance. It causes inflammation and fibrosis and leads to portal hypertension. Severe

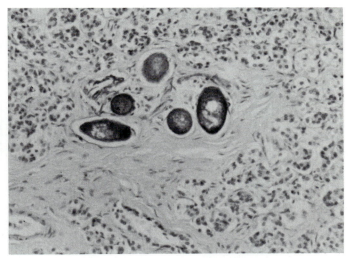

Figure 10–6 Schistosome ova in pancreas. The ova are probably dead, because they are calcified and stain deeply with hematoxylin owing to their calcium content. In spite of their being dead, they can still excite a chronic inflammatory response ($\times$250).

disease is produced by *S. japonicum;* the infection is fatal within 2 to 5 years unless treatment is instituted.

All types of schistosomiasis may also involve the lungs and central nervous system.

Present estimates of 180 million infected persons bear witness to the continued success of this parasite. Its existence is related to poor sewage disposal as well as to the popular habit of passing urine and feces into water channels that are used for bathing. The reversal of such habits is difficult, and education is all-important.

Cestodes or Tapeworms

Tapeworms possess a head (scolex) and a neck followed by a chain of segments or proglottides arranged in a ribbon, often many feet long (Fig. 10–7). Two hosts are necessary; humans are the definitive host of three common tapeworms and the intermediate host of one other (hydatid disease).

Taenia saginata. The beef tapeworm grows only in the human intestine. It has up to 2000 segments and can be 30 feet long. The mature terminal segments contain vast numbers of eggs, which are passed in the feces. As mature segments are cast off at one end, new ones are formed in the neck region. The worms are very long-lived—some have reportedly lived over 40 years.

When cattle eat the mature proglottides or isolated eggs, the embryos hatch out, penetrate the intestine, and migrate to the skeletal muscle, where they form the next larval stage, which is cystic (this stage of the tapeworm is called the *cysticercus*). Humans become infected by eating undercooked infected beef. Symptoms consist of vague abdominal pains or skin eruptions (*e.g.,* urticaria) due to hypersensitivity.

Taenia solium. This is the pork tapeworm. It has up to 1000 segments and can extend to 20 feet in length. The intermediate host is the pig. Humans acquire intestinal infection by eating undercooked pork containing cysticerci.

Occasionally humans eat the eggs of *Taenia solium,* and cysticerci develop in muscles, heart, brain, skin, and other organs. The human being then becomes the intermediate host. Symptoms of the condition known as *cysticercosis* are mainly neurologic.

Diphyllobothrium latum. This is the largest of the tapeworms, measuring up to 33 feet in length, with more than 3000 proglottides. The intermediate host is a fish, and the disease is most prevalent among the inhabitants of the fish-eating countries: Scandinavia, parts of Russia, and Asia.

Hydatid Disease. *Echinococcus granulosus* is a small tapeworm found in the intestine of dogs, wolves, and other carnivorous animals. Ova are ingested by sheep, which constitute the usual intermediate host. The cysticercal forms, called

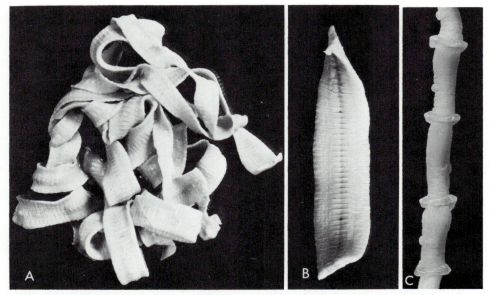

Figure 10–7 Tapeworms. *A,* Part of the tapeworm *Diphyllobothrium latum.* The total length of the worm is over 30 feet. The head is about 1 mm in diameter, and the immature segments (proglottides) are much smaller than are the segments shown (×1.5). *B,* Part of the worm shown in *A.* It is made up of many segments, each of which is wider than it is long. *C,* Part of the tapeworm *Taenia saginata.* Each segment is longer than it is wide.

hydatid cysts, develop in the liver, the lungs, and elsewhere (Fig. 10–8). Dogs become infected by eating infected sheep carcasses. Occasionally, humans ingest eggs and also develop hydatid cysts. These are most common in the liver and lungs, but they may occur in any part of the body. The disease is particularly prevalent in the sheep-raising areas of Australia.

Nematodes or Roundworms

Ascaris lumbricoides. The adult ascarides are 15 to 35 cm in length and live in the small intestine, where they usually cause no trouble except in those instances of a heavy infection, when their bulk causes obstruction (Fig. 10–9). Ova are passed in the stools and develop in soil into embryonated ova. When these are ingested, they hatch into larvae, which penetrate the gut wall and reach the lungs via the blood stream. They enter the alveoli, ascend the bronchi and trachea, and finally pass down the esophagus to reach the intestine. Why this parasite pursues this remarkable course is quite unknown. Per-

haps its ancestors had a different life cycle (*i.e.,* like that of *Ancylostoma duodenale,* described in the following), and the migrating habit has been retained by the worm for no more useful purpose than as a reminder of its heritage. During the migratory phase, the patient may experience asthmatic attacks and develop patchy pneumonic consolidation. Blood eosinophilia is common, as it is in many helminthic infections, particularly when the parasites are migrating through the tissues.

Ancylostomiasis (Hookworm Disease). This disease, which is of worldwide distribution, is caused by *Ancylostoma duodenale* in the Old World and *Necator americanus* in the New World. The worms attach themselves to the wall of the small intestine and cause bleeding. With a heavy infection, the blood loss may lead to a severe chronic iron deficiency anemia, which, when combined with undernutrition, is an important cause of chronic ill health in underdeveloped countries. Elsewhere, it is rare.

Eggs are passed in the feces and hatch in the soil into larvae that have the ability to penetrate the skin of a barefooted passerby. They migrate

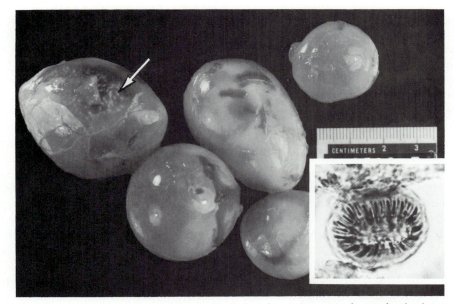

Figure 10–8 Hydatid cysts. The patient had emigrated to North America at 21 years of age after having previously lived and worked on a sheep farm in Yugoslavia. Nine years later he developed a rapidly expanding mass in the upper abdomen. Laparotomy was performed, and multiple hydatid cysts were found in the liver. The largest of these were drained, but unfortunately some of the cysts' contents were spilled into the peritoneal cavity. The parasite was thus disseminated. During the next 10 years, four further operations were necessary for removal or drainage of cysts in the peritoneal cavity, spleen, mediastinum, and pleural cavities.

Five separate hydatid cysts are shown. These have an epithelial lining from which small cysts or brood capsules develop. These are pinhead sized (see arrow), and from within them, scoleces of the head of the worm project. The inset shows one scolex with its characteristic hooklets. On being ingested by a dog or wolf, this structure will form the head of a new tapeworm.

via the blood to the lungs, penetrate the alveoli, ascend the trachea, and finally reach the gut to develop into adult worms.

Enterobius vermicularis (Pinworm or Threadworm). This nematode is very common in all parts of the world and lives in the lower gut. The females deposit their fully infective eggs around the anus, particularly at night, when their host is asleep. In so doing, they cause severe itching *(pruritus ani)*; pinworm infection should always be suspected as a cause of this condition, particularly in children. Infection is acquired by swallowing the eggs, which develop into adult forms in the intestine. The worms have a short life span (1 to 2 months), but continuous reinfection will maintain the infection unless strict personal hygiene is enforced. One cannot but admire the ingenuity of this worm: the severe anal

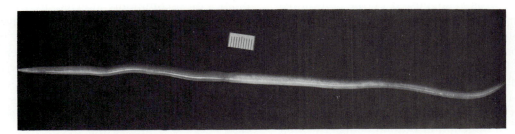

Figure 10–9 *Ascaris lumbricoides.* This worm is the largest roundworm parasite of humans and superficially resembles an earthworm (from the Latin *lumbricus,* an "earthworm"). It ranges in length from 15 to 35 cm. The specimen was approximately 20 cm (8 inches) in length. Other common roundworms are considerably smaller: *Trichuris trichiura,* 3 to 5 cm; *Enterobius vermicularis,* 8 to 13 mm; and *Ancylostoma duodenale,* up to 1 cm. (The scale above the roundworm shown is 1 cm.)

itching demands scratching and results in deposition of eggs under the nails. How many small children can refrain from sucking their fingers at some stage during the day?

Diagnosis is most easily accomplished by pressing a piece of adhesive tape or a specially prepared material against the child's perianal skin in the morning just after wakening. Ova will be found adherent to the tape.

Trichinella spiralis. The ban on eating pork imposed by some religious groups and the tradition of eating only well-cooked meat by others perhaps originated with some understanding of the life cycle of *Trichinella spiralis.*

Trichinella spiralis is primarily a parasite of rats. In the intestine, the adult male worm dies after copulation, a fate that is not uncommon in the world of worms. The pregnant female burrows into the intestinal wall and discharges hundreds of larvae into the blood stream. When these reach skeletal muscle, they curl up and form small cysts. Those larvae that reach other tissues are less fortunate—they die. When rats eat infected rat muscle, the dormant, encysted parasites awaken and develop into adult worms. Pigs and bears become infected by eating the carcasses of diseased rats, and human beings acquire infection (trichinosis) by eating undercooked pork or bear.

The symptoms of trichinosis vary. Minor infection is common, and there are no symptoms. With heavy infection, the early symptoms are gastrointestinal; these are followed by systemic symptoms such as fever, generalized edema, and muscle pains. Involvement of the respiratory muscles or heart can, on occasion, cause death. In Canada, this is an occasional sequel to an otherwise successful bear party.

The diagnosis is suggested by the clinical features (particularly muscle pains and periorbital edema combined with a marked blood eosinophil leukocytosis) and is confirmed by one of the serologic tests. Finding the parasite in a biopsy of the deltoid or gastrocnemius muscle provides the most convincing proof.

Strongyloides stercoralis. Strongyloidiasis is an intestinal infection of human beings by *Strongyloides stercoralis,* a tiny (2 mm) roundworm that resides in the mucosa of the upper jejunum. Generally, the infection is asymptomatic. The common life cycle of the parasite is similar to that of the hookworm, and infective larvae, which develop in the soil, enter the skin and return to the intestine via the lungs.

The organism is, however, remarkable for having several alternative life cycles. In one of these, the ova in the intestine develop into infective larvae that penetrate either the intestinal wall or the perianal skin. Autoinfection can thus occur. In the immunologically suppressed patient, massive infection can result in a severe illness characterized by colitis, pneumonitis, and meningitis as well as a complicating gram-negative bacteremia. Strongyloidiasis, when diagnosed, should therefore be treated even if it is asymptomatic because of this potential lethal complication.

Filariasis. Filariasis is caused by a type of nematode that invades the subcutaneous tissues and lymphatics of humans (Fig. 10–10). The female produces vast numbers of larvae, or *microfilariae,* which pass through the one intermediate host that transmits the infection to the human host.

Bancroft's Filariasis. This disease, commonly referred to as filariasis, is caused by *Wuchereria bancrofti,* which is a worm about 10 cm in length that resides in lymphatics. The females produce large numbers of microfilariae, which are liberated at night into the blood stream, where they can be sought for diagnosis. If an infected individual is bitten by a mosquito (also nocturnal), the mosquito becomes a carrier of the disease and infects persons it subsequently bites.

The adult forms of *W. bancrofti* produce little damage to lymphatics until they die. There then follows a severe chronic inflammatory reaction that results in lymphatic obstruction. The lymphatics most commonly affected are those of the groin; the leg consequently develops severe lymphatic edema. Marked overgrowth of the skin and subcutaneous tissues produces enormous swelling of the limb and sometimes the scrotum. The condition is called *elephantiasis* and occurs in many tropical and subtropical countries.

Onchocerciasis. This is a much neglected disease because it affects the peoples of the rural areas, where it is endemic. The disease occurs in Africa, Central and South America, and Yemen. Repeated infection by the bite of an infected

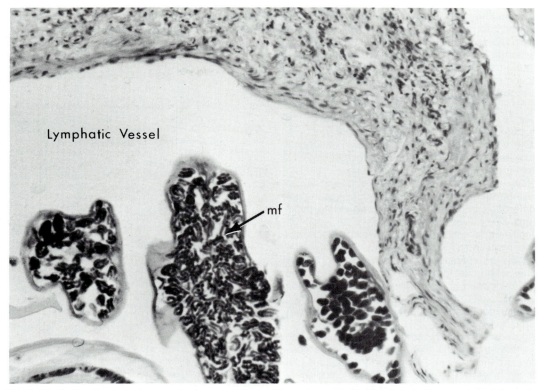

Figure 10–10 Filariasis. Section of a nodule from a patient with onchocerciasis. The lymphatic vessel contains adult worms shown in cross section. Numerous microfilariae (mf) are present in the body of the gravid female (×250).

black fly is necessary before severe clinical effects are apparent. Hence, short-term visitors and travelers tend to escape. Yet it affects about 40 million and has blinded up to one-half million persons. The disease is caused by *Onchocerca volvulus*, which resides in the subcutaneous tissues and causes an inflammatory reaction that leads to nodule formation (Fig. 10–10). The microfilariae produced by the females migrate widely and, when they die, cause a local inflammatory reaction. In the skin, this produces a dermatitis characterized by incessant itching. The most serious complication is due to involvement of the eye that can ultimately result in blindness.

This account of human helminthic diseases has included only some examples of worms that affect persons in widespread areas of the world. Many other examples are known, some restricted to particular geographic areas. Thus, a localized outbreak of infection by *Capillaria philippinensis* has been described in the Philippine Islands and

is manifested as a type of enteritis with a high mortality. It is caused by a minute whipworm and is acquired by eating infected fish and crustaceans. The crustaceans are often eaten alive in a form of "jumping salads"!

Summary

- Fungi are molds, yeasts, yeastlike fungi, or dimorphous fungi. Most are saprophytes, but some cause skin infections; others cause pulmonary or widespread infection.
- *Entamoeba histolytica* causes amebic dysentery, sometimes complicated by hepatic abscess.
- *Giardia lamblia* is a cause of diarrhea.
- Three species of *Plasmodium* cause malaria; the organisms parasitize red blood cells and are transmitted by mosquitoes. Cerebral malaria and blackwater fever are important complications.
- *Toxoplasma gondii* is a parasite of cats but causes widespread subclinical human infection. Severe ef-

fects occur in immunocompromised individuals and in the congenital form.

- Cryptosporidiosis causes diarrhea, often severe in AIDS patients. Similarly, *Pneumocystis carinii* causes severe lung infection in this group.
- Trypanosomes cause sleeping sickness in Africa, but the South American infection becomes chronic and is a leading cause of heart failure.
- Kala-azar is a serious, widespread infection of the mononuclear phagocyte system with *Leishmania donovani*. Other leishmania cause a local skin infection.
- *Trichomonas vaginalis* is a common cause of vaginitis with discharge.
- The definitive host of a helminth is the one in which the parasite reaches maturity and produces gametes.
- The trematodes or flukes have a complex life cycle and cause disease of the intestine, liver, or lung; the most important is schistosomiasis, which affects the bladder or intestine.
- Humans are the definitive host of several cestodes or tapeworms. They reside in the intestine. In hydatid (due to *Echinococcus granulosus*) disease, humans are the intermediate host and develop hydatid cysts. Occasionally this also happens with the pork tapeworm.
- The nematodes or roundworms usually parasitize the intestine (filariasis is the exception). *Trichinella spiralis*, derived from pork, is important because it spreads to skeletal muscle (trichinosis) and may cause death. Massive infection with *Strongyloides stercoralis* can spread widely, particularly in immunosuppressed subjects. Bancroft's filariasis, spread by a mosquito, invades lymphatics and ultimately causes elephantiasis. Onchocerciasis, another filarial disease, affects the skin and eye. It is an important cause of blindness in some areas.

Selected Readings

Blissingden, J. G.: *Cryptosporidium* and diarrhoea. Br. Med. J. *293*:287, 1986.

Blumenthal, D. S.: Intestinal nematodes in the United States. N. Engl. J. Med. *297*:1437, 1977.

Evans, E. G. V., and Gentles, J. C.: Essentials of Medical Mycology. Edinburgh, Churchill Livingstone, 1985.

Jeffrey, H. C., and Leach, R. M.: Atlas of Medical Helminthology and Protozoology. 2nd ed. Edinburgh, Churchill Livingstone, 1975.

An atlas giving the morphology, life cycle, and major effects of common parasite infection. Useful for parasite identification.

Koneman, E. W., and Roberts, G. D.: Practical Laboratory Mycology. 3rd ed. Baltimore, Williams & Wilkins, 1985.

Krick, J. A., and Remington, J. S.: Toxoplasmosis in the adult: An overview. N. Engl. J. Med. *208*:550, 1978.

Leading article: Toxoplasmosis. Br. Med. J. *1*:249, 1981.

Leading article: Battles against *Giardia* in gut mucosa. Lancet *2*:527, 1982.

Leading article: Pneumocystis: An orphan organism. Lancet *1*:676, 1985.

Markell, E. K., Voge, M., and John, D. T.: Medical Parasitology. 6th ed. Philadelphia, W. B. Saunders Co., 1986.

Mettrick, D. F., and Desser, S. S.: Parasites: Their World and Ours. Amsterdam, Elsevier, 1982.

Navin, T. R., and Juranek, D. D.: Cryptosporidiosis: Clinical, epidemiologic, and parasitologic review. Rev. Infect. Dis. *6*:313, 1984.

Strickland, G. T.: Hunter's Tropical Medicine. 6th ed. Philadelphia, W. B. Saunders Co., 1984.

11

Disorders of Growth

DEVELOPMENTAL ANOMALIES
  Types of Malformations
ACQUIRED DISORDERS OF GROWTH
  Quantitative Abnormalities of Cellular Growth
  Abnormalities of Cellular Differentiation
  Other Cellular Abnormalities

After studying this chapter, the student should be able to:

- Describe the causes of developmental anomalies.
- List 11 types of malformation and give an example of each.
- Describe the lessons learned from the thalidomide tragedy.
- Describe the fetal alcohol syndrome.
- Compare and contrast hypertrophy with hyperplasia.
- Define the terms atrophy, hypoplasia, aplasia, metaplasia, dyscrasia, and dysplasia.
- Classify the causes of atrophy and give examples of each.
- Discuss the use of the term dysplasia as applied to diseases of the skin, cervix uteri, and breast.

Disorders of cellular growth and differentiation most commonly occur during the period of embryonic development. This is hardly surprising, since a single cell, the fertilized ovum, can transform itself into an entire animal, albeit immature, in a short space of time—21 days in the case of a mouse, and 9 months in the case of a human

being. Errors that occur during this period of marked change can result in gross defects. Postnatal development, on the other hand, is a relatively sedate affair, and the likelihood of an error occurring is correspondingly less.

Minor variations in development are so common that the resulting abnormalities are regarded as variants of the normal. More serious errors in development result in the production of malformations that are usually present at birth but may not become evident until later in life. Gross abnormalities are often incompatible with life and result in abortion, stillbirth, or neonatal death.

The changes that are described in this chapter concern abnormalities of cell growth: too much, too little, or the wrong sort, or to use the pathologic terms *hyperplasia* and *hypertrophy, atrophy,* or *metaplasia*. In addition, *neoplasia* falls into this group. Such changes form a heterogeneous group; they often appear to bear little relationship to each other. Nevertheless, the changes are worthy of study, for they form the cellular or functional entities that are commonly encountered in many disease processes.

It is convenient to divide the abnormalities of cell growth into two groups:

1. *Developmental anomalies.* These arise before the affected part has reached its mature, adult form.

2. *Acquired anomalies.* These arise in an organ or tissue after maturity has been attained.

205

Inevitably, there is some overlap between these two groups because it is sometimes difficult to decide when maturity has been attained. Nevertheless, the classification has some merit. A "developmental anomaly" is found in an organ that has never been normal. In contrast, an "acquired anomaly" occurs in an organ that has previously attained normal adult stature.

DEVELOPMENTAL ANOMALIES

Genetic Causes. Inherited conditions, such as achondroplasia, and those associated with gross chromosomal anomalies (Chapter 3) are well-known causes of malformations. When one encounters a patient with a developmental anomaly, it is wise to carry out a chromosomal analysis and to investigate the family for a history of similar anomalies. Genetic counseling is a practical way of avoiding future abnormalities.

Environmental Causes. External agents that act on the developing fetus and cause developmental anomalies are called *teratogens*. Infections and drugs are the most important agents, but ionizing radiation and certain metabolic defects can also be teratogenic.

Infection transmitted from the mother to the fetus can cause serious damage, particularly if the transmission occurs during the first 3 months of pregnancy when development of important organs such as the heart and brain is proceeding rapidly (see also TORCH in Chapter 7).

German measles (rubella) has acquired a particularly evil reputation in this respect. Deformities, particularly congenital heart disease, cataract, and deafness, occur in as many as 25 per cent of babies born to mothers who had the infection during pregnancy. The first month of pregnancy is the most dangerous period in which to be exposed with respect to both the frequency of malformations and their severity. Women of child-bearing age who have not had rubella are potentially at risk. If there is doubt about whether they have had the disease, serum antibodies should be measured because the presence of antibodies to the virus in the blood indicates past infection and therefore immunity. Rubella vaccine should be given to those who are not immune.

Toxoplasmosis is another infection that can cross the placenta and cause serious effects. Underdevelopment of the brain and eye are common. Cytomegalovirus infection has similar effects. Human immunodeficiency virus can also infect the unborn child; malformations of the brain and impairment of the immune system result in these patients with congenital acquired immunodeficiency syndrome (AIDS).

The tragedy that followed the administration of the sedative drug thalidomide has highlighted the selective toxic effects that some drugs have on the developing embryo. The most common anomalies found in the "thalidomide babies" were absence of limbs or parts of limbs, angiomatous malformations (see hamartomas, discussed later) of lips and nose, and other malformations of the heart, alimentary tract, and genitourinary system. Because the deleterious (teratogenic) effects of a particular drug on the human fetus can be established only by testing the substance on pregnant women, it is current policy to avoid administration of any drug during pregnancy unless it is absolutely vital.

A teratogenic drug of great current interest is isotretinoin (Accutane), which is used in the treatment of severe acne vulgaris. Giving the drug to a female patient of reproductive age is hazardous. Before starting the course of treatment, a negative blood test for pregnancy must be obtained, and an effective contraception regimen must be followed during treatment. Other drugs include anticoagulants and anticonvulsants.

A common and important teratogen is alcohol. Maternal alcoholism results in the birth of infants with the *fetal alcohol syndrome*. They are short and below average weight and have a characteristic face with a long upper lip. The brain is small, and this may be associated with mental retardation.

Other teratogenic agents include antimetabolites (used in the treatment of cancer), heavy maternal tobacco smoking (associated with low birth weight), and hormones, whether administered therapeutically (*e.g.,* stilbestrol; see vaginal carcinoma) or produced by a hormone-secreting tumor.

Radiation is a potent teratogen, and exposure of the fetus during treatment for maternal malignant disease is capable of causing abnormalities of brain and bone development. Whether the low dosage received during diagnostic radiology is capable of causing fetal damage is not known, but it is a wise precaution to avoid exposing the fetus unless it is absolutely essential.

The fetal abnormalities that result from hemolytic disease of the newborn are described in Chapter 18.

Types of Malformations

Malformations can affect any part of the body, and a large number have been described. It is convenient to group them under the following 11 headings:

1. **Failure of development.** There may be a complete failure of a part to develop *(agenesis)*, or the part may remain rudimentary and never attain a full mature size *(hypoplasia)*. An example of this incomplete development has already been mentioned in the case of the thalidomide babies' limbs. Likewise, one or both kidneys can show either agenesis or hypoplasia. The possibility of this anomaly is important to the surgeon who is considering the removal of one kidney. It is essential to check that the other kidney is present and normal.

2. **Failure of fusion.** During development, many structures normally fuse together, and a failure to do so can result in abnormality. A harelip or cleft palate is a common example of this failure to fuse.

3. **Failure of separation.** A good example of this malformation is the webbing that may persist between the fingers or toes (Fig. 11–1).

4. **Failure of canalization.** Many channels in the body originate as solid cords and subsequently canalize. A failure in this process leads to a congenital obstruction, which is frequently termed *atresia*. Examples of this are esophageal atresia and imperforate anus (anal atresia).

5. **Ectopia.** Sometimes organs and tissues are found at abnormal sites. This is termed *ectopia, heterotopia,* or *aberrance.* An interesting example

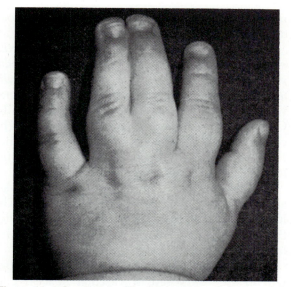

Figure 11–1 Syndactyly. The third and fourth fingers of the hand are joined together. This abnormality can easily pass unnoticed in a young baby. (Courtesy of V. S. Brookes.)

of this is the ectopic thyroid that develops at the base of the tongue. In such a case, no thyroid tissue is found in the normal location in the neck. Aberrant blood vessels are quite common. They may even be noticed by a patient and cause anxiety, such as when the radial artery runs a superficial course at the wrist and its pulsation can be seen. Aberrant renal arteries can be damaged by a careless surgeon who relies on the normality of the patient's anatomy.

6. **Heteroplasia.** Sometimes there is an anomalous differentiation of a particular tissue in an organ. For instance, tissue identical to gastric mucosa may be found in the esophagus. Sebaceous gland formation may occur in the oral mucosa; the small white dots that this produces can be seen in the buccal mucosa of many otherwise normal individuals.

7. **Local gigantism.** Occasionally, there is a simple overgrowth of an organ or tissue. Thus, there may be an enlarged limb in neurofibromatosis (von Recklinghausen's disease). Likewise, there may be enormous overdevelopment of the female breast or breasts at puberty.

8. **Supernumerary organs.** Additional or supernumerary organs are not uncommon. A good example is hands or feet that exhibit six digits (polydactyly). Supernumerary nipples are not

uncommon, and infrequently these are associated with breast tissue.

9. **Hamartomas.** *A harmartoma is a tumorlike malformation in which the tissues of the particular part of the body are arranged haphazardly, usually with an excess of one or more components.* The term was coined by Albrecht and is derived from the Greek word *hamartanein,* meaning "to err." The concept of the hamartoma is of great importance because a large number of common lesions fall into this general category.

The best-known example of a hamartoma is a simple mole or melanotic nevus of the skin. The lesion is composed of an excess of melanocytes that subsequently change into nevus cells. This lesion is described in detail in Chapter 31.

Some hamartomas (both of the skin and elsewhere) are composed of vascular spaces. Like many other hamartomas, these vascular lesions are given a name resembling that given to a neoplasm (hemangioma), even though, strictly speaking, this is incorrect, since they are not neoplasms. Hemangiomas of the skin may produce a noticeable mass (Fig. 11–2) or a flat lesion that cannot be felt but is obvious because of its bright red color. This type is called a "port-wine" stain (Fig. 11–3).

An uncommon but important hamartoma is found in the lung. This consists of a nodule of cartilage and a few spaces lined by a respiratory type of epithelium (Fig. 11–4). The lesion appears on a radiograph as a circumscribed opacity, commonly called a "coin lesion"; its discovery can

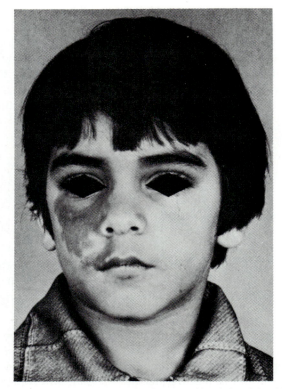

Figure 11–3 Hemangioma affecting the skin of the right side of the face in the region of the maxilla. (Courtesy of Dr. Margaret C. Grundy and the Department of Clinical Illustration, University of Birmingham, England.)

lead to the mistaken diagnosis of cancer. Radical surgery for such a lesion is a medical catastrophe.

Some hamartomas tend to be multiple. Hemangiomas of the face can be associated with similar hemangiomas of the retina or brain. The skin lesions are thus pointers to the more serious underlying condition. Another well-known but distinctly uncommon example is neurofibromatosis. This inherited autosomal dominant trait results in widespread hamartomatous overgrowths of nerve sheath tissue. These lesions closely resemble neoplasms and are generally loosely described as "neurofibromas." There is sometimes localized regional overgrowth, and gross deformity can result.

10. **Persistence of normally vestigial structures.** During the course of development, many structures are formed that are of immediate importance to the developing embryo but that ul-

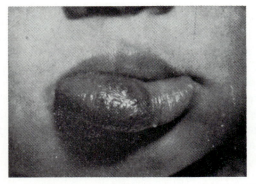

Figure 11–2 Hemangioma of the lower lip. (Courtesy of G.S. Hoggins and the Department of Clinical Illustration, University of Birmingham, Birmingham, England.)

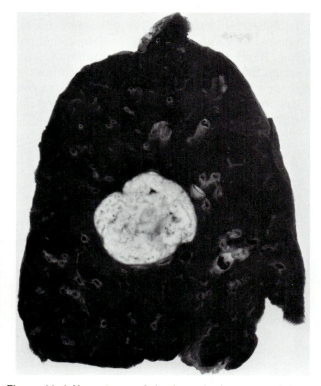

Figure 11–4 Hamartoma of the lung. In the center of the upper lobe there is a circumscribed, pearly-white, hard, round mass. It consists predominantly of mature cartilage, and there is no obvious capsule around it. (Reproduced by kind permission of the President and Council of the Royal College of Surgeons of England. Hunterian Museum specimen ER 22.1.)

11. **Complex Malformations**. Some malformations are complex and do not fit into any of the categories described. For example, there may be abnormalities in the rotation of the gut or the heart. Indeed, the whole body can develop as a mirror image of the normal (*complete situs inversus*).

ACQUIRED DISORDERS OF GROWTH

In the mature individual, all organs and tissues (with the notable exceptions of muscle fibers and neurons) show a steady turnover, with mitosis compensating for cell death. In some organs, such as the liver, the turnover is slow; in others, such as the lymphoid tissue, it is fast. The mechanism controlling this turnover is not understood, but the end result is that most organs remain at a constant normal size. Furthermore, there is a considerable reserve of tissue that can be drawn upon whenever additional work is demanded of it. Therefore, under normal conditions, no structural adjustment is necessary other than that of regulating the blood flow through the organ. Thus, tissues at rest are maintained by an intermittent blood flow through their supplying capillaries. This mechanism results in an economical use of the circulation, and it explains why noxious substances spread by the blood stream may nevertheless produce patchy effects. When more work has to be performed, the shutdown vessels dilate, and the organ shows an increased blood flow (active hyperemia). This is well illustrated by the tremendous increase in blood flow that occurs in skeletal muscle during periods of activity and in the salivary glands during eating.

Quantitative Abnormalities of Cellular Growth

Under abnormal circumstances, organs and tissues may show a change in size that is due to either an increase or a decrease in the bulk of parenchymal cells. Abnormalities of cellular growth are found in virtually all tissues, and only a few examples are given here.

timately disappear and become obliterated by the time of birth or shortly thereafter. Occasionally, such structures persist and lead to trouble. The two most important complications are neoplasia and cyst formation. Neoplasia is considered in Chapter 12. Patent ductus arteriosus is described in Chapter 20.

A good example of a *developmental cyst* is the dermoid cyst. This results from sequestration and growth of a piece of skin beneath the surface and occurs when folds of skin fuse together during development. During the complex development of the face, various folds are formed and fuse. Dermoid cysts tend to occur along the lines of these fusions, such as at the angles of the eye or mouth. Another example is persistence of a segment of the thyroglossal duct, which results in a midline cystic swelling in the neck, known as a *thyroglossal cyst*.

Hyperplasia

An increase in the number of cells of a tissue or organ that results in enlargement is called *hyperplasia*. The cause is generally related to the overaction of a tangible stimulus, which is often a basically physiologic one acting to excess. Hyperplasia is therefore often the result of an increased demand for function. For example, there is hyperplasia of the red blood cell precursors in the bone marrow after hemorrhage, whereas in infection it is the white blood cell element of the marrow that responds. In bacteremia, cells of the mononuclear phagocyte system in the spleen undergo hyperplasia, and if this is marked, there is splenomegaly.

In passing, it should be noted that enlargement of an organ is commonly denoted by the use of the suffix *-megaly*. Thus, enlargement of the spleen is described as splenomegaly. The term gives no indication of the cause of the enlargement; for example, it might be due to hyperplasia of the spleen's constituent cells, or it could equally well be caused by an abscess or a neoplasm. As always, there are exceptions to any rule; enlargement of the lymph nodes is spoken of as lymphadenopathy.

Hyperplasia is generally regarded as an adaptive mechanism by which an increased number of cells is produced as a useful response to a stimulus. Thus, chronic physical irritation of the skin results in thickening of the epidermis; calloused hands are well suited to manual work. When the physical irritation is removed, the epidermis returns to normal. This response is different from that seen in neoplasia, in which withdrawal of the stimulus does not lead to a return to normal (see Chapter 12 for further discussion). Nevertheless, there are examples of cellular overgrowth in human disease, although classified as hyperplasia, that are not produced by any known stimulus and are not necessarily self-limiting or useful. An example of this is fibrocystic disease of the breast in which there is epithelial and mesenchymal overgrowth (Chapter 28). An analogous condition is benign prostatic enlargement encountered in elderly men (Chapter 26).

Pseudomalignant Hyperplasia. In some instances, hyperplastic lesions can be very difficult to distinguish histologically from malignant neoplasms. A good example of pseudoepitheliomatous hyperplasia is the keratoacanthoma, a skin lesion that closely mimics a malignant tumor but that disappears spontaneously. Similarly, pseudolymphomas can occur at various sites, for instance, in the skin at the site of a tick bite.

Hypertrophy

Hypertrophy is defined as the increase in size of an organ or tissue due solely to an increase in the size of its constituent specialized cells. In practice, this phenomenon applies only to muscle, and the stimulus for this enlargement is almost always a mechanical one.

Any muscle that is continually stimulated by overwork tends to show enlargement. This is commonly seen in skeletal muscle, in which the bulging muscles of the athlete contrast with the slender ones of the sedentary worker. Cardiac muscle, likewise, shows enlargement if the heart is constantly forced to overwork. This is seen when the heart has to force blood through a stenosed orifice (*e.g.*, when there is left ventricular hypertrophy in aortic stenosis; Fig. 11–5) or when it has to contract against a high blood pressure (*e.g.*, in patients with left ventricular hypertrophy in systemic hypertension).

It is noteworthy that the human heart at birth weighs approximately 30 g, and thereafter no new cells are formed. The heart muscle cells steadily increase in size; by maturity, therefore, there has been a tenfold increase in weight and a tenfold increase in size of muscle fibers. Any further enlargement is due to additional increase in muscle size. Although these large fibers are initially capable of vigorous contraction, it is unfortunate that they ultimately fail. This appears to be due to an inadequate blood supply, since enlargement of muscle fiber size is not accompanied by an increase in number of blood vessels. It follows that an enlarged heart (cardiomegaly) due to hypertrophy is a diseased heart, and one that will ultimately fail to function efficiently.

Hypertrophy of smooth muscle cells is seen in the muscular coats of hollow organs that are forced to expel their contents against resistance.

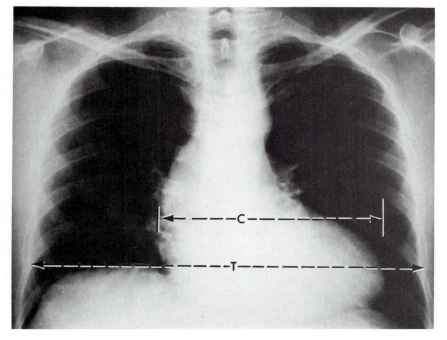

Figure 11–5 Hypertrophy of the left ventricle. This patient had aortic stenosis with enlargement of the heart *(cardiomegaly)* due to hypertrophy of the muscle of the left ventricle. It is convenient to assess the size of the heart by comparing the maximum width of the heart shadow (C) with the width of the chest cavity at the level of the highest point of the right side of the diaphragm (T). The cardiothoracic ratio, C/T, is normally less than 0.5. Here, of course, the ratio is greater than 0.5. (Courtesy of Dr. D.E. Sanders, Department of Radiology, Toronto General Division of the Toronto Hospital, Toronto.)

The muscular urinary bladder wall hypertrophies when the prostate gland enlarges and causes urethral obstruction. The intestinal muscular wall undergoes hypertrophy proximal to any stenosis (*e.g.,* the stomach wall thickens in pyloric stenosis).

Atrophy

A small organ or tissue is described as *atrophic* when its diminution in size is due to a decrease in either the size or number of its constituent specialized cells. Only in muscle is the decrease in size of cells a major factor. In all other instances, the number of cells is also reduced. Atrophy of the bone marrow is commonly called *hypoplasia*, whereas extreme atrophy is known as *aplasia*. This is unfortunate, because the term "hypoplasia" is also used by some pathologists in a different connotation to indicate an imperfect development of an organ or tissue.

Physiologic Atrophy. There are many examples of structures that are well developed at a certain time of life but subsequently undergo atrophy. Many fetal structures, such as the thy-roglossal duct and the hyaloid artery, which supplies the developing lens, completely disappear before birth. Other structures, such as the ductus arteriosus, atrophy early in postuterine life. From adolescence, the lymphoid tissues of the body undergo steady atrophy; after parturition, the uterus undergoes atrophy (commonly called *involution*); in old age, most tissues (particularly the sexual organs) sustain a generalized process of atrophy.

Pathologic Atrophy. Generalized atrophy occurs in starvation and is also a feature of the cachexia of malignant disease. Hypopituitarism results in atrophy of most of the endocrine glands. The widespread atrophy of bone, termed *osteoporosis,* is described in Chapter 30.

Local Atrophy. Local atrophy is usually the result of impaired blood supply (ischemia). An example is provided by the atrophy of the skin associated with peripheral vascular disease of the legs. Atrophy of the brain follows cerebral atherosclerosis.

A particular variant of ischemic atrophy is produced by local pressure. A steadily enlarging cyst or an expanding neoplasm produces pressure on adjacent tissues and leads to atrophy of the parenchyma. The fibrous tissue stroma tends to be more resistant; it persists and forms a capsule around the lesion.

Disuse Atrophy. It has been tritely stated that what a patient does not use, he loses. A striking example of this is the effects of immobilization of a limb. Marked atrophy of bone, ligaments, and muscle follows joint immobilization; it is the task of the physical therapist to prevent this. Atrophy of muscles and ligaments occurs around a joint that is fused *(ankylosis)* or when movement is limited by pain as in rheumatoid arthritis. There is atrophy of the kidney after complete obstruction of the ureter, and likewise disuse atrophy of an exocrine gland follows obstruction of its duct (Fig. 11–6). It is of historic interest that Banting and Best ligated the pancreatic duct to remove the exocrine portion of the pancreas so that insulin could be extracted from the endocrine component without the complicating action of trypsin on their tissue extracts.

There are a number of conditions in which tissues undergo atrophy for no obvious reason. Sometimes there appears to be a genetic defect; sometimes there appears to be an autoimmune mechanism; in most instances, however, there is no apparent cause. A distressing example of this is the atrophy of the brain that occurs prematurely in some people and leads to severe mental deterioration (dementia). Various types of this presenile dementia are known and are categorized under different names, *e.g.,* Alzheimer's disease. Idiopathic endocrine atrophy is seen in some cases of Addison's disease (Chapter 29) and in hypothyroidism and cretinism.

Abnormalities of Cellular Differentiation

Metaplasia

Metaplasia is a condition in which there is a change in one type of differentiated tissue such that it takes

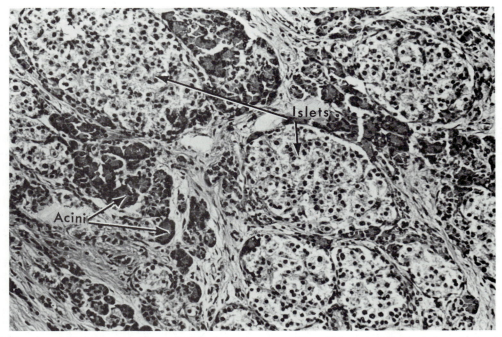

Figure 11–6 Atrophy of the pancreas. This patient had chronic pancreatitis, which caused the formation of a hard mass in the head of the organ. The mass had obstructed the main pancreatic duct. The section illustrated was taken from the body of the organ and shows atrophy of the exocrine component of the gland. Many acini have disappeared; those that remain are small. The shrinkage of the exocrine portion of the gland has resulted in condensation of the islets of Langerhans, which are themselves unaffected. At least seven are present in the field illustrated. Compare this with Figure 2–3. There is some increase in the amount of fibrous tissue and a sparse infiltration by small round cells, indicating a mild degree of chronic inflammation. This case illustrates the principle that if the duct of a secreting gland is obstructed, its parenchyma undergoes atrophy.

on the characteristics of another differentiated tissue. Two forms of this condition are described.

Epithelial Metaplasia. It is quite common for the pseudostratified columnar ciliated epithelium of the trachea and bronchi to be replaced by a stratified squamous type of epithelium that may even undergo keratinization and resemble epidermis. This *squamous metaplasia* generally seems to be the result of chronic irritation. This condition is also found in the urinary tract, particularly in association with urinary stones and infection. Sometimes metaplasia can be more subtle. The bronchial lining can be replaced by a columnar epithelium in which simple mucus-secreting goblet cells predominate. This is extremely common in chronic bronchitis and is one of the factors that results in the excessive production of mucus that is continually coughed up (expectorated). The concept of metaplasia is important because it helps explain why neoplasms of the lung can resemble those normally arising in the skin (squamous-cell carcinoma) or in a mucus-secreting gland (adenocarcinoma).

Connective Tissue Metaplasia. The fibroblasts of connective tissue and scar tissue can sometimes take on the characteristics of osteoblasts and lead to bone formation. Spicules of bone are often found in chronically inflamed tonsils, in old scars, and in the fibrous elements of goiters. Since these areas of bone formation are visible in radiographs, they are of importance in diagnostic radiography.

Other Cellular Abnormalities

The term *dystrophy* is commonly used, but it is difficult to define. It is generally applied to any condition in which there is an alteration in the structure or function of an organ or tissue that does not readily fit into the other categories (*i.e.,* agenesis, atrophy, hypertrophy, or metaplasia). For example, in *corneal dystrophy,* the cornea becomes opaque at about the time of puberty, and ultimately this results in blindness. Some varieties are inherited, and these appear to be degenerative. Dystrophy is also used to describe the crumbly, deformed nails affected by fungal infection or psoriasis. It is evident that the term ''dystrophy'' has no precise definition and is used in many specialties to describe diseases of widely differing nature.

The term *dyscrasia* is now used only by hematologists to describe some blood disorders of unknown cause and undetermined pathogenesis. The term serves no useful function and should be abandoned.

Dysplasia has been used to describe an abnormal development of tissue; like dystrophy, however, the term is also used by specialists in many fields to describe conditions of widely divergent nature. Thus, when applied to the breast (mammary dysplasia, now more commonly called fibrocystic disease of the breast), dysplasia denotes a complex condition of unknown origin in which there is irregular hyperplasia and metaplasia of breast substance. In the cervix uteri, dysplasia has acquired a completely separate meaning. It is used to describe a type of epithelial overgrowth that is thought to progress steadily to *carcinoma in situ* and ultimately to invasive cancer. In the skin, dysplasia is used in a similar context to describe the atypicality and irregular maturation seen in the epidermis in actinic keratoses and in Bowen's disease (see Figs. 12–15 and 12–16). In these organs, therefore, the term ''dysplasia'' denotes a change that is thought to precede the onset of cancer. Atypia is also used to describe this change.

From this short account, it is evident that the terms *dystrophy, dysplasia,* and *dyscrasia* are used quite arbitrarily to denote various types of conditions, the nature of which is poorly understood.

In this chapter, many different perversions of cell growth have been described. The one factor they all have in common is that they are self-limiting and reversible if the stimulus is removed. In the following chapter, *neoplasia* is discussed. With this condition, the perversion of cell growth persists even when the stimulus that produced it is eliminated.

Summary

- Developmental anomalies arise during embryonic development. Infections (rubella, toxoplasmosis, cytomegalovirus infections, immunodeficiency virus infections) and drugs (thalidomide, isotretinoin, and alcohol) are important causes.

- Types of malformation include failure of development (agenesis and hypoplasia), failure of fusion of parts, failure of separation, failure of canalization, ectopia, heteroplasia, local gigantism, supernumerary organs, hamartomas, persistence of normally vestigial structures, and complex malformations.
- Acquired disorders of growth include hyperplasia, hypertrophy, atrophy, and metaplasia.
- Dystrophy and dyscrasia are ill-defined terms. Dysplasia has several meanings; in some circumstances, it implies a premalignant condition.

Selected Readings

Clarren, S. K., and Smith, D. W.: The fetal alchohol syndrome. N. Engl. J. Med. *298*:1063, 1978.

Hill, R. M.: Isotretinoin teratogenicity. Lancet *1*:1465, 1984.

McBride, W. G.: Thalidomide and congenital abnormalities. Lancet *2*:1358, 1961.

Neoplasia

**After studying this chapter, the student
should be able to:**

- Define neoplasm, adenoma, cystadenoma, fibroma, leiomyoma, carcinoma, sarcoma, and teratoma.
- Discuss the concepts of anaplasia, dormant cancer, carcinoma *in situ,* metastasis, and the staging and grading of tumors.
- Describe the main features of benign tumors and compare them with those of malignant tumors.
- List the malignant tumors that commonly metastasize to bone.
- Discuss the concept of tumors having intermediate malignancy using basal-cell carcinoma of the skin as an example.
- Outline the classification of tumors.
- Give examples of chemical and physical carcinogenic agents, in particular those that are involved in human disease.
- Outline the steps involved in the evolution of a malignant tumor after the application of a chemical carcinogen.
- List the tumors in which there is a hereditary predisposition.
- Discuss the relationship between hormones and cancer.
- Give examples of viruses that have been incriminated as a cause of cancer in animals. Indicate the relevance to human disease.
- Describe the concept of an oncogene and its relevance to the development of cancer.
- Describe the development of cancer through the stages of atypia (dysplasia) and carcinoma *in situ.*
- Discuss the evidence that a cancer involves the overgrowth of one cell rather than in many cells simultaneously.
- Describe the genetic and the epigenetic theories of cancer.

The presence of a lump or mass is a common clinical finding, and the term "tumor" was applied at one time to such a lesion; the suffix *-oma* was used to denote it. This practice of classifying all swellings as tumors became established long before the nature of the lesions was understood, and even today this relic of medical history persists in the use of names like "hematoma," "hamartoma," "tuberculoma," and "granuloma." In due course, the swellings of known origin, especially the infective ones, were excluded from the category of tumors, and there remained a large group of swellings of unknown cause that apparently had arisen as a result of the unrestrained growth of the individual's own cells. In all other pathologic processes, the growth of cells appears to be coordinated and under strict control. A tumor is now regarded as resulting from a breakdown in this mechanism and has been defined by Willis as *an abnormal mass of tissue, the growth of which exceeds and is uncoordinated with that of the normal tissues and persists in the same excessive manner after cessation of the stimulus that evoked the change.* This definition is unsatisfactory in several respects. First, it implies that the stimulus producing a tumor need act only for a short time. Second, it implies that the regulating mechanism governing cell growth is abolished. Unfortunately, we know little of this regulating mechanism, and we are consequently not able to prove or disprove that it is nonfunctional.

Although the excessive growth of cells is often manifested by the production of a tumor mass, this does not always occur. Sometimes the migration of newly formed cells from the site of formation outweighs the bulk of abnormal proliferation, and no swelling as such exists. One excellent example of this is the diffuse infiltrating carcinoma of the stomach; another is leukemia. *Neoplasia,* which literally means "new formation or new growth," is a more suitable term. It implies that there is an abnormal type of growth that may be evident not only in the intact animal but also in cells grown in culture. Nevertheless, the terms "tumor" and "neoplasm" are commonly used synonymously and in this book are used in this manner.

CLASSIFICATION OF NEOPLASMS

A neoplasm is regarded as resulting from an unrestrained growth of cells, and it follows that one possible classification can be based on the cell of origin. Since the tissues of the body have been divided into either epithelium or connective tissue, tumors can likewise be placed into one of two groups. Furthermore, each group can be subdivided. Thus, epithelial tumors can be grouped into those arising from stratified squamous epithelium, those from columnar epithelium, and so on. This delineation, based on the cell type of origin, is an important component of our present-day classification. In itself, it is quite inadequate, because the effects of a tumor are determined not only by the tissue of origin but also by its biologic behavior. In some tumors, the dividing cells adhere to each other, and the neoplastic mass remains as a circumscribed mass. Such a lesion is termed a *benign tumor,* and its behavior can be contrasted with that of tumors in which the cells do not adhere to one another and are thereby enabled to invade the surrounding tissues. These are the *malignant tumors,* or *cancers.* Cancer cells often enter natural channels such as lymphatics or blood vessels, and groups of tumor cells are carried as emboli to other parts of the body, where they grow and set up *secondary growths,* or *metastases.* Local invasion and embolic spread are the two characteristics of malignant tumors. The term "malignant" is particularly suitable, for, with the very few exceptions of spontaneous regression, this type of tumor inevitably causes death unless effective treatment is instituted. Nevertheless, the rate of progression varies markedly from one tumor to another, as will be seen from some examples studied later.

In addition to the typical benign and malignant tumors, there are other types that show patterns of behavior not fitting into either group. There are tumors of *intermediate malignancy* in which the tumor cells invade locally but have a limited capacity to metastasize. *Carcinoma in situ* and the phenomena of *spontaneous regression* and *dormant cancer* are considered later.

The neoplastic cells are supported and nourished by a network of host connective tissue that consists predominantly of blood vessels, lymphatics, fibroblasts, and a varying amount of collagen. This network is called the stroma, and although an intimate part of the tumor, it is not considered to be involved in the neoplastic change. Both benign and malignant tumors produce a number of factors that seem to promote stroma formation. One of these encourages the ingrowth of blood vessels and is called an angiogenic factor. When the stroma is abundant and fibrous, the tumor is hard and is described as desmoplastic or scirrhous.

When the patient is first seen clinically, the organ of origin is the most striking feature of many tumors. If the cell type of origin and biologic behavior of the tumor can be determined, a satisfactory diagnosis may be obtained. In practice, however, it is not possible to assess behavior by leaving the tumor alone and awaiting development. It has been found that behavior can frequently be related to the microscopic appearance of the tumor. The ultimate classification of a particular tumor is therefore attained by establishing its site of origin, its tissue of origin, its behavior, and its microscopic appearance. An outline of the classification in current use is shown in Table 12–1.

It will be seen that the majority of tumors can be classified as arising from either epithelium or mesenchyme (connective tissue). Benign epithelial tumors are either *papillomas* or *adenomas.* Malignant tumors of epithelial tissues are termed *carcinomas.* Benign mesenchymal tumors are named after the cell type of origin, *e.g.,* fibroma, whereas malignant tumors of mesenchyme are called *sarcomas.* There are some instances in which this overall classification cannot be used.

Undifferentiated Tumors. A tumor so anaplastic that no differentiation can be seen on routine microscopy cannot be classified because neither its cell of origin nor its direction of differentiation is evident. The problem can sometimes be resolved by recourse to *electron microscopy* because minor degrees of differentiation may be apparent that are not detectable by routine light microscopy. For instance, the presence of melanosomes suggests origin from melanocytes, and neurosecretory granules indicate a diffuse endocrine type of tumor, *e.g.,* a carcinoid tumor. Electron microscopy of tumors has now developed into a major subspecialty in pathology.

Many cell types have specific antigen markers that can be detected by use of a monospecific *immunoperoxidase technique.* The finding of a particular marker in a tumor therefore suggests its cell type of origin. For example, an undifferentiated tumor of skin that stains for the protein

S100 is likely to be derived from melanocytes (melanoma), but if it is positive for cytokeratin, a diagnosis of carcinoma is more likely. When a tumor is so undifferentiated that its tissue of origin is unrecognizable by current or available techniques, a descriptive name is used: small cell, large cell, giant cell, and spindle cell are all self-explanatory terms when applied to a tumor.

Origin from Highly Specialized Tissues. Some tumors arise from certain very specialized tissues that are so distinctive as to be unlike those found elsewhere. For example, gliomas, although of connective tissue origin in the brain, are unlike sarcomas in other situations. Likewise, tumors of lymphoid tissue, although of mesenchymal origin, are best classified separately as lymphomas.

Origin from Embryonic or Placental Tissues. Certain tumors arise from cells that are not normally present in the adult body. Tumors can arise from cells that are present during development but disappear by the time adult life has been attained; this group includes the embryonic tumors of infancy. For instance, the *neuroblastoma* arises from primitive neuroblasts and not from adult nerve cells (which are incapable of dividing). Retinoblastomas and nephroblastoma (Wilms' tumor) also fall into this group. Other tumors arise from placental tissue. Both *hydatidiform mole* and *choriocarcinoma* are of fetal origin.

Origin from Germ Cells. Germ cells are totipotential, and tumors derived from them can differentiate into any of the tissues of the body; as would be expected, they occur most frequently in the ovary or testis. In some germ cell tumors, one type of differentiation predominates, *e.g.,* seminoma and choriocarcinoma of the testis. When many types of tissue are produced, the tumor is called a *teratoma.* The most commonly encountered example is the benign ovarian teratoma ("dermoid cyst"). The lining of the cyst consists of epidermis together with normal skin appendages, including hair follicles. The cyst contains sebaceous material and matted hair (Fig. 12–1). Other structures can be found in its wall, including thyroid tissue, teeth, bone, brain, and spaces lined by a variety of different types of epithelia. Teratoma of the testis is invariably malignant; it is indeed the most common malignant tumor of young men.

Table 12–1 CLASSIFICATION OF NEOPLASMS

Tissue of Origin	Behavior		
	Benign	*Intermediate*	*Malignant**
Epithelium			
Covering and protective type			
Squamous	Squamous-cell papilloma		Squamous-cell carcinoma
Transitional	Transitional-cell papilloma		Transitional-cell carcinoma
Columnar	Columnar-cell papilloma		Adenocarcinoma
Compact and secreting type	Adenoma; if cystic, cystadenoma or papillary cystadenoma		Adenocarcinoma; if cystic, cystadenocarcinoma
Others	Adenoma	Basal-cell carcinoma Pleomorphic salivary gland tumors Carcinoid tumor (argentaffinoma)	Carcinoma
Mesenchyme			
Fibrous	Fibroma		Fibrosarcoma
Nerve sheath	Neurofibroma		Neurofibrosarcoma
Adipose	Lipoma		Liposarcoma
Smooth muscle	Leiomyoma		Leiomyosarcoma
Striated muscle	Rhabdomyoma		Rhabdomyosarcoma
Synovial	Synovioma		Malignant synovioma
Cartilaginous	Chondroma		Chondrosarcoma
Bone osteoblast	Osteoma	Giant-cell tumor	Osteosarcoma
Blood vessels and lymphatics	Benign hemangioma and lymphangioma		Angiosarcoma
Neuroglia	Astrocytoma, oligodendroglioma, and ependymoma†		
Fetal trophoblast	Hydatidiform mole		Choriocarcinoma
Germ cells	Benign teratoma		Malignant teratoma
Embryonic tissue			
Pluripotential cell			
Kidney			Nephroblastoma
Unipotential cell			
Retina			Retinoblastoma
Hindbrain			Medulloblastoma
Sympathetic ganglia and adrenal medulla	Ganglioneuroma		Neuroblastoma
Melanocyte			Malignant melanoma

*Any malignant tumor may be so undifferentiated that it must be classified on a histologic basis, *e.g.*, carcinoma simplex, spindle-cell sarcoma. The lymphomas and many rare tumors are not included in this table.

†These tumors are difficult to classify. The common types are locally malignant, but some also metastasize within the central nervous system. Rarely, they appear to be benign in children.

Tumors Derived from Tissue of Debatable Origin. The best example of this problem is the melanoma, a malignant tumor derived from melanocytes. It is undecided whether the parent melanocyte is of epidermal, nervous, or mesenchymal origin.

BENIGN NEOPLASMS

The cells of a benign tumor closely resemble those of the parent tissue microscopically. They are therefore described as being "well differentiated." The cells tend to be regular in size and uniform in staining and shape; mitoses are scanty and, when present, are of normal type.

The cells of a benign neoplasm show no tendency to invade the surrounding tissues but do produce an expanding mass that has two local effects: pressure atrophy and obstruction.

The adjacent specialized parenchymatous tissue undergoes atrophy; the more resistant connective tissue survives to form a capsule. *Benign tumors are therefore usually well encapsulated* and

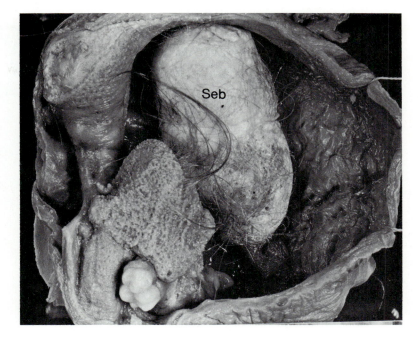

Figure 12–1 Teratoma of the ovary. The specimen shows the opened cyst. It is lined by skin, and on one side a hard mass projects into the cavity. This is covered by spongy skin containing numerous sebaceous glands, and from it is growing a tuft of hair. The mass contains bone in which a number of teeth are partially embedded. One of these is clearly shown in the photograph. The mass of tissue (Seb) contains hair but is otherwise lying free in the cyst cavity. It consists largely of sebaceous material and desquamated keratin. (Photograph of specimen courtesy of the Boyd Museum, University of Toronto.)

are not intimately connected with the surrounding tissues except at points of entry of the supplying blood vessels (see Fig. 27–1). Benign tumors can therefore be excised with relative ease; if local removal is complete, they do not recur. Nevertheless, a benign tumor cannot be dismissed as inconsequential. One within the skull or vertebral column can produce serious pressure effects and even death. The shape of a benign tumor is generally spherical, but it may be modified by firm local structures.

A benign tumor may obstruct a natural passage, causing extensive damage. Thus, blockage of a bronchus can lead to bronchiectasis and bronchopneumonia. A tumor of the intestine can produce obstruction. Benign tumors generally grow slowly and rarely ulcerate on the surface. Hence, bleeding is uncommon as a symptom, except for certain vascular surface papillomatous growths such as those of the colon or bladder.

Benign tumors of endocrine tissue occasionally produce an excess quantity of the associated hormone; this oversecretion of hormone can lead to serious and sometimes fatal effects. A good example of this is the adenoma of the islets of Langerhans, which can lead to fatal hypoglycemia as a result of the overproduction of insulin.

Therefore, it is not true that benign tumors cannot cause death.

Benign Epithelial Neoplasms

These are of two main types. Benign neoplasia of a surface or lining epithelium produces a warty tumor called a *papilloma* (Fig. 12–2). In a compact gland, such as the breast or the thyroid, the tumor is embedded in the tissue and is called an *adenoma*.

Papilloma. Papillomas may occur on any epithelial surface. Some have a broad base and are described as *sessile*, whereas others become pedunculated and are called *polyps*, a morphologic term applied to any pedunculated mass attached to a surface and not necessarily neoplastic. Papillomas are supplied by a core of connective tissue stroma containing blood vessels, lymphatics, and nerves. This is covered by a folded neoplastic epithelium composed of stratified squamous, transitional, or columnar cells, according to the type from which it has arisen. The cells show an orderly arrangement, and the epithelial basement membrane is intact unless there is distortion due to inflammation. The epithelial cells are entirely

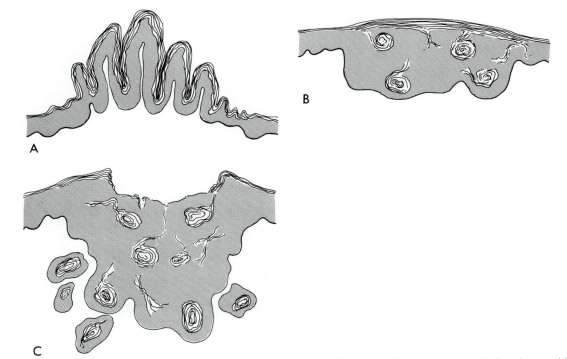

Figure 12–2 Tumors of the epidermis. Three types of neoplasia of a keratinizing stratified squamous epithelium (*e.g.*, epidermis) are shown. *A*, Benign neoplasia results in an excessive production of regular epithelium, which is thrown into a complicated folded structure in order to be accommodated. This formation is called a papilloma. The epidermal cells mature in an orderly way from the basal cells to the superficial squames. *B*, In carcinoma *in situ*, there is excessive growth of epidermis, which thereby becomes thickened (acanthosis). Maturation of the cells is disorderly; foci of keratinization are found within the epidermis instead of being present only on the surface (dyskeratosis). *C*, In carcinoma, the atypical epidermal cells break through the basement membrane and invade the underlying tissues. (Drawing by Margot Mackay, University of Toronto Faculty of Medicine, Department of Surgery, Division of Biomedical Communications, Toronto.)

restricted to the surface and do not show invasion.

Stratified squamous-cell papillomas are common on the skin; examples include warts (Fig. 12–3) and seborrheic keratoses (Chapter 31). Since the common wart (verruca vulgaris) is a squamous-cell papilloma, the term *verrucous* is commonly used to describe any papillary or wartlike lesion, whether it be on the skin or elsewhere, benign or malignant.

Adenoma. An adenoma is composed of a mass of glandular tissue that closely resembles the structure of the parent tissue. Adenomas are quite common in the colon, where they arise from the glands in the mucosa. As with papillomas, they frequently become polypoid (see Fig. 23–21).

In some adenomas, the glandular spaces enlarge to form cysts (causing a *cystadenoma*), and

papillomas can grow into these cysts (forming a *papillary cystadenoma*). Such a tumor is common in the ovary.

Benign Mesenchymal Neoplasms

A benign neoplasm, which can arise from any connective tissue, is composed of a mass of cells whose structure closely resembles that of the parent tissue. Common tumors in this group are lipomas derived from fat, leiomyomas derived from the smooth muscle (Fig. 12–4), neurofibromas (schwannomas) derived from the Schwann cells of the nerve sheaths, and fibromas derived from fibroblasts. These tumors are generally well circumscribed.

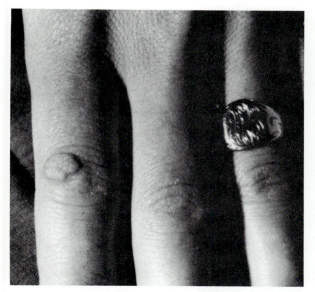

Figure 12–3 Verruca vulgaris. This patient has a common wart overlying the proximal interphalangeal joint of the left index finger. The lesion is a squamous-cell papilloma.

MALIGNANT NEOPLASMS

The cells of a malignant tumor infiltrate surrounding tissues, normal cells are enveloped and destroyed, and the edge of the tumor is poorly defined. Microscopic spread occurs beyond the naked-eye edge of the tumor, and complete excision by surgery is therefore difficult. Even if much surrounding, apparently normal tissue is included in the excision, malignant cells can often remain behind; their continued growth results in a *local recurrence.* The invading malignant cells spread in the planes of least resistance: fingerlike processes extend outward from the main tumor mass, and the growth has a fanciful resemblance to the silhouette of a crab. It is from this mode of spread that the term "cancer," from the Latin word meaning *crab,* is derived. In lay language, it is generally applied to all malignant tumors. In medical terminology, it is often used as being synonymous with *carcinoma, which is defined as a malignant tumor of the epithelial cells. A sarcoma is a malignant neoplasm derived from mesenchymal cells.*

Embolic spread of tumor cells is responsible for the production of distant metastases. Local invasion and embolic spread are the two characteristics of malignant tumors. Both are related

to the reduced cell adhesiveness that appears to be a fundamental characteristic of malignant cells, for this property is evident not only *in vivo* but also in tissue culture. The cells do not resist mechanical separation as well as do those of normal tissue (see cell transformation). The power to invade and spread, combined with the capacity for progressive growth, makes the term "malignant" particularly apt for this type of tumor. Death is inevitable in untreated cases, except for those very rare—although well-documented—cases of *spontaneous regression,* in which proven cancers have disappeared either with no treatment or with very limited palliative treatment.

Microscopic Features

Several important microscopic features should be noted. Tumor tissue may resemble the parent tissue to a considerable extent, but the similarity is not as great as with benign tumors. Differentiation is not so well developed, and recognition of the tissue of origin is often difficult or even impossible. Tumors showing little or no differentiation are called *undifferentiated.*

Malignant tumors usually show much mitotic activity. The synthesis of DNA before division results in nuclear enlargement and hyperchromatism. This synthesis, together with the formation of polyploid cells, accounts for the irregularity in size and shape *(pleomorphism)* and the mode of staining that is so characteristic of malignant tumors. Mitoses are not only numerous but also abnormal (Fig. 12–5). A number of cells may deviate from the normal complement of 46 chromosomes, and occasionally cells are seen to divide into three instead of two *(triradiate or tripolar mitosis).*

Anaplasia is a term that at first was introduced to describe new cells deviating from normal and resembling those of embryonic origin. It was at one time thought that tumors were derived from rests of embryonic cells. This concept has been abandoned, but the term anaplasia is still used to describe those cellular changes that are found in malignant tumors. Therefore, a tumor said to show a high degree of anaplasia has cells that are pleomorphic, poorly differentiated (scarcely

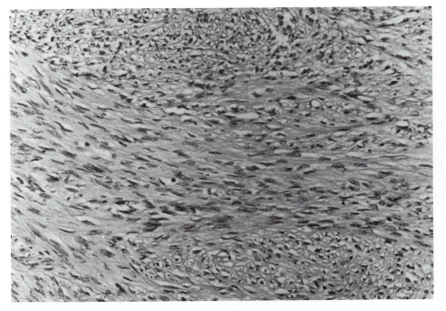

Figure 12–4 Leiomyoma of the uterus. The tumor consists of spindle-shaped smooth muscle cells arranged in sheaves, some of which are cut longitudinally, whereas others are seen in transverse section. No mitoses can be seen in this benign tumor (×250).

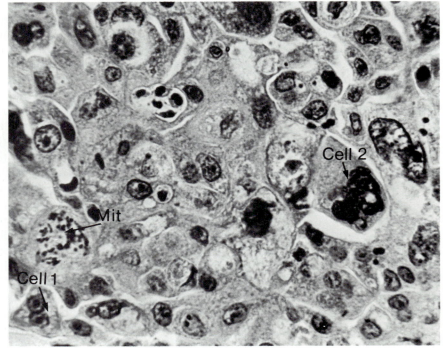

Figure 12–5 Anaplastic carcinoma of the lung. The tumor shows little evidence of differentiation, and its cells exhibit marked pleomorphism. One cell possesses two nuclei, each with a prominent nucleolus (Cell 1), whereas another has many hyperchromatic nuclei (Cell 2). In an atypical mitosis, scattered chromosomes can be identified (Mit) (×550). (From Walter, J.B., and Israel, M.S.: General Pathology. 6th ed. Edinburgh, Churchill Livingstone, 1987.)

reproducing the parent tissue), and exhibiting frequent and bizarre mitoses.

Gross Characteristics

Malignant tumors do not possess a limiting capsule, although with some very rapidly proliferating growths, such as secondary tumors in the liver, they may appear circumscribed. Microscopy, however, shows tumor extension beyond the apparent edge of the growth. Malignant tumors tend to be irregular in shape and are usually larger than their benign counterparts. As would be expected from their destructive properties, they tend to ulcerate along a free surface. Hence, any area of ulceration that fails to heal within a reasonable time should be regarded as malignant until proven otherwise. Since tumors invade and destroy blood vessels, bleeding is a frequent symptom. *Bleeding and ulceration are thus features of malignant tumors.*

Effects

Malignant tumors produce their ill effects in a number of ways.

Mechanical Pressure and Obstruction. Like benign tumors, malignant tumors cause obstruction to natural passages and lead to serious consequences. Thus, a tumor of the colon produces intestinal obstruction; a tumor of the bronchus leads to collapse and bronchopneumonia in the lung beyond it.

Destruction of Tissue. Both primary and secondary tumors infiltrate and destroy tissue. This is most obvious with cancer of the skin (Fig. 12–6) and is also well illustrated by tumors in bone, in which destruction may be so marked that minimal trauma produces a fracture. This is known as a *pathologic fracture* and may sometimes be the first symptom of a previously missed tumor.

Hemorrhage. Malignant tumors that involve any surface usually ulcerate and bleed. Repeated bleeding can cause anemia; occasionally, a fatal sudden hemorrhage can occur where a large vessel is eroded. *Clinically unexplained bleeding*

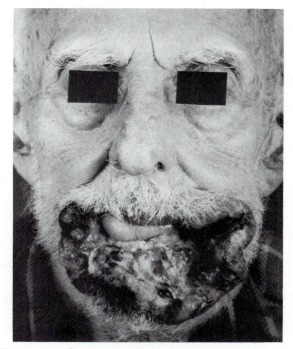

Figure 12–6 Squamous-cell carcinoma of the lower lip. This patient was a recluse and neglected himself. The carcinoma has destroyed the whole of the lower lip and part of the jaw. Cervical lymph nodes were invaded by metastatic growth. On histologic examination, the tumor was a keratinizing squamous-cell carcinoma similar to that depicted in Figure 12–10.

from any site should be treated seriously, since it is a common symptom of cancer.

Infection. All ulcerating cancers are bound to become secondarily infected with bacteria. Infection often follows in the wake of obstruction, such as bronchopneumonia with cancer of the lung and urinary tract infection with cancer of the bladder. *Repeated bouts of infection in an organ should always lead to a suspicion of an underlying malignant tumor.*

Starvation. Cancer of the mouth, pharynx, esophagus, and stomach can so obstruct the passage of food that direct starvation occurs.

Anemia. Anemia is common and is due to a variety of causes. There may be direct blood loss from an ulcerating tumor, malabsorption of essential dietary components, or bone marrow replacement if there are multiple bone metastases.

Cachexia. The emaciated appearance of patients with advanced cancer is characteristic, but it is nevertheless not uncommon for some patients to remain obese. The cause of the weight loss and the generalized body atrophy in many patients with cancer has given rise to much speculation. A polypeptide, termed *cachexin*, released from macrophages may play a part in mobilizing fat and causing weight loss. It is probably identical to tumor necrosis factor (also released from macrphages), an agent that causes tumor necrosis in experimental animals. It is too toxic for human use.

In advanced malignancy, there is usually fever, a raised erythrocyte sedimentation rate, and a neutrophil leukocytosis. In part these are effects of infection, and in part they are due to the pressure of necrotic tissue both in the tumor and in the surrounding tissues.

Hormonal Effects. Malignant tumors of the endocrine glands can sometimes produce effects by overproduction of the relevant hormone. This is less common than with benign tumors, as would be expected, because malignant tumors are less differentiated both in structure and in function.

Another curious phenomenon is the hormonal effect produced by tumors of nonendocrine origin, which are particularly common in cancer of the lung. The tumor appears to be able to secrete hormonelike substances, and symptoms of hyperadrenocorticism (Cushing's syndrome), hyperinsulinism, and hyperparathyroidism may occur. It is apparent that the atypical cells of malignant tumors can produce and secrete hormones or hormonelike substances into the circulation. This is an instance of abnormal differentiation of a malignant tumor and forms one type of paraneoplastic syndrome described in the following.

Paraneoplastic Syndromes. A variety of syndromes have been reported in association with tumors that are not explicable in terms of infiltration by either a primary tumor or its metastases. Muscle weakness, skin eruptions, signs of an intracranial tumor, and venous thrombosis are some examples of this. At necropsy, no local tumor is found to explain these features. A possible explanation is the deposition of immune complexes containing tumor antigen. For the most part, however, these strange manifestations of cancer have not been explained.

Spread of Malignant Neoplasms

Direct Spread. Tumor cells spread into the surrounding tissues, particularly along tissue planes and natural spaces. This is a feature that is used by the pathologist as an aid to the microscopic diagnosis of malignancy. Clinically, local invasion is often evident by the way in which the tumor becomes attached to adjacent structures. Thus, a carcinoma of the breast eventually becomes attached to the skin and the underlying pectoral muscles.

Invasion of Lymphatics. Carcinoma, but not sarcoma, shows a particular tendency to invade lymphatic vessels at an early stage, and the cells may grow as a long, ever-extending cord. The process is called *lymphatic permeation*, and the lymphatic obstruction it produces can cause lymphatic edema (Fig. 12–7).

Invasion of the Arteries and Veins. This is a common event and may lead to thrombosis and obstruction. There has been much study of the manner in which malignant cells adhere to vascular endothelium. They may have receptors for fibronectin and laminin, and the subsequent production of collagenase seems to aid the invasion of the vessel wall, an event that is a vital step in the establishment of a metastasis.

Spread by Metastasis. Groups of malignant cells may become detached, travel in some natural passage to a distant site, become implanted, and finally grow to produce secondary deposits, or metastases. The lymphatics, blood vessels, and serous cavities are the most important pathways.

Lymphatic Spread. Detached groups of tumor cells that have invaded lymphatic channels travel to the regional draining lymph nodes (Fig. 12–8). If the cells survive and grow, they replace the lymph node with tumor; the cells then move on to the next group of nodes. This is a common event with carcinoma and melanoma, but it is rare with sarcoma.

Blood Spread. The occurrence of blood-borne metastases is the feature of malignant disease that is responsible for death in most cases. It is the factor that limits the surgical and radiotherapeutic treatment of cancer. At first sight, the mode of production of secondary tumors is easy to understand. Malignant cells invade small ven-

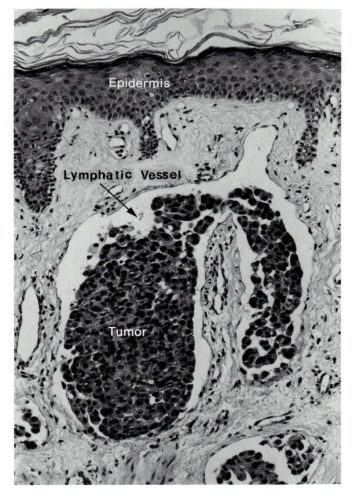

Figure 12–7 Spread of carcinoma by lymphatic permeation. Section of skin shows dilated lymphatic vessels filled with carcinoma. The specimen was taken from the skin of a woman with advanced carcinoma of the breast (×250).

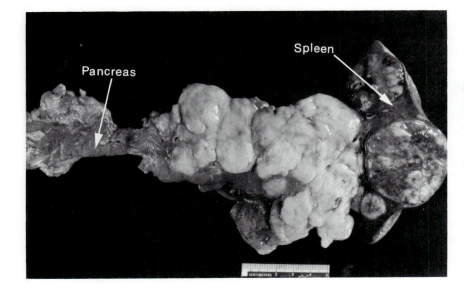

Figure 12–8 Lymph node metastases. The specimen shows a group of peripancreatic lymph nodes that are greatly enlarged by metastatic carcinoma. Several nodules of tumor are also present in the spleen. The primary growth was a small-cell (oat-cell) carcinoma of the lung.

ules, become detached, and are then carried in the blood stream until they become impacted in the next capillary network that they encounter. There the emboli take root, and the cells proliferate and develop into secondary tumors. A second route of blood-borne metastases is via the lymphatics, for all the lymph eventually drains into the venous circulation.

As would be expected, the lung is one of the most common sites of metastasis for all tumors. Primary tumors arising in an area drained by the portal vein regularly metastasize to the liver. Purely mechanical factors seem to account for this distribution, but such an explanation seems untenable upon a closer examination of the facts.

Many tumors, *e.g.*, of the breast and the kidney, give rise not only to lung metastases but also to secondary growths in the liver, bones, and other organs; such systemic metastases sometimes occur without apparent deposits in the lung. It is possible that such deposits are, in fact, present but are missed at an inadequate necropsy examination. Alternatively, one can postulate that the cells pass through the lung capillaries and travel to the systemic circulation, where they lead to secondary deposit formation.

One might expect that the distribution of metastases would be related to the blood supply of each organ. Such is not the case. Cardiac and skeletal muscle have an abundant blood supply, and yet it is rare to find metastases in muscle. The spleen also has a very large blood supply, yet splenic metastases are also quite uncommon. *Selective metastasis* is the term used to describe this distribution of metastases.

There is considerable evidence that malignant cells often reach the blood stream, where most of them die. Only a selected few are able to take root and grow into secondary deposits. In part this depends on the nature of the tumor, as experimental work on the mouse will illustrate. Isolated cells of a transplantable malignant mouse melanoma can be cloned by growth in tissue culture. When these cells are injected intravenously into other mice of the same strain, metastases predominate in one organ (lung or brain) according to the nature of the clone that has been selected. The nature of the tumor itself is therefore important in the formation of metastases.

Some examples of selective metastasis should be noted.

Liver. The most common organ in which blood-borne metastases are found is the liver, regardless of whether the primary tumor is in an area drained by the portal vein. Although massive enlargement of the liver is common, it is rare for liver failure to occur (Fig. 12–9).

Lung. This is the next most common site of metastases.

Bone. Carcinomas of the breast, lung, and prostate commonly metastasize to bone. Such spread is less frequently seen with other tumors. *Pain* is a common presenting symptom, particularly when the spine is involved and nerves are compressed.

Brain. Cancer of the lung is notorious for the frequency with which it metastasizes to brain. Indeed, secondary lung cancer is a common type of tumor to be found in the brain.

Adrenal Glands. This is a frequent site for secondary lung and breast cancer, an infrequent site for other primary growths.

Transcelomic Spread. When a malignant tumor invades the serosal layer of a viscus, it causes a local acute inflammatory response. This results in the formation of a serous inflammatory exudate in the cavity, and bleeding usually occurs. It follows that the presence of a blood-stained effusion into any serous cavity, such as that of the pleura or peritoneum, should always arouse suspicion of malignancy. Withdrawal of some fluid and an examination for malignant cells will sometimes lead to a positive diagnosis. Cells that travel in the effusion can form the basis of numerous secondary seedling growths.

Grading and Staging of Malignant Neoplasms

In order to compare the results of various forms of treatment and to assess the likely outcome of a malignant tumor (*i.e.*, to give a *prognosis*), efforts have been made to classify individual types of tumor.

Grading is an attempt to assess the biologic malignancy of a tumor by examining its microscopic appearance, taking into consideration its degree of differentiation, its number of mitoses,

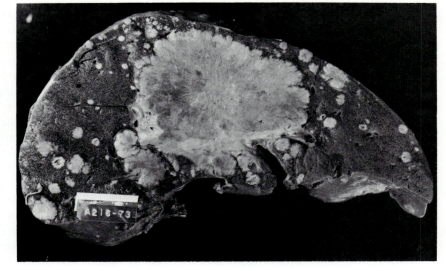

Figure 12–9 Liver with metastatic carcinoma. The liver contains numerous white nodules of metastatic carcinoma from a primary tumor in the nasopharynx. The nodules are of varying size; one of them is 13 cm in diameter.

and other factors. A grade I tumor is well differentiated, has few mitoses, and tends to have a good prognosis. A grade III tumor is poorly differentiated, has many mitoses, and tends to have a poor prognosis. Sometimes four grades are used. Unfortunately, the correlation between grade and prognosis is not good. Tumors may vary greatly from one area to another, and the assessment of the grade is very subjective.

Staging is more satisfactory and is based on the size of the primary tumor and its known extent of spread. The most widely used today is the *TNM system.* T1 to T4 describe the size of the tumor. N indicates the presence and extent of lymph node involvement; thus, N0 indicates no nodal involvement. M indicates the presence and extent of distant metastases. The details of the classification vary with each specific tumor.

Dormancy

One difficulty with staging is the tendency for some metastases to appear many years after the primary tumor has apparently been treated successfully. Patients may remain well for 10, 20, or even 30 years after removal of a primary tumor and then suddenly develop multiple secondary deposits despite the absence of any local recurrence. It is assumed that tumor cells were present in the body during the entire period, but for

reasons unknown, they remained dormant. This is one of the most mystifying aspects of malignant disease, and were we to know the factors responsible for keeping cancer cells dormant, we might well have an adequate treatment for the disease. Carcinoma of the breast and kidney and melanoma of the eye are tumors that are notorious for this tendency toward the development of metastases after a period of dormancy.

Malignant Epithelial Neoplasms

Malignant epithelial neoplasms are the *carcinomas,* the most common of all malignant tumors. Three types may be recognized: (1) squamous-cell carcinoma, (2) glandular epithelial carcinoma, and (3) transitional-cell carcinoma.

Squamous-Cell Carcinoma. This histologic type of tumor arises at any site normally covered by stratified squamous epithelium—skin, mouth, esophagus, and other similar regions. Squamous-cell carcinoma arises via the invasion of the underlying connective tissues by the germinal cells situated in the basal layer of the epithelium. Malignant cells may infiltrate separately, but more usually they form clumps and columns as they proceed into the connective tissue. The cells tend to differentiate into prickle cells and form keratin, so that in a well-differentiated tumor, clumps of cells are seen with a central whorl of keratin (Fig. 12–10). This is called an *epithelial pearl* and is in effect an attempt by the malignant cells to reproduce the stratum corneum of the normal skin. Tumors that are less well differentiated form no keratin, but they do contain prickle cells. Poorly differentiated tumors show few recognizable structures and are difficult to distinguish from poorly differentiated tumors of other types. Purely descriptive terms are used to name such tumors: giant-cell carcinoma, spindle-cell carcinoma, and large-cell carcinoma.

Squamous-cell carcinoma can also arise from columnar or transitional epithelium. This can occur in one of two ways. The normal epithelium can undergo metaplasia to squamous epithelium, and tumor growth subsequently occurs in this. A second, and more likely, explanation is that the tumor arises in the epithelium first, and then the tumor cells show squamous differentiation. One of the most common tumors of lung, arising from the bronchial mucosa, is a squamous-cell carcinoma. Likewise, squamous-cell carcinoma is also found in the urinary bladder and less frequently in the gallbladder. It should be noted that the term "squamous-cell carcinoma" is used to describe a particular microscopic appearance of a tumor showing differentiation into a keratinizing squamous type of cell. It does not always mean a tumor arising from a squamous epithelium.

Glandular Epithelial Carcinoma. This type of carcinoma may arise from a surface secreting epithelium, such as that which lines the stomach, or from a solid gland, such as liver or breast. The pattern of invasion of neoplastic epithelial cells is similar to that already described with squamous-cell carcinoma. In the case of the tumors arising from glandular epithelium, groups of cancer cells, instead of producing keratin, tend to arrange themselves into acinar structures containing a central lumen into which some secretion is poured (Figs. 12–11 and 12–12). The well-differentiated cancers showing excellent acinus formation can closely mimic the original glandular structure. If differentiation is poor, the tumor is composed of masses of cells with only

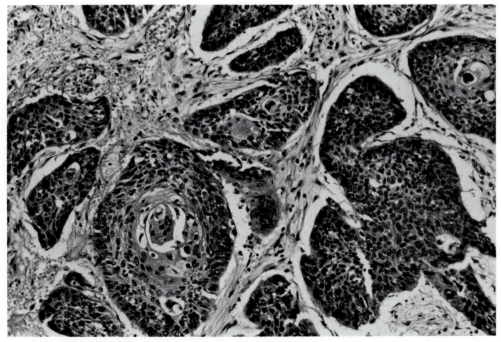

Figure 12–10 Squamous-cell carcinoma of skin. The dermis has been invaded by malignant cells that have grown to form clumps. In some areas, the central tumor cells have differentiated into keratin and have formed cell nests or epithelial pearls. This is characteristic of a well-differentiated squamous-cell carcinoma.

occasional tubule formation. A tumor derived from glandular epithelium and showing glandular differentiation is called an *adenocarcinoma.*

In poorly differentiated tumors, there are merely clumps of cells surrounded by a stroma and no evidence of central cavitation to produce an acinus. The names *carcinoma simplex, spheroidal-cell carcinoma,* and *polygonal-cell carcinoma* are applied in this type of cancer. Such tumors are particularly common in the breast and stomach.

Mucoid Cancer. Occasionally, a carcinoma derived from glandular epithelium shows such excessive production of mucus that to the naked eye the tumor appears as a gelatinous mass; on microscopic examination, there are pools of mucus in which are floating malignant cells. Sometimes the cells contain one large droplet of mucus with the nucleus pushed to one side, giving the appearance of a signet ring. This type of tumor occurs in the stomach or large intestine.

Transitional-Cell Carcinoma. This type of tumor occurs in the urinary tract and often shows areas of squamous differentiation.

Stromal Reaction to Carcinoma. The reaction of the invaded tissue to carcinoma cells varies; its growth may be so stimulated that a hard fibrotic or *scirrhous* type of tumor is produced. Most breast cancers are of this type. As with wounds, the dense fibrosis appears to be associated with a contracting tendency that is poorly understood. It is this effect that leads to obstruction with many carcinomas of the colon. The contraction causes a purse-string deformity.

When a tumor has little stroma in relation to the cell bulk, it is soft or brainlike and is described as *medullary,* or *encephaloid.* It should be noted that carcinoma cells, like normal epithelial cells,

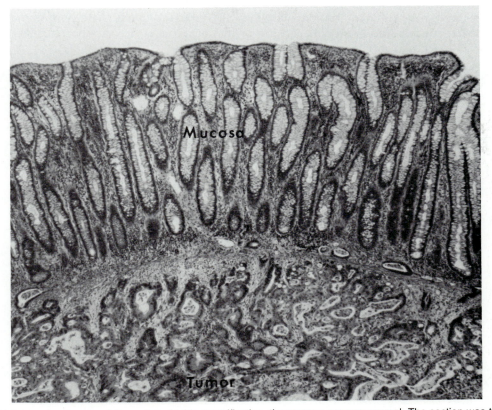

Figure 12–11 Adenocarcinoma of the colon. At this magnification, the mucosa appears normal. The section was taken from an area adjacent to a carcinoma; tumor has invaded the submucosa. Normally, this layer consists of loose connective tissue similar to that seen in the small intestine (Chapter 2) (×60).

tend to grow in solid sheets or clusters with close cell-to-cell apposition. Only with very anaplastic tumors do the cells separate, and their growth then resembles that of a sarcoma (see following).

Malignant Mesenchymal Neoplasms

These malignant tumors are called *sarcomas* and are much less common than carcinomas; like carcinomas, they occur at all ages. On the whole, sarcomas spread more rapidly than do carcinomas, and the prognosis is correspondingly more grave. The cells of a sarcoma tend to separate after mitosis and to be intimately associated with the stroma and its blood vessels. This helps explain why blood-borne metastases appear early: the lungs are often riddled with secondary deposits. Lymphatic involvement is very much less common than with carcinoma.

Fibrosarcomas can arise in any fibrous connective tissue and can vary in their degree of differentiation. A well-differentiated tumor shows some cellular irregularity and good collagen formation; distinction from a fibroma can be extremely difficult. Poorly differentiated tumors show little or no collagen formation and are then termed *spindle-cell sarcomas*. A distinction from anaplastic carcinomas is sometimes difficult.

The most common type of sarcoma of soft tissues is the *malignant fibrous histiocytoma*. It usually arises in the subcutaneous tissues or retroperitoneum. Its precise cell type of origin is undecided because the malignant cells resemble histiocytes and yet appear to make collagen. *Liposarcoma, angiosarcoma,* and *leiomyosarcoma* occur but are uncommon. *Osteosarcoma* is described in Chapter 30.

Tumors of the Lymphoreticular System

Tumors of the lymphoreticular system are the lymphomas and the tumors of the hematopoietic system such as leukemia, which is considered in Chapter 18.

The Lymphomas. The lymphomas are malignant tumors of the lymphoreticular system. They

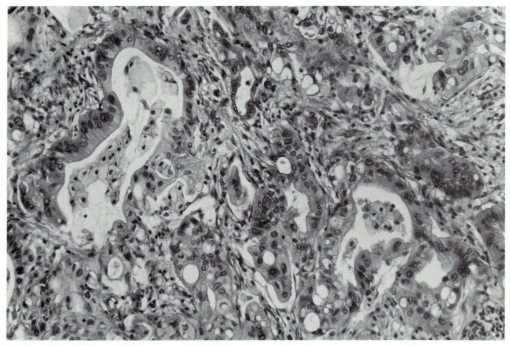

Figure 12–12 Adenocarcinoma of the colon. This section is from a lymph node metastasis of the tumor shown in Figure 12–11. Although the growth is well differentiated, the pattern of glandular formation is quite different from the normal. Some malignant cells line large spaces, whereas others form solid clumps (×250).

are the second most common malignant tumors; carcinomas occur most often. They generally start at one site—usually a lymph node—but spread to other lymph nodes and eventually become disseminated, with deposits being found in the spleen, liver, bone marrow, lungs, and elsewhere. Whether this represents metastasis or multicentric origin is debatable. Unlike many types of sarcoma, they are generally extremely radiosensitive. Sometimes a local lesion can be cured by radiotherapy, but unfortunately, recurrence and spread throughout the body are common. Two major types of lymphoma are recognized.

Hodgkin's Disease. This is the most common of the lymphomas and affects young and middle-aged adults predominantly. Lymph nodes are first affected and are replaced by tumor tissue that consists of atypical histiocytes together with lymphocytes, eosinophils, plasma cells, and often much fibrous tissue. The essential neoplastic element is believed to be the histiocytes. In particular, Reed-Sternberg cells must be identified in order to substantiate the diagnosis. These cells usually have two nuclei, each with a prominent nucleolus, and the nuclei are so arranged that the one appears to be the mirror image of the other. If the disease is treated while it is still localized, the prognosis is quite good, but when the disease has become systemic, the outlook is poor. The prognosis also depends on the histologic appearance of the tumor present. Various classifications are in vogue that relate histologic appearance to prognosis.

Non-Hodgkin's Lymphomas. Many classifications of this group of lymphomas have been proposed but none has proved satisfactory. The problem stems from the complexity of the lymphoreticular system itself. Electron microscopy and immunochemistry have revealed that there are many types of cells involved—B cells, T cells, and reticulum cells and their subtypes; but on routine microscopy, they appear very similar—they are just lymphocytes, or cells of the germinal centers! Even tumors derived from cells that were once thought to be of mononuclear phagocytic system origin have turned out to be types of lymphocytes. In an effort to lessen the confusion, the National Cancer Institute of the United States initiated a study that culminated in a "working formulation for clinical usage." On the basis of clinical features, the lymphomas are divided into three groups: low grade, intermediate grade, and high grade. Individual types are classified histologically. The various types of lymphoma will not be discussed further, except to mention one particular variant. This is Burkitt's lymphoma, a tumor that occurs extensively and almost exclusively in the low-lying moist region of Central and West Africa. It is almost entirely confined to children between the ages of 2 and 14 years and affects the jaws, ovaries, lymph nodes, and kidneys. The usual mode of presentation is an enormous facial swelling with loosening of the affected teeth. The fascination of this tumor is that it is thought to be caused by the Epstein-Barr virus.

Malignant Conditions of the Hematopoietic Tissue. The most important of these are the *leukemias,* in which the malignant cells are found circulating in the peripheral blood, and *multiple myeloma,* in which the bone marrow is replaced by plasma-cell tumors. Both conditions are considered in detail in later chapters.

Neoplasms of Intermediate Malignancy

In their behavior, tumors of intermediate malignancy are between the benign and the malignant groups. Since local invasion occurs, the tumors cannot be regarded as benign. Nevertheless, they do not show the steady, inexorable growth pattern of true malignant tumors. The victims do not inevitably die of the disease if they are left untreated. The most common tumor in this group is the *rodent ulcer,* or *basal-cell carcinoma.* This invades locally, but almost never metastasizes (Figs. 12–13 and 12–14).

Another tumor in this group is the pleomorphic salivary gland tumor. On histologic examination, this is an adenomatous growth and is unusual in that the stroma appears to consist of cartilage (see Fig. 23–7). The tumors often appear encapsulated, but the capsule is infiltrated by lateral extensions of growth. Simple enucleation is therefore followed by recurrence. Blood-borne metastases may develop, but this is a rare event.

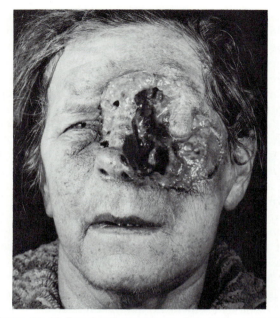

Figure 12–13 Basal-cell carcinoma. This badly neglected tumor involves a large area of the face and has invaded the orbit and nasal cavity. Tumor invasion has combined with infection to cause considerable tissue destruction. The basal-cell carcinoma almost never metastasizes. This particular tumor was cured by radiotherapy together with excision of the left eye. This picture should be remembered when one considers the effects of any invasive tumor that is not readily visible. From this picture, one can appreciate how an ulcerated carcinoma of the stomach, colon, or bladder could be accompanied by tissue destruction, infection, and bleeding. (Courtesy of the late Professor D.D. Smithers.)

In this group of tumors with erratic behavior are the carcinoid tumors of the lung (Chapter 22) and of the intestine.

THE INCIDENCE AND CAUSE OF NEOPLASMS

Observations on the incidence of tumors both in individuals and in ethnic and geographic groups have led to the unraveling of many factors that are involved in the production of tumors. These are considered under the following headings: chemical carcinogenesis; external carcinogenic physical agents; hereditary predisposition; hormonal factors; viral infection; and neoplasia following chronic disease.

Chemical Carcinogenesis

The observation by Percivall Pott in 1775 that cancer of the scrotum was common in chimney sweeps led to the conclusion that soot and its derivatives cause cancer of the skin. It has been amply confirmed both in humans and in animals that certain chemicals, termed *carcinogens*, can lead to the formation of tumors. As would be expected, the first group of chemicals to be discovered were those derived from coal tar, and of these, 1,2:5,6-dibenzanthracene and 3,4-benzpyrene are among the best known. When applied to the skin of animals, they cause squamous-cell carcinoma, and when injected into deeper tissues, they cause a variety of other tumors, including sarcomas. It has been found that when skin is painted with relatively small doses of carcinogen, no obvious change may be apparent. Nevertheless, if the skin is subsequently irritated by relatively nonspecific agents, such as croton oil, tumors can arise upon it. The supposition is that the carcinogen produced a change called *initiation*, such that relatively nonspecific stimuli can subsequently *promote* the formation of a malignant tumor.

The initiation process is thought to begin by the binding of the active carcinogen to some part of the cell, either DNA, RNA, protein, or other component. The biochemical damage so caused may be repaired enzymatically, and the cell can return to its normal state. Alternatively, the change may become fixed if cellular proliferation occurs. Thus, it is difficult to initiate tissues in which mitotic activity is normally low, *e.g.,* liver and kidney. On the other hand, it is easy to understand how hormonal stimulation or regeneration after injury (*e.g.,* viral hepatitis in the case of liver) can aid initiation. Likewise, epidermis can be initiated with ease because it normally exhibits considerable mitotic activity. The state of initiation appears to be long-lasting. By contrast, the effects of a promoting agent are of brief duration. All complete carcinogens are both initiators and promoters, but the relative potency of each activity varies. Thus, saccharin in large doses in animals is a weak initiator but a more powerful promoter in the bladder epithelium. Asbestos fibers act as a promoter in human lung previously initiated by cigarette smoking.

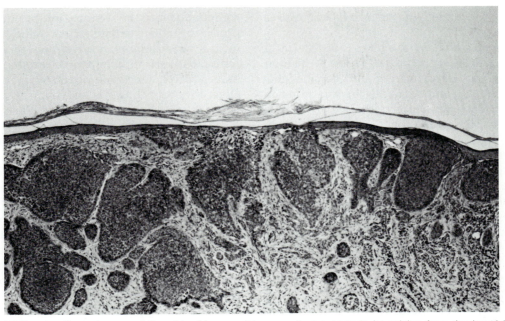

Figure 12–14 Basal-cell carcinoma of the skin. Masses of tumor cells are seen to be arising from the basal layer of the epidermis. Some still maintain their attachment to the epidermis, whereas others have become detached and are spreading deep into the dermis. This is a typical basal-cell carcinoma and shows no tendency to form keratin ($\times 60$).

The simple two-stage development of cancer described by Berenblum (initiation and promotion) has now been extended to envisage a *multistep process.* There is selective growth of the initiated cells to form focal areas of proliferation—some showing atypical hyperplasia, others dysplasia, adenomas, or papillomas. There seems to be progressive evolution of clones through the stages of hyperplasia, dysplasia, and carcinoma *in situ* to carcinoma of low malignancy and finally carcinoma of high malignancy. The whole process takes many months in the case of animals and many years in humans. The process may stop at any point, and indeed some of the stages are reversible. The probability of regression decreases as the lesions become more malignant, but even highly malignant tumors with metastases do on occasion regress—sometimes by differentiation into normal type cells. Possibly keratoacanthoma (Chapter 31) can be explained in this way. It is unfortunate that we know very little of the factors that govern the evolution of tumors.

Many hundreds of carcinogenic compounds have now been identified. Some are positively charged compounds (called *electrophilic reactants* because they react with sites on molecules that are rich in electrons). These agents (*direct acting carcinogens*) act directly on cells to induce cancer. The majority of carcinogens (*procarcinogens*), however, must be activated to form an electrophilic *ultimate carcinogen.* This activation is often accomplished within cells by enzymatic action (Chapter 4). The ultimate carcinogen may act on the cell where it is formed, or it may affect a susceptible tissue that it reaches through the blood stream or via the urine, bile, or other secretion.

The appreciation that chemicals can cause cancer has been of great significance in industry, and it is convenient at this point to mention the carcinogens of importance.

Polycyclic Aromatic Hydrocarbons. These are formed whenever organic material is heated. Hence, they are ubiquitous, being present in food, car exhaust fumes, cigarette smoke, and coal tar derivatives.

Aromatic Amines. Naphthylamine and benzidine used in the chemical and rubber industries are converted in the liver into an ultimate carcinogen that is excreted in the urine and causes *bladder cancer*.

Nitrosamines and Nitrosamides. Nitrites (used to preserve meat) and nitrates (present in food and water) can be converted into carcinogenic nitrosamines and nitrosamides in the stomach and colon. Bacterial action plays a part in this conversion. These carcinogens may well be responsible for cancer of the stomach and colon. The increasing use of refrigeration as a means of preserving meat could be a factor in the declining incidence of stomach cancer.

Naturally Occurring Carcinogens. The mold *Aspergillus flavus*, which contaminates groundnut meal, produces a toxin *(aflatoxin)* that is a powerful liver carcinogen. This may explain why liver cancer is so prevalent in Africa. *Betel nuts* commonly chewed in India are a factor in the development of mouth cancer.

Other Compounds. Many other chemicals have been incriminated as possible human carcinogens. Saccharin and cyclamates have been linked to bladder cancer; vinyl chloride, the monomer of polyvinyl chloride, to hemangiosarcoma of the liver; diethylstilbestrol (DES) given to pregnant women, to carcinoma of the vagina in their female offspring; and chromium, nickel, and asbestos, to cancer of the lung. Indeed, the list is never-ending, and other examples will be cited when the causes of individual tumors are discussed.

Carcinogenic substances may be formed within the body from its own constituents. Bile salts may be modified in the gut to produce carcinogenic chemicals.

The testing of new compounds for carcinogenic activity is an important public health undertaking. Administration to animals is expensive, time-consuming, esthetically unpleasing, and above all unreliable because the activity of a particular carcinogen shows great species variation. An alternative is the *Ames test,* in which the compound is tested for its ability to cause mutations in bacteria. Since 90 per cent of carcinogens prove to be mutagenic, this procedure, or some variant of it, is used as a quick, easily performed screening test. The ultimate proof of safety remains as before—the use of the chemical on human beings.

Inhibition of Chemical Carcinogenesis. Many compounds are known to inhibit the tumor-producing ability of chemical carcinogens. They include antioxidants, derivatives of vitamin A (retinoids), anti-inflammatory steroids, and perhaps vitamin C. These agents may have their effect by preventing the activation of procarcinogens (see earlier), or they could block the processes of initiation or promotion.

Some authorities believe that up to 80 per cent of human cancers are caused by the activity of some chemical carcinogen. Hence, there is hope that some of these carcinogens may be avoided and that the incidence of cancer will decline. Nevertheless, it is evident that the evolution of cancer is a complex process and that drastic changes in living style might have unexpected effects, for not only may carcinogens be removed from our environment, but so also may protective anticarcinogens be eliminated.

External Carcinogenic Physical Agents

The discovery of ionizing radiations was soon followed by an appreciation that these rays can cause cancer. Cancer of the skin occurred in the early radium workers and in those exposed to x-rays. The ingestion of radioactive compounds can lead to more widespread damage. The most famous example of this was recorded in female workers who painted luminous watch dials. They sucked their brushes to point them and thus ingested radioactive compounds used in the luminous paint; these compounds were deposited in the bones. The patients developed sarcoma of the bones as well as leukemia. The most recent demonstration of the carcinogenic activity of ionizing radiation has been the increased incidence of malignant disease in the survivors of the Hiroshima and Nagasaki bomb explosions. It is now appreciated that even diagnostic radiology carries a minor risk; consequently, all efforts are made to minimize the dosage received for essential radiographic procedures. Since it is believed that the embryo is particularly susceptible, the radiation of pregnant women is now carried out only for vital reasons.

Ultraviolet light is another carcinogenic agent. The common lesions it produces are solar keratoses and basal-cell carcinomas. The current increase in frequency of malignant melanoma has been linked to sun exposure.

The damage caused by both ionizing radiation and ultraviolet light can be repaired by the cell. Cancer is therefore liable to develop only if radiation is received at a rate that exceeds the cells' ability to repair the damage. Hence, individuals with little protective melanin pigment in their skin, such as those of North European stock, are particularly liable to develop malignancies of the exposed skin if they live in a sunny climate, such as that of Australia.

There is a rare inherited disorder (xeroderma pigmentosum) in which there is a defective DNA repair mechanism. The unfortunate sufferers are destined to develop multiple skin cancers and to die early unless they are adequately protected from damaging sunshine.

Hereditary Predisposition

Experimentally, there is good evidence of a strong hereditary predisposition to the development of certain tumors. It is possible to breed a strain of animals in which virtually all members of the strain will die of a particular cancer if they live long enough. Similarly, there are a number of very uncommon neoplastic diseases in humans that are inherited. For example, *familial polyposis coli* is transmitted as an autosomal dominant trait. Although it is the adenomas that are inherited, one of them sooner or later becomes malignant, and the patient dies of carcinoma of the colon, usually before the age of 40 years. Retinoblastoma, particularly if it is bilateral, is also inherited as a mendelian dominant trait; a mutant antioncogene is involved (see later). Cancer of the breast is more common in the relatives of affected women than in the female population at large. Likewise, the incidence of carcinoma of the ovary is high in certain families. Nevertheless, for many common cancers, there is little evidence of an inherited tendency.

Hormonal Factors

The observation that administration of estrogens to mice leads to an increased incidence of cancer of the breast was at first thought to indicate that hormonal imbalance could cause cancer in humans. It was soon appreciated that in mice, cancer of the breast is linked to infection by the Bittner retrovirus, and that the major effect of the estrogens was to allow the male mice to develop breasts in which cancer could develop. There have been human parallels. Some men who have been deliberately castrated and undergone "sex change operations," and who have been given estrogens for breast development, have subsequently developed cancer of the breast and have died of their disease. There seems little doubt that prolonged estrogen administration to women is a factor in the development of endometrial carcinoma.

There is indeed little evidence that hormones play a major part in the cause of most human tumors. Nevertheless, hormones are related to tumors in various subtle ways. Some teenage girls whose mothers were given the synthetic estrogen diethylstilbestrol during pregnancy have subsequently developed carcinoma of the vagina. This disease is extremely rare under normal conditions. It seems that the effect of estrogens on the developing fetus is to allow certain vestigial structures to remain; these subsequently develop into tumors during the offspring's adolescence.

Hormone-Dependent Tumors. If hormones can seldom be directly incriminated as a cause of human cancers, there are examples of tumors that appear to require the presence of hormones for their continued growth. Removal of the hormone may therefore cause regression of the tumor and relief of symptoms. A good example of a hormone-dependent tumor is carcinoma of the prostate. If patients with cancer of the prostate are castrated, or are given estrogens, there is often a dramatic relief of symptoms and regression of both the primary tumor and its metastases. Unfortunately, although there is some initial response, the tumor seems to lose its hormonal dependency.

Carcinoma of the breast is another tumor that can manifest hormone dependency. Some patients, particularly if the tumor has many estrogen receptors, show improvement if the level of estrogens is reduced by removal of the ovaries or by drug therapy. Unfortunately, the effects of therapy tend to be temporary.

Viral Infection

Fowl leukemia was shown to be transmissible by a virus in 1908 by Ellerman and Bang; a short time later, fowl sarcoma was observed by Rous to be transmissible. Since that time, tumor-producing, or oncogenic, viruses have been shown to play a part in the development of tumors in most species, including humans. The oncogenic DNA viruses have the ability to integrate their DNA into the genome of the host cell. In the case of the oncogenic RNA viruses, the action of viral enzyme reverse transcriptase leads to the formation of DNA provirus, and this integrates with the host DNA. In both instances, the effect on the cell is to cause abnormal behavior and allow it to grow continuously in culture; this is termed *cell transformation.* When implanted into a suitable host, the transformed cells grow to form a malignant tumor.

One of the most interesting RNA viruses is the virus responsible for cancer of the breast in mice. This was first described as the Bittner factor and is a virus present in the milk that infects the newborn suckling mice. When the female offspring mature, they subsequently develop cancer of the breast. Infected males are not affected unless they are given estrogens to encourage breast development, when they also develop cancer.

The DNA Oncogenic Viruses. The DNA oncoviruses of human importance fall into three groups. The first group comprises the *oncogenic herpesviruses* (Epstein-Barr virus and herpes simplex virus type 2). The second group of DNA viruses is the *oncogenic papovaviruses;* this group includes the polyoma virus and papilloma viruses. The polyoma virus causes a variety of different tumors in many species of animals but not in humans. The papilloma viruses are oncogenic in both animals and humans. The third group is the hepatitis virus types B, C, and perhaps others.

Under suitable circumstances, the DNA of an oncogenic DNA virus is integrated into the host cell's DNA, the cell undergoes transformation,

mRNA of viral type is produced, and subsequently viral type protein is synthesized by the cell. One product is the *tumor-specific transplantation antigen,* which is present on the cells' surface.

The DNA viruses require at least two genes for completing the transformation of a normal cell into a tumor (transformed) cell. The first is an immortalizing gene that enables the cell to grow indefinitely; the second, or transforming gene, induces the changes that are accompanied by loss of the remaining constraints to orderly growth.

The Epstein-Barr virus (EB virus) is the cause of infectious mononucleosis in North America and Europe. The disease is characterized by proliferation of atypical B lymphocytes; malignancy is not a complication. In Africa, infection with the virus can lead to the development of Burkitt's lymphoma. It is believed that chronic malaria and other chronic infections so impair the immune response that the B-cell proliferation, instead of being self-limiting as in infectious mononucleosis, continues unabated and results in neoplasia. The EB virus is also associated with nasopharyngeal carcinoma in humans, but the relationship is not defined.

Herpes simplex virus type 2 (HSV-2) infection is associated with carcinoma of the cervix uteri. Women with HSV-2 infection have a higher incidence of carcinoma, and patients with cervical dysplasia, carcinoma *in situ,* and invasive tumor have serologic evidence of past infection. Furthermore, viral DNA sequences have been identified in the tumor cell's genome. It is not known whether the virus plays a causative role in the development of malignancy or whether it is merely a passenger growing in the favorable soil that the malignant cells provide.

Many strains of *human papilloma viruses (HPV)* have been identified, and they are responsible for various types of warts and laryngeal papillomas. Rarely, the skin lesions, particularly those due to HPV-5 or HPV-8, progress to carcinoma. The situation is analogous to the Shope papilloma virus in rabbits, in which the virus causes papillomas that progress to squamous-cell carcinoma. In humans, there has recently been an increase in the incidence of genital infection with HPV, and this has been accompanied by an increase in the incidence of dysplastic lesions. Such lesions may progress to invasive carcinoma. The virus involved is HPV-16, less frequently HPV-18, but as with HSV-2 infections, the precise relationship between infection and tumor is not yet delineated.

The viruses of human hepatitis (HBV, HCV, and perhaps others) are associated with an increased incidence of hepatocellular carcinoma.

The Oncogenic RNA Viruses. The oncogenic RNA viruses, or oncornaviruses, are associated with leukemia and lymphoma in birds, mice, and cats; with Rous sarcoma in birds; and with mammary tumors in mice (Bittner virus).

The mode of action of the RNA viruses is quite different from that of other viruses in several respects. They contain the enzyme *reverse transcriptase* that is used to copy the viral RNA genome into DNA. The *DNA provirus* is integrated into the host nuclear DNA, where it replicates when the cell divides, and it can even be passed on to subsequent generations through the germ cells. The host cell may become neoplastic if the infecting virus carries an *oncogene,* that is, a gene capable of transforming a normal cell into a malignant cell. Only about 10 per cent of the viral RNA (*e.g.,* "src gene") is necessary to induce transformation.

Oncogenes. RNA oncogenic viruses have few genes, and the new methods of DNA research have enabled them to be identified. One of them is termed an *oncogene.* These viral oncogenes (v-onc) have been given three-letter code names derived from the animal or tumor from which they were first derived; *e.g.,* v-src was found in a virus from a sarcoma of chickens, and v-ras is a rat sarcoma. The oncogene v-src codes for nonstructural phosphoprotein. This has phosphokinase activity that leads to the phosphorylation of enzymes and alters the metabolism of the affected cell.

By use of specific DNA probes, it has been found that the DNA of normal cells contains sequences that are very similar to viral oncogenes. These are termed *cellular oncogenes* (c-onc) or *proto-oncogenes.* Thus, c-src can be identified in human cells. Oncogenes have been identified in human tumors and, if introduced into suitable cells in tissue culture, cause cell transformation.

In certain human tumors, constant chromosomal abnormalities have been discovered. The best known is the 9–22 translocation of chronic myeloid leukemia. The part of the short arm of chromosome 9 translocated to chromosome 22 contains the oncogene c-abl. The translocation appears to activate the gene and be associated with the development of leukemia. Thus, tumor transformation may be due to the activation of a cellular oncogene, caused in this instance by its relocation in a different chromosome. In this new situation, it might have escaped from some normal restraining influence of an adjacent gene. Other mechanisms for the activation of cellular oncogenes have been postulated. Mutation of the cellular oncogene might be brought about by the mutagenic action of a chemical carcinogen. A further mechanism is gene amplification, in which multiple copies of a gene are produced. Gene amplification appears to be a component of tumor progression; it is accompanied by a poor prognosis and the development of resistance to the effect of cytotoxic drugs. Finally, an oncogene might be activated by the insertion of an adjacent tumor virus in the host's DNA. This could explain the oncogenic activity of those RNA tumor viruses that do not themselves contain oncogenes.

Another mechanism that might be involved in carcinogenesis relates to the function of *antioncogenes.* Normal individuals have two allelic *Rb* genes, whereas individuals with familial retinoblastoma inherit one abnormal recessive mutated *Rb* gene on chromosome 13. Mutation of the remaining normal allele leads to the development of a retinoblastoma. The normal gene *Rb* has been regarded as an antioncogene, and a mutation or interference with its action in some way abolishes the action of the antioncogene.

Oncogenes seem to play a part in the regulation of the metabolism and growth of normal cells. They are believed to regulate the formation of growth factors, growth factor receptors, and other proteins. In normal cells, these growth-stimulating factors are probably important in regulating cell division and differentiation. A mutated or other abnormal oncogene may be responsible for the unruly growth that is the hallmark of neoplasia. Thus, there may be overproduction of growth factor, either by the cell itself (autocrine secretion) or by one of its neighbors (paracrine secretion).

Neoplasia Following Chronic Disease

Chronic irritation and chronic inflammation have been regarded as precursors of malignancy, but it seems unlikely that, acting alone, they can produce cancer. Perhaps they act as promoting agents. There are a number of conditions that can be regarded as precancerous because the development of tumors is a well-recognized complication. Examples include liver cell carcinoma in cirrhosis, squamous cell carcinoma in chronic skin ulcers and fistulous tracks, osteosarcoma in Paget's disease, and colonic carcinoma in chronic ulcerative colitis. Nevertheless, the great majority of human tumors apparently arise in previously normal tissue.

EARLY STAGES IN THE DEVELOPMENT OF NEOPLASIA

In some organs, cancer does not develop suddenly. Cancer of the epithelia of the skin and uterine cervix illustrates this well (Figs. 12–15 and 12–16). The first stage results in irregular maturation of the epithelial cells, and this *atypia* or *dysplasia* steadily progresses until the whole epithelium is replaced by atypical, pleomorphic cells that have the cytologic features of carcinoma. At this stage the basement membrane is still intact, and the condition is called *carcinoma in situ*. The final stage results in invasion of the underlying connective tissues and subsequent metastasis. The whole process probably takes several years.

The cells of the cervix uteri are shed into the vaginal secretions; a smear from these can be examined for the presence of atypical cells. This examination forms the basis of exfoliative cytology, which was pioneered by Papanicolaou. By regular examination of "Pap smears" of adult women, the early stages in the development of carcinoma can be detected, and the occurrence of invasive cancer can be prevented.

Carcinoma *in situ* is now recognized in other organs and has been studied more extensively in the skin, which is so easily examined. Bowen's disease and actinic keratoses provide good examples (Chapter 31).

THE NATURE OF NEOPLASIA

Cancer is generally assumed to be due to a change in the character of the cells, which causes them to exhibit uncontrolled growth. The possibility that the connective tissue stroma plays some part cannot be entirely ignored, because there are many examples in the embryologic development in which the epidermis relies on the connective tissue for its stimulation and maintenance, and vice versa. The possibility that the essential change in cancer lies in the connective tissue has not been completely excluded. Nevertheless, it is generally assumed that the essential changes are in the cancer cell itself. The results of years of research have given us a vast amount of knowledge concerning the properties of such cells. These may be summarized as follows.

Morphologic Abnormalities. The pleomorphic and bizarre appearances of malignant cells have already been described. It is by recognizing these changes that a pathologist is able to diagnose cancer from the Pap smear or a tissue section.

Membrane Changes. Many chemical differences in the cell membrane of malignant cells as opposed to normal cells have been catalogued, but little insight into the fundamental nature of neoplasia has been attained. Some changes, such as loss of surface fibronectin, release of plasminogen activator, and secretion of hyaluronidase, may be correlated with the lack of cell adhesion and possibly the invasive tendency of malignant cells. Other changes include increased surface mobility of cell receptors and increase in number of receptors to growth factors.

Biochemical Abnormalities. Malignant cells produce lactate at a higher rate than do most normal cells. At the time of this discovery by Warburg, this was thought to be a unique property of malignant cells, but it is now regarded as an expression of rapid growth rather than malignancy.

Many other biochemical changes can be cited. Some tumors produce substances normally

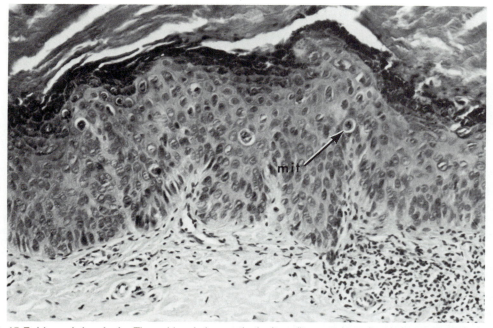

Figure 12–15 Epidermal dysplasia. The epidermis is acanthotic. Its cells are enlarged and show irregularity in size and shape. Mitoses can be identified (mit), and the keratin layer shows occasional remnants of nuclei, a condition termed parakeratosis (×250).

found only in the fetus. The formation of alpha-fetoprotein by some liver cell cancers is an example of this reversion to a more primitive behavior. Likewise, carcinoembryonic antigen is produced by many colorectal carcinomas. Some tumors produce enzymes or hormones that their parent cells were incapable of producing. These events all point to the conclusion that malignant cells can display a behavior that suggests *gene derepression.* Sometimes the detection of the abnormal product is useful in clinical diagnosis or in the detection of metastases after removal of the primary growth. However, there is no specific change such as the production of a chemical marker by which cancer can be detected. The changes described all appear to be differences from the normal quantitatively but not qualitatively. Hence, no specific "biochemical cancer test" is available.

Changes in Behavior in the Intact Animal. The usual relentless progressive growth, invasion of tissues, and metastases characteristic of malignant tumors have already been described.

Changes in Behavior in Vitro. Many changes have been observed in tissue culture. The cells appear to have attained potential immortality, since they can be grown indefinitely if subcultured at suitable times into an appropriate medium (see HeLa cells, Chapter 1). Normal cells tend to die after a limited number of mitoses. Malignant cells tend to pile up when grown on a glass surface because they show *decreased sensitivity to both contact inhibition* and *density-dependent inhibition of growth.* Furthermore, malignant cells grow in a semisolid or fluid medium, whereas normal cells will grow only on a surface in a monolayer. This is described as *loss of anchorage dependence.*

Cells that exhibit these characteristics *in vitro* are termed *transformed cells,* and if implanted into a suitable intact animal, they behave in a malignant manner.

Antigenic Change. The immunologic aspects of cancer have been extensively investigated. Some tumors appear to lose tissue-specific antigens because of their poor differentiation, and it has been proposed that they thereby escape the immunologic surveillance activity of lymphocytes. There is indeed some increase in the incidence of malignant tumors in patients who are

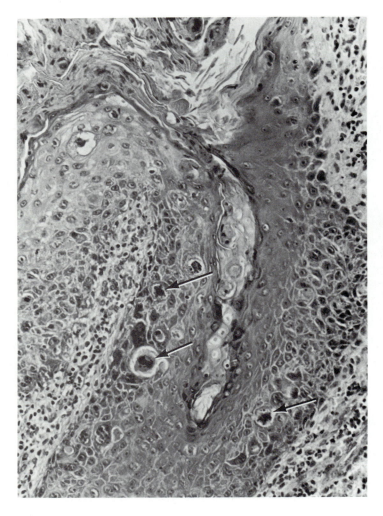

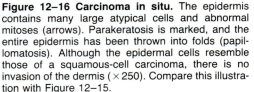

Figure 12–16 Carcinoma in situ. The epidermis contains many large atypical cells and abnormal mitoses (arrows). Parakeratosis is marked, and the entire epidermis has been thrown into folds (papillomatosis). Although the epidermal cells resemble those of a squamous-cell carcinoma, there is no invasion of the dermis (×250). Compare this illustration with Figure 12–15.

immunodeficient, but the tumors are usually of the lymphoreticular system and to a lesser extent the skin. There is no appreciable increase in the common types of malignant tumors.

Some tumors develop new antigens. These have been best documented in experimentally induced animal tumors. The most important are the tumor-specific transplantation antigens. These may be individual for tumors produced by chemical carcinogens, or they may be shared by all tumors produced by an oncogenic virus. If tumors express new antigens, it might be expected that a specific immune response would develop. The presence of a lymphocytic infiltration in some tumors suggests the development of a cell-mediated immune reaction. Indeed,

there is experimental evidence that specific cytotoxic lymphocytes can kill cancer cells. Moreover, other types of lymphocytes are able to kill tumor cells without prior sensitization. One group is the natural killer (NK) cells; others are called natural cytotoxic (NC) cells and lymphokine-activated killer (LAK) cells, both of which can be stimulated by interleukin-2. Finally, macrophages can kill tumor cells.

A humoral antibody response to tumor-associated antigens can be demonstrated, and the formation of immune complexes may account for some of the curious manifestations of cancer that are not directly explicable by the presence of tumor cells themselves. In theory, immunoglobulins could damage tumor cells by the process of antibody-dependent cell-mediated cytotoxicity and complement activation.

In summary, there is much evidence of an immune response to tumor antigens, but there is little evidence to support the once popular theory of cancer being due to breakdown of immunologic surveillance. However, the fact that an immune response does occur has encouraged research workers to test methods of stimulating the response. Interferon, interleukin-2, and bacille Calmette-Guérin have all been used, but with very limited success.

Changes in Karyotype. In tumor cells, there is often a great range in chromosomal abnormality in regard to number (aneuploidy), translocations, ring chromosomes, and many other complex deviations from the normal. Nevertheless, there is no constant change found in all tumors that can be used as a tumor marker. In some neoplasms, however, there is a constant karyotypic change. The first to be discovered, and the best known, is the Philadelphia chromosome found in most cases of chronic myelogenous leukemia. There is a balanced reciprocal translocation between the short arms of chromosomes 22 and 9. Likewise, in Burkitt's lymphoma there is a translocation between chromosomes 8 and 14. High-resolution banding techniques have revealed many other chromosomal abnormalities in neoplastic disease. Much of the work and consequently most of the correlations have been done in the leukemias. In some instances, several different patterns have been found in one disease, *e.g.,* in acute nonlymphocytic leukemia, there are 17. In Burkitt's lymphoma, three translocations can be found, and they all involve the long arm of chromosome 8 at the site of the myc oncogene.

THEORIES OF CARCINOGENESIS

Whether a tumor commences in one cell or begins simultaneously in many cells has been argued for years. Recent studies of tumors in women have provided a partial answer. It has been found that with most tumors, all the tumor cells contain either the paternal X chromosome or the maternal X (see the Lyon hypothesis, Chapter 2). If the malignant change spreads from

cell to cell like an infection, one would expect both types of cells to be involved. Thus, the tumor appears to be a clone of cells derived either from one cell or from a limited number of cells in one area. It seems likely that during the development of a tumor new clones evolve, each showing changes that enable it to replace its predecessors. Ultimately, the clone of malignant cells appears. Thus, cancer is a disease that evolves slowly, and it is not surprising that in those areas that have been intensively studied, a sequence of premalignant changes can be found that ultimately progress through dysplasia to malignant tumor formation.

The nature of the change within the cancer cell is poorly understood, but two major theories have evolved:

1. *Epigenetic theory*—aberrant differentiation.
2. *Genetic theory*—somatic mutation.

The *epigenetic theory* presupposes that the basic genetic material of cancer cells is normal but the abnormality is in the expression of this genetic material. The cancer cell is assumed to result from the aberrant differentiation of the cell, with the defect lying anywhere from the transcription of DNA to RNA to the translation at the cytoplasmic level. The interposition of viral nucleic acid could upset this mechanism of differentiation. Chemicals likewise could modify the effect of genetic material by either turning off or modifying the effect of repressor genes. This theory would explain why some mutagens are not carcinogenic and vice versa. It also explains why some tumors produce fetal antigens and ectopic hormones by suggesting that the normal genetic material is not basically altered but merely misused. This theory also explains why the evolution of a tumor is not an all-or-nothing affair but can proceed through a series of intermediate stages as genetic material is differently interpreted.

Further evidence in favor of the epigenetic theory of cancer comes from two different sources. It is possible to obtain early embryos of two separate strains of mice, fuse them together so that one embryo results, and finally allow this to develop within the uterus of another pregnant female. Such animals (termed allophenic) consist of clones derived from each of the separate strains. If mice of black and white hair strains are used, the resultant allophenic mouse has alternating black and white stripes, giving a tigroid appearance! This experiment has been extended to include fusion of a normal developing fetus of one strain of mouse with malignant tumor cells derived from a different strain of mouse. Completely normal baby mice are the result, and they contain differentiated cells derived not only from the normal embryo of one strain but from the malignant cells of the other. Hence, the malignant cells may be presumed to contain normal genetic material capable of supervising the normal development of all parts of the body.

A second piece of evidence in favor of the epigenetic theory of cancer is the observation that certain cases of neuroblastoma (a highly malignant tumor derived from primitive neuroblasts) can on occasion differentiate into a benign ganglioneuroma containing mature neurons. Indeed, sometimes the tumor shows spontaneous regression and self-cure. Again, this evidence suggests that the malignant tumors possess a normal genome but that differentiation is at fault. It is possible that these examples supporting the epigenetic theory are merely isolated rare events. On the other hand, they may indicate a more general principle that neoplastic, and particularly malignant, change is merely an example of aberrant differentiation much in the same way as metaplasia and hyperplasia are now regarded. This gives considerable hope for the future because it is conceivable that means may be found to persuade malignant cells to differentiate along normal lines and bring the neoplastic process to a halt. Such a line of treatment would be vastly superior to the modes of therapy currently used.

The *genetic theory* of cancer is currently favored. It supposes that there is a change or mutation in the DNA of normal cells to form tumor cells. This change is inherited by all the progeny of the altered cells, and the clone so produced forms the tumor. Further mutations could occur, and more malignant types of cell are produced and become the dominant cell type; this may explain tumor progression. The postulated alteration in DNA can be inherited, as appears to be the case in certain rare inherited tumors, *e.g.*, retinoblastoma, or it can be due to the insertion of viral DNA containing an oncogene. A mutation in the host DNA, possibly in a proto-oncogene, is another possibility.

The present treatment for cancer consists of the radical removal of tumor by using either surgical resection or radiotherapy. These measures are effective only when the tumor is localized, but there is much evidence that cancer is not simply a local disease. Even if removal of the entire area is feasible, the presence of secondary deposits represents an unknown hazard. Since these deposits may remain dormant for many years, it is evident that an assessment of the effects of local treatment is very difficult. When the disease is clinically generalized, many cytotoxic drugs are available for use either separately or in various combinations. Often this holds tumor growth in check for many months, but complete cure is difficult to attain. Hormone therapy can produce some alleviation of symptoms in particular cases. Attempts to stimulate the body's immune response constitute another approach, but as noted previously, this has met with limited success.

The most successful approach to the control of cancer at the present time lies in its prevention. Many known physical and chemical carcinogenic agents have already been described, and their avoidance can appreciably reduce the incidence of cancer. Each tumor must be considered separately; for instance, a reduction in the amount of cigarette smoking and atmospheric pollution would undoubtedly reduce the incidence of lung cancer; avoidance of intense sunlight would reduce the incidence of malignant skin tumors; ionizing radiation is a known factor in the cause of leukemia.

A second method of cancer prophylaxis is the treatment of known precancerous lesions. A regular Pap smear can reduce the incidence of uterine cancer; once again, each individual type of tumor must be considered separately.

Summary

- Tumors or neoplasms are classified on the basis of their tissue of origin, their behavior, and sometimes their cellular morphology.
- Benign tumors never spread or metastasize. If epithelial, they are termed papillomas or adenomas. If connective tissue or mesenchymal, they are named

after the tissue of origin, *e.g.*, fibroma. Benign tumors are often encapsulated and produce their effects mechanically, *e.g.*, by causing obstruction.

- Malignant tumors invade local tissues, and embolic spread leads to metastases in regional lymph nodes and, when the blood stream is invaded, to distant organs. Malignant tumors cause mechanical pressure and obstruction but also destroy tissue, leading to ulceration, infection, and hemorrhage. Malignant epithelial tumors are called carcinomas and further subdivided depending on their differentiation: squamous-cell carcinoma, adenocarcinoma, and so on. Malignant mesenchymal neoplasms are called sarcomas. Various paraneoplastic syndromes may occur with either; these include hormonal effects and other syndromes not explicable on the basis of the presence of tumor cells or their secretion. Malignant tumors are also classified by grading and staging.

- Tumors of intermediate malignancy invade locally but have limited metastatic ability. Basal-cell carcinoma of skin and carcinoid tumors are in this group.

- Tumors of special tissues are classified separately, *e.g.*, germ-cell tumors such as teratomas, tumors of chorionic tissue, melanomas, and lymphomas.

- Electron microscopy and immunochemical marker studies can help identify the origin of some poorly differentiated tumors.

- Chemical carcinogens may act directly on cells to cause tumors but often require activation (often in the liver) to an ultimate carcinogen. The actual development of a tumor is a multistep process.

- Physical carcinogenic agents include ionizing radiation and ultraviolet light (skin cancers and melanoma).

- Hereditary factors play a part in the development of certain tumors.

- Hormones are involved in the development of certain tumors and in the maintenance of hormone-dependent tumors such as carcinoma of the prostate.

- Oncogenic DNA viruses include herpesviruses (EB virus and HSV-2) and papovaviruses (particularly HSV in genital cancer).

- Oncogenic RNA viruses are retroviruses and often contain oncogenes that are closely related to normal cellular or c-oncogenes or proto-oncogenes.

- Malignant tumors evolve through a series of steps that result in cellular atypia (dysplasia) and culminate in carcinoma *in situ* and finally invasive tumor. Recognition and treatment of these lesions is used to prevent development of tumors, *e.g.*, Pap smears in the prevention of cervical cancer.

- Many features of malignant cells have been described; these involve abnormalities in morphology, cell membrane, biochemical properties, behavior in the intact animal and in culture, antigenicity, and karyotype. None is diagnostic.

- Present evidence suggests that tumors are monoclonal and originate in one cell; a change in the cells' DNA is involved: by inheritance, insertion of a viral oncogene, or a mutation of a c-oncogene.

Selected Readings

Ames, B. N.: Dietary carcinogens and anticarcinogens. Science *221*:1256, 1983.

Beutler, B., et al.: Identity of tumor necrosis factor and macrophage secreted factor cachectin. Nature *316*:552, 1985.

Broder, J. E.: Hormone production by bronchiogenic carcinoma. A review. Pathobiol. Annu. *9*:205, 1979.

Editorial: Metastatic fundamentals. Lancet *1*:1052, 1989.

Farber, E.: Chemical carcinogenesis. N. Engl. J. Med. *305*:1379, 1981.

Hart, I. R., and Fidler, I. J.: Cancer invasion and metastasis. Q. Rev. Biol. *55*:121, 1980.

Hobbs, J. R.: Immunotherapy of human cancers. Br. Med. J. *299*:1177, 1989.

Howley, P. M.: On human papillomavirus. N. Engl. J. Med. *315*:1089, 1986.

Illmensee, K., and Mintz, B.: Totipotency and normal differentiation of single teratocarcinoma cells cloned by injection into blastocytes. Proc. Natl. Acad. Sci. *73*:549, 1976.

Knudsor, A. G.: Hereditary cancer, oncogenes and anti-oncogenes. Cancer Res. *45*:1437, 1985.

Lachmann, P. J.: Tumor immunology: A review. J. R. Soc. Med. *77*:1023, 1984.

Leading article: Multistage carcinogenesis. Lancet *1*:395, 1980.

Leading article: Reversal of cancer. Lancet *1*:799, 1983.

Leading article: Human virus, hepatic cancer. Lancet *2*:134, 1981.

Leading article: Molecular mechanisms of tumour evolution. Lancet *1*:780, 1986.

Leading article: Growth factor and malignancy. Lancet *2*:317, 1986.

Leading article: Gene amplification in malignancy. Lancet *1*:839, 1987.

Lebovitz, R. M.: Oncogenes as mediators of cell growth and differentiation. Lab. Invest. *55*:249, 1986.

Melnick, S., et al.: Rates and risks of diethylstilbestrol-related clear-cell adenocarcinoma of the vagina and cervix. N. Engl. J. Med. *316*:514, 1987.

Vile, R.: Tumour suppressor genes. Br. Med. J. *298*:1335, 1989.

Zetter, B. R.: The cellular basis of site-specific tumor metastasis. N. Engl. J. Med. *322*:605, 1990.

Ionizing Radiations and Their Effects

**After studying this chapter, the student
should be able to:**

- Distinguish between the direct and indirect action of
  ionizing radiations.
- Describe the effects of irradiation on a cell and
  relate them to the stages of the mitotic cycle.
- Describe the relative sensitivities of cells when they
  are irradiated in the intact animal.
- Describe the effects of ionizing radiation on skin,
  gonads, lung, and bone.
- Describe the effects of total body irradiation with
  (a) 500 cGy;
  (b) 800 to 5000 cGy;
  (c) more than 5000 cGy.
- Describe two important late effects of total body
  irradiation.
- List the factors that enable one to predict the
  radiosensitivity of a tumor.

The nature of ionizing radiations is now the domain of the physicist, and no detailed account will be given. It has taken many years for the damaging effects of these radiations to become generally accepted. The local effects first became apparent when the early physicists who handled radium and other radioactive substances developed chronic radiodermatitis and skin cancers of the fingers. The use of ionizing radiation for the treatment of cancer and other diseases reinforced the conclusion that the treatment was not without risk—witness the incidence of cancer of the thyroid in adults who as children were given radiation to the upper chest for "thymic asthma" and apparent enlargement of the thymus, or the increased incidence of leukemia in patients whose spines were irradiated for ankylosing spondylitis. The full importance of the hazards of radiation did not finally become apparent to the general population until the late effects of the atomic explosions at Hiroshima and Nagasaki were observed. The effects of accidents, particularly large ones such as occurred at Chernobyl in which there were leaks of radioactive material into the environment, are now matters of widespread public concern. The physical properties of ionizing radiations have been well studied, and it would be expected that the damage they produce in living tissues would be easy to understand. Such has not been the case because the fundamental processes that occur in cells are poorly understood. Cancer produced by ionizing radiation is no easier to explain than that which evolves spontaneously or is produced by a chemical carcinogen.

CHANGES INDUCED IN MATTER BY PASSAGE OF IONIZING RADIATION

When ionizing radiation passes through matter, energy is absorbed. This leads to a variety of physicochemical events. Some molecules are excited, and ions and free radicals are formed. The changes vary with each particular variety of radiation.

Particulate Radiation. The density of ionization for charged particles is *directly proportional to the square of their charge and inversely proportional to their velocity.* Thus, electrons and protons of equal velocity produce the same ion density; as they slow down, however, the density increases. Alpha particles (with their double charge and slow velocity) produce very dense ionization—hence, more damage.

Beta Particles. Because of their charge and negligible mass, beta particles are rapidly slowed down and give up energy to atoms through which they pass. They therefore have little power of penetration and can be used in the treatment of superficial tumors. Beta particles or artificially produced beams of electrons are used therapeutically in certain forms of skin tumors. Electrons generated at 2 MeV (million electron volts) have a maximum range of about 1 cm in soft tissues.

Alpha Particles. These have a double positive charge and a mass of 4. Their high charge and slow velocity means that they have little penetrating power. Alpha particles are readily stopped by the superficial layers of the epidermis; therefore, there is little danger of damage from an external radiating source. If taken internally, however, radioactive elements that emit alpha particles can cause serious damage.

Electromagnetic Radiation. Gamma rays and x-rays have much greater penetrating power than do the particulate radiations. The shorter the wavelengths, the greater their penetration. It should be noted that the particulate radiations have a definite range of penetration, whereas the electromagnetic radiations are merely reduced in quantity. Thus, a particular thickness of a sheet of material (the half-value thickness) will reduce the intensity by half, a further thickness will reduce it by another half, and so forth. When gamma and x-rays traverse matter, they give up a quantity of energy and cause atoms to emit high-velocity electrons, which then behave like beta particles. Gamma and x-rays of high energy (short wavelength) produce fewer ionizations than do low-energy x-rays. They are therefore less destructive, since damage is caused by energy that is absorbed.

BIOLOGIC EFFECTS OF IONIZING RADIATION

The net effect of these various changes is that molecules become more reactive, causing chemical changes to occur. Large molecules such as DNA and proteins can be affected by two separate processes.

Direct Action. Chemical change may be caused by energy absorbed in the molecule itself.

Indirect Action. Alternatively, chemical change may be induced in a large molecule from the action of an adjacent ion or radical that had been produced by the effect of ionizing radiation on a nearby water molecule. Many of the biologic effects of ionizing radiation are due primarily to the effects on water. Highly reactive ions are formed, in particular the free radicals OH^- and H^-, which are electrically neutral but highly unstable. They react with water, particularly in the presence of oxygen, to form powerful damaging oxidizing substances such as HO_2^- and H_2O_2.

It is generally supposed that ionizing radiations initially produce an intracellular chemical change and that this leads to a *biochemical lesion,* which in turn produces morphologic and functional changes in the affected cells. The nature of this biochemical lesion is poorly understood.

Effects on the Cell

Although it would be desirable to explain cellular damage in terms of known physicochemical changes, this is not yet possible. With very high dosages, *e.g.*, on the order of 10,000 cGy* or more, cells die regardless of their stage in the mitotic cycle. With a lower dosage of radiation, DNA synthesis is inhibited and mitosis is delayed. When DNA synthesis is resumed, it may not be followed by mitosis, resulting in the formation of giant nuclei. When mitosis does occur, various chromosomal abnormalities become apparent. Breaks in chromosomes are characteristic, and the fragments may reunite in an abnormal way or join other chromosomes. Sometimes these abnormalities are incompatible with life, and the cell dies.

Fractionated doses of radiation do not produce a strictly cumulative effect, and an intracellular mechanism seems to exist to correct radiation damage.

The sensitivity of cells to damage varies according to the stage in the mitotic cycle at which the radiation is given. Maximum sensitivity occurs in most cell types during mitosis itself. It follows that normal tissues with a high mitotic rate, *e.g.*, lymphoid and hematopoietic, are more sensitive than are those in which mitosis rarely or never occurs, *e.g.*, skeletal and cardiac muscle. Likewise, as a general principle, malignant tumors are more sensitive than are either benign tumors or the parent tissue of origin.

Two main theories have been proposed to explain the mechanism of cellular damage.

The Target Theory. This supposes that damage to cells is related to injury of a specific sensitive spot in the cell. Attractive as it may be to visualize a chromosome or a particular organelle as a target, there is little evidence to support this theory.

The Poison Theory. This supposes that ionization leads to the production of poisonous substances—usually powerful oxidizing agents—that then cause the cellular damage. There is considerable evidence that oxidizing substances are indeed formed in irradiated tissues. Thus, chemicals with a reducing action, *e.g.*, cysteine, give some degree of protection against ionizing radiation if they are present at the time of the initial irradiation. Furthermore, if tissues are irradiated in the absence of oxygen, they show considerably more resistance. This is probably because free oxygen is necessary for the production of oxidizing substances by ionizing radiation. This observation is of some importance in clinical radiotherapy, because many areas of a tumor are relatively hypoxic and conceivably could be protected during radiation therapy. Attempts have been made to overcome this by allowing patients to breathe pure oxygen under pressure during the actual administration of radiotherapy.

Effects on the Intact Animal

This important aspect of radiobiology is also the most difficult and least well understood. A remarkable feature is the delay in the appearance of radiation lesions. The actual damage caused by radiation must be almost instantaneous, and yet the effects may not be apparent for days, months, or even years. An experiment with amphibians has helped explain this phenomenon. Frogs can be given a dose of radiation that will kill them within 6 weeks. If irradiated animals are kept at 5°C, they remain alive for several months, but on being warmed up, they die within 6 weeks. The experiments indicate that radiation damage manifests itself only when cells are active. This lends strong support to the concept that a biochemical lesion is produced. Such a lesion is not in itself harmful, but it produces effects when cellular activity commences. This goes some way toward explaining two of the phenomena of radiation damage.

Relative Sensitivity of Cells. In the human, the germinal cells of the ovary are the most sensitive. Then, in order from most to least sensitive, are the seminiferous epithelium of the testis, the lymphocytes, the erythropoietic and myeloid marrow cells, the intestinal epithelium, the muscle cells, and the nerve cells. This order of sensitivity to some extent parallels the rate of mitoses seen in the various tissues. Thus, the highly active intestinal epithelium is sensitive, and this explains the necrosis with its attendant gastrointestinal symptoms that follows total body exposure to ionizing radiation. Neurons, on the

---

*A unit commonly used is the gray: 1 gray equals 100 rad; 1 rad equals 1 cGy (centigray).

other hand, never divide and are relatively resistant.

The Chronic Nature of Radiation Lesions.
When tissue is irradiated, several phases of damage occur. This is probably because different tissues have different rates of division and metabolic activity and therefore exhibit damage at different times. Hence, an irradiated area shows changes that persist for many weeks or months and have the characteristics of chronic inflammation. This inflammation can follow a single exposure of ionizing radiation.

When studying the action of radiation on any tissue, one must consider two main effects: (1) *the primary effect* of radiation on the tissue concerned; and (2) *the secondary effect,* which is due to damage to adjacent tissues. The most important example of this is damage to blood vessels, which generally results in thrombosis or gradual obliteration due to endarteritis obliterans. The ischemia that follows either event leads to necrosis. Some authorities attribute much of the beneficial effects of radiotherapy in cancer to this mechanism.

Effects of Irradiation on Individual Tissues

Skin. After a single dose of ionizing radiation to the skin, there is a phase of erythema beginning at about 10 days and showing all the features of acute inflammation. This phase is followed by pigmentation, due to melanin formation, causing the skin to acquire a dusky hue. With a heavy dosage, necrosis follows and an ulcer is produced. This heals slowly, and even when healed, the scar may subsequently break down after only trivial injury. With a lower dose of irradiation of skin, a smoldering chronic inflammation ensues. This is made evident by fibrosis and endarteritis obliterans. Giant fibroblasts are often seen in the dermis. The hair follicles and sebaceous glands are more sensitive than is the epidermis, and these structures tend to disappear. After several years, the area of irradiation appears atrophic. There is disturbance of pigmentation, and the area—although ischemic—shows the presence of dilated blood vessels (telangiectasia). The disturbed pigmentation

(areas of hyperpigmentation and hypopigmentation) combined with atrophy and telangiectasia is called *poikiloderma* (Fig. 13–1). This is an unfortunate end result that is sometimes seen when a tumor such as a basal-cell carcinoma is treated by radiotherapy.

Case History I

As a teenager and young woman, the patient had atopic dermatitis that was treated by local radiation and by many doctors. From repeated exposure to radiation, the patient developed severe radiodermatitis. During the previous 10 years, several basal-cell carcinomas had appeared and had been treated by curettage or excision. Figure 13–1 shows that a new tumor has developed and that necrotic facial bone is visible.

This patient's history illustrates many points:

1. It is dangerous to treat benign conditions with radiation, particularly in young people.
2. A patient can go from one physician to another, each being unaware of the treatment administered by

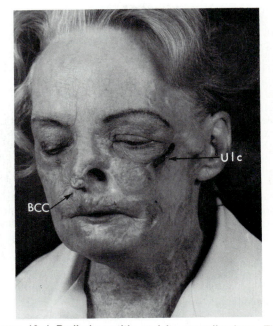

Figure 13–1 Radiodermatitis and its complications. This patient has severe dermatitis as a result of repeated radiation treatments for atopic dermatitis. A new basal-cell carcinoma (BCC) is present just above the right upper lip. A chronic indolent ulcer (Ulc) is present on the left cheek. The black tissue in the base of the ulcer is necrotic facial bone. Several attempts to close this defect by skin grafting have failed. Note that part of the nose has been lost. (For further information, see Case History I.)

the other. It was estimated that parts of this patient's face had received a total dose of over 11,000 cGy. This is two to three times the dose commonly given to treat a malignant tumor.

3. Chronic ulceration is a feature of radiodermatitis.

4. Healing of radiation ulcers is slow, and skin grafting is often unsatisfactory because of the local ischemia.

5. Multiple tumors can develop in radiation-damaged tissues.

Gonads. The ovaries and testes are particularly susceptible to irradiation damage; with a dose of over 500 cGy, the germinal cells are destroyed, and permanent sterility results.

Lungs. Irradiation of the lungs produces interstitial pneumonitis that culminates in fibrosis. This is a complication of radiotherapy applied in the treatment of cancer of the lung or cancer of the breast (Fig. 13–2).

Bone. Irradiation of bone produces inflammatory changes that can persist for years and be punctuated by episodes of painful radionecrosis. Doses of over 1000 cGy inhibit the growth of bone at the epiphyses, leading to stunted growth of the part affected.

Case History II

The patient was a 39-year-old woman whose left breast had been removed for carcinoma. Because several axillary lymph nodes had been found to contain metastatic tumor, postoperative radiotherapy was given. She remained well for 2 years but then began to experience fever, night sweats, and shortness of breath. A lung infection had been suspected, but in spite of extensive investigations, no definite diagnosis could be made. Thoracotomy and open-lung biopsy were performed in the hope that some treatable condition was present. The specimen showed extensive fibrosis consistent with radiation damage; in addition, however, carcinoma cells were present in lymphatic vessels. Death occurred 3 days later from respiratory failure. Necropsy revealed metastatic carcinoma in the lungs, mediastinal lymph nodes, liver, and vertebrae. No tumor was present in the mastectomy scar or the right breast. Radiation damage was marked in the left upper lobe of the lung (Fig. 13–2).

Effects of Irradiation on the Whole Body

When the whole body is exposed to irradiation, the effect is the sum total of the damage to all tissues. This is called the *radiation syndrome*. It has been studied extensively in animals, but in humans, experience is limited only to those occasional accidents such as occurred at Chernobyl and to those individuals involved in the Japanese atomic explosions. It is convenient to describe the effects of total body irradiation under two headings: (1) those occurring during the first 2 months (immediate effects) and (2) those occurring later (late effects).

Immediate Effects of Total Body Irradiation

Very Heavy Dosage. (over 5000 cGy per single exposure)—*the cerebral syndrome.* Death usually occurs within a day or two, with the patient developing shock, convulsions, and coma. The effects are due to a direct action on the central nervous system, since a similar syndrome results when the head alone is irradiated.

Moderate Dosage. (800 to 5000 cGy per single exposure)—*the gastrointestinal syndrome.* An initial phase occurs shortly after irradiation and is manifested as loss of appetite, nausea, and vomiting. The explanation for this is not known. The symptoms usually abate, only to recur some 2 to 3 days later with intractable severity. Vomiting and diarrhea dominate the picture, and death occurs from dehydration and shock. These serious effects are due to necrosis of the intestinal epithelium.

Low Dosage. (less than 800 cGy per single exposure)—*the hematopoietic syndrome.* The initial phase of nausea and vomiting is less severe, and the subject may then appear to make a complete recovery. Two to 3 weeks later, the results of bone marrow aplasia become apparent. The serious effects of irradiation of this type are due to damage to the hematopoietic tissues. The granulocyte count falls after about 1 week and subsequently reaches very low levels. This predisposes the person to infection, particularly of the mouth and lungs. The lymphocytes show the earliest drop, and there is marked lymphopenia within a day or two. This is associated with an impaired immune response. The platelets also decrease in number, and there is marked thrombocytopenia within 4 weeks. This condition predisposes the victim to severe hemorrhage, often into the lungs. Although the red blood cell precursors are highly radiosensitive, the mature red blood cells are resistant, and the effects of bone marrow aplasia on the peripheral count are delayed. Thus, the anemia is of gradual onset and

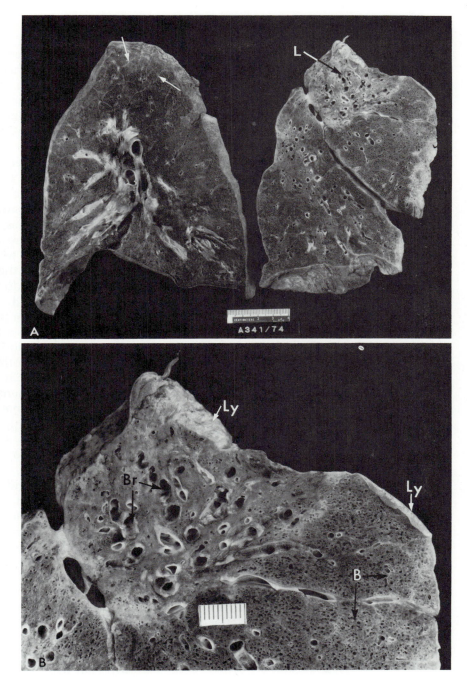

Figure 13–2 Radiation fibrosis of lung. Specimens of lung taken at necropsy from a patient who had died of respiratory failure. *A,* The cut surface of both lungs. The right lung exhibits prominent septa (arrows) that outline the lung lobules. On microscopic examination, these septa are shown to contain tumor. The apex of the left lung (L) is shrunken. *B,* The lung parenchyma is seen to have been destroyed and replaced by fibrous tissue. The bronchi (Br) are dilated, a condition called *branchiectasis.* Below this, the lung is consolidated, but some dilated bronchioles (B) can be seen. Lymphatic vessels (Ly) on the pleural surface contain tumor. (For a more complete description, see Case History II.)

is maximal at 6 to 8 weeks in those individuals who survive the effects of agranulocytosis and thrombocytopenia. If the patient survives, the blood counts return to normal over a period of many months. In humans, 450 cGy is generally taken as the dose that will kill 50 per cent of those exposed.

Late Effects of Total Body Irradiation. Those exposed to a sublethal dose may suffer from the following aftereffects.

The Carcinogenic Effect. Widespread irradiation of the bone marrow leads to an increased incidence of leukemia. This has been recorded in the survivors of the Nagasaki and Hiroshima atomic explosions and in patients with ankylosing spondylitis treated with radiotherapy. Likewise, local irradiation is followed by an increased incidence of malignant tumors at that site. Thus, carcinoma of the skin was reported as early as 1902 in workers who handled radioactive material or who were exposed to x-rays. Other examples are carcinoma of the thyroid that follows accidental irradiation of the gland for treatment of mediastinal lesions and osteosarcoma that follows local irradiation of bone lesions. Tumors have also been reported after the ingestion of radioactive substances such as radium and mesothorium, which are stored in the bones.

Genetic Effect. The ability of ionizing radiation to increase the rate of mutation is well established in microorganisms, plants, and animals. Mutations in the germ cells are of potential significance, since the new factor is handed down to subsequent generations. In clinical practice, it is usual to protect the genitalia as much as possible during routine radiography for this reason.

RADIOTHERAPY

The destructive effects of ionizing radiation on living cells, particularly those in an active state, have led to its widespread use in the treatment of malignant disease. Radiotherapy plays an important part in the curative treatment of some primary cancers as well as in the palliation of those that have metastasized and are beyond the scope of surgical removal.

Factors Influencing Response

Tumors differ widely in their response to radiotherapy, and it is only after treatment has commenced that the effects can be assessed. Nevertheless, there are some guidelines that help one to predict the probable local results. The following factors are of importance.

Tissue of Origin

The relative sensitivity of the normal tissue is often related to the radiosensitivities of the tumors derived from it. Thus, the lymphomas, like the parent lymphoreticular system, tend to be highly radiosensitive. Fibrosarcomas, on the other hand, are relatively radioresistant, like the normal fibroblast.

Degree of Differentiation and Mitotic Activity. It is generally taught that within any tumor group, the most undifferentiated tumors are also the most radiosensitive. As a generalization, this is true; nevertheless, the histologic features of a tumor are no sure guide to its sensitivity in practice. Thus, a well-differentiated squamous-cell carcinoma of the tongue or skin is usually highly responsive to treatment.

The Tumor Bed. The nature of the stroma supporting a tumor is also a factor of importance. If it is avascular as a result of previous radiation, the tumor tends to be more resistant. This has been attributed to the effects of hypoxia. It has been suggested that the stroma, particularly its lymphoid component, plays a part in restraining the growth of some tumors. Excessive irradiation, by destroying the stroma, might have a deleterious effect, since those tumor cells that survive are able to grow and subsequently metastasize.

Nature of the Individual Tumors. In practice, it has been found that certain tumors respond well, whereas others are resistant. Thus, most basal-cell and squamous-cell carcinomas of the skin are sensitive to treatment, whereas squamous-cell carcinoma of the lung is less responsive.

The Cure Rate

As with surgical treatment, the cure rate to be expected from radiotherapy must be considered in relation to the general properties of the tumor. Many malignant tumors (*e.g.*, the lymphomas) cannot be regarded as local diseases; although a tumor mass may respond remarkably well, the clinical course is characterized by the recurrence of the disease at other sites. Likewise, the oat-cell carcinoma of the lung is highly radiosensitive, and the local tumor masses in the chest melt with remarkable rapidity. Nevertheless, this tumor nearly always metastasizes widely, and death occurs from this generalized spread.

Radiotherapy is often effective as a palliative treatment because it can reduce the size of a tumor mass and produce relief of symptoms. A mediastinal mass, such as that produced by oat-cell carcinoma or lymphoma, can obstruct the major blood vessels and trachea, producing grave respiratory difficulty: this condition can be alleviated by local irradiation. Bone metastases are often extremely painful, and the pain can be relieved by treatment. With relatively slow-growing tumors (*e.g.*, cancer of the breast and Hodgkin's disease), radiotherapy can hold the disease in check for long periods and give the patient several years of useful life. It may well be that radiotherapy and surgery are both forms of palliation that allow the body to retard the growth of a tumor; depending on whether the malignant cells stay dormant for a short or long period, one may speak of a "5-year cure," a "10-year cure," and so forth.

Summary

- Penetration and damage produced by particulate radiation depend on the square of the charge and the velocity of the particles. With electromagnetic radiation, the wavelength is important. With x-rays, this is related to the voltage used to generate them.
- Radiation damage to molecules is by either direct action or indirect action. Indirect action involves formation of damaging free radicals. On cells, the damage may be to some target or by the formation of damaging poisons, probably oxidizing agents.
- Damage to cells and tissues is related to metabolic and mitotic activity; gonads and lymphoid tissue are most sensitive.
- Total body irradiation may produce the cerebral syndrome (heavy dosage, with early death), the gastrointestinal syndrome (moderate dosage, with later death), or the hematopoietic syndrome (low dosage, with effects due to low red and white blood cell counts and thrombocytopenia).
- Late effects of total body irradiation include malignant disease and genetic effects due to gonadal damage.
- The sensitivity of tumors to radiation depends on the tissue of origin, the type of tumor, its degree of differentiation and mitotic activity, and the tumor bed.

Selected Readings

Committee for the Compilation of Materials on Damage Caused by the Atomic Bombs in Hiroshima and Nagasaki. Translated by Eisel Ishikawa and David L. Swain. New York, Basic Books, 1981.

Finch, S. C.: The study of atomic bomb survivors. Am. J. Med. *66*:899, 1979.

Mettler, F. A., Jr., and Mosely, R. D., Jr.: Medical Effects of Ionizing Radiation. Orlando, Fla., Grune & Stratton, 1985, pp. 1–288.

Pizzarello, D. J., and Witcofski, R. L. (eds.): Medical Radiation Biology. 2nd ed. Philadelphia, Lea & Febiger, 1982.

Prosnitz, L. R., Kapp, D. S., and Weisserberg, J. B.: Radiotherapy. N. Engl. J. Med. *309*:771 and 834, 1983.

Fever and Hypothermia

**After studying this chapter, the student
should be able to:**

• Describe the physiologic mechanisms by which the
  body's temperature is maintained within narrow
  limits.
• Define fever and hyperpyrexia.
• List ten causes of fever.
• Describe the central heat-regulating center and
  outline its mode of action
  (a) under normal conditions;
  (b) in a patient with pneumonia;
  (c) in a patient with heat stroke.
• Describe the role of interleukin-1 in the pathogenesis
  of fever.
• Describe the circumstances under which malignant
  hyperpyrexia is usually encountered.
• Define hypothermia and describe the common
  causes and effects in infants and in adults.
• Give two examples of the value of induced
  hypothermia in medicine.

A rise in the body's temperature is so commonly found in illness that this response has
been recognized since ancient times. Indeed, the
term "fever" is sometimes used as being synonymous with disease. "Hay-fever" and "cat-
scratch fever" bear witness to this association,
because in neither disease is fever an important
feature. To avoid this confusion, the term "pyrexia" is commonly used in clinical medicine.

Before considering fever itself, one must understand the normal body temperature and the
mechanism of its control.

THE NORMAL BODY TEMPERATURE
AND ITS CONTROL

The most reliable method of taking the body's
temperature is by placing a thermometer under
the tongue with the lips closed. The temperature
taken in this way varies from 36.1° to 37.4°C (97°
to 99°F) and accurately reflects the temperature
of the inside of the body (the *core temperature*).
The maximum temperature is generally attained
at about 6:00 P.M., whereas it is at its lowest at
about 3:00 A.M. In women, there is an elevation
of the temperature during the middle of the
menstrual cycle; its onset is thought to herald
ovulation, and this rise in temperature has been
utilized in the rhythm system of contraception.
In unconscious patients, it is convenient to take

the temperature by placing a thermometer in the rectum; the readings obtained in this way are about 0.3°C higher than those taken by mouth. Measurement of temperature by placing the thermometer in the axilla or groin is quite unreliable, since it does not accurately reflect the core temperature. The surface skin temperature fluctuates widely and may approximate that of the external environment.

The maintenance of a constant body temperature is one aspect of homeostasis, and in humans it has obtained a high degree of efficiency. The importance of this is obvious when it is remembered that cellular activity involves many chemical reactions that are largely dependent on enzymatic activity and therefore very susceptible to changes in temperature. The body's temperature is regulated by a heat-regulating center that initiates the various mechanisms to increase or decrease heat loss.

The constancy of the body's temperature is maintained by balancing the amount of heat produced in the body with that lost to the environment.

Heat Gain and Loss in the Body

The major source of heat is the body's metabolic activity. Heat production under fasting conditions with the individual at complete mental and physical rest is called the *basal metabolic rate,* which ranges from 1400 to 1800 kcal* per day. The heat released by the operation of the sodium pump (Chapter 2) in all cells is an important source of heat. In addition, heat is produced by other essential metabolic activity, *e.g.,* the beating of the heart and contraction of the diaphragm.

Under normal active conditions, additional heat is produced by exercise, which can be quite modest with sedentary workers (*e.g.,* 1000 kcal) or rather high in those engaged in heavy manual labor (*e.g.,* 6000 kcal). The heat produced by metabolism raises the temperature of the blood through the relevant organs. Thus, the blood

---

*The unit used in metabolic studies is the kilocalorie (kcal), which equals 1000 calories. One calorie is the quantity of heat required to raise the temperature of 1 gram of water 1°C.

leaving the brain and the liver is warmer than that entering them. Likewise, during manual work, blood leaving the skeletal muscles is heated. The warm blood from these centers of heat production is distributed to the organs of heat loss. Of these, the skin is the most important.

Heat is lost from the blood as it perfuses the skin. Convection, radiation, and evaporation of sweat all play a part in the loss of heat. Evaporation is particularly important when the ambient temperature exceeds that of the body. The blood supply to the skin is regulated by the sympathetic division of the autonomic nervous system, which plays a dominant role in the maintenance of a constant body temperature. Some heat is also lost from the respiratory tract and mouth. In humans, this is a relatively constant amount, but in animals it can be increased considerably by panting.

The Temperature-Regulating Mechanism

When there is a change in body temperature, mechanisms come into play in response to impulses from temperature-sensitive receptors that are situated both centrally within the nervous system and peripherally in the skin. A change of as little as 0.2°C can be detected and set the compensatory mechanisms in motion in response to impulses from the temperature-sensitive receptors.

The *central receptor,* situated in the preoptic area of the hypothalamus, is a group of nerve cells that is sensitive to the temperature of the arterial blood reaching it. When the temperature of the blood changes, impulses pass from this area to other parts of the hypothalamus. There are two main areas: (1) an anterior *heat-losing center,* which, when stimulated, leads to changes in the rest of the body, causing increased heat loss; and (2) a posterior *heat-promoting center,* which, when stimulated, leads to increased production, conservation of heat, and a rise in body temperature (Fig. 14–1).

The *peripheral temperature receptors* are situated mainly in the skin. When the body's temperature falls, impulses pass to the heat-promoting hy-

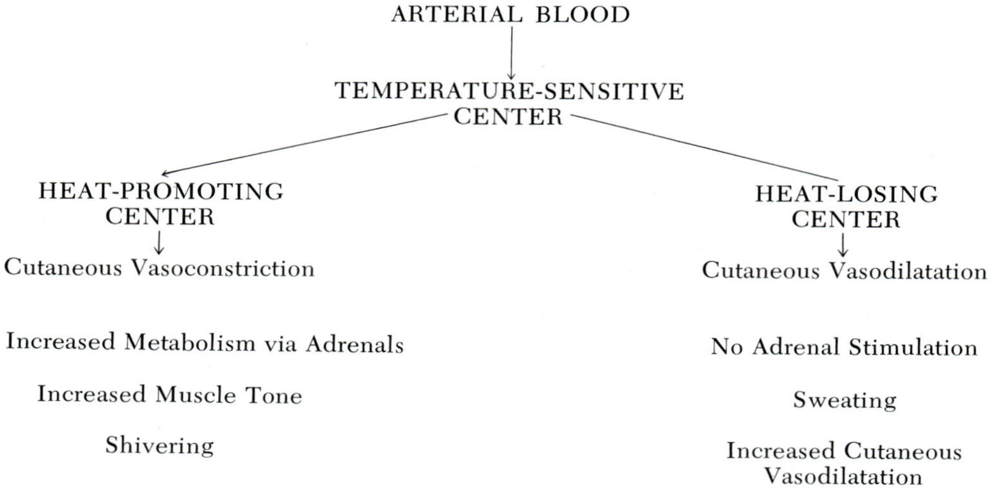

ARTERIAL BLOOD

TEMPERATURE-SENSITIVE
CENTER

HEAT-PROMOTING
CENTER

Cutaneous Vasoconstriction

Increased Metabolism via Adrenals

Increased Muscle Tone

Shivering

HEAT-LOSING
CENTER

Cutaneous Vasodilatation

No Adrenal Stimulation

Sweating

Increased Cutaneous
Vasodilatation

Figure 14–1 Diagram illustrating the principal heat-regulating mechanisms.

pothalamic center and lead to conservation of heat.

Mechanism for Increasing Body Temperature. The heat-promoting center acts mainly through the sympathetic division of the autonomic nervous system. Cutaneous vasoconstriction reduces the amount of heat lost from the skin, and blood diverted to the internal organs is insulated from the exterior by the subcutaneous fat. Furthermore, as the skin becomes cooler, the subject feels cold and may take appropriate voluntary action such as putting on extra clothing.

The increased sympathetic outflow causes an increased output of epinephrine and norepinephrine from the adrenal glands. These hormones increase the metabolic rate of all cells through a mechanism that is not well understood. Metabolism is further increased by a *generalized increase in muscle tone*. If these mechanisms are inadequate, muscle tone increases to the extent that stretch reflexes are elicited and *shivering* commences. As one group of muscles contracts, a stretch reflex of the antagonistic group is set in motion and initiates a fresh stretch reflex of the first group. This continuous shaking greatly increases the rate of heat production.

Mechanism for Decreasing Body Temperature. When the body's temperature tends to rise, there is a withdrawal of sympathetic vasoconstriction activity, the skin becomes warm, and heat is lost. The subject feels hot and may remove

clothing, retire to the shade, or take other appropriate action. If this regulating mechanism is inadequate, the heat-losing center initiates sweating from the eccrine glands. Evaporation of this fluid requires heat, but an additional effect of sweating is the local release of bradykinin from the glands. This induces further vasodilation and heat loss.

FEVER

Fever, or *pyrexia*, may be defined as an elevation of the body's temperature that follows a disturbance of the regulating mechanism. When the temperature reaches or exceeds 40°C (104°F), the condition is called *hyperpyrexia*.

Common Causes of Fever

The following common causes should be noted.

Infection. Infection is the most common cause of fever; the pattern of the temperature chart is sometimes characteristic of a particular disease. The relapsing course of malaria and brucellosis is an example of this. So also are the two phases of fever that characterize dengue. With some acute infections, particularly if there is an initial septicemia as in urinary tract infections and lobar pneumonia, the onset of fever is sudden. The following stages are recognized.

The Cold Stage. At the onset of the illness, the patient experiences an intense feeling of cold. There is peripheral constriction evident as pallor, and the patient starts to shiver. The teeth chatter, and the patient shakes all over with the familiar "rigor." The increased muscular activity combined with reduced heat loss causes the temperature to rise. The blood pressure and pulse rate also rise. In general, there is an increase in pulse rate of about 18 beats per minute for each 1°C rise in temperature (10 beats per minute for each 1°F). In children, the rigor may be replaced by a convulsion.

The Hot Stage. As the temperature approaches its peak, the peripheral vasoconstriction relaxes, and the patient feels dry and warm. The amount of heat loss now balances that formed, and the temperature remains constant. The thermostat of the heat-regulating mechanism is still functioning but is set to maintain the temperature at a level higher than normal. The normal daily variation in temperature is seen, so that the highest levels occur during the evening. This phase can last for several hours or days. If hyperpyrexia occurs, the heat-regulating mechanism ceases to function.

The Sweating Phase. The temperature begins to fall, and the patient soon experiences a sensation of intense heat and sweats profusely. Bedclothes are thrown off, and the temperature returns to normal. When this phase occurs over a short period, as in lobar pneumonia and malaria, the termination is described as the *crisis.* If the pyrexia subsides slowly, as in typhoid fever, the termination is described as *lysis.*

The response to infection is marked in young children, and a trivial infection can cause a high fever. Sometimes there is a seizure. In old age and in debilitated subjects, no fever may occur even with severe infections.

Chronic infections frequently cause fever, and the prolonged rise in metabolic rate combines with loss of appetite to produce weight loss. Chronic pulmonary tuberculosis provides an example of this, and the emaciated appearance of the patients earned the terms "consumption" and "phthisis" for the disease. The terminal stage of AIDS is now a more familiar example.

Infarction. A mild fever is commonly encountered in patients with infarction, particularly of the lung or the myocardium.

Venous Thrombosis. A mild fever may be the only clinical evidence of deep vein thrombosis of the leg.

Tumors. Some tumors are particularly liable to be associated with pyrexia, even in the absence of a complicating infection. It is a well known feature of clear-cell carcinoma of the kidney and Ewing's tumor of bone. Acute leukemia is often accompanied by fever, and this can be severe enough to mimic an infection. A low-grade fever is common in chronic leukemia and lymphoma. In any patient with pyrexia (fever) of unknown origin, the possibility of malignant disease should always be remembered.

Hemorrhage. Fever may follow bleeding, particularly bleeding into the gastrointestinal tract or the peritoneal space. Sudden hemorrhage from a ruptured ectopic pregnancy, for example, can produce acute abdominal pain, abdominal distention, and fever, a combination of signs and symptoms that might easily be mistaken for an infection such as acute appendicitis.

Brain Damage. Any cause of brain damage (*e.g.,* bleeding, infection, or infarction) can lead to an upset of the central heat-regulating mechanism either by damaging the hypothalamus directly or by interfering with the outflow of autonomic nervous impulses.

Injury. Fever is a feature of the catabolic phase that follows injury.

Severe Anemia. During phases of acute hemolysis, fever is sometimes prominent.

Heat Syndromes. There are three syndromes associated with a high environmental temperature.

Heat Stroke. Some rise in body temperature normally occurs during extreme exercise because the heat-eliminating mechanisms cannot immediately keep pace with the excessive heat production in the muscles. When the environment is hot and humid, even mild exercise can cause a marked rise in body temperature, particularly in elderly individuals with pre-existing chronic disease. Sometimes the heat-regulating mechanism breaks down under these circumstances and the temperature rises excessively. This is the condition of *heat stroke* or *sunstroke,* and unless it is promptly treated efficiently, the body's temperature continues to rise, reaching 43°C (109.4°F) or even higher. Patients become comatose, have convulsions, and may have permanent brain damage if they survive. Heat stroke must therefore be treated most energetically by immersion in cool water until the temperature approaches normal.

Heat Cramps. Heat cramps are characterized by painful cramps of the voluntary muscles of the limbs and usually follow strenuous exercise. The spasms are apparently due to local loss of sodium and chloride.

Heat Exhaustion. Heat exhaustion or heat collapse is the most common heat syndrome. It usually affects elderly individuals who are unable to adapt to a high external temperature. The pathogenesis is not clear. Weakness, headache, nausea, and vomiting are followed by collapse and hypotension. The body's temperature is either normal or low, as it is in other forms of shock. Patients with heat exhaustion are generally depleted of salt and water owing to prolonged sweating combined with inadequate fluid and salt intake. Whether this is the major cause of the condition is not clear, but certainly fluid and electrolyte imbalance should be corrected as part of the treatment of the condition.

Malignant Hyperthermia. Malignant hyperthermia is one of the most common causes of anesthetic-induced deaths. It is characterized by a rapid rise in temperature during the administration of a general anesthetic. In many cases, halothane and suxamethonium have been given. Tachycardia, tachypnea, instability of the blood pressure, and acidosis develop. In some cases, skeletal muscular rigidity is noted; instead of the expected muscular relaxation, there is muscle stiffness. Progress of the pyrexia is extremely rapid, and unless the condition is recognized and vigorously treated, the patient may die.

The exact pathogenesis is unclear, but a familial incidence has been noted and in some families a type of myopathy is present. An elevation in the plasma levels of creatine phosphokinase might be present, but a more reliable test is muscle biopsy. A history of other family members having died under anesthesia should alert the anesthetist to the possibility of the development of malignant hyperthermia and forewarn of possible trouble.

Miscellaneous Conditions. Fever is a prominent feature of acute gout and some of the collagen diseases (*e.g.,* lupus erythematosus and rheumatic fever). An adverse reaction to a drug is another important cause. Occasionally, fever is present in syndromes of obscure nature, *e.g.,* cyclical fever.

Fever or Pyrexia of Unknown Origin. Sometimes fever is present for no apparent reason. It is a common clinical problem, and accurate diagnosis demands considerable clinical skill combined with laboratory aids. A good history combined with a knowledge of epidemiology will sometimes suggest the correct diagnosis (see Case History I and Fig. 14–2).

Case History I

The patient was a 69-year-old man who had gone on an African safari for 1 month. While there, he had occasional attacks of diarrhea and had developed a chronic cough, which was productive of a large amount of sputum. He gave a history of having had such severe night sweats on several occasions that the whole bed had been soaked. Before leaving Africa, he developed a superficial skin infection between the fourth and fifth fingers of his right hand. Two days after arriving in Canada, he was brought into the emergency ward, having collapsed at home while unpacking a suitcase. He had struck his head and had lost consciousness for about 20 minutes. He complained of a mild headache, had a temperature of 38.9°C (102°F), and had a laceration of the left frontal area of the scalp. Infection was noted on the hand, and the fever was attributed to this infection. He was given penicillin and sent home. The next day he felt quite well, but the following day he was found by a friend to be drowsy, although still responsive and able to watch a hockey game. The next morning he was found unconscious and was again admitted to a hospital, this time in a coma. Blood and urine were obtained for culture, and numerous biochemical tests were ordered. In view of the history of cough and drenching night sweats, the possibility of pulmonary tuberculosis was considered; a radiograph of lung, however, revealed no evidence of disease. Cerebrospinal fluid was obtained by lumbar puncture and revealed an elevated protein content (0.56 g/L). The patient was noted to be slightly jaundiced. Before the results of the various tests were obtainable, a blood film was examined and was found to contain a large number of malaria parasites (Fig. 14–2). A diagnosis of malignant malaria with cerebral involvement was made, and emergency treatment with the antimalarial

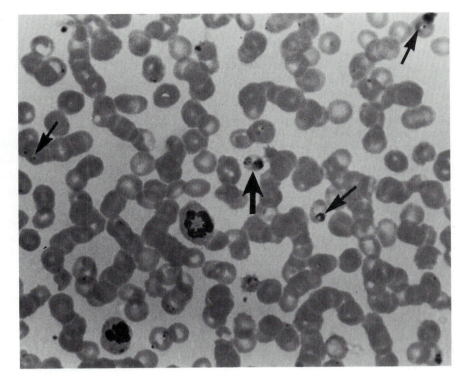

Figure 14–2 Blood film from a patient with malignant tertian malaria. Numerous ring forms (small arrows) of *Plasmodium falciparum* are present in the blood film. Particularly characteristic is the presence of two or more organisms in one red cell (large arrow). Blood film stained by Giemsa stain (× 1000).

drug chloroquine was undertaken. Nevertheless, the patient rapidly deteriorated, developed hypotension, and died within 4 hours. This case illustrates how a good history and a knowledge of diseases endemic to particular geographic locations can help in arriving at a diagnosis. Attributing fever and loss of consciousness to a minor skin infection was a mistake that cost this patient his life.

A fever combined with a heart murmur suggests bacterial endocarditis; repeated blood cultures must be performed for an accurate diagnosis. Pulmonary tuberculosis can be remarkably silent but will be revealed by a radiograph. Fever in a patient past the age of 40 years should lead to a search for occult cancer; fever in a child might suggest leukemia; and fever in a young adult might cause suspicion of infectious mononucleosis. In the diagnosis of pyrexia of unknown origin, the physician's skills and knowledge can thus be taxed to the extreme (see Case History II).

Case History II

A 30-year-old male was admitted to the hospital for the investigation of fever. Five weeks before admis-

sion, he had developed severe pain in the back, which had been relieved by aspirin. Two weeks later, the pain recurred and radiated toward the sternum. Although a heart attack was suspected, an electrocardiogram showed no abnormality; his serum enzymes were also normal. He had several bouts of fever during the next 3 weeks. On examination in the hospital, he was found to be a pale, sallow, somewhat overweight man who was sweating profusely and in moderate distress. His temperature on admission was 40.5°C (105°F), and his pulse was 120 beats per minute; blood pressure was 115/65 mm Hg. A murmur was heard over the precordium, and bacterial endocarditis was considered a possible cause. Numerous blood cultures were performed, all of which were sterile. Analysis of the urine was normal; culture was sterile. No obvious site of infection could be found clinically. The fever dropped to 38.8°C (100°F) with aspirin but recurred each evening while the patient was in the hospital. Numerous other investigations were performed, including radiographs of the chest and vertebrae and an intravenous pyelogram. Blood was taken for the Widal, Weil-Felix, and brucella agglutination tests. Radiographs of the abdomen revealed no evidence of a subphrenic abscess such as might occur after a perforation of appendix, peptic ulcer, or diverticulum of the colon. All agglutination tests were negative, as was the VDRL test. A blood count was, however, unusual. In spite of the patient's having a fever, he had a total white blood cell count of 4.4 × 10⁹/L with 95 per cent neutrophils and 4 per cent band forms. The platelet count was 95 × 10⁹/L. Systemic lupus erythematosus was first considered, but since no anti-DNA antibodies were present in the blood, this condition was eliminated from consideration. In view of the unusual blood findings, a bone marrow puncture was performed, and the smear revealed almost complete replacement of normal marrow cells by primitive blast cells. There were a few normal erythroid precursors and virtually no megakaryocytes. In cases such as this, at times it is not possible to decide whether the cells are lymphoblasts or myeloblasts. The terms *stem-cell leukemia* or *blast-cell leukemia* are therefore convenient. About a week after admission, the patient still had a fever at night, and he developed ulceration of the mouth. He was treated with a variety of chemotherapeutic agents in courses over the next few months, but he died 8 months after the first admission with bronchopneumonia. This case illustrates how malignant disease—in this case, leukemia—can closely mimic infection by virtue of fever that is a presenting and constant feature.

Pathogenesis of Fever

The intravenous injection of gram-negative organisms produces a rigor and a sharp rise in temperature due to the release of bacterial lipopolysaccharides called bacterial pyrogens. They cause white blood cells, particularly macrophages, to release interleukin-1, previously called endogenous pyrogen. Interleukin-1 stimulates an increased synthesis of prostaglandin E2 (PGE2) from arachidonic acid; in turn, PGE2 has two important actions. It acts directly on the hypothalamus to cause an increase in body temperature and on muscle to cause increased protein catabolism. Cyclo-oxygenase inhibitors, such as aspirin and indomethacin, act as antipyretic drugs by blocking prostaglandin formation from arachidonic acid.

Macrophages also release interleukin-1 during phagocytosis; this explains how fever is a feature of noninfective inflammatory conditions, *e.g.,* acute gout and lupus erythematosus.

The bacterial pyrogens are heat stable and are of importance because they can produce febrile reactions if they are present in the fluids used in intravenous therapy, which, although sterile, may still cause a sharp rigor on intravenous injection. Pyrogen-free fluids used for injection are prepared by distillation to ensure that all bacterial products are excluded.

Certain steroid hormones can produce a rise in body temperature, and it is believed that the release of progesterone is responsible for the temperature rise that occurs during the menstrual cycle.

In the fully anesthetized patient, the heat-regulating mechanism is not functioning. The body therefore becomes poikilothermic (like the body of an amphibian) and equates with the temperature of the surrounding atmosphere. The patient must therefore be protected against hyperpyrexia as well as hypothermia.

Recent work has shed some light on the pathogenesis of fever, but the value of a rise in temperature in infection is not clear. Interferon production by infected cells is increased, and this is presumably of value in limiting viral infection. Little is known of any possible advantage in other infections.

HYPOTHERMIA

Hypothermia may be defined as a body temperature below 35°C (95°F). It is an important cause of death in cold climates, especially of infants and the aged, and it has been utilized as an adjunct to anesthesia.

Hypothermia in Infants

Newborn infants are particularly susceptible to cold because of the relatively high ratio of surface area to body mass, the paucity of subcutaneous fat, and the low production of heat by physical means because of the inability to exercise or shiver. Furthermore, the thermoregulatory mechanism is relatively inefficient at birth and remains so for several hours.

During the first few weeks of life, infants need constant warmth, especially when ill. In cold countries, open windows, lukewarm baths, and power cuts can cause inconvenience to adults but can be fatal to infants.

The early signs of cold injury are lethargy and difficulty in feeding. Indeed, the child has a still, serene appearance, and the cheeks, nose, and extremities have a flush that deludes the on-looker into believing all is well. The cry is like a whimper, and the body feels cold. Later, brady-cardia and edema of the eyelids and extremities occur. In the worst cases, the subcutaneous fat becomes hard.

Hypothermia in Adults

Hypothermia can occur in adults in a number of circumstances. Immersion hypothermia is one of the lethal factors in shipwreck. Hypothermia is an important complication of myxedema and hypopituitarism, and it also occurs in patients with widespread eczema and generalized eryth-roderma. In widespread skin disease, the passive diffusion of water through the epidermis is greatly increased, and heat is lost by both evap-oration and convection.

The most important example is the sponta-neous hypothermia that occurs in old people—usually women—who live alone in poorly heated rooms and are poorly clothed. Undernutrition is often an additional factor; in persons who are in both calorie- and protein-deficient states, the basal metabolic rate is decreased. Hypothermia in the aged is sometimes a complication of senile dementia or the effects of depressant drugs like alcohol and chlorpromazine that have dulled the mind. There is sometimes a severe precipitating infection such as pneumonia.

The patient with hypothermia looks ill. There is a corpselike chill of the body, and the rectal temperature can be as low as 21°C (70°F). The skin is pale, and the subcutaneous tissue is pliant and doughy. The patient remains still; muscles are rigid, and shivering is absent. The tendon reflexes are sluggish, and there is bradycardia, sometimes with atrial fibrillation. Since periph-eral edema and puffiness of the eyelids are com-mon, myxedema may be simulated. Oliguria (di-minished urine output) is common, respiration is depressed, and death often occurs from cardiac arrest.

It is easy to overlook hypothermia, in both infants and adults. Clinical thermometers that register as low as 24°C (75°F) should be available and used if the circumstances raise the possibility of hypothermia.

Induced Hypothermia

Some animals have acquired the ability to hi-bernate for long periods in a state of hypothermia as a useful adjunct to survival in winter. From experimental work carried out on small animals, it has been found that they can be cooled below 0°C (32°F) if they are made first to ingest propyl-ene glycol. Mice can be kept in suspended ani-mation for about 1 hour and then reanimated by artificial respiration and microwave diathermy. Larger animals do not tolerate this treatment so well and usually die within a few days. A lesser degree of hypothermia has been used as an adjunct to cardiac surgery. If the body's temper-ature is lowered, cardiac arrest can be tolerated for about 1 hour. The development of extracor-poreal circulatory systems has allowed profound hypothermia to be used in open-heart surgery. In one method, the blood is cooled rapidly by passage through a heat exchanger and the cir-culation is maintained extracorporeally. At the temperature of 12.7° to 15°C (55° to 59°F), the circulation is stopped, and the heart is opened in a bloodless field. When the operation is fin-ished, the blood is rewarmed, the heart is defi-brillated, and a normal circulation is restored. Extracorporeal circulations are now so efficient that hypothermia is less commonly used or is merely used as an adjunct to this procedure.

Local Hypothermia

Extreme cold causes tissue damage; when the part is rewarmed, an acute inflammation follows and blisters occur. Direct damage to the capillar-ies is prominent, and vascular occlusion contrib-utes to tissue necrosis. This type of cold injury is called frostbite and in cold climates is not uncommon after accidental exposure to cold. Usually, the toes, fingers, ears, and nose are affected. Deliberate application of extreme cold (cryosurgery) is used therapeutically in surgical practice. Solid carbon dioxide and liquid nitrogen are commonly applied to warts and other skin tumors. Various types of probes that are refrig-erated by liquid nitrogen have been devised for applying cold to deeper tissues. They have been used to treat eye tumors as well as in intracranial surgery. At present, the use of cold is confined to special centers; the late effects are still being assessed.

Summary

- The normal body temperature is maintained by balancing heat gain with heat loss. Impulses from temperature-sensitive receptors in the skin and hypothalamus reach hypothalamic centers that set compensatory mechanisms in motion.
- Fever occurs with infection; with acute infection, fever passes through a cold stage, a hot stage, and finally a sweating stage as it subsides by crisis.
- Other causes include infarction of heart or lung, deep vein thrombosis, tumors, internal hemorrhage, brain damage, acute gout, and the catabolic phase that follows severe injury. Until the cause is found, the terms fever or pyrexia of unknown origin are used.
- The heat syndromes include heat pyrexia, heat cramps, and heat exhaustion.
- Malignant hyperthermia is an important cause of death during anesthesia (commonly using halothane and suxamethonium). Increased skeletal muscle activity is the source of the heat, and a muscle abnormality appears to be the basic abnormality. Some cases are familial, and a family history warns of danger.
- Bacterial pyrogens produce fever indirectly. They cause the release of interleukin-1 from white blood cells, and this mediator stimulates the synthesis of prostaglandin E2, which acts directly on the hypothalamus. Aspirin acts by blocking PGE2 formation.
- Hypothermia is most common in infants and the aged; it may also complicate conditions with generalized cutaneous hyperemia.
- Therapeutic hypothermia is used as an adjunct to surgery.

Selected Readings

Britt, B. A.: Malignant hyperthermia: A review. *In* Milton, A. S. (ed.): Handbook of Experimental Pharmacology. Vol. 60. Berlin, Springer-Verlag, 1982.

Dinerello, C. A., et al.: New concepts in the pathogenesis of fever. N. Engl. J. Med. *319*:397, 1988.

Guyton, A. C.: Textbook of Medical Physiology. 7th ed. Philadelphia, W. B. Saunders Co., 1986.

See, in particular, Body Temperature, Temperature Regulation, and Fever.

Nelson, T. E., and Flewellen, E. H.: The malignant hyperthermia syndrome. N. Engl. J. Med. *309*:416, 1983.

Rae, D.: Accidental hypothermia. Can. Nurse *76*:28, 1980.

Root, R. K., and Petersdorf, R. G.: Alterations in body temperature. *In* Wilson, J. D., et al. (eds.): Harrison's Principles of Internal Medicine. 12th ed. New York, McGraw-Hill, 1991, pp. 125–133.

15

Disorders of Nutrition

After studying this chapter, the student should be able to:

- Describe the metabolic effects of starvation.
- Distinguish between nutritional marasmus and kwashiorkor.
- Define obesity and describe the differences between lifelong obesity and adult-onset obesity.
- List the endocrine disorders that are associated with obesity.
- List the complications of obesity.
- Classify and list the vitamins that are required by humans.
- Describe the sources of vitamin A and discuss the effects of vitamin A deficiency and excess.
- Describe the sources of vitamin C and give an account of scurvy.

- Classify beriberi according to its several forms and describe the features of each type.
- Outline the main features of pellagra.
- Describe the effects of pyridoxine deficiency.
- Describe what is meant by a trace element.
- Describe the syndromes that are known to be caused by a deficiency of a trace element.

The most important disorders of nutrition relate to a deficiency or an excess of those components of the diet that provide both energy and the materials for the synthesis of proteins, carbohydrates, and fats. *Starvation* and *obesity* are described first. The role of *vitamins* is then considered. Finally, a note has been added concerning the *trace elements;* the note is short, for although these elements are probably of great importance in the human body, remarkably little is known about their role in health and disease.

STARVATION

With the world population expanding at an estimated rate of 70 million each year, it is likely that malnutrition will become increasingly common. The effects of total starvation are described first.

Metabolic Changes

The body's store of glucose and glycogen is sufficient for only 1 day's metabolic needs. The protein supply and triacylglycerols of adipose tissue could provide enough energy for 2 to 3 months, but in practice, when 18 to 20 per cent of body weight is lost, other factors, such as gastric intolerance of fluid and general weakness, can terminate life.

The starving person is particularly susceptible to intercurrent infections. Gastroenteritis, dysentery, and tuberculosis take their toll, particularly in children and in poverty stricken communities.

Immediate Changes. The brain normally uses only glucose as fuel; after the first day of starvation, the blood glucose level is maintained by new glucose formation in the liver, in which amino acids are used as fuel. The amino acids are provided by the breakdown of protein. Because the nitrogen component is excreted as urea, the body is in negative nitrogen balance.

The triacylglycerols of adipose tissue are broken down to glycerol and fatty acids. Fatty acids are converted into ketone bodies in the liver, and these are used directly by most organs of the body instead of glucose.

Later Changes. After the first week of starvation, the breakdown of protein declines rapidly. A change occurs in the brain's metabolism such that it is able to utilize ketone bodies, particularly beta-hydroxybutyrate, instead of glucose. Starvation can now continue until all the stores of body fat are utilized. When the supply of fat has been exhausted, only protein remains. The muscle masses decline, and death soon follows.

During starvation, the body conserves energy by reducing energy output. The starved individual is apathetic and lacks interest in life. Hypothermia is a danger in cold climates.

Starvation is also a feature of *anorexia nervosa*, a condition usually encountered in psychoneurotic adolescent girls that is characterized by an obsessive aversion to food. Extreme wasting and amenorrhea are the main features and are secondary to starvation. Unlike the patients with enforced starvation, patients with anorexia nervosa are restless and hostile. They usually deny hunger, and if obliged to eat by circumstances, they induce vomiting as soon as they can be alone in a bathroom. The precise cause of this distressing disease is unknown. Its treatment is unsatisfactory, and there is a significant mortality. *Bulimia nervosa* is allied to anorexia nervosa but is more common. The patient has an abnormal fear of obesity but engages in episodes of binge eating followed by the employment of various techniques, such as self-induced vomiting, use of large doses of diuretics and laxatives, strict dieting, or vigorous exercise, in an attempt to avoid digestion of the food and weight gain.

Loss of water is a characteristic feature of early starvation. Its cause is unknown. For individuals who try weight-reducing diets, this loss provides false encouragement during the first few days of the regimen. In starvation, the kidney is unable to concentrate urine, and polyuria results.

The edema of starvation affects the dependent parts and appears to be due to the laxity of the subcutaneous tissues.

The wasted appearance of the starving person is all too familiar. The lax, dry skin and wasted muscles are matched by wasting of the internal organs. In particular, with advanced starvation, the intestine becomes increasingly thin; hence, when treating a starving patient, one must give frequent small feedings if the person's life is to be saved.

The starving person is particularly susceptible to infections. The functions of T and B lymphocytes, macrophages, and neutrophils have been reported as showing defects. Tuberculosis, dysentery, and other infections often complete the lethal process initiated by starvation. This is particularly evident in protein-calorie malnutrition in childhood.

Protein-Calorie Malnutrition in Childhood

Protein-calorie malnutrition is regarded as a spectrum of disease with marasmus at one end and kwashiorkor at the other end.

Nutritional Marasmus

Marasmus is the name given to starvation in infants. It is due to deficiency of both protein and calories and is encountered in infants under 1 year of age. It is a common condition in the developing countries and is usually due to cessation of breast feeding when the mother again becomes pregnant. The child exhibits the wasted appearance of starvation and in addition shows lack of growth. In those who survive, dwarfism is a frequent complication.

Kwashiorkor

This is a syndrome observed in children between the ages of 1 and 3 years. Its name is derived from a local African word denoting illness in a child displaced from the breast by a subsequent pregnancy.

Kwashiorkor is due to a low protein intake and the presence of a reasonably adequate carbohydrate supply. It is characterized by a fatty liver and marked edema of the subcutaneous tissues. The inadequate protein supply leads to defective pigment formation; consequently, the hair becomes pale and even red in African children, and the skin is often depigmented and shows hyperkeratosis and flaking.

OBESITY

Obesity has been a problem of mankind since time immemorial, for evidence of it has been found in the relics of the Stone Age, in ancient Egyptian mummies, and in Greek sculptures. It is now rampant in the affluent world, as a walk down any main street in North America will bear witness. It has been estimated that approximately 20 per cent of middle-aged males and 40 per cent of middle-aged females are obese.

There is no precise definition of obesity, since there is no sharp cut-off from those individuals who are well covered and considered normal to those who are obese. For practical purposes, an obese individual can be defined as one having a body weight over 20 per cent above mean ideal body weight based on height, build, and age. Life insurance companies have compiled tables giving such mean ideal body weights. The measurement of skin fold thickness over various parts of the body with the use of simple calipers

provides another guide. Skin fold thickness at the triceps greater than 23 mm for men and greater than 30 mm for women indicates obesity.

Pathology and Pathogenesis

The number and variety of published weight-reducing diets and the existence of weight-losing clinics and spas bear witness to our lack of comprehension of this topic and the ineffectiveness of treatment.

Clinical Types

Two clinical types of obesity can be recognized.

Lifelong Obesity. Although of normal weight at birth, these individuals tend to be heavy as children and to have large spurts of weight gain during puberty and, in women, during pregnancy. Fat tends to be widely distributed, affecting limbs as well as trunk. Eventually, these individuals tend to be grossly overweight, and weight reduction is a lifelong losing battle. A possible explanation for this type of obesity is that there is an increased number of fat cells (adipocyte hyperplasia). In the normal individual, adipose cell proliferation occurs during the first 2 years of life and again at puberty. In obese children, the number of adipose cells continues to increase throughout childhood.

There is probably a genetic basis for childhood obesity. There are strains of rats that invariably develop adipose cell hyperplasia and become obese. The situation in humans is difficult to assess because environmental influences may override genetic trait. Even adipose cell hyperplasia may not be the primary cause of the obesity; it can be induced by overfeeding in childhood.

Adult-Onset Obesity. These individuals are of normal weight until the age of 20 to 40 years and then steadily become obese. This "middle-aged spread" is associated with deposition of fat, predominantly in a central location. Hence, the increase in thickness of a scapular skin fold is greater than that of measurements taken over the triceps or ulna. The number of fat cells is normal, but they are overdistended with neutral fat. This is in contrast to persons with lifelong obesity, in whom there is fat cell hyperplasia.

The reasons for developing "middle-aged spread" are poorly understood: too little exercise, social customs, overeating, and overdrinking may all play a part. The key to the answer must be a knowledge of the mechanism by which food intake is adjusted to energy output. The presence in the hypothalamus of a feeding center and a satiety center has been postulated, but these centers are ill-defined and their regulation is not understood. Eating habits, emotional state, social custom, olfactory impulses, and visual temptations all influence an individual's desire to start eating and indicate when to stop. There can be no doubt that excess of calorie intake over energy expenditure results in excess fat deposition. When a steady state is attained, energy input again equals output, but the adipose cells remain overloaded and the feedback mechanism by which overfilled adipocytes inhibit appetite is defective. Unfortunately, we are ignorant of the mechanism involved.

Other Causes

There are strains of rats that are genetically destined to develop obesity due to adipose cell hyperplasia. A human counterpart is possible, but the situation is obscured because environmental influences may override genetic traits. Obesity in a family may be the effect of adipose cell hyperplasia induced by overfeeding in childhood.

Obesity is a feature of hypothalamic lesions, hyperinsulinism (associated with an islet cell tumor), hypothyroidism, and hypogonadism. It is also a feature of Cushing's syndrome, but in this condition the distribution of the fat is quite characteristic.

Effects of Obesity

The effects of obesity are severe, for not only is life expectancy reduced but so also is the quality of life. Complications of obesity may include:

1. *Diabetes mellitus.* In obese individuals, there is insulin resistance due to tissue insensitivity to this hormone. It appears that there is a decreased number of insulin receptors on the adipocytes. Hyperinsulinemia results, and eventually diabetes mellitus of the insulin-independent (maturity-onset) type develops.

2. *Atherosclerosis.* Obese individuals develop hyperlipoproteinemia of a pattern that predisposes them to develop atherosclerosis.

3. *Systemic hypertension.* This coupled with atherosclerosis renders the obese person particularly vulnerable to ischemic heart disease and cerebrovascular accidents.

4. *Osteoarthritis.* This degenerative disease affects particularly the large weight-bearing joints.

5. *Hypoventilation (Pickwickian syndrome).* This syndrome is discussed in Chapter 22.

6. *Operative risks.* The obese person is at risk following surgery not only because of ventilatory problems but also because of the purely mechanical factors that the surgeon encounters when trying to enter an obese abdomen.

7. *Miscellaneous.* Intertrigo, varicose veins, gallstones, hernias, and toxemia of pregnancy are all more common in the obese than in the normal subject.

THE VITAMINS

Vitamins are organic substances that the body cannot manufacture and that are necessary for normal metabolism; only ten such substances are known. If these substances are present in insufficient quantity, disease results. The ten vitamins essential for good health are listed in Table 15–1.

Table 15–1 THE ESSENTIAL VITAMINS

Fat-Soluble	Water-Soluble
Vitamin A	Vitamin C
Vitamin D	Vitamin B complex
Vitamin K	Thiamine
	Riboflavin
	Niacin
	Pyridoxine
	Cobalamin (B_{12})
	Folate

Vitamin A (Retinol)

Vitamin A is one of the fat-soluble vitamins. In herbivorous animals, the colored pigments (carotenoids, such as carotene) of plants and vegetables are converted into vitamin A in the intestine, are absorbed, and subsequently are stored in the liver. Humans acquire their supply either directly from the carotenoids in vegetable matter (*e.g.*, carrots, beet root, and green vegetables in general) or indirectly from animal or dairy products. The concurrent absorption of fat and the presence of bile salts in the intestine favor vitamin A absorption.

Vitamin A Deficiency

This is usually due to a deficient diet. This nutritional problem usually occurs in Indonesia, parts of Asia, India, the Middle East, and Latin America; it is almost unknown in North America and Europe. Vitamin A deficiency does, however, occur as a complication of the malabsorption syndrome; indeed, the blood level of carotene or vitamin A is used as a measure of the degree of malabsorption occurring.

Effects of Vitamin A Deficiency. The eye and the skin are the organs that suffer the most.

The Eye. Vitamin A forms an essential component of rhodopsin, a pigment in the rods of the retina. By absorbing light, rhodopsin initiates an electrical impulse that is transmitted to the brain and is interpreted as light. The first sign of vitamin A deficiency, therefore, is *night blindness*. Apart from this known biochemical action of vitamin A, its other functions remain a mystery in spite of much research. It is known that vitamin A regulates the structure of certain epithelial cells. In vitamin A deficiency, the epithelia of the genitourinary tract, the trachea, the nose, and the conjunctiva tend to undergo *squamous metaplasia*. The most important effect is in the eye. The conjunctival epithelium loses its mucus-secreting goblet cells and becomes keratinized, thereby taking on the characteristics of epidermis. The lacrimal ducts are affected in the same way, so that the eye becomes dry and subject to cracking and infection. The condition is called *xerophthalmia*. In due course, the cornea becomes cloudy; with infection it can soften (*keratomalacia*), causing the globe to be perforated. The lens can be extruded, and blindness results. Indeed, vitamin A deficiency is a leading cause of blindness in the world.*

The Skin. Phrynoderma, a toadskin appearance, has been attributed to vitamin A deficiency. It is associated with dryness of the skin with plugging of the hair follicles by keratin.

Other Effects. The replacement of respiratory epithelium (with its goblet cells and cilia) by keratinized squamous epithelium is a factor in the production of respiratory infections. Nevertheless, in the presence of a normal amount of vitamin A, there is no evidence that an excessive intake can prevent respiratory infections. The time-honored tradition of administering children large quantities of vitamin A (in cod-liver oil) to prevent colds and respiratory infections appears to be quite ill-founded. Indeed, such a practice can cause toxic effects (see later).

In spite of the dramatic changes seen in epithelium in vitamin A deficiency, the biochemical nature of the defect is quite unknown. If a small piece of skin is grown in organ culture and is subjected to vitamin A deficiency, it soon shows hyperkeratosis. If an excess quantity of vitamin A is now added to the medium, the epithelium changes to a goblet-cell, mucus-secreting type. There is no evidence, however, that excess vitamin A in humans can convert normal keratinized epidermis into mucus-secreting epithelium.

Toxicity of Vitamin A

Acute Toxic Effects. Very large doses of vitamin A are toxic and can cause an increase in intracranial pressure with headache, blurring of vision, and vomiting. This effect has been noticed by Arctic explorers after eating the livers of polar bears or bearded seals, which are very rich sources of vitamin A.

Chronic Toxic Effects. Chronic poisoning is sometimes encountered in children given the

---

*Other common causes are trachoma, diabetes mellitus, onchocerciasis, gonococcal ophthalmia, injury through accidents, cataract, and glaucoma. Although smallpox has now been eradicated, blindness caused by past cases of the disease is still common.

vitamin for treatment of acne or prevention of colds. The condition is easily overlooked because the symptoms are vague and include loss of hair, dry skin, hyperpigmentation of the skin, liver damage, bone pains, raised intracranial pressure, and psychiatric symptoms.

Vitamin E

Vitamin E includes a group of fat-soluble substances (tocopherols) that act as antioxidants. Various vitamin E deficiency states are recognized in animals. In humans, vitamin E deficiency has been described in premature infants and in patients having cystic fibrosis with severe steatorrhea (Chapter 23). There is unfortunately no good evidence that excess vitamin E can ward off old age, coronary disease, or the other ills that are associated with the aging process.

Vitamin D

The main action of vitamin D is on calcium metabolism; it is discussed in Chapter 30.

Vitamin K

Vitamin K is described in Chapter 18 in relation to blood coagulation.

Vitamin C (Ascorbic Acid)

Humans share with other primates and the guinea pig the feature of being among the few mammals that cannot synthesize vitamin C. The main dietary sources are citrus fruits, currants, berries, green vegetables, and potatoes.

Vitamin C is needed for the synthesis of collagen; a deficiency of this vitamin causes *scurvy*. The effects in adults are different from those encountered in children.

Adult Scurvy. The outstanding feature is swelling and bleeding of the gums. This is seen only in those who have teeth, and it is associated with infection. Wound healing is impaired (Chapter 5). Bleeding into the skin is character-istic and is first detected around the hair follicles. Bleeding may also occur into the joints, the gastrointestinal tract, and elsewhere.

In the past, scurvy has plagued sailors on long sea voyages, because the disease first becomes manifest after a person has been on a deficient diet for about 2 months. For example, Vasco da Gama is reported to have lost 100 men of his 160-man crew on his trip around the Cape of Good Hope (1497). Lind, a British naval surgeon, introduced oranges, limes, and lemons into his sailors' diet in 1747, and he thereby earned the nickname of "limey" for his countrymen.

Infantile Scurvy. Milk and milk products are often a poor source of vitamin C; consequently, scurvy can develop in infants at about the age of 8 months. There is impaired osteoid formation, and the epiphyses can become dislocated. An outstanding feature is subperiosteal hemorrhages, which are extremely painful. Bleeding can occur elsewhere, but gum lesions are not seen unless the teeth have erupted.

Vitamin B Complex

Thiamine

Thiamine is a coenzyme necessary for several steps in carbohydrate metabolism. In the absence of this vitamin, lactic and pyruvic acids accumulate rather than enter the Krebs cycle. The vitamin is widely distributed in foodstuffs. Thiamine deficiency was once prevalent in the Orient, where polished (highly milled) rice formed the staple diet (the process of milling removes most of the thiamine from the rice). Thiamine deficiency is now much less common in the world, but it is still encountered in the Orient, particularly in persons of all ages living in isolated communities, in infants, and in pregnant women. In North America, it is sometimes encountered in chronic alcoholics.

Effects of Thiamine Deficiency. The early symptoms of thiamine deficiency (called beriberi) are vague: weakness, swelling of the ankles, "pins and needles" (paresthesia), and numbness of the legs. At any time, one of the two major severe forms may develop.

Wet Beriberi. In this form, it is theorized that

the accumulation of lactic acid and other vasodilator chemicals causes so much vasodilation that a form of high-output heart failure develops. The outstanding features are extensive edema and accumulation of fluid in the serous sacs. Sudden death from heart failure is not uncommon.

Dry Beriberi. The outstanding feature of this form is degeneration of nerve fibers, particularly of the peripheral nerves (polyneuropathy). Numbness and anesthesia are the results of sensory nerve damage, whereas weakness and muscle wasting are the effects of motor nerve involvement. The patient eventually becomes bedridden.

Two other effects of thiamine deficiency are noteworthy.

Infantile Beriberi. Infants with a low thiamine intake can develop acute beriberi between the ages of 2 and 6 months. The sudden development of heart failure, which is often fatal, is characteristic.

Wernicke's Encephalopathy and Korsakoff's Psychosis. These conditions, described in Chapter 33, may occur with other forms of beriberi, but in Europe and North America they are invariably encountered in alcoholics.

Beriberi responds promptly to thiamine administration; with the wet form, early treatment is essential, since sudden death is common. Likewise, in Wernicke's encephalopathy, delay may lead to irreparable brain damage.

Riboflavin

Riboflavin is a constituent of many foods and is a component of several enzymes that play a vital role in metabolism. Yet the lesions associated with its deficiency are ill-defined. A sore mouth is an early symptom. The angles of the mouth become macerated and later develop cracks *(angular stomatitis or perlèche);* the lips become sore, dry, and cracked *(cheilosis);* and the tongue becomes smooth and sore *(glossitis).* A scaly dermatitis, resembling seborrheic dermatitis, develops later and affects the face and the scrotum or vulva.

Niacin

Niacin* is a generic term that includes nicotinic acid and nicotinamide. As with thiamine and riboflavin, this vitamin is widely distributed in plant and animal food and is also a component of important enzymes.

Effects of Niacin Deficiency. Deficiency of niacin causes *pellagra,* a disease so named because of the rough skin (from the Italian *pelle agra,* or "rough skin") that is present. Pellagra is a disease of poor peasants who subsist chiefly on maize (American corn). Although this cereal contains niacin, the vitamin is in a bound form. Furthermore, maize is deficient in tryptophan, an amino acid from which the body can manufacture niacin. Indeed, pellagra is probably caused by a lack of niacin, tryptophan, and riboflavin, perhaps combined with an excess of toxic or antivitamin substances.

Pellagra was once common in Spain and Italy. It became widespread in the United States in the early 1900s, but it has been largely swept away by improved economic circumstances. Nevertheless, it is still sometimes encountered in chronic alcoholics. The symptoms of pellagra are most easily remembered as the *four D's.*

Dermatitis. Erythema, superficially resembling a sunburn, is present on the sun-exposed areas. This may progress to blistering and a chronic type of dermatitis.

Diarrhea. Diarrhea is common, as is a smooth, sore tongue of "raw beef" appearance.

Dementia. Mental symptoms are common; they may be in the form of acute delirium or a chronic manic-depressive state followed by progressive dementia.

Death. Death was a common end result of pellagra before the advent of vitamin therapy.

Pyridoxine (Vitamin B₆)

Pyridoxine is also a component of important coenzymes. Dietary deficiencies are unusual, but

---

*Strictly speaking, niacin should not be labeled a vitamin, since it can be manufactured from tryptophan in the body. However, 60 mg of tryptophan is needed to produce 1 mg of niacin, and by convention niacin is always included in the list of vitamins necessary for humans.

pyridoxine deficiency has been reported as a complication of drug therapy, particularly with the administration of isoniazid, which is used in the treatment of tuberculosis. It has also been reported as a complication of taking the birth control pill. A seborrheic type of facial dermatitis, angular stomatitis, sore tongue, and anemia are the main effects.

It is evident from this short account that thiamine, riboflavin, niacin, and pyridoxine are widely distributed in food and that deficiencies are due to an unbalanced or inadequate diet. Such dietary deficiencies are generally the effect of poverty, ignorance, or alcoholism. It follows that multiple deficiencies are often present in the same patient. Hence, it is common and acceptable practice to treat a patient with a prescription containing a mixture of all members of the vitamin B complex.

Cobalamin (Vitamin B₁₂) and Folate

These vitamins are necessary for red blood cell maturation. The absence of these substances leads to a megaloblastic anemia (Chapter 18).

MINERALS

Electrolytes

Sodium, potassium, magnesium, and chlorine are generally available in abundance. Calcium metabolism is considered in Chapter 30.

Trace Elements

Inorganic elements that are present in the tissues in trace amounts (micrograms to picograms per gram of wet tissue) are termed trace elements. The following are thought to be essential to life: chromium, cobalt, copper, fluorine, iodine, iron, manganese, molybdenum, nickel, selenium, silicon, tin, vanadium and zinc. Iodine is essential in the synthesis of thyroid hormone, and the effects of deficiency are discussed in Chapter 29. Iron is an essential component of

hemoglobin; the anemia that follows its deficiency is described in Chapter 18.

The precise role of other trace elements is incompletely understood. The metals are often involved in the activation of enzymes or are part of the enzyme molecule itself. Disease can occur as a result of a direct excess or deficiency of a trace element, or more often there is an imbalance among several metal ions wherein an excess of one affects the function of another. Hence, simple measurement of the concentration of one ion does not necessarily reflect its activity *in vivo*. Furthermore, the actual measurement of trace elements is technically difficult and not within the expertise of most pathology laboratories. It is therefore not surprising that, with the exceptions of iodine and iron, the syndromes of trace element excesses or deficiencies are not well documented.

Zinc deficiency has been reported in childhood as a cause of retarded growth and hypogonadism. A better documented syndrome is *acrodermatitis enteropathica,* which is characterized by severe diarrhea, loss of hair (alopecia), and ulceration around the body orifices and on the extremities. The disease is apparently caused by zinc deficiency in patients with an autosomal recessive defect. The possible role of zinc in wound healing is mentioned in Chapter 5.

Copper deficiency is rare in humans but has been reported as a cause of anemia and leukopenia.

Summary

- In starvation, the brain adapts to use ketone bodies instead of glucose; hence, protein breakdown for glucose production, initially marked, is no longer needed after the first week.
- Protein-calorie malnutrition in childhood leads to marasmus or kwashiorkor.
- Obesity may be lifelong and probably related to adipocyte hyperplasia or may be of adult-onset type, the cause of which is unknown. Its chief complications are diabetes mellitus, atherosclerosis, systemic hypertension, and osteoarthritis.
- Vitamin A deficiency leads to night blindness, xerophthalmia, and phrynoderma. In large doses it is toxic.
- Vitamin C deficiency causes scurvy with bleeding gums associated with infection and impaired wound healing due to defective collagen formation. In infantile scurvy, bone formation is impaired, and painful subperiosteal hemorrhages are characteristic.

- The water-soluble vitamin B complex includes thiamine, riboflavin, niacin, and pyridoxine.
- Thiamine deficiency leads to beriberi with heart failure in the wet form and polyneuropathy in the dry form. Wernicke's encephalopathy and Korsakoff's psychosis are complications most often encountered in chronic alcoholics with thiamine deficiency.
- Riboflavin deficiency causes sore lips and sore, red tongue.
- Niacin deficiency causes pellagra characterized by dermatitis, diarrhea, and dementia.
- Pyridoxine deficiency leads to dermatitis, soreness of the mouth and tongue, and anemia.
- Trace elements are needed in minute amounts, and deficiency can cause severe effects. The effects of lack of iron, iodine, and zinc are the best documented.

Selected Readings

Bistrian, B. R., et al.: Prevalence of malnutrition in general medical patients. JAMA *235*:1567, 1976.

Cahill, G. F.: Starvation in man. N. Engl. J. Med. *282*:667, 1970.

Fairburn, C. G.: Bulimia nervosa. Br. Med. J. *300*:485, 1990.

Goldbloom, D. S., et al.: Anorexia nervosa and bulimia nervosa. Can. Med. Assoc. J. *140*:1149, 1989.

Hirsch, J., and Leibel, R. L.: New light on obesity. N. Engl. J. Med. *318*:509, 1988.

Mann, G. V.: The influence of obesity on health. N. Engl. J. Med. *291*:178, 1974.

Trustwell, A. S.: A B C of nutrition. Vitamins I and Vitamins II. Br. Med. J. *291*:1033 and 1103, 1985.

Van Itallie, T. B.: Bad news and good news about obesity. N. Engl. J. Med. *314*:239, 1986.

Metabolic Disorders

After studying this chapter, the student should be able to:

- Describe the concept of an inborn error of metabolism with particular reference to sickle cell anemia, galactosemia, glucose 6-phosphate dehydrogenase deficiency, phenylketonuria, alpha₁-antitrypsin deficiency, and the lysosomal storage diseases.
- Describe how the level of blood glucose is regulated.
- Classify the types of diabetes mellitus.
- Distinguish between insulin-dependent and non–insulin-dependent diabetes mellitus with respect to age of onset, etiology, and pathogenesis.
- List the complications of diabetes mellitus.
- Describe the causes and effects of hypoglycemia.
- Describe the clinical and pathologic features of gout.
- Distinguish between primary gout and secondary gout.

There are many diseases in which the mechanism causing the basic lesion is a metabolic disorder, often the absence or functional deficiency of a single protein, often an enzyme. These are genetically determined biochemical lesions, or *inborn errors of metabolism.* The diseases are important because they demonstrate how a simple biochemical error can affect many tissues and often produce severe disease. An abnormal allele can occupy the locus of a structural gene or a gene that exercises control, such as an operator gene. When a structural gene is involved, the effects can vary. The protein formed in the body, being of abnormal composition, may differ in chemical or physical properties; a good example is HbS that causes sickle cell disease. In the case of enzymes, their specific activity may be lessened or abolished altogether. Defective enzyme activity can be due to several mechanisms, and it is not surprising that apparently simple enzyme deficiency states, such as glucose 6-phosphate dehydrogenase deficiency or alpha₁-antitrypsin deficiency, are not simple disease entities but constitute a group of similar diseases; in general they resemble each other in the metabolic defect, but the clinical effects often vary widely.

INBORN ERRORS OF METABOLISM

A very large number of inborn errors of metabolism are now known; only some interesting, instructive, or common examples are described.

Galactosemia

This is a condition in babies who fail to thrive and who develop mental retardation, cataract, and cirrhosis of the liver. The defect is usually due to an absence of the enzyme that is responsible for converting galactose 1-phosphate to glucose 1-phosphate (Fig. 16–1). It follows that galactose (from the lactose of milk) cannot be utilized; it accumulates and is excreted in the urine. Galactose itself is not toxic, but galactose 1-phosphate probably interferes with some metabolic process that is essential for the proper development of the infant. The avoidance of galactose in the diet from an early age is the treatment.

Glucose 6-Phosphate Dehydrogenase Deficiency

This defect is inherited as a sex-linked factor and is common in black Africans and their American descendants. The defect comes to light when the subject takes certain drugs (*e.g.*, primaquine or sulfonamide); the lack of the enzyme in the red blood cells leads to an acute hemolytic anemia. A large number of variants of glucose 6-phosphate dehydrogenase deficiency are now known.

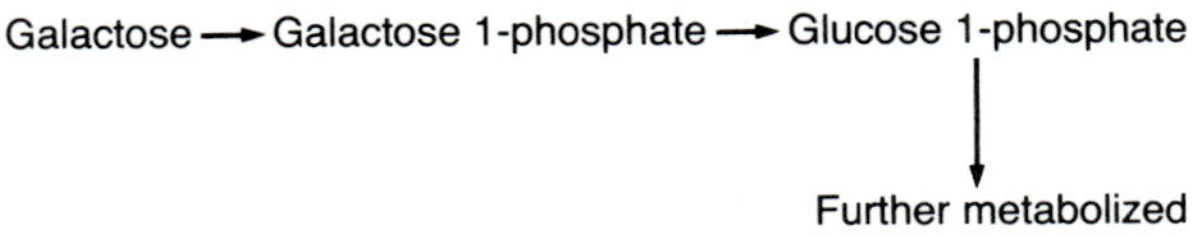

Galactose → Galactose 1-phosphate → Glucose 1-phosphate
↓
Further metabolized

Figure 16–1 Outline of the metabolic pathway of galactose utilization. In galactosemia, there is a defect in the enzymatic conversion of galactose 1-phosphate to glucose 1-phosphate.

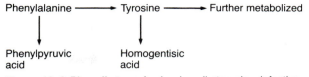

Figure 16–2 Phenylketonuria. In phenylketonuria, defective enzymatic conversion of phenylalanine to tyrosine results in accumulation of phenylalanine and its metabolites in the blood. One of these, phenylpyruvic acid, can easily be detected in the urine.

Phenylketonuria (PKU)

Subjects with this defect lack the enzyme that converts phenylalanine into tyrosine (Fig. 16–2). Phenylalanine derived from the diet therefore accumulates in the blood, and either it or one of its derivatives causes retardation of mental development. Between three and five persons per 100,000 of the population exhibit this condition. If the disease is detected early by testing the urine for phenylalanine derivatives, the infant can be given a diet low in phenylalanine content, and brain damage can be largely averted. PKU is inherited as an autosomal recessive trait; 1 per cent of the population are heterozygotes and can be detected by the administration of a dose of phenylalanine, when the blood level rises. This does not occur in a normal individual.

Alpha₁-Antitrypsin Deficiency

Individuals who have marked deficiency of alpha₁-antitrypsin develop panacinar emphysema, but the severity of the lung damage is variable presumably because emphysema is related also to other factors, particularly smoking and atmospheric pollution. Alpha₁-antitrypsin is a serum protease inhibitor and is synthesized in the liver. A single allele is inherited from each parent, and the phenotype is the result of codominant expression. At least 33 variant alleles have been identified.

Lysosomal Storage Disease

Lysosomes play a vital part in the removal of effete cytoplasmic components within a cell.

Hence, if a particular lysosomal enzyme is absent, its natural substrate accumulates in the cell and may damage it. The following groups of disease are included under the heading of lysosomal storage disease.

Glycogenosis (one type). In this disease, there is accumulation of glycogen.

The Lipidoses. The best known member of this group is Gaucher's disease. There is massive splenomegaly due to the accumulation of a lipid.

The Mucopolysaccharidoses. In this uncommon group of diseases, there is a deficiency of enzymes involved in metabolism of glucosaminoglycans of the extracellular matrix. This leads to skeletal defects and sometimes opacity of the cornea. The best known member is Hurler's syndrome, also known as "gargoylism" because of the grotesque appearance of the head of its sufferers.

The Gangliosidoses. Tay-Sachs disease is the most common member of this group. It is inherited as an autosomal recessive trait.

The disease is most frequent in Ashkenazic Jews; in some communities, one in 30 of the population is a heterozygote. The defect is absence of the lysosomal hexosaminidase A; this results in ballooning and degeneration of neurons secondary to an accumulation of ganglioside. Motor and mental deterioration beginning between 3 and 6 months of age is obvious at 1 year and results in death by the age of 3 years. It should be possible to eliminate this disease because heterozygotes can be detected and therefore counseled. In addition, a prenatal diagnosis can be made by examining the amniotic fluid or, preferably, its cells. Tay-Sachs disease emphasizes the value of studying the inborn diseases of metabolism; if the enzyme defect is known, prenatal diagnosis is possible, and heterozygote carriers can be detected and counseled. Possibly in the future, new genetic material can be introduced into the patients' cells so that the disease can be cured.

The Glycogenoses (Glycogen Storage Diseases)

There are a number of inherited disorders in which there is an excessive accumulation of glycogen in various tissues owing to an abnormality of glycogen metabolism. Each is related to a defective enzyme activity in the synthesis or degradation of glycogen. At least eight separate conditions are described; in one of the types, the defect is of a lysosomal enzyme. The conditions are uncommon and will not be described.

Disorders of Collagen Synthesis

Disorders of collagen synthesis are not common but include the interesting group of diseases known as the Ehlers-Danlos syndrome.

Ehlers-Danlos Syndrome. This syndrome constitutes a group of at least nine diseases in which the collagen is defective so that it can be unduly stretched with ease. The biochemical defect has been identified in some types. Subjects who are "double-jointed," being able to hyperextend their joints, have a mild form of the disease. In more severe types of Ehlers-Danlos disease, the hypermobility of the skin and joints produces the "India-rubber men" of the circus ring. In types with defective type III collagen formation, excessive fragility of blood vessels and the intestine can lead to rupture.

OTHER METABOLIC DISEASES WITH A STRONG GENETIC BASIS

There are many other diseases in which the basic defect is less clear and it seems that both genetic and environmental factors are at work; diabetes mellitus is a prime example. A feature common to all these diseases is the widespread nature of the lesions so that many organs and tissues are involved. In the remainder of this chapter, some important examples are described. First and foremost, there is diabetes mellitus.

Diabetes Mellitus

The study of diabetes mellitus has centered around the details of glucose metabolism. This is outlined before the disease itself is described.

Glucose Metabolism

Glucose is used as a fuel by many cells of the body and is the only substance used by the brain under normal circumstances. Hence, the maintenance of a blood glucose level within narrow limits (3 to 5 mmol/L [55 to 90 mg/dl] in the fasting subject) is an important homeostatic mechanism. The blood level is mainly regulated by the balance between the production of insulin, which lowers the blood glucose level, and the activity of the liver, which can either store glucose as glycogen or produce glucose from glycogen (*glycogenolysis*) or noncarbohydrate sources (*glyconeogenesis*). After the absorption of glucose from the intestine, the rise in the blood glucose level stimulates the secretion of insulin from the pancreatic islets by a direct action. Furthermore, various intestinal hormones are released, and these also act on the pancreatic islets to promote secretion. Insulin enhances the entry of glucose into cells by aiding its transport across cell membranes. This is particularly important in resting muscle and fat cells, which are the *insulin-dependent tissues*. After the ingestion of 100 g of glucose, only about 15 per cent enters these tissues along insulin-dependent pathways. An additional 25 per cent escapes from the splanchnic bed and is utilized to meet the ongoing glucose needs of insulin-independent tissues, especially the brain. From 55 to 60 per cent of the glucose absorbed is retained in the liver, for there is no barrier to its entry into liver cells, and this organ is well situated anatomically to intercept glucose from the portal vein and prevent it from entering the systemic circulation. In the liver, glucose is utilized in the synthesis of glycogen and triglycerides. It follows that in the normal person, even after a carbohydrate meal, the blood glucose does not rise above 9 mmol/liter; this forms the basis of the glucose tolerance test.

In the glucose tolerance test, a fasting subject previously on an adequate carbohydrate diet is given 100 g of glucose by mouth. The blood glucose should not exceed 5 mmol/L at the start of the test nor 9 mmol/L an hour later. It should have returned to normal after 2 hours. When the blood level of glucose exceeds 10 mmol/L, glucose escapes into the urine because the renal tubules are no longer able to reabsorb the excessive amount that is present in the glomerular filtrate. *Glycosuria* therefore results.

In the fasting state, the liver and insulin-dependent tissues (resting muscle and fat) show little glucose uptake. The insulin-independent tissues, particularly the brain, show a continued glucose uptake, and the normal blood glucose level is maintained by release of glucose from the liver.

Secretion and Actions of Insulin. Insulin is synthesized in the rough endoplasmic reticulum in the B cells of the islets of Langerhans. The initial product is a precursor molecule called *proinsulin,* a large polypeptide, the head and tail of which are joined by two disulfide bonds. By the action of peptidases, the middle segment (termed the *C peptide*) is excised, leaving the head and tail of the molecule to form the A and B chains of the insulin molecule; these remain united by the original disulfide bonds. The excretion of C peptide in the urine is used as a measure of the rate of insulin synthesis. The insulin itself, after passage through the Golgi complex, is released in membrane-bound secretory granules into the cytoplasm and is finally secreted by a process of exocytosis. Hyperglycemia is the major stimulus for both insulin synthesis and release, but glucagon, gastrin, and other intestinal hormones also play some part. The release of these intestinal hormones that follows oral administration of glucose plays a minor role in promoting insulin secretion.

Adipose and muscle cells are the major targets for insulin; both types of cell have specific insulin receptors; the action of insulin is to enhance the transport of glucose into the cell, increase the synthesis of glycogen, promote the synthesis of protein from amino acids, and inhibit the breakdown of neutral fat (lipolysis).

Insulin has two important actions on the liver: in small doses, insulin inhibits the breakdown of glycogen to glucose (glycogenolysis); larger concentrations inhibit glucose formation from noncarbohydrate sources such as amino acids (gluconeogenesis).

The various actions of insulin combine to lower the blood glucose level; the hormone has a very short half-life (3 to 4 minutes), and the continuous and varying secretion of insulin is the main regulatory mechanism whereby the blood glucose level is normally maintained within narrow limits.

Other Hormones Affecting Glucose Metabolism. Four other hormones are involved in glucose metabolism, but their action in normal homeostasis is much less important than that of insulin.

Glucagon. This hormone is the secretion of the A cells of the islets of Langerhans and its actions are to oppose those of insulin. It is released whenever the blood glucose level drops below 4 to 5 mmol/liter; its actions cause a rise in blood glucose and increased formation of ketone bodies in the liver.

Epinephrine. Epinephrine raises the blood glucose level by promoting glycogenolysis in the liver and muscles.

Pituitary Growth Hormone. This hormone opposes the actions of insulin, thereby raising the blood glucose level.

Adrenal Glucocorticoids. These corticosteroids cause a rise in the blood glucose level by decrease of glucose utilization in muscle and fat. Gluconeogenesis in the liver is stimulated.

Diabetes Mellitus—The Disease

Diabetes mellitus is a disease of great antiquity. The disease affects about 3 per cent of the population; although its great frequency has stimulated a vast amount of research into the metabolism of glucose, even today there are many aspects that are incompletely understood. The discovery of insulin by Banting and Best appeared to provide both an explanation of the pathogenesis of diabetes mellitus and an effective treatment. Ironically, this outstanding discovery retarded further research into the true nature of the disease. It has become evident that insulin deficiency is only one factor in the disease. Many diabetic subjects require injections of insulin in quantities far in excess of those required by a totally pancreatectomized individual. Some diabetics have a blood insulin level that is normal or even above normal. Finally, one must admit that although insulin therapy can prolong the life of some diabetic subjects, it fails to prevent premature death from the cardiovascular complications or the onset of blindness. The life expectancy of a diabetic patient is still below that of the normal individual.

Diabetes mellitus can be regarded as a syndrome characterized by a relative or absolute deficiency of insulin. Three major types of the disease can be recognized: *spontaneous diabetes mellitus, diabetes mellitus associated with other endocrine disorders,* and *diabetes mellitus associated with pancreatic disease.*

Spontaneous Diabetes Mellitus

Over 90 per cent of diabetics fall into this group. Since the earliest descriptions of diabetes mellitus, it has been recognized that the disease is familial and that it could occur either in a severe lethal form or as a mild affliction associated with gluttony, obesity, and somnolence. It is now evident that spontaneous diabetes mellitus is not a single entity but a group of separate entities with a similar upset in glucose metabolism. For simplicity it can be divided into two main types, but this division must not be regarded as absolute (Table 16–1).

Type I or Insulin-Dependent Diabetes Mellitus (IDDM). This type of diabetes generally begins abruptly, before the age of 30 years, and is often called juvenile-onset diabetes. The symptoms are thirst (polydipsia), increased production of urine (polyuria), weight loss in spite of a good appetite, blurring of vision, general lassitude, and sometimes a craving for sweet beverages. Nausea, vomiting, coma, and death follow within weeks or possibly months. Only insulin therapy can save these patients.

Etiology. Type I or IDDM is strongly associated with certain HLA haplotypes (*e.g.*, DR3 and DR4). There are several explanations for this association:

1. The haplotypes are closely linked with other, as yet unidentified, genes that are responsible for the disease.

2. The haplotypes render the subject susceptible to certain viral infections that cause the destruction of the islets (see MHC restriction of antibody response, Chapter 6). Infection with a coxsackie B virus is the best documented.

Table 16–1 COMPARISON BETWEEN INSULIN-DEPENDENT AND NON–INSULIN-DEPENDENT DIABETES

	Insulin-Dependent Diabetes (Type I)	Non–Insulin-Dependent Diabetes (Type II)
Age of onset	Usually under 30 years	Usually over 40 years
Ketoacidosis	Common	Rare
Body weight	Thin	80% are obese
Prevalence	0.5%	2%–4%
Genetics	HLA-associated in 40%–50%	Familial but not HLA-associated
Circulating islet cell antibodies	50%–85%	Less than 10%
Treatment with insulin	Necessary	Usually not required

Modified from Felig, P., Baxter, J. D., Broadus, A. E., and Frohman, L. A.: Endocrinology and Metabolism. New York, McGraw-Hill, 1981. Reproduced with permission of McGraw-Hill, Inc.

3. The haplotypes predispose to the formation of autoantibodies against islet tissue. Damage to the islets by viral infection or possibly by some as yet unidentified poison could trigger an autoimmune reaction. The autoimmune hypothesis is supported by the observation that 60 to 85 per cent of recently diagnosed patients have autoantibodies in their sera that react to islet cell components.

The islets in IDDM show cell degeneration and an infiltration by lymphocytes. The changes are not marked and could be due to either a viral infection or an autoimmune process.

Pathophysiology. The blood level of insulin is very low in fully developed type I diabetes mellitus. The uptake of glucose by muscle and fat cells is low, and the liver manufactures glucose from glycogen and noncarbohydrate sources— mostly amino acids derived from the skeletal muscles, which therefore waste.

In this type of severe diabetes mellitus, there is hyperglycemia even in the fasting state. The blood glucose level rises even higher after a carbohydrate meal because, in the absence of insulin, storage of glycogen in the liver is inhibited. The patient becomes dehydrated and thirsty because of the loss of water and electrolytes that accompanies the osmotic diuresis secondary to the heavy glycosuria. Blurring of vision results from the osmotic effects in the lens and humors of the eye produced by the fluctuating levels of blood glucose.

Lipolysis in the adipose tissue is accelerated in the presence of a low insulin level. The released fatty acids are utilized by the liver to form acetylcoenzyme A. Although normally this could enter the Krebs cycle, in the presence of an increase in the ratio of glucagon to insulin it is converted into ketone bodies (beta-hydroxybutyrate, acetoacetate, and acetone). The use of these ketone bodies as a fuel by peripheral tissues is inhibited by the low levels of insulin, and hyperketonemia and ketonuria result. These changes combined with a metabolic acidosis are responsible for diabetic coma and death.

It is evident that in diabetes mellitus of this type, the body's metabolism is geared to the maintenance of a high blood glucose level, even though this exceeds the renal threshold. The body literally starves in the midst of plenty, as fats and proteins are converted into glucose, only to be passed in the urine and lost from the body. Loss of weight and hunger are therefore characteristic symptoms.

Type II or Non–Insulin-Dependent Diabetes Mellitus (NIDDM). This type of diabetes mellitus is most common after the age of 40 years and it is therefore commonly called maturity-onset diabetes. The onset is insidious, and the symptoms are generally mild. Ketoacidosis is uncommon. The disease is often uncovered by the detection of glycosuria or hyperglycemia during the performance of a routine medical check-up. This emphasizes the importance of periodic medical examinations.

Etiology. Type II diabetes mellitus is a familial disease, but the precise mode of inheritance is not known. Hence, the disease is usually described as being multifactorial, with genetic and environmental factors playing a part. There is no association with HLA types as in type I diabetes mellitus.

Pathophysiology. In type II diabetes mellitus, the blood insulin levels may be low, normal, or high. In the early stages of the disease, the pancreas is slow to respond to the rise in blood glucose that follows a carbohydrate meal. Hence, hyperglycemia results but is transient because it stimulates the islets of Langerhans to produce excess insulin, and this results in *hypoglycemic attacks*. This phase of the disease is temporary.

Histologic examination of the pancreas gives no clues to the nature of the defect. The islets may appear normal; or, in the later stages of the disease, they may be atrophic with fibrosis or infiltration by amyloid tissue.

Because absolute lack of insulin does not seem to be the cause of type II diabetes mellitus, some other factor must be in operation. The presence of insulin antagonists and excess of secretion of glucagon have been proposed but appear not to be major factors.

Insulin resistance of tissues is the major abnormality. This may be due to the peripheral tissues having fewer insulin receptors per cell; alternatively, the attachment of insulin to its receptor somehow fails to lead to the usual intracellular response. A complicating factor is obesity in type II diabetes because for reasons that are unclear, it is associated with insulin resistance. For this reason, patients who are obese are greatly helped if they can lose weight. Often their disease can be managed by drugs or diet alone, and insulin is not needed. Nevertheless, the situation is complex because 20 per cent of type II diabetics are not obese, and some other cause for insulin resistance must operate. Pregnancy is another factor that can cause such insulin resistance.

In conclusion, it may be supposed that some individuals have a genetic fault that prevents the islets from producing adequate insulin when the demand for this hormone increases. This increased demand may occur when the patient becomes obese. Possibly the tendency to develop obesity in diabetes mellitus is itself inherited. The relationship to obesity is complex, however, because in type II diabetes there is sufficient insulin in the blood to prevent breakdown of lipids in the fat cells. Obesity could therefore be an effect of the disease and not a prime factor in its pathogenesis. Certainly, wasting is not a feature of this type of the disease. The differences between the two types of diabetes are summarized in Table 16–1.

The Anatomic Lesions of Diabetes Mellitus. Patients with diabetes mellitus exhibit a wide range of pathologic lesions. Most of these are related to vascular changes, particularly of the small vessels of kidneys and the retina. These are described under the heading of complications.

The Islets of Langerhans. The islets show surprisingly few changes, and indeed there is often no abnormality. As described previously, a lymphocytic infiltrate may be present in early-onset diabetes. Amyloid or fibrous tissue replacement of the islet tissue may be found in long-standing cases.

Complications of Diabetes Mellitus. The complications are summarized below.

Diabetic Ketosis and Coma. This complication is most common in the juvenile-onset type of the disease and may be precipitated by the patient's failure to administer the prescribed amount of insulin. Vomiting and abdominal pain may be severe enough to mimic a perforated peptic ulcer or appendicitis. This emphasizes the necessity of performing a routine urinalysis in all seriously ill patients.

Hyperosmolar Nonketogenic Coma. This condition is generally encountered in patients with type II diabetes and may be precipitated by an acute illness, such as myocardial infarct or pneumonia. The plasma glucose level is very high (over 55 mmol/liter), and the osmotic diuresis that follows leads to hyponatremia and hypovolemic shock, with effects most marked in the central nervous system; coma is characteristic, and seizures occur in about one third of cases. Ketosis is not a feature.

Cardiovascular Disease. Diabetic subjects are liable to develop more severe atherosclerosis than are nondiabetic subjects of like age. Indeed, among diabetics, myocardial infarction is the most common cause of death. Involvement of the major vessels of the legs contributes to peripheral vascular disease. This may culminate in gangrene of the feet. The pathogenesis of the arterial disease in diabetes is poorly understood, and its severity does not seem to be related to the severity of the diabetes or to the efficiency of the treatment. Systemic hypertension, microangiopathy of the vasa vasorum, obesity, and hypertriglyceridemia may all be causative factors.

Diabetic Microangiopathy. There is thickening

of the basement membrane and later occlusion of small vessels in the skin, muscles, kidney, retina, and other parts of the body. The effects are particularly important in the kidney, the retina, and the nerves.

Diabetic Nephropathy. The microangiopathy affects both the arterioles supplying the glomeruli and the vessels in the glomeruli themselves. The nephrotic syndrome may develop in some patients. Ultimately the vessels become thickened, basement membrane–like material accumulates between the capillaries, and the whole glomerulus becomes converted into an eosinophilic hyaline mass. This is associated with the development of chronic renal failure, and indeed this is a common mode of death in diabetes mellitus. *Papillary necrosis* may occur and is clinically characterized by hematuria and the rapid onset of renal failure.

There has been much argument in the past as to whether these vascular changes are caused by the hyperglycemia and other effects of the disease or whether they are associated with the primary defect. The matter is undecided, but there is little firm evidence that the methods of controlling diabetes now available can prevent the development of microangiopathy, particularly as it affects the kidneys and leads to renal failure.

Changes in the Eye. In diabetic retinopathy, there are ischemic changes in the retina due to thickening of the walls of the small retinal vessels. Characteristically, there are also focal dilations of the vessels with the formation of microaneurysms.

Bleeding may occur into the vitreous; subsequent organization of the hematoma can result in retinal detachment. *Cataract formation* is another important complication of diabetes; it is little wonder that the disease is one of the leading causes of blindness in the world.

Changes in the Nerves. The microangiopathy causes ischemic changes in the peripheral nerves, thereby producing the common peripheral polyneuropathy of diabetics. It results in a symmetric loss of sensation of the hands and feet, giving the so-called stocking-and-glove effect; paradoxically, it is sometimes associated with spontaneous pain. The lack of pain sensation in the feet can lead to unnoticed injuries, and these can be

the initiating factors that result in infection and gangrene. Neuropathy of the autonomic nervous supply to the gut can cause constipation or diarrhea and the malabsorption syndrome. Involvement of the bladder with difficulty in emptying the bladder can contribute to urinary tract infection.

Susceptibility to Infection. Diabetic subjects are particularly liable to recurrent infections of various types. Recurrent boils of the skin and recurrent cystitis, particularly in women, should always alert one to the possibility of underlying diabetes mellitus. Pruritus vulvae is a common complaint of patients with diabetes and may be associated with candidal vaginitis. It is an old observation that diabetics are particularly susceptible to tuberculous infection of the lungs.

Surgery and Diabetes Mellitus. The balance between insulin and glucose requirements is easily upset by trauma and infection. Any diabetic patient who is subjected to surgery should therefore have skilled medical treatment.

Diabetes Mellitus Associated with Other Endocrine Disorders

In this group, there is an overabundant production of hormones that counteract the action of insulin. Examples include Cushing's disease, acromegaly, and pheochromocytoma.

Diabetes Mellitus Associated with Pancreatic Disease

Diabetes is occasionally encountered as a complication of chronic pancreatitis, hemochromatosis, cystic fibrosis, and total pancreatectomy performed for carcinoma.

Hypoglycemia

If the blood glucose is below 3 mmol/liter, particularly if its fall is rapid, symptoms of hypoglycemia develop. These consist of sweating, hunger, mental confusion, and—in severe cases—coma, convulsions, and death. Common causes of hypoglycemia include

1. *Insulin overdosage.* All diabetic subjects on insulin therapy should be warned of the effects of hypoglycemia.

2. *Diabetes mellitus.* In the early stages in the development of diabetes mellitus, the hyperglycemia that follows a meal may lead to such a delayed and excessive secretion of insulin by the pancreas that hypoglycemia follows.

3. *Tumors of the islets of Langerhans.* An islet-cell tumor (adenoma or carcinoma) can cause periodic attacks of hypoglycemia.

Purine Metabolism—Gout

Clinical Features

Gout is a disease of great antiquity and is characterized by a high blood uric acid level *(hyperuricemia)* accompanied by recurrent attacks of acute arthritis. Deposits of urates are found in the joint cartilages, and these lead to chronic arthritis. Nodular deposits of monosodium urate are also found in connective tissues around the joints as well as in some nonarticular cartilages, particularly those of the external ear, where they are called *tophi.* The clinical features of gout were well recognized by Hippocrates; the classic features were described by Sydenham, who himself was a sufferer. The initial attack invariably affects the great toe and is characterized by the sudden onset of severe pain and inflammation. Rigors and fever accompany the attack, which usually subsides within a few days. It responds well to the administration of colchicine, a drug introduced into North America by Benjamin Franklin, who was yet another famous sufferer of gout, and still used today. Repeated attacks of arthritis occur and affect other joints; ultimately, a chronic arthritis develops in all four limbs, particularly in the distal joints. Urates are also deposited in the kidney, leading to renal damage and ultimately to renal failure. About one third of the patients develop kidney stones composed of urates.

Pathogenesis

Uric acid is the end product of the metabolism of the purines derived from nucleic acid. Most of this uric acid is of endogenous origin, but some is exogenous, being derived from the diet. Two types of gout are recognized.

Primary Gout. This is a heterogeneous group of inborn errors of metabolism. In some types, there is an overproduction of uric acid that is sometimes accompanied by a failure to recycle purines in the formation of new nucleic acid. In other types, there is impaired renal excretion. Primary gout is familial and tends to affect males more often than females. The precise biochemical error causing most familial forms of gout is not understood. There are, however, some rare types of gout in which the enzyme defect is known.

Secondary Gout. As in primary gout, the secondary variety can be due either to increased production of uric acid or to decreased excretion of uric acid. Widespread malignant disease, such as leukemia and polycythemia (particularly if treated with cytotoxic drugs), is a common cause of secondary gout; this is due to overproduction of uric acid. Chronic renal failure, particularly if it is due to hypertension, and chronic lead poisoning can lead to typical attacks of gout through retention of uric acid.

The precise reason for the deposition of urates in joints, tendons, and cartilages is not understood. The acute attacks are believed to be due to the deposition of urate crystals in the joint spaces. These crystals are phagocytosed by polymorphs. Lysosomal enzymes are then released and mediate the local inflammatory reaction as well as the rigors and fever.

Summary

- In the inborn errors of metabolism, there is an abnormal gene that leads to the formation of an abnormal protein, frequently an enzyme. In galactosemia, phenylketonuria, and the lysosomal storage diseases (the lipidoses, mucopolysaccharidoses, and gangliosidoses), accumulation of the substrate of the normal enzyme leads to the effects of the disease. Glucose 6-phosphate dehydrogenase deficiency is more complex and is associated with hemolytic anemia. Alpha,-antitrypsin deficiency is associated with pulmonary emphysema.
- In the glycogenoses, an increased amount of glycogen is laid down in the tissues.

- In the Ehlers-Danlos syndrome, the genetic defect leads to abnormalities in collagen synthesis.
- In some diseases (such as diabetes mellitus), both genetic and environmental factors play a vital role.
- Spontaneous type I diabetes mellitus, or insulin-dependent diabetes mellitus (IDDM), is associated with HLA haplotypes DR3 and DR4. An acute viral infection and an autoimmune response seem likely precipitating events. The onset is acute, and there is an absolute lack of insulin. Hyperglycemia, glycosuria, and loss of weight culminate in ketotic coma and death unless insulin is supplied.
- Spontaneous type II diabetes mellitus, or non–insulin-dependent diabetes mellitus (NIDDM) is familial, occurs in older people, and is associated with obesity. Insulin levels may be high, and the tissues show insulin resistance. Insulin therapy is not always necessary.
- Complications of diabetes mellitus include susceptibility to infection, coma (ketotic or hyperosmolar nonketogenic), atherosclerosis and its sequelae, cataract, microangiopathy causing diabetic nephropathy (including papillary necrosis), retinopathy, and peripheral neuropathy.
- Diabetes mellitus can be caused by other endocrine disorders and total pancreatic destruction or loss.
- Primary gout is a group of inborn errors of metabolism with overproduction or underexcretion of uric acid. Arthritis, tophi, and renal damage are its main features.
- Secondary gout results from malignant disease or renal failure.

Selected Readings

Byers, P. H., Barsh, G. S., and Holbrook, K. A.: Molecular pathology in inherited disorders of collagen metabolism. Hum. Pathol. *13*:89, 1982.

Clements, R. S., and Bell, D. H. S.: Complications of diabetes: Prevalence, detection, current treatment, and prognosis. Am. J. Med. *79*(Suppl. 5A):1, 1985.

Eisenbarth, G. S.: Type 1 diabetes mellitus. N. Engl. J. Med. *314*:1360, 1986.

Foster, D. W., and McGarry, J. D.: The metabolic derangement and treatment of diabetes ketoacidosis. N. Engl. J. Med. *309*:159, 1983.

German, D. C., and Holmes, E. W.: Gout and hyperuricemia: Diagnosis and management. Hosp. Pract. *21*:119, 1986.

Leading article: Lysosomal storage diseases. Lancet 2:898, 1986.

Scriver, C. R., and Clow, C. L.: Phenylketonuria: Epitome of human biochemical genetics. N. Engl. J. Med. *303*:1336 and 1394, 1980.

Stanbury, J. B., Wyngaarden, J. B., Fredrickson, D. S., Goldstein, J. L., Brown, M. S., and Scriver, C. R. (eds.): The Metabolic Basis of Inherited Disease. 6th ed. New York, McGraw-Hill, 1989.

Truglia, J. A., et al.: Mechanisms of insulin resistance in non-insulin dependent diabetes. Am. J. Med. *79*(Suppl. 3B):12, 1985.

Wolf, E., Spencer, K. M., and Cudworth, A. G.: The genetic susceptibility to Type 1 (insulin-dependent) diabetes: Analysis of the HLA-DR association. Diabetologia 24:224, 1983.

17

The Plasma Proteins: Amyloidosis

After studying this chapter, the student should be able to:

- Describe five methods used to separate the plasma proteins.
- List the causes of hypoalbuminemia.
- Classify the types of hypergammaglobulinemia.
- Outline how the erythrocyte sedimentation rate test is performed, give the normal values, and indicate its usefulness.
- Describe the forms in which lipid is carried in the blood and indicate how they are formed and metabolized.
- Describe the complications of an abnormal blood lipid level.
- Classify amyloidosis and outline the main features of each group.
- Describe the effects of amyloid infiltration on the
　(a) heart;
　(b) kidney;
　(c) liver.
- Outline what is known about the formation and composition of amyloid.

THE PLASMA PROTEINS

The blood stream forms the major route by which the secretions of one organ can travel to distant parts of the body and influence other organs and tissues. It is not surprising, therefore, that an analysis of the blood itself has proved to be a rewarding pursuit and has shed light on many body functions. The plasma proteins are readily available for examination, and their study has been especially fruitful. They have been classified in various ways; unfortunately, the terminology is quite complex. In order to understand the classification, it is essential to have an elementary knowledge of the physicochemical properties of the proteins, because the name attached to a particular member is often a reflection of the method used in its identification.

Knowledge of the evolution of the present rather complex system is instructive. *Fibrinogen* presents no great problem; it is a protein that forms an insoluble fibrin clot during coagulation. Until the middle of the last century, the remaining serum was thought to contain a single protein called albumin. It was then shown that by half-saturation of the serum with ammonium sulfate, part of the protein could be precipitated (now called *globulin*), leaving the remainder in solution (the *albumin*). Estimation of these three fractions is a useful first step in clinical investigation. The normal levels are the following:

Albumin	40–50 g/L
Globulin	25–35 g/L
Fibrinogen	1.5–3.5 g/L
Total	65–80 g/L

In aqueous solutions at a suitable pH, the proteins have a negative charge, so that when they are placed in an electric field, they migrate toward the anode. Individual proteins move at a particular rate dependent, to a great extent, on their size and electric charge. The test, called *electrophoresis*, is conveniently performed on strips of filter paper, starch gel, or cellulose acetate; an electric current is passed for a suitable time, the strip is dried, and the separated proteins are stained (Fig. 17–1). When serum undergoes electrophoresis, the albumin travels fastest as one large band. The globulins, on the other hand, separate into three major groups, which have been designated alpha globulin, beta globulin, and gamma globulin. In fact, each of these bands can be resolved into numerous smaller bands, each composed of a distinct protein. It is the separation and identification of the globulins that is carried out by immunoelectrophoresis, illustrated in Figure 17–2. The protein fractions are separated by electrophoresis and then identified immunologically.

Another method of plasma protein separation uses a high-speed ultracentrifuge. Large molecules tend to settle quickly, whereas small ones can be spun down with greater difficulty. The various fractions that can be obtained are measured in *Svedberg units*. The large globulin molecules, termed *macroglobulins*, are spun down in the 19S fraction. This fraction contains an important group of antibodies, which are therefore designated IgM. The more abundant IgG forms the 7S fraction.

Some proteins precipitate out in the cold. These are called *cryoglobulins*; an abnormal in-

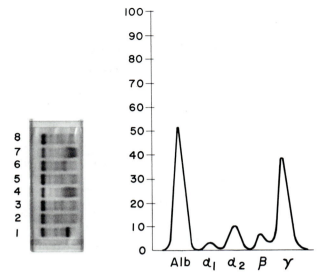

Figure 17–1 Cellulose acetate electrophoresis of serum. On the left, electrophoretic strips from eight separate sera are shown. The anode is on the left, and the dense band that has moved farthest to the left is due to albumin. No. 8 is normal serum, whereas No. 4 and No. 7 show a diffuse increase in the gamma globulins. Each shows the picture of a polyclonal gammopathy. No. 1 shows a dense band in the gamma globulin area. The density of the bands of strip No. 1 is depicted in graphic form on the right. The various serum proteins are in the same relative positions on both the strip and the graph. The sharp spike in the region is characteristic of a monoclonal gammopathy. (From Hall, C.A.: Neoplasms of the blood. *In* Halsted, J.A., and Halsted, C.H. [Eds.]: The Laboratory in Clinical Medicine. 2nd ed. Philadelphia, W.B. Saunders Company, 1981.)

crease in concentration (*cryoglobulinemia*) can cause trouble because of vascular obstruction when the hands are exposed in cold weather. Finally, some proteins contain either lipid or carbohydrate. The former are called *lipoproteins*, and the latter are termed *glycoproteins*.

It is evident that an individual chemical protein can be described in a number of ways. Thus, a single protein may be a macroglobulin in the 19S range, a gamma globulin, and also a glycoprotein. This protein may also be an antibody and therefore an immunoglobulin. The function of a particular protein is yet another way in which it may be described.

Albumin

Albumin, like most of the plasma proteins (with the notable exception of the immunoglobulins), is produced in the liver.

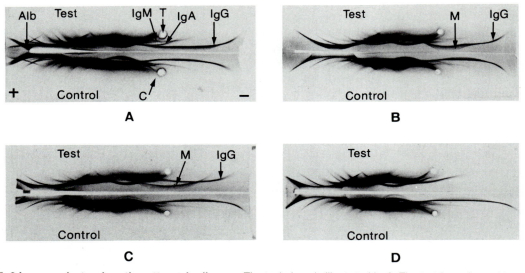

Figure 17–2 Immunoelectrophoretic patterns in disease. The technique is illustrated in *A*. The test is performed in an agarose gel. Test serum is placed in well T, and a control normal serum is placed in well C. A current is passed for a suitable period, and the proteins tend to migrate toward the anode (+). Albumin (Alb) migrates most quickly, whereas IgG moves most slowly; under the conditions of the test, some IgG actually moves toward the cathode. The separated plasma components are demonstrated by placing antiserum to whole plasma down the central strip. From there, the antibodies diffuse to form precipitin lines with each separated protein. The sheet is stained and photographed.

A, The IgG band is heavier than that of the control and is closer to the central strip. Serum tested here was from a patient who had systemic lupus erythematosus with a polyclonal hypergammaglobulinemia. The IgA and IgM bands are clearly shown.

B, An M protein is present and distorts the normal IgG band. The serum is from a patient with multiple myelomatosis and an IgG M protein.

C, An M protein is present and is in the position of the normal IgA band. Note how the normal IgG band crosses the M protein. The serum is from a patient with multiple myelomatosis producing an IgA M protein.

D, Note the deficiency of the IgG band. The serum is from a patient with congenital hypogammaglobulinemia.

(Courtesy of Dr. K.C. Carstairs, Toronto General Division of the Toronto Hospital, Toronto.)

Hypoalbuminemia. Chronic liver disease, especially in the terminal phases, is often accompanied by hypoalbuminemia resulting from underproduction of this protein. Similarly, during starvation, the plasma albumin level tends to fall rather more quickly than the other plasma protein levels do. The plasma level of albumin falls in acute infections and after severe trauma. This is a component of the acute phase response and is described in Chapter 19. Although the response is quite nonspecific, it forms the basis for a common pathologic test, the erythrocyte sedimentation rate, which is discussed later in this chapter.

Hypoalbuminemia also occurs whenever there is excessive loss of albumin from the body. This is seen under several circumstances:

1. With the *nephrotic syndrome,* when large quantities are lost in the urine.

2. With *chronic loss of inflammatory exudate* from the body. Common examples are draining abscesses, extensive burns, and severe, infected wounds.

3. With *protein-losing enteropathy,* which is an uncommon cause of hypoalbuminemia and is due to loss of protein into the intestine. This syndrome is associated with a variety of gastrointestinal lesions, including gastric cancer, Crohn's disease, and ulcerative colitis.

Effects of Hypoalbuminemia. Albumin is a small molecule (molecular weight 70,000) and is in high concentration in the plasma. It therefore constitutes the major noncrystalloid component of plasma. As would be expected, hypoalbuminemia leads to edema (Chapter 19).

Hyperalbuminemia. This occurs whenever there is hemoconcentration due either to lack of water intake or to excessive water loss.

The Globulins

The globulins include a wide array of plasma proteins. The immunoglobulins form a major component: mostly they are present in the gamma fraction, but they are also found to a lesser extent in the beta fraction. The normal level appears to be maintained by the body's contact with microorganisms, particularly those in the intestine. Thus, in germ-free animals the gamma globulin level is maintained at about one fifth of normal. When the intestinal flora of such animals is restored, the plasma proteins return to normal.

Hypergammaglobulinemia. Hypergammaglobulinemia is invariably due to an increase in the level of immunoglobulins. Two major patterns are described.

Polyclonal Gammopathy. An increase in the gamma globulins is seen in many chronic infections when there is a prolonged and marked immune response. Chronic tuberculosis, lepromatous leprosy, and kala-azar can be singled out as typical examples. It is also characteristic of those diseases in which the production of autoantibodies is a major component. Systemic lupus erythematosus is the prototype of this type of disease. Hypergammaglobulinemia is also characteristic of sarcoidosis; the pathogenesis, however, is complex. The electrophoretic pattern in these conditions is that of a broad-based elevation of the gamma globulins. There is an elevation in the levels of all classes of immunoglobulins, and it is assumed that many clones of antibody-forming cells are stimulated: hence, the term *polyclonal gammopathy.*

Monoclonal Gammopathy. In some cases of hypergammaglobulinemia, it is found that the increase in gamma globulin is due entirely to an increase in one particular protein belonging to *one* of the major classes—IgA, IgG, IgE, IgM, or IgD—and furthermore consists of either the lambda or the kappa variety. The supposition is that the globulin is produced by one particular clone of antibody-forming cells. Monoclonal gammopathy is usually associated with malignancy of the lymphoreticular system. The most common example is that of multiple myelomatosis, which is described elsewhere, but it is also seen in a variety of other malignant lymphomas and occasionally other malignant tumors. The term *M protein* (derived from *Multiple Myelomatosis; Malignant lymphoma; Malignant tumor)* is applied to an abnormal homogeneous protein, which appears as a spike on electrophoresis, in contrast to the broad-based increase seen in the polyclonal gammopathies (see Fig. 17–1). The finding of such a spike in a case of hypergammaglobulinemia leads the physician to search for malignancy—particularly malignant lymphoma—in the patient.

The Lipoproteins

The lipids of the plasma are carried in the blood as complexes with each other and with *apolipoproteins,* a group of proteins that form complexes with the water-insoluble lipids to form the lipoproteins of the plasma and the chyle (Fig. 17–3). Some tissues have receptors for the apoproteins, and in this way the lipoproteins are taken up by endocytosis and metabolized.

Free fatty acids are derived from the adipose tissues, carried in the blood combined with albumin, and transported to the liver and muscles for metabolism.

Chylomicrons are formed in the intestine after the absorption of dietary fat. Chylomicrons are particles, over 1 μm in diameter, that have a high neutral fat (triglyceride) content. Chylomicrons adhere to endothelial cells in muscle and adipose tissues. In the presence of the enzyme *lipoprotein lipase,* the triglyceride content is hydrolyzed, and the fatty acids so formed are absorbed by the cells for oxidation or re-esterification. The remainder of the chylomicrons are released as *remnant particles* now rich in cholesterol. This fraction is taken up by the liver, which has specific remnant receptors, and is utilized for bile formation as well as for other purposes.

Triglyceride is synthesized in the liver from carbohydrate and lipid sources; it is released in the form of *very-low-density lipoproteins (VLDL).* This is the form of triglyceride that is present in the blood under fasting conditions. By the action of endothelial cell–derived lipoprotein oxidase, there is progressive metabolism of the triglyceride core of the VLDL. This leads to the formation of intermediate-density lipoproteins and finally

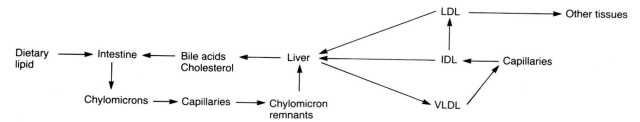

Figure 17–3 Metabolism of lipoproteins. Dietary lipid absorbed in the intestine is carried in the circulation as chylomicrons. In capillaries, the action of lipoprotein lipase causes the triglyceride content to be hydrolyzed and removed, leaving chylomicron remnants rich in cholesterol. These are taken up by the liver. The liver produces very-low-density lipoproteins (VLDL) rich in triglyceride. The triglyceride is hydrolyzed in the capillaries, leaving the intermediate-density lipoproteins (IDL) to re-enter the circulation. Some of these are taken up by the liver; the rest lose their remaining triglyceride content and form the low-density lipoproteins (LDL). These are rich in cholesterol and are taken up by the liver and other cells that have LDL receptors. (Adapted from Goldstein, J.L., Kita, T., and Brown, M.S.: Defective lipoprotein receptors and atherosclerosis. Reprinted by permission of *The New England Journal of Medicine, 309:288, 1983.)*

the *low-density lipoproteins (LDL).* Cholesterol is its major lipid, and over 70 per cent of the plasma cholesterol is normally present in this form. LDL is taken up by cells that have LDL receptors and is the transport form for delivering cholesterol to tissues.

High-density lipoproteins (HDL) are alpha-lipoproteins and contain both triglyceride and cholesterol.

Abnormalities in the lipoproteins of the blood are closely related to atherosclerosis, a disease that is responsible for about 50 per cent of all deaths. It is believed that a high blood cholesterol level (high LDL and VLDL) or a low HDL level predisposes to the development of atherosclerosis, whereas a high HDL level is protective. The blood level of the various lipoproteins is determined in part by genetic factors and in part by environmental factors.

Abnormalities of the Plasma Lipoproteins

The plasma lipoproteins have been intensively studied in the hope of solving the pathogenesis of atherosclerosis. There are two major groups of hyperlipoproteinemia: the *primary* or *familial hyperlipoproteinemia* and the *secondary hyperlipoproteinemia.*

In the primary group, there is an inherited defect in an apoprotein or a specific enzyme. In the secondary group, the lipid abnormality is associated with some acquired metabolic abnor-

mality, *e.g.,* alcoholism or diabetes mellitus. The division between the two groups is not rigid, because the effects of an inherited trait may become apparent only under certain circumstances—a particular diet or the development of some disease.

The current classification of the hyperlipidemias is based on the pattern of lipid abnormality in the blood. Five patterns are recognized, and so far as the primary groups are concerned, examples of the five groups have been recognized. Two of these are described.

Familial Lipoproteinase Deficiency. This is a rare autosomal dominant condition in which chylomicrons are not metabolized to remnants (Fig. 17–3). The plasma has a creamy appearance due to the accumulation of chylomicrons. The disease illustrates the effects of hyperchylomicronemia. The subjects are prone to develop attacks of *acute pancreatitis* and develop *eruptive xanthomas* of the skin; these are deposits of foamy xanthoma cells that appear as yellow or orange papules because of their carotene content.

Familial Hypercholesterolemia. In this disease, there is a marked elevation of the LDL owing to the presence of an abnormal LDL receptor. Normally these receptors bind LDL and facilitate its uptake by cells. In familial hypercholesterolemia, there is decreased removal of LDL from the plasma, and the excess is taken up by phagocytic cells. The result is the formation of *tendinous xanthomas* and the development of *severe atherosclerosis,* particularly of the coronary arteries. Subjects homozygous for the abnormal gene generally die of ischemic heart disease by the age of 20 years; the heterozygotes are affected by the age of 30 years. This disease should always be remembered when there is a family history of young persons dying of ischemic heart disease.

It must be stressed that the lipoprotein pattern in the blood is greatly influenced by the diet. Abnormal patterns can be produced by abnormal diets even in the absence of genetic or associated disease. Hence, lipid estimations must be performed under close dietary control.

In *secondary hyperlipoproteinemia,* the same spectrum of lipoprotein patterns is found. Abnormal patterns are common in diabetes mellitus, obstructive jaundice, acute alcoholism, pancreatitis, hypothyroidism, and the nephrotic syndrome.

Lipoprotein Deficiency Syndromes. A number of syndromes are known in which there is absence of a particular apoprotein, or the protein is in an abnormal form. In one form, there is a low HDL and a high incidence of coronary disease.

THE ERYTHROCYTE SEDIMENTATION RATE

When a column of blood rendered incoagulable with an anticoagulant such as citrate or oxalate is allowed to stand vertically, the red blood cells steadily gravitate downward because their density is greater than that of the plasma. The speed at which this sedimentation occurs is dependent on several factors, the most important of which are the degree of rouleaux formation and the extent of sludging. In *rouleaux formation,* the red blood cells pile one on the other like an orderly pile of plates; in *sludging,* the massing of red blood cells with mutual adhesion is much more irregular and more closely resembles that of agglutination, except that the clumps of cells can be readily separated. Any increase in the plasma content of high-molecular-weight substances (*e.g.,* the macroglobulins and fibrinogen) is found to increase the erythrocyte sedimentation rate (ESR). The low-molecular-weight albumin *delays* red blood cell sedimentation. For this reason, a raised ESR is particularly characteristic of the acute reaction to stress (noted on page 327), macroglobulinemia, and hypoalbuminemia.

The ESR is normally higher in women than in men, and it shows a significant rise with age. The upper limits of normal based on the commonly performed Westergren method* may be taken as 15 mm for men and 20 mm for women under the age of 50 years, and 20 mm and 30 mm, respectively, for those over that age. It is usually raised during infection and after tissue necrosis, *e.g.,* myocardial or pulmonary infarction. Presumably, an alteration in the balance between the plasma components is responsible, but the precise alterations concerned are ill-defined and rarely investigated. The nonspecific nature of the ESR limits its value in diagnosis; nevertheless, it is a useful investigation. It is of interest to note that the ESR was once introduced as a test for pregnancy because it is elevated in this condition.

The presence of a raised ESR must always be taken to indicate disease, provided anemia and pregnancy are first excluded. Also, administration of birth control pills is reported to raise it slightly. However, a normal ESR does not rule out organic lesions. A patient with a small carcinoma of the breast or lung often has a normal ESR. The ESR is of value in following the course of a known disease, such as tuberculosis and rheumatoid arthritis. Sequential measurements provide a useful indication as to the activity of the disease and its response to treatment. In the Wintrobe method of measuring ESR, the tube contains 1 ml of undiluted oxalated blood and is graduated from 1 to 100. The method has the advantage that after the ESR is read, the tube can be centrifuged and the packed cell volume can be measured. The normal level is 0.40 to 0.54.

It should be noted that the precise values of the ESR depend very much on the technique employed. The Westergren and Wintrobe meth-

---

*In the Westergren method, the column of citrated blood is 200 mm in height. As the red blood cells sediment, a clear zone of plasma appears on top of the red blood cell mass. The ESR is reported as the distance from the top of the plasma to the top of the red blood cell mass at the end of 1 hour. The Wintrobe method uses a smaller tube (100 mm in height) and oxalated blood. It is less accurate but has the advantage of permitting the hematocrit to be measured by centrifuging the tube after a reading of the ESR at 1 hour. Partial clotting of a blood sample and other errors in technique can influence the ESR. An unexpected result should always be checked by repeating the test.

ods give different figures. When using a laboratory, one must learn to appreciate the normal range of its findings.

The ESR is paralleled by the blood level of C-reactive protein; measurement of this protein is now commonly used as an alternative investigation to the more troublesome ESR.

AMYLOIDOSIS

Amyloid is an eosinophilic, hyaline material that is deposited in the extracellular spaces. It reacts with iodine in acid solutions to give a blue color; this superficial resemblance to starch led Virchow to call it starchlike or "amyloid." At a neutral pH, it stains a mahogany-brown color with iodine. Amyloid is commonly identified in histologic sections by the fact that it takes up the stain Congo red. When viewed under ordinary light, the amyloid is pink in color, but with polarized light this changes to apple green. The characteristic fibrillar appearance under the electron microscope is the most reliable method of identifying amyloid.

Amyloid is not normally present in the body in detectable amounts; its deposition in the tissues constitutes the condition of amyloidosis. Amyloidosis is currently classified on the basis of the chemical nature of the amyloid itself and the clinicopathologic features of the condition in which it is found.

Under the electron microscope, the major component of amyloid appears as nonbranching fibrils. These are composed of polypeptide chains arranged in beta-sheet formation. The polypeptide chains are formed by digestion of a precursor protein. Commonly, this protein is either the light chains of immunoglobulin, serum amyloid A (SAA) (an acute phase reactant), or prealbumin. In the generalized types of amyloidosis, these precursor proteins in the blood are broken down by proteolytic enzymes, probably in mononuclear phagocytic cells, and the polypeptide chains so formed circulate in the blood. They polymerize to produce the amyloid fibrils that are deposited at many sites.

In the localized type of amyloidosis, the polypeptide chains are derived from local protein, *e.g.*, calcitonin or keratin, and synthesis of amyloid occurs locally. The types of amyloidosis are summarized in Table 17–1.

Immunocyte-Derived Systemic Amyloidosis

This type may be idiopathic (primary) or occur secondary to a B-cell dyscrasia, particularly multiple myelomatosis.

Primary Systemic Amyloidosis. Primary amyloidosis is a disease of the elderly, and deposits tend to occur in the mesenchymal tissues such as the tongue, respiratory tract, and heart. Liver and spleen may be affected, and renal involvement can lead to uremia. Death generally follows within 1 year of onset.

Immunocyte Dyscrasia-Associated Amyloidosis. The generalized amyloidosis that complicates about 10 per cent of cases of multiple myelomatosis closely resembles the primary amyloidosis described in the preceding text. It is also encountered in other B-cell dyscrasias, *e.g.*, Waldenström's macroglobulinemia and light-chain disease. The amyloid fibrils are derived from the immunoglobulin light chains, usually of the gamma type. An excess of the corresponding light chain is usually present in the blood and is found in the urine as "Bence-Jones protein."

Reactive Systemic Amyloidosis (Secondary Amyloidosis)

This is the common type of generalized amyloid disease. At one time it was encountered in tertiary syphilis, chronic pulmonary tuberculosis, and chronic suppurative disease such as osteomyelitis and bronchiectasis. These conditions are

Table 17–1 CLASSIFICATION OF AMYLOIDOSIS

Immunocyte-derived systemic amyloidosis (AL amyloidosis)
   Primary systemic amyloidosis
   Immunocyte dyscrasia-associated amyloidosis
Reactive systemic amyloidosis (AA amyloidosis)
   Secondary systemic amyloidosis
Heredofamilial amyloidosis
Localized amyloidosis
   Endocrine-associated, senile, and others

now uncommon, and amyloidosis is more often a complication of rheumatoid arthritis, ankylosing spondylitis, Crohn's disease, lepromatous leprosy, the decubitus ulceration and suppurative pyelonephritis found in paraplegic patients, and malignant disease, particularly clear-cell carcinoma of the kidney and Hodgkin's disease. The amyloid deposits that occur in reactive systemic amyloidosis are widely distributed and affect particularly the kidneys, liver, spleen, lymph nodes, and intestine. Renal involvement causes proteinuria; this is followed in due course by the development of the nephrotic syndrome accompanied by hepatosplenomegaly. Nevertheless, involvement of any tissue may be the outstanding or presenting feature, *e.g.,* heart failure or even involvement of the joints. The fibrils that make up the bulk of the deposits in this type of amyloidosis consist of amyloid A (AA), a protein (molecular weight 8000 to 14,000 daltons) that has an amino acid sequence in common with part of a serum protein, SAA, which has a molecular weight of about 180,000 daltons). The amyloid is thought to be derived from it by proteolytic cleavage, perhaps by the activity of macrophages or polymorph proteinases. SAA is an apolipoprotein of high-density lipoprotein and, like C-reactive protein, is greatly elevated in the acute phase reaction.

Heredofamilial Amyloidosis

Several hereditary syndromes are known. Each has its characteristic features and affects particular organs, such as the heart or nerves.

Localized Amyloid Deposits

Endocrine-Associated Amyloidosis. An extensive deposition of amyloid in the stroma of medullary carcinoma of the thyroid is characteristic of this tumor. The amyloid is derived from calcitonin, the hormone produced by this C-cell tumor.

Amyloid deposition is common in the islets of Langerhans in association with diabetes mellitus in advancing age and is also found in the stroma of some islet-cell tumors, particularly those pro-

ducing insulin. The amyloid indeed is produced by proteolysis of insulin or its prohormone.

Senile Amyloidosis. Deposits of amyloid are common in the aged and are found in the heart and brain; they form the senile plaques that are common in Alzheimer's disease. The precursor protein is prealbumin.

Other Localized Deposits of Amyloid. Amyloid deposits may be restricted to a particular site or organ. They may be microscopic in size or form large nodular masses. Such amyloid "tumors" are most often encountered in the lung and larynx but may occur in other sites—skin, bladder, eye, and tongue.

The amyloid consists of AL protein in most cases that have been investigated.

Specific Organ Involvement in Amyloid Disease

Spleen. Amyloid is laid down in the walls of the malpighian arterioles, and the cut surface of the organ therefore presents a characteristic appearance of *sago spleen* with numerous scattered, firm, translucent nodules (Fig. 17–4). A diffuse type of amyloidosis of the spleen is also recognized in which the amyloid is deposited in the walls of the sinuses.

Case History I

The patient was a 62-year-old woman who had suffered from rheumatoid arthritis for many years. The disease had first become evident at the age of about 35 years when she noticed stiffness and pain in the fingers. The arthritis steadily progressed in spite of treatment with aspirin and gold injections. Ultimately there was great deformity of the hands and feet. During the last few months of her life, she developed the nephrotic syndrome (albuminuria, hypoalbuminemia, and edema). She died of bronchopneumonia. At necropsy, heavy deposits of amyloid were found in the liver, spleen (see Fig. 17–4), and kidneys. Smaller amounts were present in the intestine, lung, thyroid, and adrenal glands.

Liver. The organ is enlarged, heavy, pale, and firm. The amyloid is laid down in the walls of the sinuses between the endothelium and the liver cells (Fig. 17–5).

Kidney. The organ is large and pale. The amyloid is deposited in the glomeruli, in the

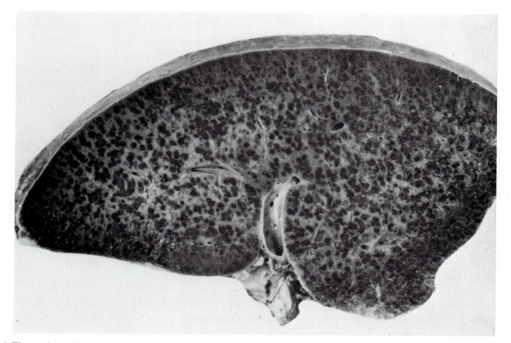

Figure 17–4 The spleen in amyloidosis. The cut surface of the spleen has been treated with an iodine solution. Many dark, firm, semitranslucent nodules of amyloid material can be seen, each surrounding a central arteriole of the white pulp. The deposits have been likened to grains of sago. This type of splenic involvement, therefore, is commonly referred to as a sago spleen. See Case History I for clinical details.

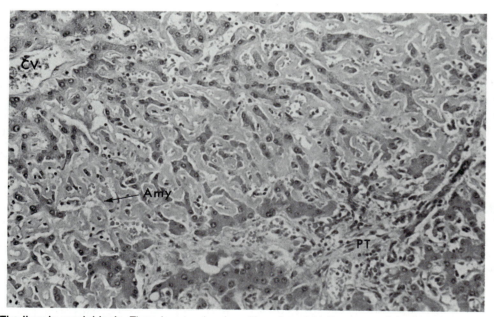

Figure 17–5 The liver in amyloidosis. There is extensive deposition of amyloid (Amy) around the liver sinusoids. The deposits have compressed the liver cells, many of which are small; others have disappeared completely. The liver cells around the central vein (CV) and the portal tract (PT) present a more normal appearance. A liver with this degree of involvement is enlarged, hard, and easily palpable. Nevertheless, clinical evidence of liver failure is generally lacking, such is the reserve capacity of this organ (×250).

walls of the arterioles, and in the interstitial tissue between the tubules. Renal amyloidosis causes hematuria and albuminuria; the albuminuria may be sufficiently severe to produce the nephrotic syndrome. Renal vein thrombosis is a well-recognized and fatal complication.

Other Sites. Adrenal glands, lymph nodes, lung, and gut may all be affected. Deposits in the intestine may cause diarrhea, and rectal biopsy is sometimes used as a diagnostic procedure. Amyloid is also laid down in the gingiva, and again biopsy may be employed to facilitate diagnosis.

Effects of Amyloid

The deposition of amyloid generally excites no inflammatory reaction, but there is atrophy of the parenchyma. In an organ with an abundant reserve like the liver, this is of little functional significance, but in nerves and kidney, the effects may be severe. Renal failure is a common cause of death in amyloidosis. An affected organ becomes rigid, and this is important if it has a mechanical function to perform, *e.g.*, the heart and tongue. Affected vessels are brittle, and therefore hemorrhages are a feature, *e.g.*, into the skin or kidney, causing hematuria. Since almost any tissue can be involved in amyloidosis, the clinical picture can be extremely varied, and the diagnosis should always be kept in mind whenever one is confronted with an unusual case.

Pathogenesis of Amyloidosis

Amyloid fibrils can be formed *in vivo* from a variety of polypeptide fragments, derived either from immunoglobulin or from other protein. In chronic destructive diseases such as osteomyelitis or tuberculosis, it is possible that the tissue proteins themselves provide the raw material for the formation of amyloid protein. Some polypeptide fragments are more amyloidogenic than are others; thus, the L light chains form amyloid fibrils more readily than do the K chains. Under some circumstances, the formation of amyloid appears to be a local affair and may be related to

the partial breakdown of proteins by local mononuclear phagocytic cells. Thus, the localized deposits of amyloid in medullary carcinoma of the thyroid are derived from calcitonin, whereas the amyloidosis of the islets of Langerhans and that found in some islet-cell tumors could be explained by the formation of fibrils from polypeptide fragments of either insulin or glucagon.

In generalized amyloidosis, an amyloidogenic protein (immunoglobulin light chains, SAA, or prealbumin) is present in the blood stream, and a polypeptide fraction of it is deposited in various sites. Even under these circumstances, it is possible that the mononuclear phagocyte system plays some part, for the cells of this system could take up the precursor protein and produce the necessary polypeptides for the formation of amyloid fibrils. Amyloidosis is therefore not a disease entity but rather a variety of different diseases—the amyloidoses or the beta-fibrilloses—that have in common the deposition of an abnormal type of fibril with characteristic properties.

Summary

- The plasma proteins consist of albumin, fibrinogen, and a wide array of globulins.
- Hypoalbuminemia is a feature of the nephrotic syndrome, chronic sepsis, and protein-losing enteropathy. It leads to edema.
- Hypergammaglobulinemia may be polyclonal or monoclonal; the monoclonal gammopathy is associated with an M protein.
- The lipoproteins consist of lipids combined with apoproteins. The relative amount of each type of lipoprotein in the blood depends on genetic factors, the presence of other disease, and diet. A high level of those that contain much cholesterol (low-density lipoprotein and remnants from the degradation of chylomicrons) is associated with an increased incidence of atherosclerosis (particularly of the coronary arteries) and the formation of xanthomas. The high-density lipoproteins are protective, and subjects with a low level have a high incidence of coronary disease.
- The erythrocyte sedimentation rate is raised in many diseases as a component of the acute phase response. It is paralleled by a raised C-reactive protein level.
- Amyloid is an abnormal protein of beta-pleated structure and has characteristic microscopic appearances and staining properties. It is derived from breakdown products of immunoglobulin light chains, serum amyloid protein A (SAA), prealbumin, endocrine secretions, or local protein.

- Immunocyte-derived systemic amyloidosis may be primary or associated with a B-cell dyscrasia such as myelomatosis. It is derived from light chains of immunoglobulin.
- Reactive systemic amyloidosis complicates chronic inflammatory disease. The amyloid is of unknown origin (AA derived from SAA).
- Other types of amyloid are the heredofamilial type (usually derived from prealbumin), endocrine-associated (*e.g.*, from calcitonin), senile amyloid, and localized amyloid.
- Generalized amyloidosis commonly affects spleen, liver, intestine, liver, and kidney. The renal involvement is the most serious.

Selected Readings

Benson, M. D.: Hereditary amyloidosis. Disease entity and clinical model. Hosp. Pract. *23*:125, 1988.

Brown, M. S., and Goldstein, J. L.: The hyperlipoproteinemias and other disorders of lipid metabolism. *In* Wilson, J. D., et al.: Harrison's Principles of Internal Medicine. 12th ed. New York, McGraw-Hill, 1991, pp. 1814–1825.

Cohen, A. S., and Connors, L. E.: The pathogenesis and biochemistry of amyloidosis. J. Pathol. *151*:1, 1987.

Editorial: The ESR: An outdated test? Lancet *1*:377, 1982.

Glenner, G. G.: Amyloid deposits and amyloidosis: The B-fibrilloses. N. Engl. J. Med. *302*:1283 and 1333, 1980.

Halsted, J. A., and Halsted, C. H. (eds.): The Laboratory in Clinical Medicine. 2nd ed. Philadelphia, W.B. Saunders Co., 1981.

See pages 124–127 for a description of the hyperlipoproteinemias, and pages 575–577 for a discussion of the erythrocyte sedimentation rate.

Levo, Y., Livni, N., and Laufer, A.: Diagnosis and classification of amyloidosis by an immune-histological method. Pathol. Res. Pract. *175*:373, 1982.

Special Pathology

18

Blood

After studying this chapter, the student should be able to:

- Outline the stages in the formation of the red blood cells and the white blood cells and indicate the sites of hematopoiesis.
- Describe the mature red blood cell and the abnormal forms that are encountered in disease.
- List the normal values of the red blood cell count, the hemoglobin content of blood, the packed cell volume (PCV), the mean corpuscular hemoglobin concentration (MCHC), and the white blood cell count.
- List the requirements for red blood cell formation and describe the fate of old, worn-out red blood cells.
- Indicate the clinical features of anemia and describe the five main types of this condition (as outlined in this chapter) in terms of the following factors:
  (a) causes;
  (b) blood picture;
  (c) pathologic changes in organs other than blood.
- Describe the main features of the red blood cell fragmentation syndrome.
- Define polycythemia and distinguish between the primary and secondary forms.
- Define the following terms and give at least one cause of each: leukocytosis, leukopenia, neutropenia, lymphocytosis, monocytosis, eosinophilia, and pancytopenia.
- Classify the leukemias and describe the salient features of each type.
- Describe the outstanding features and important causes of the following conditions:
- (a) bone marrow aplasia;
  (b) hypersplenism;
  (c) leukoerythroblastic anemia;
  (d) myelodysplastic syndrome.
- Describe the clotting mechanism and differentiate between the intrinsic system and the extrinsic system.
- Classify the bleeding diseases and give examples of each type.

- Briefly describe the following tests and indicate the value of each in assessing the cause of a bleeding disease: platelet count, clotting time, bleeding time, capillary fragility test, partial thromboplastin time, and prothrombin time.
- Describe the ABO and Rhesus blood groups, and outline the way in which a sample of blood is typed.
- List the hazards of blood transfusion and indicate how they may be avoided.

The formed elements of the blood consist of the red blood cells (erythrocytes), the white blood cells (leukocytes), and the platelets. In the fetus, blood formation (hematopoiesis) takes place in the bone marrow (in the medullary cavity of the bones), liver, spleen, and other organs. After birth, the extramedullary sites disappear, so that within a few weeks, blood formation occurs only in the bone marrow. As the child develops, the blood-forming tissue in the long bones is replaced by fatty marrow, so that by the time adulthood is reached, the main source of blood cells is the red marrow of the ribs and the vertebral column. The marrow of the long bones is available for extension of hematopoietic tissues should a need arise for increased production.

In adult life, the ultimate precursor cell or stem cell of all blood cells is the *totipotential hematopoietic stem cell*. This cell is inconspicuous in the bone marrow because it does not divide often under normal circumstances but provides a reserve in times of need. It gives rise to stem cells of more restricted potential. One such cell gives rise to the T lymphocytes, another to the B lymphocytes. A third forms the *pluripotent myeloid stem cell*, and this in turn gives rise to other stem cells of even more limited potential; they provide cells for maturation into polymorphs, monocytes, red blood cells, and platelets. The various stem cells divide both to replace themselves and to provide cells that differentiate into recognizable blood cell precursors that ultimately differentiate into mature blood cells.

The Red Blood Cells

The first recognizable red blood cell precursor is termed a *pronormoblast;* its cytoplasm contains many ribosomes but no hemoglobin. As hemoglobin is formed, the cytoplasm becomes more eosinophilic, and the nucleus becomes condensed (a process called pyknosis). Such a cell is termed a *normoblast;* early, intermediate, and late stages are recognized. Ultimately, the nucleus is extruded, and the cell assumes the flattened shape of the mature erythrocyte.

The Mature Erythrocyte

The red blood cell is a biconcave disk and is conveniently examined by making a smear of blood on a glass slide and staining with one of the Romanowsky stains* (Fig. 18–1). The average diameter of a red blood cell when examined in this manner is 6.7 to 7.7 μm. Young red blood cells have a faint basophilia in the cytoplasm that is due to remnants of rough endoplasmic reticulum. Such cells are termed *reticulocytes*. Normally, less than 2 per cent of the total red blood cells are reticulocytes, and an increase in their number generally indicates a more rapid production of cells such as occurs in hemolytic anemia or after a hemorrhage. Reticulocytosis is also seen whenever an anemia is treated successfully, such as when an iron deficiency anemia is treated with iron. Under normal conditions, the nucleated red blood cells are prevented from leaving the bone marrow; however, with extremely rapid erythropoiesis, particularly if it is occurring in abnormal sites such as the liver and spleen, nucleated red blood cells can appear in the circulation. A good example of this phenomenon is *hemolytic disease of the newborn.*

Examination of the Red Blood Cell. The normal red blood cell count is 4.5 to 6.5 × 10^{12}/L in males; the normal hemoglobin content is 140 to 180 g/L. In women, the red blood cell count is

---

*These stains, which include Leishman, Jenner, and Giemsa, consist of blended mixtures of methylene blue and eosin.

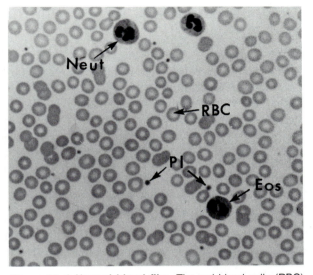

Figure 18–1 Normal blood film. The red blood cells (RBC) are of uniform diameter and evenly stained. The central, pale-staining area is due to their biconcave shape. Also shown are two neutrophil polymorphs (Neut), one eosinophil (Eos), and several platelets (Pl) (×600).

3.9 to 5.6 × 10^{12}/L, and the hemoglobin level is 120 to 160 g/L. A useful and accurate measurement is the hematocrit reading, or packed cell volume (PCV). In this test, a thin, cylindrical, graduated Wintrobe tube is filled with blood and centrifuged for half an hour at 3000 revolutions per minute. In the adult male, the PCV is 0.42 to 0.52 for males (0.37 to 0.47 for females), meaning that 42 to 52 per cent of the blood volume consists of red blood cells. There are three *absolute values* in common use:

Mean corpuscular volume (MCV), which is obtained thus:

$$\frac{\text{Volume of packed red blood cells (L/L)} \times 1000}{\text{Red blood cell count } (\times\ 10^{12}/\text{L})}$$

The result is expressed in 10^{-15} L or femtoliters (fl). The normal is 80 to 95 fL.

Mean corpuscular hemoglobin (MCH), which is obtained thus:

$$\frac{\text{Hemoglobin (g/L)}}{\text{Red blood cell count } (\times\ 10^{12}/\text{L})}$$

The result is expressed in 10^{-12} g or picograms (pg). The normal is 27 to 36 pg.

Mean corpuscular hemoglobin concentration (MCHC), which is obtained thus:

$$\frac{\text{Hemoglobin (g/L)}}{\text{Volume of packed red blood cells (L/L)}}$$

This is expressed in grams of hemoglobin per liter of packed red blood cells (g/L).

The MCHC is an index of the concentration of hemoglobin in the red blood cells. The normal range is 320 to 360 g/L, and a value less than 320 g/L indicates underhemoglobinization of the cells and suggests impaired hemoglobin synthesis, a condition often caused by iron deficiency. The normal absolute values are summarized in Table 18–1.

With experience, it is possible to get a great deal of information merely by microscopic examination of a well-stained blood film. The normal red blood cell is described as *normocytic* and *normochromic*. If it is smaller than normal, it is called *microcytic*; if larger than normal, *macrocytic*. If the cell is poorly hemoglobinized, it looks pale and is termed *hypochromic*. The normal cell is fully saturated with hemoglobin, and therefore hyperchromia cannot occur. If the cells vary greatly in size, the term *anisocytosis* is used. The presence of irregularly shaped cells is called *poikilocytosis*. *Burr cells* have projections or spikes arising from their surface; *sickle cells* have an elongated shape; *spherocytes* are spherical, rather than being flat disks. Spherocytes look abnormally small and stain darkly in a blood film. Another interesting pathologic variant is the *target cell*, in which a small central dot of hemoglobin is seen; this is separated from the outer rim by a wide clear area (Fig. 18–2).

Table 18–1 CHARACTERISTICS OF THE NORMAL RED BLOOD CELL

Packed cell volume (PCV)	0.42–0.52 (male), 0.37–0.47 (female) (no unit is necessary, but liter/liter is implied)
Mean corpuscular volume (MCV)	80–95 fL
Mean corpuscular hemoglobin (MCH)	27–36 pg
Mean corpuscular hemoglobin concentration (MCHC)	320–360 g/L
Mean corpuscular diameter (MCD)	6.7–7.7 μm

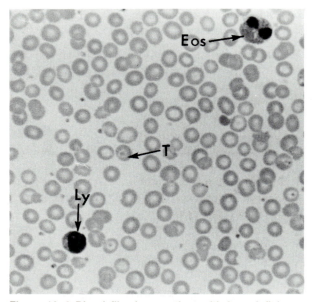

Figure 18–2 Blood film from patient with iron deficiency anemia. The red blood cells are hypochromic, and the central pale-staining area is more pronounced than normal. The cells that exhibit a central dot are called target cells (T). Also shown is an eosinophil (Eos) with a typical bilobed nucleus and a small lymphocyte (Ly) (×600).

Requirements for Red Blood Cell Formation

Hemoglobin consists of protein (globin) combined with heme, an iron-containing porphyrin.

In starvation, inadequate globin production can result in anemia. Under most circumstances, however, it is the formation of heme and maturation of the cells that are most important for the formation of healthy red blood cells; for this, the following components are required (Table 18–2).

Iron. Each heme molecule contains one atom of iron; without this, hemoglobin cannot be formed. Iron is absorbed from food in an ionic form by the mucosal cells of the duodenum and

upper small bowel. Heme, derived from hemoglobin and myoglobin in the diet, can be absorbed directly.

The manner in which iron is absorbed is complex, and there is a mechanism by which the amount absorbed can be regulated. Thus, in iron deficiency states, if there is accelerated erythropoiesis, the amount of iron absorbed in the gut is increased. On the other hand, if the body is overloaded with iron, the amount absorbed is decreased.

Once absorbed, iron combines with an iron-free protein (termed *apoferritin*) to form *ferritin*, the storage form of iron in the body. Much of this is stored in the cells of the mononuclear phagocyte system, where it is available for hemoglobin and myoglobin synthesis.

Vitamins. The most important vitamins essential for blood formation belong to the B complex vitamins: *folic acid* and *vitamin B$_{12}$*. Both are necessary for the proper development of the normoblast. If either substance is deficient, the normoblast develops abnormally; that is, it remains large, and the nucleus has an abnormal stippled appearance of its chromatin. Such a cell is termed a *megaloblast*, and the red blood cell that it produces is large (a *macrocyte*). Both vitamins are present in the diet and are absorbed in the small bowel. The two vitamins differ in that folic acid is absorbed directly, whereas vitamin B$_{12}$ cannot be absorbed unless it is bound to a complex mucoprotein secreted by the gastric mucosa. This substance is called *intrinsic factor*. It follows that gastric secretion is essential for the absorption of vitamin B$_{12}$.

Vitamin C. Although this vitamin is also required for red blood cell production, deficiency is rarely a factor in human disease.

Other Substances. These include *copper* and *cobalt*, but although deficiency in the experimen-

Table 18–2 REQUIREMENTS FOR RED BLOOD CELL FORMATION

Requirement	Marrow Changes	Blood Changes	Other Changes
Iron	Normoblastic hyperplasia	Hypochromic microcytic anemia	Oral mucosal atrophy
Folic acid	Megaloblastic hyperplasia	Normochromic macrocytic anemia	Oral mucosal atrophy
Vitamin B$_{12}$	Megaloblastic hyperplasia	Normochromic macrocytic anemia	Oral mucosal atrophy; subacute combined degeneration of cord

tal animal causes anemia, their role in human disease is debatable. *Thyroxine* is necessary for red blood cell formation, and it is not surprising that anemia is encountered in myxedema. Likewise, *androgens* stimulate erythropoiesis and are used in the treatment of some types of aplastic anemia. *Glucocorticoids* can also stimulate red blood cell formation. Anemia is seen in hypopituitarism, and polycythemia is a feature of Cushing's syndrome (Chapter 29). Erythropoietin is a hormone formed in the kidney as well as in other organs, and increased production leads to increased erythropoiesis. The stimulus for its formation is hypoxia.

Disposal of the Red Cell

The normal life span of the red blood cell is about 120 days. As cells age, they become fragmented and are taken up by the mononuclear phagocyte system (Fig. 18–3). Hemoglobin is split into globin and heme. The globin is degraded and returned to the body's pool of amino acids. The iron portion of the hemoglobin is split off and combined with apoferritin to form ferritin, which is stored for further use. The porphyrin nucleus is metabolized to bilirubin, which passes into the blood stream, becomes attached to albumin, and is excreted by the liver. Normally there is very little free hemoglobin in the plasma, and any that does appear is immediately removed by combination with a globulin component of the plasma called *haptoglobin*. Any large excess of hemoglobin in the circulation is oxidized to heme and combined with albumin to form *methemalbumin*. Both the haptoglobin and the albumin complexes are removed by the mononuclear phagocyte system so that none escapes into the urine. It is only when both these binding proteins are exhausted that free hemoglobin appears in the blood (*hemoglobinemia*) and in the urine (*hemoglobinuria*). Massive sudden destruction of red blood cells must occur before

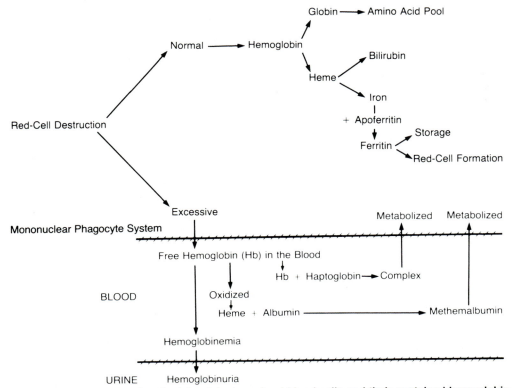

Figure 18–3 Diagram showing the fate of destroyed red blood cells and their contained hemoglobin.

this is evident (see Blackwater Fever, Chapter 10).

THE ANEMIAS

Anemia is defined as a condition in which there is *a fall in the quantity of either red blood cells or hemoglobin in a unit volume of blood in the presence of a low or normal total blood volume.* The question of blood volume is important in relation to pregnancy. A moderate fall in the level of the red blood cell count and hemoglobin is common during the last part of pregnancy and is followed by a slow recovery in the puerperium. There is a raised blood volume in pregnancy, and it is probable that much of the "physiologic anemia" is due to simple hemodilution. Nevertheless, iron deficiency can also occur.

The main clinical features of anemia are the following.

1. *Pallor,* best detected in the conjunctiva, nail bed, or mucous membrane of the mouth. Pallor of the skin, particularly of the face, is a deceptive sign. It can be absent in some patients with anemia and yet present in many pale-skinned normal people.

2. *Tiredness, easy fatigability,* and *generalized muscular weakness* are common symptoms; the pathogenesis, however, is not clear. Such symptoms are also common in psychoneurotic patients who are not anemic.

3. *Shortness of breath* and *palpitations* are common. They are related to tissue hypoxia and an increased cardiac output. *Heart failure* can occur.

4. *Angina pectoris, intermittent claudication,* and *giddiness* are due to tissue hypoxia in organs in which the blood supply is already impaired by arterial disease.

The pathologic effects of anemia are attributable to cellular hypoxia. At necropsy, there is severe fatty change of the liver, heart, and kidneys, and death is usually attributed to heart failure.

The classification of the anemias is somewhat unsatisfactory, but for practical purposes, the following groups can be recognized (Table 18–3): acute posthemorrhagic anemia; iron deficiency

Table 18–3 THE ANEMIAS

Type	Blood Picture	
Posthemorrhagic	Normochromic	Normocytic
Iron deficiency	Hypochromic	Microcytic
Megaloblastic	Normochromic	Macrocytic
Hemolytic	Normochromic	Normocytic
Anemia of bone marrow failure	Normochromic	Normocytic

anemia; megaloblastic anemia; hemolytic anemia; and anemia of bone marrow failure.

Acute Posthemorrhagic Anemia

The pathogenesis of the anemia that results from a sudden hemorrhage is described in Chapter 19. The anemia is normocytic and normochromic, provided the patient is not iron deficient as a result of previous blood loss or other disease. Within a few days a reticulocytosis occurs, and recovery proceeds to completion within about 6 weeks.

Iron Deficiency Anemia

Chronic blood loss is the most important cause of iron deficiency anemia, because although the red blood cells can easily be replaced, the body soon runs out of iron. Common examples are bleeding from a chronic peptic ulcer, gastrointestinal cancer, or hemorrhoids. In women, menorrhagia is an important cause of blood loss, whereas in underdeveloped countries, ankylostomiasis takes its toll.

Another important cause of iron deficiency anemia is inadequate absorption from the intestine. This may be secondary to dietary deficiency and is quite common in infants. It should be remembered that milk contains very little iron. Nutritional deficiency combined with the increased demand for iron by the growing fetus is a common cause of anemia in pregnancy. In the elderly, an inadequate diet can also lead to iron deficiency anemia.

Defective iron absorption is a feature of the malabsorption syndrome (Chapter 23). Thus, it accompanies many intestinal diseases and is also a common feature after gastrectomy because of the "intestinal hurry" that follows this operation.

Pathologic Changes

The bone marrow undergoes hyperplasia of the normoblastic type. Red marrow extends into the shafts of the long bones. In the peripheral blood, there is a moderate anemia in which the red blood cell count is relatively less reduced than is the hemoglobin level. *The red blood cells are markedly microcytic and hypochromic,* and target cells may be present (see Fig. 18–2). The reticulocyte count is low, unless there has been a recent hemorrhage.

Other features of iron deficiency sometimes accompany the anemia. Sometimes there is diffuse hair loss. The *nails* tend to become brittle and spoon-shaped. The most common *oral manifestation* is loss of the filiform papillae of the tongue, which consequently appears smooth and red. Mucosal atrophy can extend into the pharynx. Both in the mouth and pharynx, this atrophy is sometimes complicated by the development of squamous-cell carcinoma (see Plummer-Vinson syndrome, Chapter 23).

Megaloblastic Anemia

Megaloblastic anemia is due to a deficiency of folic acid, vitamin B_{12}, or both. It is characterized by an abnormal type of erythropoiesis in the marrow.

Causes

Dietary Deficiency. This is quite common in underdeveloped countries, where the anemia is often due to an inadequate intake of folic acid.

Pregnancy. Folic acid deficiency resulting from poor diet is sometimes precipitated by the extra demands of the fetus in pregnant women.

Gastric Disease. The intrinsic factor of the stomach is necessary for vitamin B_{12} absorption from the bowel. Therefore, total resection of the stomach leads to a megaloblastic anemia, but this does not occur for several years, so great are the body's stores of vitamin B_{12}.

By far the most important cause of megaloblastic anemia is pernicious anemia. This familial disease is accompanied by chronic fundal gastritis that is probably inborn. Before the anemia develops, the stomach gradually loses the ability to secrete pepsin and hydrochloric acid (achylia gastrica). Pernicious anemia is regarded as an autoimmune disease; the blood contains *antibodies to the parietal cells,* the cells of the stomach that secrete hydrochloric acid. More specific for the disease is a *blocking antibody* that blocks the binding of vitamin B_{12} to the intrinsic factor. Absorption of the vitamin B_{12}–intrinsic factor complex is hindered by yet another antibody (*binding antibody*) that binds to the complex.

Intestinal Malabsorption. Failure to absorb folic acid and vitamin B_{12} is a feature of the malabsorption syndromes. The defect may be related either to the bowel disease itself or indirectly to an alteration in the intestinal flora.

Drugs. Certain drugs, particularly anticonvulsants used in epilepsy treatment and the antimetabolites of the antifolic acid type used in cancer treatment (*e.g.,* methotrexate), can cause megaloblastic anemia if they are given over a prolonged period.

Pathologic Changes

The peripheral blood shows a severe anemia in which the *red blood cell count is relatively more reduced than is the hemoglobin level.* The red blood cells are conspicuously large (a condition called *macrocytosis*) and appear normally colored; they show marked *poikilocytosis* and *anisocytosis.* It is common to find both the white blood cells and platelets reduced in number. The bone marrow is markedly hyperplastic and contains many megaloblasts (Fig. 18–4).

The other effects depend on the cause of the anemia. Vitamin B_{12} is essential for the proper functioning of the central nervous system; without it, *subacute combined degeneration* of the spinal cord can occur. With this form of degeneration, there is demyelination of the posterior and lateral columns of the cord. It does not occur in pure folic acid deficiency.

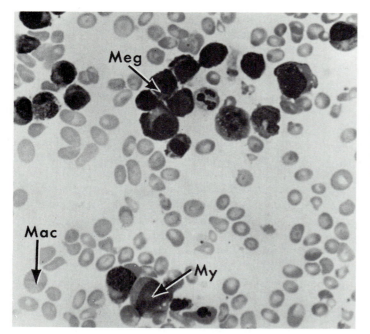

Figure 18–4 Bone marrow smear from patient with megaloblastic anemia. The red blood cells show great variation in size. Some are large (Mac), whereas others are small and are irregularly shaped. The number of nucleated red blood cell precursors is increased, and a group of megaloblasts is present (Meg). Also shown are a number of myelocytes (My) (×600).

There is sometimes a superficial stomatitis; the tongue is smooth and denuded of papillae, having a characteristic raw, beefy appearance.

Hemolytic Anemia

The term *hemolytic anemia* is applied to those conditions in which there is an increased rate of red blood cell destruction. This destruction is due either to an intrinsic defect in the red blood cells themselves or to some extracorpuscular factor acting on normal red blood cells. If the defect is primarily corpuscular, the red blood cells of a patient will have a diminished life span when transfused into a healthy normal recipient; on the contrary, normal cells transfused into a patient survive normally. If the cause of the hemolysis is extracorpuscular, normal red blood cells will be eliminated in the same way as are those of the patient, whereas the patient's red blood cells will survive well in a normal recipient.

The increased red blood cell destruction stimulates new red blood cell formation, which is manifested by a reticulocytosis.

Causes

Two groups may be recognized, depending on whether the defect is in the red blood cells themselves (corpuscular defects) or whether it is extracorpuscular.

Corpuscular Defects

Hereditary Spherocytosis. In northern European races, the most important cause is a spherical malformation of the red blood cells that causes the condition of *hereditary spherocytosis.* The abnormal cells are liable to become trapped and destroyed in the spleen so that splenectomy is usually effective in allaying the anemia but has no effect on the spherocytosis.

Abnormal Hemoglobin Structure or Synthesis. Abnormal hemoglobin formation is responsible for two groups of disease, the hemoglobinopathies and the thalassemias.

The Hemoglobinopathies. In this group, there is synthesis of an abnormal form of hemoglobin. The most important member is sickle cell disease, in which the abnormal hemoglobin S (HbS) is formed.

Sickle Cell Anemia. The formation of HbS, in which valine replaces the normal glutamic acid in one of the two beta-polypeptide chains of the globin molecule, is determined by the presence of an abnormal codominant gene. Homozygotes produce much HbS and have sickle cell anemia, whereas heterozygotes produce both normal hemoglobin and HbS and suffer from the sickle cell trait. In sickle cell anemia, the red blood cells, containing HbS, become sickle shaped, particularly under conditions of low oxygen tension. This tends to occur in the spleen, where the abnormal cells are removed and broken down. Splenic infarction is common, and the resultant splenic atrophy is associated with an increased susceptibility to infection. The sickle cell trait, which affects about 8 per cent of the black population in the United States, is generally asymptomatic unless the subject becomes hypoxic.

Many other abnormal types of hemoglobin have been found, their presence sometimes leading to a hemolytic anemia. The best known is hemoglobin C, which leads to an anemia that is less severe than that of sickle cell disease.

It should be noted that the hemoglobinopathies can occur in combination to produce complex syndromes. Thus, it is not uncommon to find sickle cell defect and hemoglobin C disease in the same person.

Thalassemia. In the *thalassemia syndromes,* the red blood cells of a patient contain various types of hemoglobin that are normally present only in the fetus. Many different types of hemoglobin are known, and the corresponding thalassemias are complex. A common example is Mediterranean anemia or beta-thalassemia in which there is absent or minimal synthesis of the beta chain of the globin molecule. The red blood cells contain much fetal hemoglobin (HbF), which contains no beta chains. The disease is common among Mediterranean, Middle Eastern, and Far Eastern populations. In the homozygous form of the disease, the anemia is severe.

Enzyme-Deficient Red Blood Cells. It was the finding that some black Americans were very likely to have a severe hemolytic anemia after the administration of certain drugs (*e.g.,* the antimalarial pamaquine) that led to the discovery that certain individuals have hereditary enzyme defects. The most important defect is a deficiency of glucose 6-phosphate dehydrogenase (G6PD) in their red cells. Many variants of G6PD deficiency have been described; these are inherited as dominant X-linked characteristics. Occasionally they lead to a chronic anemia, but more usually the defects become apparent as acute hemolytic anemia after ingestion of drugs or contact with a particular substance, such as the fava bean. The latter phenomenon is seen in some Mediterranean races; the anemia that follows contact with the bean is reputed to be the reason that Pythagoras counseled his followers never to walk in bean fields.

Extracorpuscular Defects

Autoimmune Hemolytic Anemia. The most important antibodies that act on red blood cells are autoantibodies that usually occur idiopathically but may on occasion develop during the course of some other disease. Two types of antibody are involved.

Warm Antibodies. These IgG antibodies react with red blood cells at 37°C (98.6°F). They do not agglutinate the cells in saline solution but coat the cells. This can be detected by the Coombs test.* *In vivo,* red blood cells coated with antibody are rapidly taken up by the spleen and destroyed. Clinically, this type of antibody is responsible for most cases of severe autoimmune hemolytic anemia. This is usually idiopathic but may occur as a complication of systemic lupus erythematosus or lymphoma.

Cold Antibodies. These are IgM antibodies and react with red blood cells at 4°C (39°F); they cause agglutination and often hemolysis if complement is present. This type of antibody is sometimes formed in patients with mycoplasmal pneumonia or lymphoma. Exposure to cold precipitates an anemia and sometimes Raynaud's syndrome.

Alloantibodies. The blood group can also cause a hemolytic anemia under special circumstances. For example, in Rh-hemolytic disease of the newborn, an Rh-negative woman married to an Rh-

---

*In the *direct Coombs test,* a sample of a *patient's red blood cells* that have been washed in saline is mixed with Coombs reagent (antihuman gamma globulin). A positive test is indicated by agglutination due to the presence of a coating of antibody on the red blood cells. In the *indirect Coombs test,* a sample of a *patient's serum* is mixed with a suspension of suitable red blood cells. These are washed in saline and then mixed with Coombs reagent. Agglutination indicates the patient's serum contains antibodies capable of adhering to the red blood cells. In Rh sensitization of pregnancy, the mother's serum is tested for antibodies (the indirect Coombs test), whereas the baby's cells are submitted to a direct Coombs test.

positive man produces an Rh-positive fetus. During the last part of pregnancy, and particularly during labor, a leak of fetal red blood cells into the maternal circulation is quite common. The mother is thereby stimulated to produce Rh antibodies. Although the first child escapes damage, future Rh-positive fetuses may be attacked by maternal Rh antibodies that cross the placenta. The fetus develops a severe hemolytic anemia, characterized by numerous nucleated red blood cells in its circulation (*hemolytic disease of the newborn*). In severe cases, the fetus is stillborn; generalized edema due to heart failure is a prominent feature. Less severely affected infants survive but are jaundiced and may suffer brain damage (kernicterus; see Hemolytic Jaundice, Chapter 24).

An advance of great importance was the discovery that the administration of human gamma globulin containing anti-Rh antibody of high activity can prevent sensitization of Rh-negative mothers by Rh-positive fetal cells, provided it is given within 72 hours of delivery or abortion. The passively administered anti-Rh antibodies probably coat the Rh-positive fetal cells and prevent them from providing an adequate antigenic stimulus. In this way, sensitization does not occur.

Infections. In *Clostridium perfringens* infections, the powerful toxins of the organism cause red blood cell lysis. In malaria, there is red blood cell destruction by the parasite; in blackwater fever, the hemolysis is massive.

Drugs. Some drugs cause red blood cell destruction, an effect particularly marked in patients with enzyme-deficient red blood cells. Drugs can also cause hemolytic anemia by an immune-mediated mechanism, *e.g.,* by acting as a hapten, combining with red blood cells or other proteins, and stimulating specific antibodies.

Burns. Severe burns damage red blood cells directly.

Red Blood Cell Fragmentation Syndrome. Red blood cells that are subjected to excessive physical trauma in the circulation may undergo premature fragmentation and destruction. The presence of fragmented, bizarre-shaped red blood cells (schistocytes) in the peripheral blood is characteristic. The condition is encountered with abnormalities of the heart valve and great ves-sels, particularly if prosthetic valves or intracardiac patches have been inserted. Extreme turbulence appears to be the damaging factor.

Fragmentation is also seen in association with small vessel disease (*microangiopathic hemolytic anemia*). This occurs in disseminated intravascular coagulation, and a particular example of this is the *hemolytic uremic syndrome*, which is an acute condition occurring in the great majority of cases in infants and young children. There is an acute hemolytic anemia, a low platelet count, and acute renal failure. The cause of this disease is not known, but it commonly follows *Escherichia coli* or viral infection.

Pathologic Changes

In hemolytic anemia, the red blood cells are typically normochromic and normocytic. The outstanding feature of the disease is a high reticulocyte count, which indicates active erythropoiesis. The reticulocyte count may even reach 30 per cent of the total cell count. The bone marrow shows marked normoblastic hyperplasia.

In hemolytic anemia, there is overproduction of bilirubin; jaundice is present in most patients. When the hemolytic process is sudden and severe, hemoglobinemia may occur, leading to hemoglobinuria. This response is unusual, except in the most severe cases such as in patients having blackwater fever. The presence of much free hemoglobin in the blood, particularly when the hemolysis has been caused by an immunologic reaction, may cause renal vasoconstriction, oliguria, and renal failure.

Anemia of Bone Marrow Failure

Anemia is frequent in many chronic diseases such as rheumatoid arthritis, leukemia, renal disease, and chronic suppurative infections. *The anemia* found with these diseases *is normocytic* and *normochromic* and is not attended by any significant reticulocytosis. Some deficiency or toxemia probably impairs red blood cell production, but the mechanism is not known.

Two other types of anemia come into this category and are described later: bone marrow aplasia (aplastic anemia) and bone marrow replacement (leukoerythroblastic anemia).

POLYCYTHEMIA

Polycythemia is a condition in which the red blood cell count is raised in a unit volume of blood in the presence of an increased total blood volume. It must be distinguished from hemoconcentration, such as that occurring in patients with burns, in which the red blood cell count is increased because of a decrease in the plasma volume.

Polycythemia may be secondary to chronic hypoxia. It is therefore a feature of chronic lung disease and cyanotic congenital heart disease. Some degree of polycythemia is normal in those who live at a high altitude. The stimulus under these circumstances appears to be excess produc-tion of erythropoietin, secondary to the hypoxia. Occasionally, polycythemia is encountered in renal disease, *e.g.*, a clear-cell carcinoma. Excess production of erythropoietin by the tumor is the probable mechanism.

As a primary condition *(polycythemia vera)*, there is a neoplastic proliferation of the normo-blastic component of the bone marrow. The red blood cell count can reach 10×10^{12}/L, and there is often a considerable increase in both white blood cell and platelet counts, a change not encountered in secondary polycythemia. Indeed, some cases terminate as myeloid leukemia, and it is reasonable to classify the disease as one example of a myeloproliferative disorder (p. 309). Polycythemia vera is generally a disease of middle-aged or elderly people, and thrombotic complications are common because of the high viscosity of the blood. Mesenteric venous thrombosis, coronary artery thrombosis, and cerebral thrombosis are common terminal events.

The White Blood Cells

Important white blood cells are the granulocytes, the lymphocytes, and the monocytes (Figs. 18–5 and 18–6).

Development

The precursor cell of the granulocyte is the *myeloblast*, a cell that closely resembles the pronormoblast. As it matures, it loses its nucleoli and is then termed a *promyelocyte*. When specific cytoplasmic granules—neutrophilic, eosinophilic, or basophilic—appear, the cell is called a *myelocyte*. The indented nucleus of the late or metamyelocyte is ultimately drawn out into two or more discrete lobes joined by fine chromatin threads. This is the mature *polymorphonuclear granulocyte* ("polymorph"), so called because of the shape of its nucleus. Most granulocytes have fine lilac-colored granules and are called *neutrophils*. A few are *eosinophils*, which have large red granules, and the least common is the *basophil*, which has very large purple granules. The de-velopment of the granulocytes occurs in the bone marrow; under normal conditions, only mature cells appear in the peripheral blood.

The precursor cells of lymphocytes and monocytes are called *lymphoblasts* and *monoblasts*. As these cells mature, they lose their nucleoli; in the case of the lymphocyte, the cytoplasm becomes sparse as the nucleus condenses and becomes hyperchromatic.

Normal White Blood Cell Count and Its Variations in Disease

The total white blood cell count in the blood is 4 to 11×10^9/L (4000 to 11,000/μl).* The range of the differential count for the adult is as follows:

---

*The white blood cell count has commonly been expressed in number of cells per cubic millimeter (cu mm or μl) of blood. In the SI units now in common use, it is expressed in number of cells $\times 10^9$ per liter (L). Thus, the normal white blood cell count is 4 to 11×10^9/L or, in the previous system, 4000 to 11,000/cu mm or 4000 to 11,000/μl.

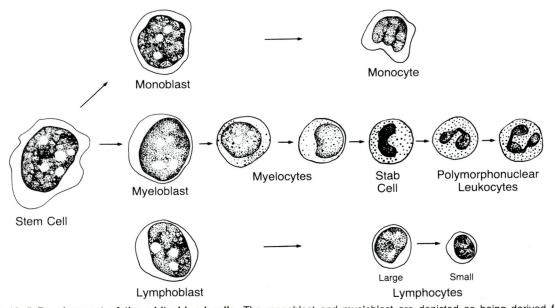

Figure 18–5 Development of the white blood cells. The monoblast and myeloblast are depicted as being derived from a common pluripotential cell called a stem cell. The lymphoblast is derived from its own stem cell. The three blast cell types cannot be distinguished easily from each other on morphologic grounds. The myelocyte matures to a stab- or band-form; the nucleus of the mature polymorph is formed by subsequent lobulation. (Drawn by Margot Mackay, University of Toronto, Faculty of Medicine, Department of Surgery, Division of Biomedical Communications, Toronto.)

Neutrophils 40% to 75% (2.0 to 7.5 $\times$ 10^9/L)
Eosinophils 1% to 5% (0.05 to 0.4 $\times$ 10^9/L)
Basophils 0% to 1% (up to 0.1 $\times$ 10^9/L)
Lymphocytes 20% to 45% (1.5 to 4 $\times$ 10^9/L)
Monocytes 3% to 7% (0.2 to 0.8 $\times$ 10^9/L)

The suffix -*cytosis* implies an excess of cells, *e.g., leukocytosis* indicates an increased total white blood cell count, and *lymphocytosis* indicates an increase in the number of lymphocytes. The suffix -*penia* means a decrease in the relevant cells, *e.g., leukopenia* means a decrease in the number of white blood cells, and *lymphopenia* is a decrease in the number of lymphocytes. *Neutrophilia* is sometimes used as an alternative to neutrophil leukocytosis. Likewise, *neutropenia* denotes a reduction in the total number of neutrophil polymorphs, and the term *agranulocytosis* is commonly used as a synonym. The figures in parentheses in the range listed indicate the absolute number of cells present. This is a more useful figure than is the percentage. Thus, if there is a drop in the number of neutrophils, the percentage of lymphocytes increases, a condition called a *relative lymphocytosis*. The term, however, is misleading, since the actual number of lym-

phocytes can remain unchanged. The main variations in the white blood cell count are as follows.

Neutrophil Leukocytosis (Neutrophilia). This common condition is usually due to infection. The highest counts are seen when the organism concerned is one of the pyogenic bacteria, *e.g.,* staphylococci, pneumococci, and coliforms.

Other important causes are *massive tissue necrosis,* such as after a myocardial infarct; *uremia; acute gout, severe hemorrhage,* and *hemolysis; rapidly growing malignant tumors* and *neoplastic disease of the marrow,* such as chronic myelocytic leukemia and polycythemia vera.

At one time, a classification of the maturity of neutrophils based on their nuclear segmentation was very much in vogue. The results were expressed in tabular form, with the left-hand side of the page listing the most primitive cells and the more differentiated cells being on the right-hand side. Although this detailed accounting is now obsolete, the term "a shift to the left" is still useful in denoting an increase of young forms of polymorphs in the blood, such as occurs in the leukocytosis of infection. In extreme cases, met-

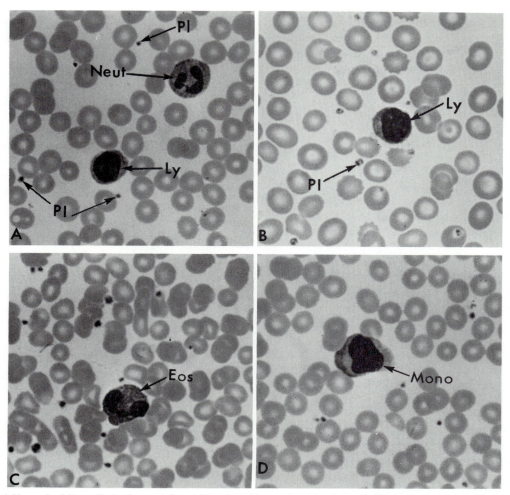

Figure 18–6 Normal white cells in the peripheral blood. *A,* The neutrophil polymorph (Neut) has a typical lobed nucleus and fine cytoplasmic granules. The small lymphocyte (Ly) has a deeply staining nucleus and scanty cytoplasm. A number of platelets (Pl) are present. *B,* Typical small lymphocyte. *C,* Eosinophil with coarse granules (Eos). *D,* Monocyte (Mono). The cell is larger than a lymphocyte and has more abundant cytoplasm (×960).

amyelocytes and even myelocytes may enter the blood. This *leukemoid blood picture* can sometimes closely mimic leukemia itself.

Neutropenia. A reduction in the number of neutrophils is seen in some infections, *e.g.,* typhoid fever and malaria. It is also a common feature of the prodromal period of many viral diseases. Any overwhelming infection, whatever the cause, also reduces the neutrophil count.

Other causes of neutropenia are hypersplenism, bone marrow aplasia, and acute leukemia.

Regulation of the Neutrophil Count. The neutrophil count can be altered by two regulatory mechanisms.

1. *Release of neutrophils from the reserves.* Of the neutrophils in the blood, over half are in a "marginated pool" adherent to the walls of the blood vessels, particularly in the lungs. These can be released rapidly; this release accounts for the leukocytosis that occurs during exercise and after the administration of epinephrine. The second reserve is in the bone marrow, where the number of neutrophils sequestered is about ten times the total number of cells present in the blood. The mechanism of their release is poorly understood, but various neutrophil-releasing factors have been described.

2. *Increased production of neutrophils in the bone*

marrow. Various growth stimulating factors and inhibitory factors (chalones) have been described. Their role, if any, in the regulation of the neutrophil count in health or disease is not clear.

Lymphocytosis. An absolute lymphocytosis is not common. It is seen in *whooping cough* and in *infectious mononucleosis.* In infectious mononucleosis, the lymphocytes are atypical. This disease, which is common in young adults, is caused by the Epstein-Barr virus. The illness usually commences with a sore throat, followed by enlargement of cervical lymph nodes and later by the appearance of the characteristic cells in the blood. An interesting feature is the presence in the serum of antibodies that agglutinate sheep's red blood cells to high titer. These antibodies may be detected by the *Paul-Bunnell test.* A variant of this test utilizing horse red blood cells is in common use and is termed the monospot test. During convalescence, specific antibodies to the Epstein-Barr virus appear in the blood as well as the heterophilic antibodies. An illness clinically resembling infectious mononucleosis can occur in cytomegalovirus infection and in toxoplasmosis. In such cases, the Paul-Bunnell test is negative.

Another important cause of lymphocytosis is chronic lymphocytic leukemia.

Monocytosis. An increased number of monocytes is typically seen in some protozoal diseases, *e.g.,* malaria and leishmaniasis. It is a feature of monocytic leukemia and also of some chronic bacterial infections, *e.g.,* tuberculosis.

Eosinophilia. This condition, which is characterized by the formation and accumulation of a large number of eosinophils in the blood, is encountered in atopic conditions, particularly bronchial asthma, hay fever, and urticaria. It is also a feature of helminthic infections, particularly when the parasites are migrating through the blood stream and tissues.

THE LEUKEMIAS

Leukemia is a condition in which there is a widespread proliferation of white blood cells and their precursors throughout the tissues in the body. There is usually an increase in the number of circulating white blood cells also. The cause of leukemia is unknown, but it has been found that there is an increased incidence after exposure to ionizing radiation. In birds and mice, the cause appears to be viral.

Classification of Leukemia

The leukemias are traditionally classified, as shown, according to the rapidity of progression of the disease and the type of cell involved. The more acute the process, the more primitive the cell type involved.

Chronic leukemia
   chronic myelogenous (myeloid or myelocytic) leukemia (CML)
   chronic lymphocytic leukemia (CLL)
Acute leukemia
   acute myelogenous (myeloblastic) leukemia (AML)
   acute lymphoblastic leukemia (ALL)

It has been noted previously that the cells of the blood are derived ultimately from stem cells, and that several cell types share a common stem cell, *e.g.,* red blood cells, granulocytes, monocytes, and platelets are derived from the pluripotential myeloid stem cell. Hence, it is not surprising that in acute leukemia, several cell types may be present in the same patient, *e.g.,* myeloblasts and monoblasts, or that the cell type may change during the course of the disease, *e.g.,* polycythemia vera may terminate as myeloid leukemia. These variants of myeloid leukemia, sometimes called nonlymphocytic leukemia, are recognized in the French-American-British (FAB) classification. Thus, seven types of AML are recognized, M1 to M7. The classification is based on the morphology and histochemical properties of the involved cell.

Many subtypes of normal lymphocytes are known, and this is reflected in the number of variants of AML and CLL. The recognition of these variants of leukemia is based on detection of specific markers and gene rearrangement in the leukemic cells.

These new classifications are of importance because many types have characteristic clinical features and respond differently to treatment.

The details of these classifications are complex, and diagnosis, like the clinical management of the patient, is best delegated to the specialist.

Chronic Myelogenous Leukemia. This is a disease of middle life and is characterized by an enormous leukocytosis, the white blood cell count reaching 1000×10^9/L on occasion. The predominant cell is the neutrophil polymorph, but metamyelocytes and myelocytes are also present. Coincidental with the leukocytosis is a progressive anemia and a gradual fall in the platelet count.

Clinically, the patient has immense enlargement of the spleen and, to a lesser extent, the liver. Death usually occurs within 3 to 5 years and may be heralded by an acute exacerbation of the disease (*accelerated phase*); this may be accompanied by a *blast crisis,* in which blast cells (usually myeloblasts, but occasionally monoblasts, erythroblasts, or even megakaryoblasts) are found in large numbers in the blood.

Chronic Lymphocytic Leukemia. This is usually a disease of later life, and there is a marked lymphocytosis with a total white blood cell count ranging up to 250×10^9/L. Most of the cells in the blood stream are mature lymphocytes, but there are a varying number of lymphoblasts. There is a progressive anemia and thrombocytopenia.

Because the condition affects lymph nodes primarily, the patient usually presents with generalized lymphadenopathy. The spleen and liver are enlarged, but to a lesser extent than with myeloid leukemia. As with myeloid leukemia, death usually occurs within 5 years and is due to anemia and secondary infection.

The leukemic cells in the majority of cases of CLL have B-cell markers. Several subsets can be distinguished by morphology and cell markers. *B-cell prolymphocytic leukemia* has a poor prognosis. *Hairy-cell leukemia* is so named because the surface of the leukemic cells has hairlike projections. The disease is of considerable interest because it is associated with HTLV-2 infection.

Acute Leukemia. The two types of acute leukemia are best considered together because they resemble each other very closely. In the acute leukemias, the white blood cell count may vary from less than 1×10^9/L to over 100×10^9/L.

When there is a raised count, the blood is invariably flooded with primitive blast cells, and it is often difficult or even impossible to be sure whether these are myeloblasts or lymphoblasts. Sometimes the cells have the features of monocytes, and the disease is labeled *acute myelomonocytic* or *monoblastic leukemia.* The monocyte and myeloblast have a common stem cell of origin, and "acute monocytic leukemia" is now regarded as a variant of acute myeloblastic leukemia.

Occasionally the cells have features of erythroblasts (acute erythroleukemia) or megakaryocytes (acute megakaryocytic leukemia), or the cells are so primitive that they cannot be classified and the condition is termed stem-cell leukemia. As noted previously, these variants are incorporated in the FAB classification of AML. ALL is also a heterogeneous group. The common type (C-ALL) has pre–B-cell markers. Others have surface B-cell markers, T-cell markers, or no identifiable markers.

In acute leukemia, the primitive white blood cells replace the mature ones, and the polymorph count is invariably reduced (agranulocytosis). This leads to an impaired defense against infection, so that gingivitis and bronchopneumonia are common.

In acute leukemia, there is rapidly progressive normocytic, normochromic anemia and severe thrombocytopenia.

Acute leukemia occurs at all ages. In childhood, it is usually lymphoblastic, but in adult life, the myeloblastic variety is more common. Clinically, it is not possible to distinguish between the two types. The onset is usually sudden, the main features being high fever, a generalized bleeding tendency, progressive anemia, and necrotic infective lesions of the mouth and throat. Acute leukemia can therefore closely mimic an acute infectious disease.

Most patients with acute leukemia die within 6 months, usually as a result of infection or bleeding into vital areas such as the central nervous system. Intensive modern therapy has increased the average survival considerably. As many as 50 per cent of patients may survive 5 years, and perhaps one third of children with acute lymphoblastic leukemia can now be cured.

Changes in the Organs in Leukemia

The pathologic course of leukemia is a monotonous infiltration of leukemic cells into numerous organs, which become enlarged, soft, and pale. Lymph nodes, spleen, and bone marrow are particularly involved and are crowded out by the responsible cells. No organ is exempt from this infiltration; massive local involvement is particularly characteristic of acute leukemia. Other changes found are those associated with infection and hemorrhage.

Myelodysplastic Syndromes

The myelodysplastic syndromes are a group of conditions in which the bone marrow is replaced by an abnormal clone of cells that differentiate into abnormal myeloid, erythroid, and megakaryocytic cells. In addition to showing abnormal morphology in the bone marrow, there is defective formation of mature cells resulting in anemia, granulocytopenia, and thrombocytopenia. Chromosomal abnormalities are frequent in the abnormal hematopoietic cells, and about one third of cases terminate in acute leukemia, generally AML.

Bone Marrow Aplasia

When the bone marrow ceases to release mature elements into the circulation, there is a serious drop in the blood count, and the condition is described as *aplasia*. Sometimes the failure of division occurs at the "blast" stage; in such cases, no mature elements are present either in the peripheral blood or in the bone marrow. At other times there is a failure in division at a later stage of hematopoiesis, so that the marrow, although crowded with maturing cells, is unable to release them into the circulation. This is called *maturation arrest*.

Aplasia of the marrow may involve all three elements, thereby leading to a diminution of all cells of the blood *(pancytopenia)*, or it may affect only one of these elements. *Pure red blood cell aplasia* is very uncommon, but aplasia of the granulocytes *(agranulocytosis)* is an important condition. Whether a *pure platelet aplasia* occurs is doubtful; in immune thrombocytopenic purpura (p. 311), the platelets are destroyed after they have been released from the bone marrow.

Pancytopenia

Aplasia affecting all the formed elements of the marrow can be due to ionizing radiation or drugs, of which the most important are chloramphenicol, the sulfonamides, phenylbutazone (used in the treatment of arthritis), gold salts (used in the treatment of rheumatoid arthritis), and the cytotoxic drugs (used in the treatment of cancer). It is also a rare complication of miliary tuberculosis. In some patients, no cause can be found, and the condition must be termed idiopathic. Some instances of the last group eventually turn out to be leukemia. An occasional cause is hypersplenism, which is described later in this chapter.

On hematologic examination, there is an anemia with no reticulocytosis, a leukopenia, and a thrombocytopenia. If the bone marrow is found to be hypocellular, the prognosis is poor. On the other hand, cases of maturation arrest have a better prognosis.

Agranulocytosis

Aplasia of the white blood cell elements is a serious complication of therapy with certain drugs, particularly thiouracil (used in the treatment of thyrotoxicosis), phenylbutazone, and chlorpromazine (used as a tranquilizer). Agranulocytosis also occurs as a result of the use of anticancer drugs. Some cases occur with hypersplenism, whereas others are idiopathic.

The chief effect of agranulocytosis is a tendency for infection to develop; consequently, ulcerating infective lesions occur in the mouth and throat, gastrointestinal tract, and vagina. Overwhelming infection with bronchopneumonia is the usual end result.

Hypersplenism

The function of the spleen in relation to blood formation is ill-understood. It is active in removing defective and aging red blood cells from the circulation, and it is possible that it exerts an inhibitory effect on the formation of white blood cells and platelets in the marrow.

Occasionally conditions leading to gross splenomegaly give rise either to marrow aplasia affecting any or all of the formed elements of the blood or to a hemolytic anemia. If the blood disorder abates after removal of the spleen, the condition is diagnosed as hypersplenism. The precise mechanism is not understood, and the condition is described in the splenomegaly of many conditions, *e.g.*, cirrhosis of the liver, schistosomiasis, and leishmaniasis.

The Syndrome of Bone Marrow Replacement

The normal bone marrow is sometimes crowded out by foreign elements such as metastatic carcinoma or myeloma. This results in a typical blood picture of *leukoerythroblastic anemia*. This consists of a normocytic, normochromic anemia in which there are many nucleated red cells (normoblasts) in the blood. There is a moderate to considerable polymorph leukocytosis, and many myelocytes and metamyelocytes are also present in the blood.

In a number of instances, a leukoerythroblastic anemia is present in the face of fibrosis of the bone marrow (*myelosclerosis*). This condition has been grouped with polycythemia vera and leukemia under the all-embracing heading of *myeloproliferative disorder*.

The Platelets and Clotting Factors

Platelets are small disks devoid of a nucleus that are formed in the bone marrow by fragmentation of the cytoplasm of large multinucleate cells termed *megakaryocytes*. Platelet adhesion and aggregation are described in Chapter 19 in relation to thrombosis. In this section, we shall consider the platelets and the clotting mechanism, particularly in relation to the defects that lead to a bleeding tendency.

THE CLOTTING MECHANISM

Blood clotting itself is a very complex mechanism (Fig. 18–7). In essence, it consists of a conversion of *fibrinogen (factor I)* to fibrin by the action of thrombin. This enzyme exists normally as an inert precursor, *prothrombin (factor II)*, which is activated to thrombin by *prothrombinase*, which itself is generated by the interaction of activated *factor X* (designated *factor Xa*) with *factor V*, platelet factor 3, and calcium ions (*factor IV*). This sequence is called the common pathway and can be initiated by two completely separate mechanisms, the intrinsic (blood) system and the extrinsic (tissue) system (Figs. 18–7 and 18–8).

The Intrinsic System. In the intrinsic (blood) system, contact with an abnormal surface leads to the activation of *factor XII* to factor XIIa. This activates *factor XI*, and factor XIa activates *factor IX*. Factor IXa in conjunction with factor VIII and platelet phospholipid activates factor X.

The Extrinsic System. In the extrinsic (tissue) system, tissue damage results in the release of a tissue factor rich in phospholipid. It is called *factor III*. This in conjunction with *factor VII* activates factor X, which, as already described, is involved in the production of prothrombinase via the common pathway.

The tissue factor is found in large amounts in the brain, extracts of which are used as a source of it in various laboratory tests, such as the prothrombin time. The venom of the Russell viper is also rich in it.

The two pathways of blood clotting are both important, for a derangement of either leads to a serious defect in hemostasis. The intrinsic system develops much more slowly than does the extrinsic one, but both are initiated by tissue damage, either by releasing tissue factor or by providing an abnormal surface. In both systems,

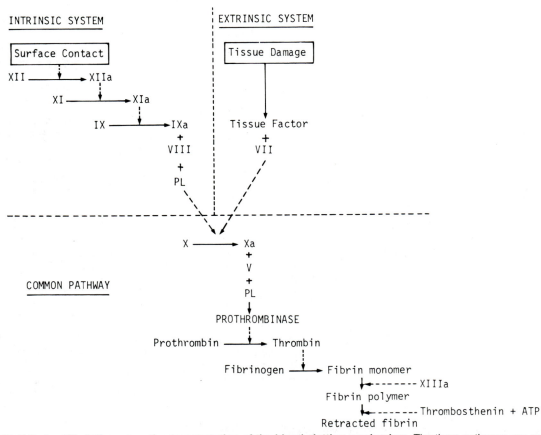

Figure 18–7 A simplified diagrammatic representation of the blood clotting mechanism. The three pathways are separated by interrupted lines. Solid arrows indicate transformation; interrupted arrows denote actions. PL denotes platelet factor 3. Not shown in the diagram is the calcium that is required for most of the steps shown. (After Marcus, A.J.: Reprinted by permission of The New England Journal of Medicine, *280:*1213, 1969.)

there is activation of factor X; from then on, there is a final common pathway involving factor V, platelet factor 3, calcium ions, prothrombin, and fibrinogen.

It should be noted that factors II, VII, IX, X, XI, XII, and XIII are all enzymes; they are of a class called *serine esterases.* Digestive enzymes and complement enzymes are also members of this class. Characteristically, they are all stored as an inactive precursor, activated by a given stimulus, and then undergo a cascadelike activation. Thus, the activation of the various factors involved in clotting is believed to follow a *cascade sequence,* many of the factors being substrates that are activated by a preceding enzyme.

The earliest phase of the intrinsic system is slow, but once thrombin is formed, the process is greatly accelerated; indeed, there is a real cascade, for thrombin potentiates the activity of factors V and VIII. It also causes platelets to aggregate and so increases the amount of lipid factor 3. This is called the *autocatalytic action of thrombin.* Interestingly, thrombin also destroys factors V and VIII after potentiating their reactivity; in this way, fibrin formation is stopped when a high concentration of thrombin has been achieved.

It should be noted that the plasma clotting factors (all globulins) are given Roman numerals. They are also given alternative names: factor VIII is antihemophilic factor; factor IX is Christmas factor; and factor XII is Hageman factor. The personal names refer to the surnames of the patients in whom a deficiency of the particular

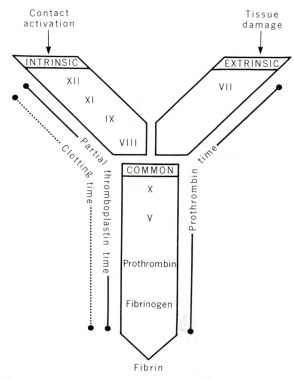

Figure 18–8 The interpretation of screening tests of blood clotting. (Modified from Bithell, T.C., and Wintrobe, M.M.: *In* Wintrobe, M.M., et al. [Eds.]: Harrison's Principles of Internal Medicine, 7th ed. New York, McGraw-Hill, 1974. Reproduced with permission of McGraw-Hill, Inc.)

factor was first described. The latest factor described is *factor XIII* (fibrin-stabilizing factor), which converts soluble fibrin into insoluble, or stabilized, fibrin.

THE BLEEDING DISEASES

When small blood vessels are damaged, the injured vessels are sealed by a mass known as a *hemostatic plug.* At first this consists of platelets, but soon this is consolidated by fibrin formation. Finally the entire aggregate contracts, probably owing to the contractile protein in the platelets called *thrombosthenin.* Thrombin released during clotting causes further platelet deposition as well as fibrin formation. Defects in the intrinsic system of blood clotting, such as in hemophilia, do not prevent the formation of a hemostatic plug, and therefore the bleeding time is normal. How-

ever, the plug is not stable, and rebleeding occurs later. Serious bleeding can therefore follow the infliction of a wound such as that caused by dental extraction. A third cause of bleeding is some abnormality in the vessels themselves.

Bleeding Due to Vascular Disease

This type of bleeding usually takes the form of purpura, but more extensive bleeding can occur into the tissues as well as into organs to produce hematuria and hematemesis.

A common form of vascular damage is vasculitis associated with deposition of immune complexes. This occurs in immune-complex disease and is also a feature of certain infections (*e.g.,* gonococcal) and other types of septicemia. Ingestion of drugs is another cause of vascular damage mediated by an immunologic mechanism.

Bleeding Due to Platelet Deficiency

The normal platelet count is 150 to 440 × 10^9/L, with an average of 250 × 10^9/L. It is raised after injuries and operations (especially splenectomy). A count below 100 × 10^9/L is designated *thrombocytopenia.*

A low platelet count (thrombocytopenia) leads to spontaneous bleeding into the tissues with the production of small petechiae. In the skin, the condition is called *purpura.* Spontaneous hemorrhage also occurs into the gastrointestinal and urinary tracts.

Immune thrombocytopenic purpura is due to the presence of an IgG autoantibody that is directed against platelets and causes them to be destroyed in the spleen. In young children, it occurs about 3 weeks after an acute viral infection (*e.g.,* chickenpox, measles, infectious mononucleosis) as an acute, self-limiting disease. In adults, the course is chronic, and unless a good response is obtained with glucocorticosteroid therapy, splenectomy is necessary.

As a secondary condition, thrombocytopenia occurs in leukemia (especially the acute variety), in marrow aplasia, in hypersplenism, and after the administration of certain drugs.

Bleeding Due to Defects in the Clotting Mechanism

Clotting mechanism defects are manifested by massive bleeding into the tissues and from the body orifices. Purpura is unusual, but intractable postoperative hemorrhage is characteristic and serious: fatal bleeding can occur even after a trivial operation or injury.

The following disorders are important.

Hemophilia A. A hereditary disease characterized by spontaneous or traumatic hemorrhages, this is due to a deficiency of factor VIII. The classic form of the disease affects males only because it is inherited as an X-linked recessive trait. However, the disease is more heterogeneous than is commonly supposed. The disease may be mild in some families and severe in others. Female carriers may show some bleeding tendency. In the classic severe case, bleeding is severe; a special feature is bleeding into joints (hemarthrosis), which is usually recurrent and leads to extensive damage to the affected joints. The disease can now be treated by giving the patient preparations of plasma containing concentrated factor VIII.

Hemophilia B or Christmas Disease. This condition is due to a deficiency of factor IX. Its mode of inheritance and clinical manifestations are indistinguishable from those of hemophilia A.

Von Willebrand's Disease. This is a common hereditary clotting disorder, but its manifestations vary from one family to another. There is a defect in factor VIII, but its precise nature has eluded detection, for in addition to affecting clotting, there is a platelet defect. The clinical features reflect this combined clotting and platelet defect. Bleeding from the mucous membranes is more common than in hemophilia, but like that disease, there is a tendency for bleeding to occur into joints as well as postoperatively.

Deficiencies of the Vitamin K–Dependent Coagulation Factors. The two common causes are liver failure and a deficiency of vitamin K. This vitamin is used by the liver for the synthesis of prothrombin as well as for the synthesis of other clotting factors. The vitamin is fat soluble, and its absorption is aided by the presence of bile salts. Consequently, it is poorly absorbed in obstructive jaundice, and this is one of the factors in the bleeding tendency that complicates obstructive jaundice and chronic liver disease.

Vitamin K deficiency also occurs in the newborn because of an inability of the infant to synthesize the vitamin in its bowel. If the mother's intake is also deficient, a serious bleeding state may occur, *hemorrhagic disease of the newborn*. Another cause of hypoprothrombinemia is the administration of dicumarol anticoagulants, which inhibit the synthesis of clotting factors in the liver. These drugs are used as a treatment of phlebothrombosis and myocardial infarction.

Hypofibrinogenemia. A deficiency of fibrinogen is usually acquired as a result of tissue factor entering the circulation. Such an event sets up intravascular clotting, causing the residual blood to become incoagulable. In addition, there is usually an activation of plasminogen so that fibrinolysis and fibrinogen destruction occur together with the clotting. The condition is called *disseminated intravascular coagulation, consumptive coagulopathy,* or the *defibrination syndrome* and is characterized by severe bleeding. It is encountered most commonly as a complication of pregnancy, when amniotic fluid enters the circulation and sets up both clotting and fibrinolysis. It also follows severe trauma, lung operations, and incompatible blood transfusions. The condition is an uncommon feature of widespread disseminated cancer.

IMPORTANT TESTS IN BLEEDING DISEASES

Platelet Count. The normal platelet count is 150 to 440 × 10^9/L.

Clotting Time. This is the time taken for a specimen of whole blood to clot *in vitro* at 37°C (98.6°F). The normal time is 5 to 10 minutes. The clotting time is prolonged if there is a deficiency in any of the factors involved in the intrinsic clotting system or in the common pathway. The test is insensitive, and a normal result can be obtained even in the presence of a very low level of some clotting factors. The clotting time is prolonged when a circulating anticoagulant such as heparin is present in excess. The test is therefore widely used to control heparin therapy. The

Table 18–4 THE BLEEDING DISEASES

Disease	Platelet Count	Clotting Time	Bleeding Time	Capillary Fragility Test	Partial Thromboplastin Time	Prothrombin Time
Primary thrombocyto-penic purpura	↓	N	↑	↑	N	N
Hemophilia	N	↑	N	N	↑	N
Christmas disease	N	↑	N	N	↑	N
Deficiency of the vita-min K–dependent coagulation factors	N	N	N	N	↑	↑
Disseminated intravas-cular coagulation	↓	↑	↑	↑	↑	↑

clotting time is greatly prolonged in hemophilia A and Christmas disease.

Bleeding Time. The time taken for a small skin puncture to stop bleeding is termed the *bleeding time.* It varies from 1 to 9 minutes and is prolonged when there is a lack of platelets. It is normal in hemophilia, but it is prolonged in thrombocytopenia.

Capillary Fragility Test. A sphygmomanometer (blood pressure) cuff is placed around the arm and inflated to a pressure of 100 mm Hg for 5 minutes. If the test is positive, the skin of the arm below the cuff shows a petechial eruption. A positive test indicates platelet deficiency, because normally the platelets seal off any defects caused by a sudden rise in blood pressure. The test is also positive if the vessels themselves are abnormal, *e.g.,* in scurvy.

Partial Thromboplastin Time (PTT). This is the time required for plasma to clot in a glass tube when an extract of brain, called *cephalin,* is added in the presence of calcium chloride. The cephalin provides excess phospholipid and makes the test independent of the platelet count.

The PTT is a sensitive measure of the factors concerned in the intrinsic and common pathways.

Prothrombin Time (PT). In this test, equal amounts of brain extract containing tissue factor, calcium chloride, and plasma are incubated, and the time required for clotting to occur is recorded. The test is measured against the time needed for a normal sample of plasma to clot. The prothrombin time is a measure of the factors concerned in the extrinsic system (factor VII) and in the common pathway (factors X, VII, and prothrombin). The intrinsic system is bypassed.

The PT and PTT together can give a fair indication of the nature of a clotting defect (Fig. 18–8 and Table 18–4). If both PTT and PT are normal, the defect is probably in the vessels or in the platelets. If either PTT or PT is prolonged, there is probably a defect in the clotting system. If both PTT and PT are abnormal, the defect is most likely in the common pathway. If the PTT is prolonged and the PT is normal, the defect is probably in the intrinsic system. The combination of a prolonged PT and a normal PTT is rare and indicates a deficiency of factor VII.

The Blood Groups and Blood Transfusion

THE BLOOD GROUPS

The red blood cells contain many antigens, but for practical purposes, those concerned with the ABO and Rhesus blood groups are the most important.

The ABO System

Antigens of the ABO system are glycoproteins and are derived from a basic antigen called the H substance. Under the influence of the *A* or *B* gene, the H substance is converted into either A or B antigen. At birth, there are no corresponding antibodies in the plasma, but within 6 months, the antibodies corresponding to the antigens not present in the red blood cells make their appearance. These antibodies, called *alloantibodies,* are capable of agglutinating the red blood cells of normal people who are of a different blood group and of not agglutinating the red blood cells of persons having the same blood group as that of the individual tested. The following table describes the distribution of ABO antigens and antibodies.

Blood Group	Antibodies Normally Present in Plasma
A	anti-B
B	anti-A
AB	none
O	anti-A and anti-B

The naturally occurring antibodies probably develop as a result of blood group–specific substances that are produced by bacteria in the intestine. The infant presumably forms antibodies against those antigens to which it is not immunologically tolerant.

To perform a blood grouping, one must treat a suspension of red blood cells with anti-A and anti-B sera, each derived from a donor with a high titer of these antibodies. If anti-A serum alone agglutinates the cells, the sample is of blood group A; if anti-B serum alone does it, the sample is of blood group B. If the cells are agglutinated by both anti-A and anti-B, the sample is of group AB, and if by neither anti-A nor anti-B, the sample is of group O. Similarly, with stock suspensions of cells of known blood group, it is possible to detect the appropriate antibodies in the patient's serum and to do the "reverse grouping."

The Rhesus System

About 85 per cent of the white population of the world has a red blood cell antigen that was first noted in Rhesus monkey red cells. This is called the Rh antigen; cells containing it are called Rhesus-positive (or Rh-positive). Rh-negative individuals do not normally have Rh antibodies in their plasma, but if they are immunized by Rh-positive cells, they may form antibodies very easily. Such immunization can follow a mismatched blood transfusion or can occur after the pregnancy of an Rh-negative woman bearing an Rh-positive fetus. Many Rhesus antigens have been discovered: C, D, E, c, among others. The most important of these is D; cells containing it correspond to the original Rh-positive cells.

Other Blood Groups

Human red blood cells contain many antigens other than those belonging to either the ABO or the Rh systems. Occasionally, antibodies to these antigens are a cause of transfusion reaction.

BLOOD TRANSFUSION

Indications

Blood transfusion is an essential and common procedure in clinical practice. Not only is it mandatory for restoring the blood volume after severe hemorrhage, but it is also used extensively in major operative procedures. In anemia, packed cells should be given rather than whole blood, which contains unwanted plasma. Surplus plasma can always be used by blood banks for other purposes, such as the preparation of factor VIII concentrates. Whenever possible, it is desirable to treat anemia with the specific agent in short supply, *i.e.,* iron or vitamin B_{12}, unless the patient's life is in danger.

Various blood components are available from transfusion centers; these are useful in restoring deficient clotting factors, such as factor VIII in hemophilia A.

Cross Matching

The important elements to consider are the donor's red blood cells and the recipient's plasma. As a general rule, the donor's plasma is not important because, with rare exceptions, the antibodies it contains are so diluted by the recipient's plasma that they are not likely to react with the recipient's cells. It is always preferable to use the blood of exactly the same ABO and

Rh groups as those of the recipient, but group O Rh-negative blood can be given in an acute emergency in which delay might lead to death from exsanguination (extensive blood loss). Under all other circumstances, a cross matching is essential. To do this matching, cells of the donor are mixed with the serum of the recipient; no agglutination should occur.

Hazards of Blood Transfusion

Incompatibility Reactions. These are usually due to the rapid destruction of the donor's red blood cells by the recipient's plasma such as when group A cells are transfused into a group O patient. The antigen-antibody reaction leads to agglutination of the red blood cells, causing blockage of capillaries, the release of vasoconstrictor substances, and widespread vascular phenomena. There is initial pain along the vein, followed by facial flushing, headache, a sense of constriction around the chest, and backache. In severe cases, renal vascular spasm combined with free hemoglobin in the blood leads to acute renal failure and death from uremia.

Bacterial Contamination of the Blood. This is usually due to the accidental introduction of coliform organisms in the transfusion fluid.

Diseases Introduced from the Donor. The most important of these are human immunodeficiency virus (HIV), viral hepatitis, syphilis, and malaria.

Febrile Reactions. These are usually due to the presence in the recipient of anti–white blood cell antibodies that have been formed as a result of previous transfusions or pregnancy. This type of febrile reaction may be quite severe, but it generally responds to simple treatment such as the administration of aspirin. Although febrile reactions themselves are of little importance, each must be investigated; fever, although not dangerous in itself, may be a component of an incompatible transfusion. Future transfusions can be given with blood from which the white blood cells have been removed in order to avoid additional febrile reactions.

Febrile reactions may be also due to the presence of gram-negative endotoxin present either in the transfusion fluid or in the apparatus.

Modern disposable apparatus and properly prepared fluids have largely eliminated this complication.

Allergic Reactions. These are usually urticarial and are due to some antigen present in the donor's plasma to which the recipient is hypersensitive.

Overloading the Circulation. Transfusing an excess volume of blood can lead to heart failure and can be avoided by slow transfusion. Pulmonary edema is the usual manifestation of this complication.

Air Embolism. With modern equipment, this is a rare event.

Thrombophlebitis. This response (inflammation of a vein with associated thrombus formation) follows the local irritation of the vein by the needle or cannula.

Transfusional Hemosiderosis. Repeated transfusions are liable to lead to iron overload with hemosiderin deposited in many tissues, including the liver, where it may set up fibrosis.

Sensitization. The transfusion of blood carrying antigens not present in the recipient may stimulate the production of alloantibodies against the foreign antigens. These alloantibodies to red blood cells, white blood cells, platelets, or plasma protein antigens may complicate future transfusions or pregnancies (see also hemolytic disease of the newborn, mentioned earlier).

Graft Versus Host Reaction. This uncommon complication occurs when viable white blood cells are transfused into an immunologically deficient host.

In modern centers, blood transfusion is a lifesaving procedure, but it must never be forgotten that the possible complications are numerous and occasionally fatal. Except under emergency conditions, transfusion should never be attempted without expert supervision. Any patient receiving a blood transfusion must be carefully and repeatedly watched so that the early signs of any complication can be detected. The nursing attendants play a vital role in the teamwork that transfusion requires. A particular function that deserves special stress involves the correct identification of specimens. More serious complications of blood transfusion result from giving a unit of blood to the wrong patient than are due to errors of grouping or cross matching. The wrong Smith can soon become a dead Smith!

Summary

- The blood cells are all derived from a totipotential common stem cell, but each normally arises from a stem cell of more restricted potential.
- Red blood cell abnormality is detected by measuring absolute values and examining a well-stained blood film for atypical shape, staining, or immaturity.
- Anemia may be acute posthemorrhagic, iron deficiency (dietary, chronic blood loss), megaloblastic (dietary, malabsorption, gastric defect with pernicious anemia), or hemolytic.
- Hemolytic anemia may be due to corpuscular defect (the hemoglobinopathies, thalassemia syndromes, enzyme-deficient red blood cells) or extracorpuscular defect (autoimmune, infections, drugs, burns, red blood cell fragmentation syndrome).
- Polycythemia may be secondary to hypoxia or primary.
- Measurement of the white blood cell count is helpful in diagnosing many diseases. A neutrophil leukocytosis is common in infection, a lymphocytosis may indicate infectious mononucleosis, a monocytosis occurs in protozoal and chronic infections, and an eosinophilia occurs in atopic diseases and helminthic infections.
- Leukemia may be chronic (myelogenous or lymphocytic) or acute. Many subdivisions are now recognized, and each type has characteristic findings.
- The myelodysplastic syndromes are related to leukemia and show abnormal maturation of myeloid cells, erythroid cells, and megakaryocytes.
- Bone marrow aplasia may cause pancytopenia or affect one element only, *e.g.*, agranulocytosis. Drugs are an important cause.
- The clotting mechanism involves an intrinsic system, an extrinsic system, and a common pathway. Defects may occur at any point and often result in a bleeding disease. Hemophilia A and B and von Willebrand's disease are important inherited diseases. Disseminated intravascular coagulation is a common acquired example.
- Bleeding can also be due to abnormalities of the blood vessels or platelets (usually thrombocytopenia).
- Blood transfusion involves matching the cells of the donor (with respect to ABO and Rhesus groupings) with the plasma of the recipient. Complications include febrile reactions and hemosiderosis, but incompatibility reactions as a result of giving blood of the wrong group are generally due to a clerical error.

Selected Readings

Beck, W. S. (ed.): Hematology. 2nd ed. Boston, MIT Press, 1990.

Lee, G. R., et al.: Wintrobe's Clinical Hematology. 9th ed. Philadelphia, Lea and Febiger, 1990.

Williams, W. J., et al. (eds.): Hematology. 4th ed. New York, McGraw-Hill, 1990.

19

The Circulation:
General Considerations

**After studying this chapter, the student
should be able to:**

• Describe the three major fluid compartments of the
  body and indicate the volume of each in an average
  normal adult human being.

• Give an account of the factors that maintain the
  body's content of water at a constant level.
• Describe the causes and effects of the following
  conditions:
  (a) pure water deficiency;
  (b) pure water excess;
  (c) combined salt and water deficiency;
  (d) combined salt and water excess.
• Define ascites, hydrothorax, and anasarca.
• List the types and causes of localized edema.
• List the types and causes of generalized edema.
• Describe the effects of an acute hemorrhage and
  the compensatory mechanisms that ensue.
• List seven important types of shock and describe
  their pathogenesis.
• Discuss the concept of irreversible shock and
  describe its pathogenesis.
• Describe the acute phase response.
• Distinguish between primary and secondary
  systemic hypertension.
• List the complications of systemic hypertension.
• Describe the main pathologic and clinical features of
  malignant hypertension.
• Distinguish between platelet aggregation and platelet
  adhesiveness.
• Define thrombosis and distinguish it from blood
  clotting.
• Describe how endothelial cell damage leads to
  thrombosis.
• Outline the mechanism by which plasmin is formed.
• Describe the common causes of thrombosis in an
  artery and list the possible effects on the tissue
  supplied.
• Compare phlebothrombosis with thrombophlebitis in
  terms of their causes and effects.

- List the circumstances under which thrombosis can occur in the heart.
- Describe the possible fate of a thrombus.
- Define hypoxia and list the four types.
- Define ischemia and classify its causes.
- Define embolus and classify emboli according to their composition.
- Describe the effects of pulmonary emboli.
- Define pyemia and describe its causes and effects.
- Outline the causes and effects of fat embolism.
- Define infarction and describe the process as it occurs in the following organs:
  (a) heart;
  (b) spleen;
  (c) brain;
  (d) intestine.
- Give examples of complications caused by arterial spasm.

The function of the circulatory system is the maintenance of an adequate perfusion of blood to all tissues of the body. Each ventricular contraction ejects a quantity of blood into the aorta and causes a rise in systemic blood pressure. The aorta and its major branches are composed largely of elastic tissue; their expansion prevents an undue rise in pressure with each ventricular contraction (systole). The branches of these elastic vessels are the muscular arteries. It is by variation in the tone of their smooth muscle walls that the amount of blood supplied to the various organs and tissues can be altered. The muscular arteries subdivide repeatedly, with blood next reaching the arterioles. These small muscular vessels provide the final mechanism by which blood is distributed to the tissues in response to their individual needs. The distribution of blood is in part regulated by the autonomic nervous system that acts on the smooth muscle of the arteries and arterioles, and in part by local mechanisms by which chemical agents, such as bradykinin, are released and act locally.

The blood flow in the major arteries is pulsatile. The elasticity of these vessels and the high resistance provided by the arterioles reduce the pulsation, so that in the capillaries and veins, the blood flow is constant. It follows that blood escaping from damaged capillaries oozes out constantly, whereas blood from a cut artery spurts out.

The important features of the circulation are the presence of fluid, blood vessels that can retain the fluid, and a pump to ensure that the blood circulates and is maintained at a pressure adequate for ensuring its proper distribution. Diseases of the heart and blood vessels are described in the chapters that follow. This chapter describes some general features of the circulation and conditions that may affect it. Four topics are covered:

1. General considerations of water balance in relation to the volume of the circulating blood and fluid in the interstitial tissues.
2. The effects of hemorrhage and shock.
3. Hypertension.
4. Local abnormalities of the circulation leading to ischemia and thrombosis.

FLUID BALANCE

Water is the principal component of the body and forms about 70 per cent of the lean body weight. Since adipose tissue contains little water, it follows that the water content of the average person is about 60 per cent of the body weight. The body can be discussed in terms of three "compartments" (intracellular space, interstitial space, and plasma), which are illustrated in Figure 19–1. Each compartment is contained within a membrane that forms a barrier with particular permeability properties. Water is freely diffusible across these barriers so that the volume of each compartment is adjusted by osmotic, electrochemical, and hydrostatic forces. With regard to osmosis, potassium, phosphate, and protein are important in the intracellular compartment. The normal endothelium provides a smooth lining that aids the unhindered flow of blood and plays a vital part in governing the composition of the blood and the interstitial fluid.

The total water content of the body is maintained at a constant level by balancing intake with output. Water is derived mainly by drinking fluid, although some is contained in food and about 300 ml is derived from oxidative processes of metabolism. Fluid is lost in the urine (about 1500 ml per day); some is lost in the expired air (about 700 ml per day); some is lost in the feces (about 200 ml per day); and a moderate quantity is lost by transpiration from the skin (300 to 500 ml per day). The mechanism by which fluid

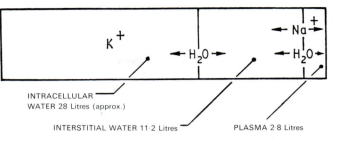

Figure 19–1 The fluid compartments of the body. This diagram shows the three compartments in which the body's water is accommodated. An excess or deficiency of water, which is freely diffusible, produces the greatest effects in the largest compartment—the intracellular space. Changes in sodium levels affect mainly the interstitial compartment.

INTRACELLULAR WATER 28 Litres (approx.)

INTERSTITIAL WATER 11·2 Litres

PLASMA 2·8 Litres

balance is attained can be considered under three headings.

Indirect Control. This includes the mechanisms that regulate sodium balance. Sodium cannot be retained without water (Fig. 19–2).

Aldosterone, a hormone secreted by the adrenal cortex, has the effect of increasing sodium reabsorption from the distal tubule of the kidney and thereby causes water retention as well. Sodium reabsorption from the proximal tubule is dependent to a large extent on the total glomerular filtrate. When the volume is reduced, as in shock and heart failure, sodium absorption is more complete, and water is also retained.

Renal Control. There are mechanisms that regulate the output of water by the kidney. The antidiuretic hormone from the posterior lobe of the pituitary gland is important in this regulation. It acts by increasing water reabsorption from the collecting tubules of the kidney.

Figure 19–2 Sodium retention. This diagram shows the means by which the body retains sodium after a sudden reduction in blood volume, *e.g.,* following a severe hemorrhage.

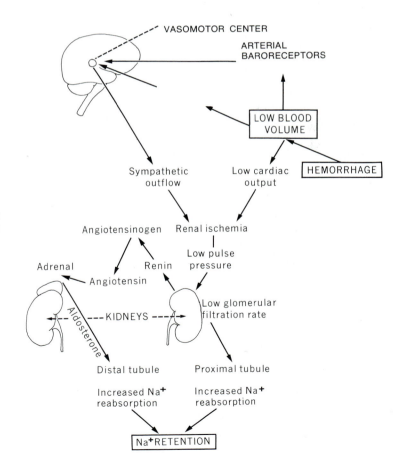

Thirst. Water intake is regulated by the sensation of thirst.

Water and sodium metabolism are so closely interrelated that it is convenient to consider them together.

Disturbances in Water and Sodium Balance

Pure Water Deficiency. This condition follows deprivation of water. It is seen in enforced starvation and in patients who are unable to swallow because of dysphagia, esophageal obstruction, or coma. It may complicate diabetes insipidus, a disease due to lack of antidiuretic hormone. Patients with this disease pass enormous quantities of urine, often 20 liters a day instead of the normal 1 to 1.5 liters.

Effects. Since water can easily cross the membranes that separate the various fluid compartments, each is depleted in volume. The intracellular space, which is the largest compartment, is the most severely affected. Cellular dehydration causes intense thirst and eventually death.

Pure Water Excess. Excessive retention of water is called *water intoxication* and causes intracellular edema. It is encountered in patients who are given too much water too quickly. Rapid intravenous infusion of glucose solution is the common culprit, but even a large enema can lead to water intoxication in a susceptible patient, such as one in renal failure or in the immediate postoperative period, when water excretion is impaired. The effects of water excess are serious. Intracellular edema of brain and muscle causes vomiting, muscle cramps, headaches, convulsions, and—ultimately—death.

Combined Salt and Water Deficiency. Salt, or salt and water, deficiency is a common condition that is seen when there is a loss from the gastrointestinal tract, such as after severe vomiting or diarrhea; the skin, such as after prolonged excessive sweating; and the kidney, such as after prolonged administration of diuretics for heart failure.

Effects. The effect of salt—or salt and water—deficiency is a reduction in the volume of the extracellular fluids. The interstitial fluid volume is reduced in amount, and the patient shows the clinical features of dehydration. The eyeballs are sunken, the skin is wrinkled, the tongue is dry, and the face is haggard. Surprisingly, thirst is often absent. The plasma volume is decreased, but vasoconstriction compensates for this. Since the veins are poorly filled, the blood pressure ultimately drops. Little urine is passed, and renal failure may be superadded. The reduction in plasma volume is detectable by a rise in the hemoglobin concentration (hemoconcentration). Unless relieved, this condition rapidly terminates in circulatory failure.

Combined Salt and Water Excess. This is invariably an artificially induced condition that is seen in patients with defective renal function who are given excessive amounts of saline solution, such as during the early postoperative period or during the course of acute renal failure.

Effect. The excess fluid is distributed mainly in the extracellular compartments, which therefore expand. The manifestations of this are an increased venous pressure and edema, both systemic and pulmonary.

EDEMA

As usually used, the term "edema" can be defined as an excessive accumulation of fluid in the interstitial tissues. Fluid is also particularly liable to collect in the various serous sacs, giving rise to *ascites, hydrothorax,* and *hydropericardium* (terms applied to effusions into the peritoneal, pleural, and pericardial sacs, respectively). When edema is generalized, it is called *dropsy* or *anasarca*. Of course, it is possible to have intracellular edema, as in hydropic degeneration of cells and in pure water intoxication. The remainder of this section, however, is devoted to types of interstitial edema.

It is necessary first to understand the normal mechanisms regulating the distribution of fluid in the body.

Starling postulated that the movement of fluid between vessels and the extravascular spaces was determined by the balance of the hydrostatic and osmotic forces acting upon it (see Fig. 5–1).

Forces tending to move fluid out of the blood vessels are the following:

1. *The hydrostatic pressure within the vessels.*

2. *The colloid osmotic pressure of the interstitial fluid.*

Since the vascular wall is completely permeable to water and crystalloids, the only effective osmotic forces acting across the vessel wall are due to colloids—mainly protein—to which the vessel wall is not permeable. The interstitial fluids normally have a low protein content, and this is therefore not an important factor in the formation of the extravascular fluids under normal circumstances. Furthermore, those proteins that do escape from the blood vessels into the interstitial tissue spaces are removed by the lymphatic vessels.

Forces tending to move the fluid into the blood vessels are the following:

1. *The tissue tension.* This is normally low (3 to 4 mm Hg). Tissue tension is important in determining the distribution of edema. Thus, edema readily occurs in lax tissues such as the eyelids, over the sacrum, and in the genital area (Fig. 19–3). Tense tissues like the palms and soles do not readily become edematous. A rise in tissue tension is an important factor in limiting interstitial tissue fluid formation in the legs under normal conditions as well as in acutely inflamed parts.

2. *The osmotic pressure of the plasma proteins.* This pressure is normally about 25 mm Hg and is due mainly to albumin. Since albumin does not normally pass through the vessel walls, the vascular permeability is important in regulating the distribution of fluids between the intravascular and extravascular compartments. In the event of an increase in the permeability, such as that occurring in acute inflammation, an exudate rich in protein is formed.

There are two types of edema:

Exudate. This is an accumulation of fluid in acute inflammation and is due to an increased vascular permeability. The fluid contains a high percentage of protein and has virtually the same composition as plasma.

Transudate. This is an accumulation of fluid due to hydrostatic imbalance between the intravascular and extravascular compartments. Since it occurs in the presence of a normal vascular permeability, the protein content of the fluid is low.

The importance of the lymphatic vessels

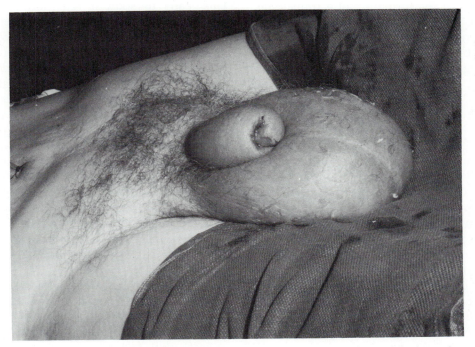

Figure 19–3 Severe edema of the scrotum and penis. The patient shows severe edema of the loose tissues of the scrotum and penis, whereas the more compact tissues of the thigh and abdominal wall are less affected.

should be remembered in any discussion of edema. They form an elaborate closed network in most tissues, and their function is to drain away fluid and protein.

Types of Edema

When considering the cause of any type of edema, one should realize that the process is usually due to a combination of factors. Starling, who appreciated this, stated that dropsy was probably never due to the derangement of a single mechanism acting alone.

Edema can be classified into local and generalized types. The localized varieties are the simplest to understand because there are fewer factors involved in their pathogenesis.

Local Edema

Acute Inflammatory Edema. This condition has been described in Chapter 5.

Hypersensitivity. Edema is present in the lesions of type I and type III hypersensitivity reactions and in severe type IV reactions. It is due to an increase in vascular permeability.

Venous Obstruction. A rise in venous pressure leads to an increase in capillary pressure, which in turn results in the formation of a transudate. Edema of the gut occurs in a strangulated hernia and in mesenteric venous thrombosis. It is this edema that causes further vascular impairment later resulting in infarction.

Lymphatic Edema. Extensive lymphatic obstruction can produce an edema of high protein content. Because chronic lymphatic edema of the limbs stimulates connective tissue overgrowth, in due course there is such enlargement of the skin and subcutaneous tissues that the part becomes grossly distorted. This resulting grotesque deformity is called *elephantiasis.* It occurs in the legs as a complication of the lymphangitis from any cause but is particularly severe in the lymphangitis associated with filariasis (Chapter 10). A similar condition can occur as a result of congenitally deformed lymphatics. Lymphedema of an arm is occasionally encountered as a complication of cancer of the breast when the lymphatic vessels are blocked either by tumor or by the fibrosis induced by radiotherapy.

Generalized Edema

Cardiac Edema. In congestive heart failure, there is retention of sodium and water that is first evident as an increase in body weight and later as a detectable edema. The distribution of this fluid is influenced by gravity. When the patient is ambulant, the legs are affected first, and swelling of the ankles is often the initial symptom. When the patient is in bed, the edema appears in the sacral and genital areas (Fig. 19–3). Firm pressure by a finger in an edematous area results in the formation of a pit that remains when the finger is removed. This "pitting edema" is characteristic of most forms of edema. Lymphedema is a major exception.

Renal Edema
Acute Glomerulonephritis. Edema is often the first symptom of acute post-streptococcal glomerulonephritis (Chapter 25). The edema is often most apparent on the face and eyelids, but ankles and genitalia may also be affected. The reduced glomerular blood flow leads to a reduction in glomerular filtration rate, and this in turn causes sodium and water retention.

Nephrotic Syndrome. The marked edema of the nephrotic syndrome is to a large extent due to the low plasma albumin level. In addition, there is a reduced blood volume, which stimulates the secretion of aldosterone from the adrenal cortex. This leads to sodium retention and therefore water retention. Hence, a salt-free diet, especially combined with a diuretic, causes considerable reduction in the amount of edema present.

Famine Edema (Nutritional Edema). The edema that is seen after prolonged starvation is usually confined to the legs. At first sight, it would seem explicable in terms of the marked hypoalbuminemia that is usually present; on closer examination, however, one finds that there is no close correlation between the level of plasma proteins and the presence of edema. The precise explanation of famine edema is not known. An important factor appears to be loss of compact tissue—mostly fat—and its replacement by a loose connective tissue in which fluid can accumulate readily without any undue rise in tissue tension.

Marked edema is a feature of kwashiorkor.

Unexplained Edema. Generalized edema sometimes occurs in the absence of any known cause. Although such cases are uncommon, they indicate that factors other than those already discussed may operate even in the common types of edema. A well-recognized condition, *cyclical* *periodic edema*, presents with recurrent attacks of edema involving skin, mucous membranes, and even internal organs. When the area involved is delimited to the subcutaneous tissues, it is called *angioedema*. The immediate cause of edema appears to be an increase in vascular permeability, but the precise cause is not known. In chronic urticaria, there is edema of the dermis; again, the cause is rarely discovered.

Generalized edema is sometimes seen in terminal states, particularly in cirrhosis of the liver. The blood pressure is often low, and attempts to raise it and maintain an adequate urinary output by the administration of fluid only worsen the situation and increase the amount of edema. The mechanisms involved are complex and are not well understood.

Pulmonary Edema. This condition is considered in Chapter 22.

HEMORRHAGE

Hemorrhage is defined as the escape of blood from the vascular system. The extravasated blood may escape to the exterior, or it may remain internal.

Effects of Acute Hemorrhage

The effects of blood loss depend on the quantity of blood lost and the speed at which the loss occurs. If a small quantity of blood is lost suddenly, there is scarcely any effect on the circulation because the large venous system acts as a reservoir for blood. Consequently, when a small amount is lost, an increase in venous tone reduces the capacity of the venous system, so that there is no reduction in the volume of blood reaching the heart (the venous return). Thus, there is no reduction in the cardiac output. When a larger volume of blood is suddenly withdrawn, this reserve mechanism of the venous reservoir is inadequate. The venous return is diminished, the cardiac output falls, and the blood pressure would also fall were there no other compensatory mechanisms available. The next response to hemorrhage is a series of reactions designed to prevent any fall in blood pressure.

Mechanisms for Maintenance of the Blood Pressure

After severe hemorrhage, the fall in blood pressure is detected by the pressure-sensitive carotid sinus and other baroreceptors; these reflexly initiate a sympathetic outflow from the central nervous system (Fig. 19–4). The result is an increase in heart rate and constriction of the arterioles of the *skin, kidneys,* and *splanchnic area* both by direct action and by the indirect action of the adrenal medulla, which is stimulated to secrete epinephrine and norepinephrine. In addition, the reduced blood pressure acts on the kidney directly and causes a release of renin. These mechanisms lead to an overall increase in the peripheral resistance, so that even with a reduced cardiac output, the systemic blood pressure is maintained at normal or near-normal levels. The maintenance of an adequate blood pressure allows the blood flow to the brain, the heart, and the respiratory muscles to remain virtually unaltered. However, the areas affected by arteriolar vasoconstriction tend to suffer; for example, the *skin* is cold and pale, the *kidneys* show a reduced urinary output *(oliguria)*, and salivary gland secretion decreases, resulting in dryness of the mouth. Thus, the vasomotor response to acute hemorrhage causes a redistribution of blood, a mechanism that may be regarded as an emergency measure designed to keep the essential organs supplied with blood.

Restoration of Blood Volume

During the first few hours after bleeding, the extravascular fluids pass into the blood stream, thereby restoring the blood volume. This can be demonstrated quite easily by checking the hemoglobin levels at intervals. Immediately after a sudden hemorrhage, the hemoglobin level is normal. During the next 8 hours, it falls as dilution occurs. This process is largely complete by the end of 48 hours, by which time the hemoglobin level is a good guide to the extent of a previous blood loss. The transfer of extracellular fluid to the blood stream occurs as a result of the reduced capillary hydrostatic pressure, which is secondary to arteriolar vasocon-

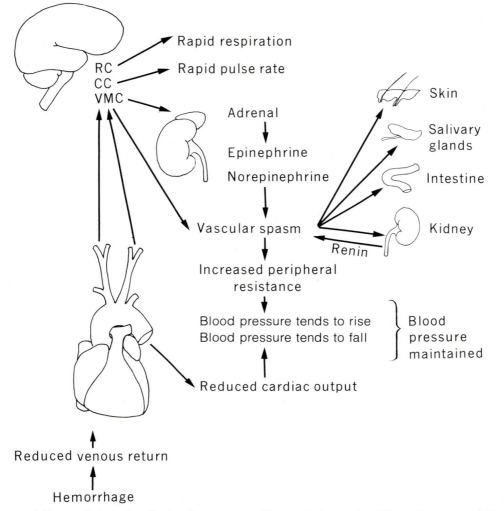

Figure 19–4 The cardiovascular effects of hemorrhage. (RC, respiratory center; CC, cardiac center; VMC, vasomotor center.)

striction. Complete restoration of the plasma volume is dependent on replacement of the lost plasma proteins. These are manufactured for the most part in the liver and enter the circulation via the thoracic duct.

Changes in the Blood

Within a few minutes of bleeding, the clotting time is considerably decreased; during the next few hours, there is an increase in the level of platelets and neutrophils, which persists for several days. The restoration of the red blood cell count is a slow process, since the body has no reserve store of erythrocytes. New red blood cells have to be manufactured, and a normal count is not attained until 4 to 6 weeks later, regardless of the severity of the blood loss.

A normal adult can lose 500 ml of blood quite rapidly with little discomfort, a fact attested to by millions of blood donors. A sudden loss of 30 to 50 per cent of the blood volume (1.5 to 2.5 liters) can be fatal. However, such a loss spread over a day or so can be tolerated if the compensatory mechanism keeps pace with the blood loss. When the compensatory mechanisms are inadequate for this purpose, the patient sinks into a state described as shock, and this may be fatal.

Shock

Shock is seen after many forms of injury; it may occur immediately, or it may happen after a period of comparative well-being. The patient lies still and listlessly; the temperature is subnormal, the skin cold and clammy, and the face ashen. Obvious cyanosis is often present, the blood pressure is low, and the pulse is rapid and thready. Little or no urine is passed.

In shock, there is an inadequate blood supply to many tissues, leading to tissue hypoxia, metabolic acidosis, and defective function of the tissues concerned. Liver, lungs, heart, and kidneys are commonly affected, but under particular circumstances, the effects of ischemia of other tissues (*e.g.*, retina, pituitary, and pancreas) may dominate the situation.

The clinical picture of shock may occur in a variety of conditions, and not surprisingly, these have all been assembled under the all-embracing title of "shock." Conditions that lead to a state of shock include *loss of blood, trauma, loss of plasma* (*e.g.*, following burns), *loss of fluid and electrolytes, overwhelming infection, acute heart failure, and generalized anaphylaxis.* The inclusion of so many diverse conditions under the one heading of shock has tended to obscure our understanding of the condition. They all produce a similar clinical picture, but it is hardly to be expected that the mechanisms involved would be the same in each case. Furthermore, a state of shock can occur as a terminal event under many other circumstances, *e.g.*, after electrocution, overdose of drugs, drowning, or massive total body irradiation. To attempt to understand shock, one must consider each condition separately.

Hemorrhagic Shock. If the compensatory mechanisms that follow bleeding are inadequate to maintain an effective perfusion of the tissues of the body, a state of shock ensues (Fig. 19–5). Recovery may occur spontaneously or as a result of efficient treatment, such as transfusion; such shock is therefore said to be *reversible*. Occasion-

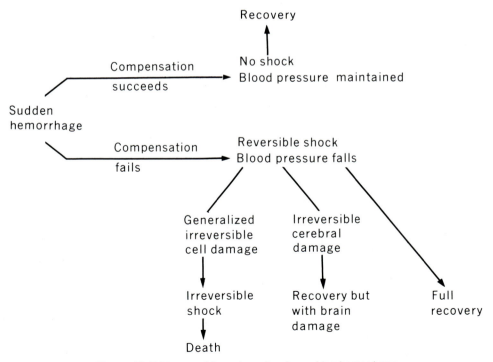

Figure 19–5 The possible end results of a sudden hemorrhage.

ally, in spite of efficient, vigorous treatment, the blood pressure continues to fall, the patient's clinical condition deteriorates, and death ensues. This response, termed *irreversible* (or *decompensated*) *shock,* is considered later.

Traumatic Shock. The circulatory changes that follow trauma are very similar to those seen after hemorrhage. The possible mechanisms are the following.

Hemorrhage. It is often not appreciated that there is considerable bleeding into the tissues after any injury, even closed injuries such as a fractured femur. Much of the swelling that is seen around the fracture is due to blood that has poured into the adjacent tissues; some is due to inflammatory exudate, itself derived from the blood.

Infection. There is little doubt that the powerful exotoxins of the pathogenic clostridia exert a profound shocking effect. Gas gangrene, even in the absence of substantial tissue damage, causes shock and death.

Endotoxic Factor. The intravenous injection of endotoxins of the gram-negative bacilli leads to a shocklike state in animals. This is particularly marked following a second injection 24 hours after a previous one. The mechanism is not well understood, and the phenomenon is known as the Shwartzman phenomenon. Patients whose wounds are infected with gram-negative coliforms can suddenly develop shock as a result of endotoxemia or septicemia (*"septic shock"*).

Inflammatory Exudate Formation. The outpouring of fluid into inflamed tissues is responsible for some of the swelling around injured parts and adds its quota to that of bleeding as a cause of reduction in blood volume.

In summary, *blood loss is the single most important factor in causing traumatic shock.*

Shock Following Thermal Burns. The severe shock that follows burns is largely related to the tremendous loss of plasma in the inflammatory exudate. At a later stage, bacterial infection, such as that with *Pseudomonas aeruginosa* and other coliforms, may play a part. An important point of difference from hemorrhagic shock is that there is concentration, rather than dilution, of blood. The hemoglobin level rises owing to this hemoconcentration.

Shock due to Loss of Water and Electrolytes.

Loss of water or sodium can lead to such depletion of the extracellular tissue fluids that unless replacement therapy is instituted, shock can develop as a result of an inadequate volume of circulating plasma. This condition is seen after persistent vomiting due to pyloric stenosis or intestinal obstruction, in cholera, and in any severe diarrhea (particularly in children).

Shock in Infection. Shock is seen in a variety of infections. It is prominent in infections with the toxic organisms of diphtheria and gas gangrene, and it is also a feature of many other severe infections: pneumonia, peritonitis, typhoid fever, typhus, and others of a similar nature. In recent years, a new syndrome—endotoxic shock—has been recognized; it is caused by the sudden entry of gram-negative coliform organisms or their endotoxins into the circulation. It is a complication of any coliform infection and is usually a sequel to urinary tract infection. There is a sudden onset of profound shock; unless treated expeditiously, it causes high mortality.

The shock of infection has a complex pathogenesis: at least three factors must be considered:

1. *Pooling of blood.* Blood is sequestered in the splanchnic area because of vasodilation. The effective blood volume is thereby reduced.

2. *Loss of fluid in inflammatory exudate.* In gas gangrene, the profuse loss of protein-rich exudate is in part responsible for the hemoconcentration and the reduction of blood volume.

3. *Heart failure.* Some bacterial toxins (*e.g.,* diphtheria toxin) damage the myocardium, and an element of heart failure may further embarrass an already failing circulation.

Cardiogenic Shock. Extensive myocardial infarction, sudden severe cardiac dysrhythmias, rupture of a valve cusp, and the sudden accumulation of fluid or blood in the pericardium can sometimes lead to a state of shock resembling shock that follows trauma. This condition results from a low cardiac output, for it leads to underperfusion of tissues as an initial effect, and the resulting metabolic acidosis (see following) causes peripheral vasodilation and pooling of blood. The shock that follows massive pulmonary embolism has a similar pathogenesis.

Anaphylactic Shock. Generalized anaphylaxis

occurs when an individual, already sensitized by IgE, encounters the specific sensitizing antigen. See Chapter 6 for a more complete discussion.

The Metabolic Upset During Shock

A patient in shock shows a profound reduction in metabolic rate (the nature of which is not well understood), but this reduction appears to be related to a block in carbohydrate utilization. In spite of cutaneous vasoconstriction, and therefore a reduction in heat loss, the patient's temperature tends to fall. An important effect of shock is that the underperfusion of tissues results in anaerobic glycolysis with the release of pyruvic and lactic acids into the circulation. A *metabolic acidosis* is characteristic of shock.

The Acute Phase Response. Whenever there is tissue damage and inflammation, changes occur in the blood that are known as the acute phase response. There is a dramatic rise in the blood levels of C-reactive protein and serum amyloid A protein. A lesser rise occurs in fibrinogen, whereas the albumin falls. These changes are reflected in a rise in the erythrocyte sedimentation rate. The acute phase response results from the release of interleukin-1 by macrophages. It acts on the liver, where these proteins are manufactured; it also acts on muscle to increase protein metabolism and the hypothalamus to cause fever. These changes are all seen in shock.

Summary of the Pathogenesis of Shock

It is evident that shock is essentially a state in which there is underperfusion of tissues. Shock may be mediated by the following.

Hypovolemia. A low blood volume can occur after hemorrhage (external or internal); external loss of water and electrolytes (resulting from vomiting, diarrhea, diabetes insipidus, or the excessive use of diuretics); rapid accumulation of inflammatory exudate (from burns and infection); and dehydration (heat exhaustion and inadequate fluid intake). If there is hemoconcentration, the increase in blood viscosity further impedes the peripheral circulation.

Reduction of Effective Blood Volume due to

Internal Sequestration. Peripheral vasodilation can result in pooling of blood so that the effective volume of circulating blood is decreased. The splanchnic area and skeletal muscle are the sites where vasodilation commonly occurs. This state has been called *peripheral circulatory failure* and is encountered particularly in endotoxic shock and metabolic acidosis.

Cardiac Factors. A state of low output can result from acute heart failure or from mechanical problems such as cardiac tamponade.

Sludging. If the flowing blood of a patient in shock is observed with a microscope, it will be seen that the red blood cells tend to flow in clumps rather than as individual cells. When this phenomenon was first described, the blood was said to be converted into a "mucklike sludge," from which comes the name *sludging*. The process differs from true agglutination in that the masses of red blood cells can be broken up mechanically *in vitro*. The cause of sludging appears to be an increase in the high-molecular-weight substance of the blood, and its effect is to impede the blood flow through tissues. Sludging therefore contributes to the poor perfusion of tissues in shock.

Irreversible Shock

Some patients with shock recover either spontaneously or as a result of treatment. Others steadily deteriorate in spite of all efforts to save them. It is commonly believed that there is a stage from which recovery becomes impossible. This is called *irreversible* or *decompensated shock*. The phenomenon can be demonstrated experimentally. If an animal is bled, it passes into a state of shock. It can be allowed to stay in a state of hypotensive hypovolemic shock for a few minutes and then be resuscitated by returning its own lost blood through a catheter. If the animal is allowed to stay in a state of shock for too long, the transfusion fails to reverse the shock, and its condition steadily deteriorates until death ensues.

The present concept of shock is that the major abnormality is the underperfusion of certain vital organs. If the state of shock is allowed to persist too long, there is permanent damage to tissues,

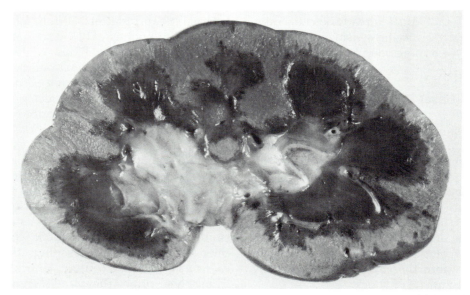

Figure 19–6 Cortical necrosis of the kidney. Specimen from a 40-year-old woman who died in renal failure shows necrosis of the outer two thirds to three fourths of the cortex. The inner layer of the cortex and the medulla are congested. This is the most severe type of ischemic renal damage encountered in shock. The condition affects both kidneys equally and is similar to the changes seen in the rabbit in the generalized Shwartzman phenomenon. For a more complete description, see Case History I. (From Walter, J. B., and Israel, M. S.: General Pathology. 6th ed. Edinburgh, Churchill Livingstone, 1987.)

and recovery is therefore impossible. The concept of irreversible shock as an entity is currently downplayed. One cannot deny that some patients reach a stage from which recovery is impossible, but the cause for this varies from case to case and is due to the summation of biochemical abnormalities, such as metabolic acidosis, and damage sustained by many tissues. Organs that show damage are the following.

Liver. It is common to find centrilobular necrosis in patients dying of shock.

Heart. Patchy myocardial infarction is common, and acute heart failure can be added to a state of shock produced by other mechanisms.

Lung. The important changes that take place in the lung are described in Chapter 22 (see Acute Adult Respiratory Insufficiency Syndrome).

Kidney. Oliguria and anuria are characteristic of shock. Acute tubular necrosis, which can become extensive, may lead to irreversible renal damage (Fig. 19–6).

Case History I

The patient was a 40-year-old woman who had had a normal pregnancy until the thirty-first week of ges-

tation. She was then found to be hypertensive (blood pressure raised to 240/120); she also developed abdominal pain and began to bleed from the vagina. Her condition was diagnosed as abruptio placentae (premature detachment of the placenta). An emergency cesarean section was performed, but it failed to save the child; there was also considerable loss of blood during the operation. The patient went into shock, developed anuria, and, in spite of peritoneal dialysis, experienced a rise in blood potassium to 7.0 mEq/liter (normal level is 3.5 to 5.5 mEq/liter). Her blood urea nitrogen also rose to 100 mg/dl (normal level is 10 to 20 mg/dl). She died in renal failure 8 days after the onset of symptoms (see Fig. 19–6).

Gastrointestinal Tract. Although the gastrointestinal tract is congested in shock, the blood flow through it is decreased. Patchy mucosal necrosis can occur in both the small and large intestine; the resultant bleeding may be severe and further complicate the clinical situation. Acute stress ulcers in the stomach and duodenum can cause further blood loss.

Pituitary. Infarction of the pituitary is best known as a complication of shock after labor.

Eye. Retinal ischemia can result in blindness.

Pancreas. Patchy pancreatitis is not uncommon, but it is usually silent clinically.

It is evident that death from shock may occur for many reasons, either as a result of damage to some organ or from a metabolic upset secondary to this damage. From a practical point of view, the efficiency of treatment is of overriding importance, because many of the potentially lethal causes and effects of shock can be counteracted. Irreversible shock must be regarded as being almost always due to inefficient treatment.

Syncope

Syncope is described before the important topic of shock is concluded because in the past it has been termed primary shock. However, except that it follows trauma, it has little in common with shock as previously described.

Syncope, or a vasovagal attack, is better known as the common faint. The subject is invariably standing up; the initial symptoms are giddiness and lightheadedness. Shortly after this, consciousness is lost and the subject falls to the ground. Pallor of the skin is a striking feature; the body is bathed in a cold sweat. The blood pressure is low, and the pulse is weak, with its rate either slowed or normal. Syncope can occur after blood loss, but it can also be caused by pain or psychological factors. The very thought of having an injection or having blood withdrawn is enough to send some people into a faint. It is believed that syncope is caused by sudden autonomic overactivity that leads to vasodilation in the muscles and pooling of blood there. The venous return is suddenly reduced and with it the cardiac output, blood pressure, and blood supply to the brain. The loss of consciousness in syncope is brief, and if the subject is laid horizontally, or attains that position spontaneously, recovery soon occurs. In rare cases, death may occur; at least this is one suggestion for the rare cases of sudden death that occur unexpectedly, such as when a needle is introduced into the pleural cavity or during an attempted abortion. It has been reported that syncope occurring during induction of anesthesia may be fatal if the anesthetic is administered with the patient in the upright position, such as in a dental chair.

SYSTEMIC HYPERTENSION

High blood pressure, or systemic hypertension, is a common condition that is often discovered accidentally during a routine medical examination. It is normal for the systemic blood pressure to rise as a response to emotion and physical exercise. If a raised pressure is discovered, it is wise to check the measurement after the patient has been at rest for some time and has grown accustomed to the surroundings. Another factor to consider is the age of the patient. As people get older, the aorta becomes less elastic; with each ventricular contraction, the systolic blood pressure rises rapidly. However, the blood drains away normally through the arterioles to the venous system, and the diastolic blood pressure remains normal. In systemic hypertension, the diastolic blood pressure rises. A rough guideline is that the systolic blood pressure should be less than 100 mm Hg plus age in years. There is, however, no sharp cut-off above which a patient may be regarded as having hypertension. A systolic pressure over 160 mm Hg with a sustained diastolic pressure over 95 mm Hg is usually taken as indicative of hypertension. The precise incidence of the disease is difficult to determine, but probably around 20 per cent of the population suffer from the disease to some extent or another.

Types of Hypertension

For practical purposes, two types of hypertension can be recognized: primary hypertension and secondary hypertension.

Primary, or Essential, Hypertension. This is the common form of high blood pressure, and it accounts for about 90 per cent of the cases. By definition, its cause is unknown. Although an increase in cardiac output may play some part in the pathogenesis of hypertension, it is generally assumed that the cause of the increased blood pressure is an increase in peripheral resistance to blood flow. It is a condition that is more common in women than in men, and it is especially prevalent in North American blacks. Primary renal or adrenal abnormalities have been postulated as causing this hypertension, but no conclusive evidence has been obtained.

Secondary Hypertension. About 10 per cent of cases of hypertension fall into this secondary group. Renal disease is by far the most common cause, but it is also a feature of pheochromocytoma, a rare tumor of the adrenal gland, and is due to the effects of epinephrine and norepinephrine, which are secreted by the tumor. The hypertension is characteristically episodic. Hypertension is also a feature of some adrenal cortical tumors.

Pathogenesis of Hypertension

As noted previously, it is generally assumed that the cause of the increased blood pressure is an increase in peripheral resistance to blood flow. Many experimental models have been investigated in attempts to elucidate the nature of this resistance to blood flow in essential hypertension.

The classic experiments of Goldblatt proved that in the dog, an obstruction to the renal artery blood flow could produce hypertension. This response is due to the release from the ischemic kidney of a proteolytic enzyme (called *renin*) that acts on a plasma globulin, angiotensinogen, to convert it into angiotensin I. Another plasma enzyme converts angiotensin I into angiotensin II, a peptide that induces vascular spasm and produces hypertension. Angiotensin II also stimulates the adrenal cortex to increase its secretion of aldosterone. This causes retention of sodium and water.

In humans, hypertension sometimes, but not always, occurs in acute and chronic glomerulonephritis, pyelonephritis, and other renal diseases. The mechanism producing the hypertension may or may not be similar to that operating in the Goldblatt experiment; present evidence is against such a pathogenesis because the plasma renin level is not elevated in the majority of cases. In chronic renal failure, retention of sodium and water leads to a rise in blood volume and cardiac output. Removal of sodium and water from the body by diuretics lowers the blood pressure. Hypertension with unilateral renal lesions, such as obstruction to the renal

artery, is sometimes relieved either by unilateral nephrectomy or by correction of the arterial stenosis. Unfortunately, this treatment is not always successful, presumably because secondary vascular events have taken place in the other kidney by the time diagnosis is made.

The pathogenesis of primary systemic hypertension is not known. Retention of sodium, increased blood volume, and a rise in cardiac output have been postulated. Peripheral vasoconstriction is assumed to be secondary to this. Alternatively, a primary increase in the peripheral resistance may be the mechanism. Evidence for this being mediated by the renin-angiotensin mechanism is poor. A primary defect in the autonomic nervous system has been postulated, but its nature is not known. Perhaps stress triggers the mechanism, as suggested by the finding that hypertension is more common in individuals exposed to a high level of stress. Another possibility is that an abnormal sensitivity of the vascular smooth muscle leads to excess constriction in response to normal levels of vasoconstrictor substances such as epinephrine and angiotensin. A high level of sodium in the cells may be involved. It is known that hypertension is more common in individuals and races that have a high dietary sodium intake. Finally, there is the possibility that genetic influences are of importance. These are not well defined, and it is generally stated that the tendency to develop hypertension is multifactorial.

Effects and Complications of Hypertension

These are summarized in Figure 19–7.

Hemorrhage. Weakened blood vessels tend to rupture more commonly in the hypertensive than in the normal subject; dissecting aneurysm of the aorta, ruptured berry aneurysm of the circle of Willis, and cerebral hemorrhage are all more common in the hypertensive subject.

Atherosclerosis. Atherosclerosis, with all its complications, is more common in patients with hypertension. Myocardial infarction and strokes bedevil the patient with hypertension.

Arteriolosclerosis. The small arteries of many organs show thickening of their walls, particu-

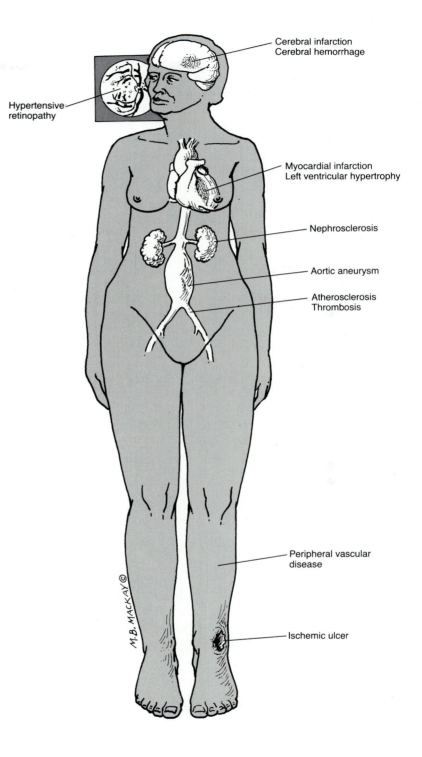

Figure 19–7 Complications of hypertension.

larly the tunica intima, with hyaline material. This thickening is most marked in the arterioles of the renal glomeruli; gradually, as these vessels close down, the glomeruli and tubules that they supply become atrophic and are replaced by fibrous tissue. This scarring of the kidney is termed *nephrosclerosis*.

The arterioles of the retina share in this generalized process. The thickening of their walls and resulting ischemic changes in the retina constitute the features of *hypertensive retinopathy*.

Heart Failure. Systemic hypertension causes left ventricular hypertrophy and ultimately left ventricular failure.

Malignant Hypertension

Hypertension, whether primary or secondary, may occasionally evolve into a malignant phase. The disease may also arise without pre-existing hypertension. The blood pressure becomes very high, causing necrosis of the arteriolar walls. Two organs are especially affected: the kidney and the brain. In the *kidney*, the vascular changes cause hematuria and culminate in uremia. In the *brain*, the changes cause hemorrhage and edema. Swelling of the optic disks (papilledema) is a useful sign of raised intracranial pressure; symptoms include mental confusion and epileptiform seizures. The syndrome of malignant hypertension usually progresses rapidly over a period of several weeks and, unless treated expeditiously, results in death from uremia, from an intracranial vascular catastrophe, or from heart failure.

The pathogenesis of malignant hypertension is not understood. Blood renin levels are high, and presumably angiotensin causes vasoconstriction as well as retention of sodium and water via aldosterone secretion. The severe renal damage causes further renal ischemia, and a vicious circle ensues that ends in death.

COAGULATION AND THROMBOSIS

In the vascular system, the normal endothelium provides a smooth lining that aids the unhindered flow of fluid and plays a vital part in governing the composition of the blood and the interstitial fluid. Should the endothelium be injured, deposition of platelets and later the formation of fibrin effectively seal minor defects and guard against the danger of hemorrhage.

The platelet deposit is initially unstable, but with the formation of a fibrin meshwork, the mass is stabilized and forms a *hemostatic plug*. Unfortunately, this intravascular deposition of platelets and fibrin can sometimes become excessive, a process called thrombosis, and lead to obstruction of the damaged vessel, causing local ischemia. Widespread intravascular fibrin formation can lead to even more widespread, severe damage. The importance of this finely balanced homeostatic mechanism has led to much research into the coagulation mechanism, the properties of platelets, and the role of the endothelium.

The Coagulation Mechanism. Coagulation, or clotting, involves the conversion of fibrinogen to fibrin. The mechanism is described in Chapter 18, and it is sufficient to note here that coagulation can be initiated by clotting factors derived either from the blood (intrinsic clotting system) or from damaged tissue (extrinsic clotting system). There are several mechanisms that counter excess fibrin formation. Thus, antithrombin-III and its cofactor heparin are naturally occurring anticoagulants, and the constant bathing of the area by a flow of blood removes excessive accumulation of clotting factors. Nevertheless, small quantities of fibrin are probably formed even under normal conditions, and there exists a fibrinolytic system for its removal. The active agent plasmin is formed on the fibrin threads and leads to their dissolution (Fig. 19–8).

Platelets. Platelets are small, nonnucleated structures present in the blood and have the property of sticking to each other (displaying *aggregation*) and of adhering to abnormal surfaces (showing *adhesiveness*).

Platelet Aggregation. Platelets aggregate immediately in the presence of adenosine diphosphate (ADP). This mechanism may be demonstrated *in vitro* by the addition of ADP to a platelet-rich preparation of plasma that is kept agitated. The aggregation can be detected by measuring the ensuing decrease in optical density of the plasma. An important property of thrombin is that it causes the release of ADP from platelets, and it therefore soon causes aggregation.

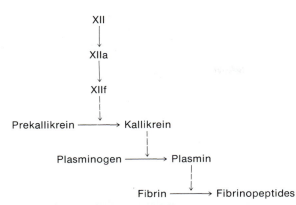

Figure 19–8 The blood fibrinolytic system. Plasmin is a fibrinolytic enzyme that digests fibrin to polypeptides (fibrino-peptides). It is formed from a precursor (plasminogen) by the action of the enzyme kallikrein, which itself is formed from a precursor by the activity of an activated component (factor XIIf) of factor XII (Hageman factor). Note that factor XII activation also initiates the intrinsic clotting mechanism, and that kallikrein is one of the important components of the chemical mediators of acute inflammation. Transformations are depicted as solid lines, and enzymatic activities are shown as interrupted lines.

Platelet Adhesiveness. Experimentally, platelets are found to adhere to a variety of foreign surfaces. Thus, if a platelet-rich fluid is passed through a column containing glass beads, the platelets are found to adhere to the beads, and few are contained in the fluid that issues from the column. Since platelets also adhere to the walls of damaged blood vessels, it is believed that exposure of collagen in the vessel wall is an important factor in the ready adhesion of these structures; platelets readily adhere to collagen when tested *in vitro.* Adherent platelets swell and release a variety of chemicals *(platelet release reaction),* including phospholipid (platelet factor 3, which plays a part in clotting), heparin-neutralizing substance (platelet factor 4), 5-hydroxy-tryptamine (5-HT), ADP, and thromboxane A2 (TXA2). TXA2 is a powerful agent that causes vasoconstriction and promotes platelet aggregation.

The Vascular Endothelium. Normal endothelial cells inhibit coagulation and the deposition of platelets. After injury to the vessel wall, a small hemostatic plug is formed; but endothelial cells soon cover it, and continued deposition of platelets and fibrin is brought to an end. Endothelial cells therefore play a vital role in preventing thrombosis. A number of mechanisms are involved. Endothelial cells secrete heparin-like substances and promote the formation of protein C, a proteolytic agent that inactivates factors V and VIII. They also form prostaglandin I2 (PGI2 or prostacyclin), which inhibits platelet aggregation. Prostaglandins are believed to play an important role in normal vascular homeostasis and thrombosis in addition to acting as inflammatory mediators. It is therefore relevant to review their properties.

Prostaglandins. The prostaglandins are potent agents derived from 20-carbon polyunsaturated fatty acids that are present in the phospholipids of all cell membranes. They have been named by letter (approximately in order of discovery) and by figures 1 to 3 (according to the number of double bonds in the molecule). They are synthesized from *arachidonic acid,* which is released from cell membrane phospholipid by the action of phospholipase A2. The enzyme cyclo-oxidase converts arachidonic acid into the two unstable *prostaglandin endoperoxides.* In platelets, these endoperoxides are converted into *thromboxane A2* (TXA2).

When platelets adhere to a vessel wall, TXA2 is formed, platelet aggregation is encouraged, and a platelet thrombus is formed. However, the endoperoxides formed by the platelets can also be used by cells of the vessel walls; these cells convert the endoperoxides into *prostacyclin* (PGI2), which is a vasodilator and can inhibit platelet aggregation. A balance between the formation of thromboxane A2 by the platelets and prostacyclin by the vessel wall may well be an important factor in determining the extent of thrombus formation. Damage to a vessel wall may impede prostacyclin formation and thereby encourage thrombus formation.

The vessel wall synthesizes prostacyclin from its own precursors as well as from endoperoxides released by platelets. Thus, the continuous formation of prostacyclin may be an important homeostatic mechanism by which platelets that are forced onto the vascular endothelium (or onto areas of minimal damage) are prevented from building up an abnormal platelet thrombus. Prostacyclin in the circulation, partially derived from the lungs, appears to be an additional protective mechanism. When it is remembered that platelet deposition on arterial walls is thought to be a major factor in the pathogenesis of arteriosclerosis, it will be readily understood why research into the formation and properties of the prostaglandins is currently so active.

Pathogenesis of Thrombosis

Thrombosis may be defined as the formation of a solid mass in the circulation from the constituents of the streaming blood. The mass itself is called a thrombus. Thrombosis involves two distinct processes.

Deposition of Platelets on a Vascular Surface. As noted previously, normal endothelium has properties that prevent platelet deposition. However, it can occur under several circumstances: (1) when the endothelial lining is damaged or removed; (2) with vascular stasis, when the platelets fall out of the axial stream and impinge on the wall; or (3) in association with turbulence, when eddy currents deflect the platelets to an area on the wall.

Whenever any of these three factors operates to an excessive extent, an abnormal mass of platelets is formed. This is a *pale,* or *platelet, thrombus.* The small platelet thrombus that forms first is quite unstable, and platelets may break off and return to the circulation. The addition of a fibrin clot causes the thrombus to become stable.

The Formation of a Clot of Fibrin in Which the Blood Cells Are Trapped. If the platelet thrombus is not speedily endothelialized, or if there is stasis, a blood clot is formed, and red and white blood cells are trapped in its meshes. Thrombin is potent in causing platelets to adhere to each other, and its liberation during the process of coagulation readily leads to a further deposition of platelets. In this way, a large mass is built up. When blood clot is the major component, it is called a *red,* or *coagulation, thrombus.* Frequently the thrombosis is made up of both red clot and pale platelet components, and it is then called a *mixed thrombus* (Figs. 19–9 and 19–10).

The crucial feature of thrombosis is the deposition of platelets on a vascular surface. This can occur only in the presence of a flowing stream and is therefore produced spontaneously only in

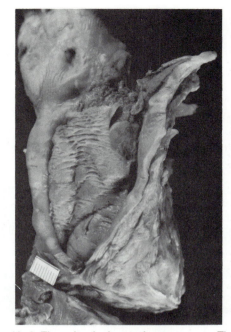

Figure 19–9 Thrombosis in aortic aneurysm. The aortic aneurysm has been opened to show adherent thrombus. The thrombus has a characteristic ribbed, or corrugated, appearance; this is quite different from the smooth, shiny surface of a postmortem clot.

the living animal. The clotting is a secondary phenomenon. It follows that the terms "clot" and "thrombus" are quite distinct; a thrombus contains a variable amount of clot, but the important feature is a platelet scaffold, which is lacking in a clot; it can be formed only *in vivo.* Clotting, on the other hand, may occur as part of thrombosis and is also seen in a column of static blood *in vivo* or *in vitro.*

Since the cardinal process in thrombosis is the deposition of platelets on an intimal surface, it is evident that the integrity of the vascular system is all-important in preventing it. Two features of the vascular system that are important in preventing thrombosis are (1) the smooth endothelial lining, which diminishes frictional resistance between the wall and the circulating blood, and (2) the streamline of blood along the complex circulatory pathways, which moves the formed elements in a central axial stream (Chapter 5).

The speed of flow prevents local stasis, and the absence of irregularities in the walls does not allow the development of eddy currents. The

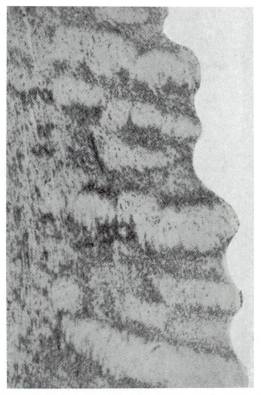

Figure 19–10 The structure of a thrombus. This is a photomicrograph of a thrombus and includes its free surface on the right. The thrombus consists of pale platelet laminae between which there is coagulated blood. Many white cells are adherent to the platelet laminae. Retraction of the clot leaves the laminae projecting from the free surface, and this is responsible for the ribbed appearance noted in Figure 19–9. The organized structure, with platelet laminae alternating with coagulated blood, distinguishes a thrombus from a blood clot, because it indicates that the structure has been formed from the elements of a flowing stream of blood. (From Hadfield, G.: Annals of the Royal College of Surgeons of England, *6:*219, 1950.)

streamline of blood can be threatened in a variety of ways, which are illustrated in Figure 19–11. These lesions all lead to local stasis as well as to the formation of eddy currents, and the platelets that cover them are actually performing a remedial function. They serve to smooth out the contours of the wall and restore the streamline of blood in the vessel. The small amount of clotting factors that they generate is dissipated in the flowing blood, and they themselves are rapidly endothelialized. It is when this process is retarded that the platelet mass grows, clotting factors accumulate, much fibrin is produced, and thrombosis proceeds even to the extent of obliterating the vessel lumen.

General Causes of Thrombosis

Three factors *(Virchow's triad)* must be considered in regard to the mechanism of thrombosis.

The Vessel Wall. The various types of anatomic changes in the vessel wall that may lead to thrombosis are depicted in Figure 19–11. In general, these abnormalities play an important part in thrombosis involving the heart valves and ventricles. In the arteries, atheroma is by far the most common cause of thrombosis. In the veins, changes in the vessel wall are usually of much less importance.

The Flow of Blood. The formation of *eddy currents* is important, for whenever the stream of the blood is disturbed, the flow becomes turbulent, and platelets are thrown against the vessel wall and are deposited as a thrombus. This mechanism is important in fast-moving streams, *e.g.,* over the heart valves and in arteries. Slowing of the blood, or *stasis,* is the most important cause of excessive thrombosis involving veins. It is also a factor in inducing thrombosis in the sac of an aneurysm as well as in the atria of the heart.

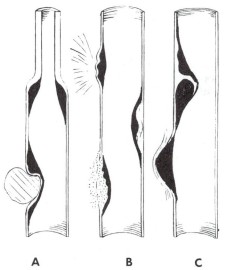

A   B   C

Figure 19–11 Vascular abnormalities that lead to thrombosis. This diagram shows seven different causes of a disruption of the normal streamlining of the blood flow and the manner by which platelets (shown in black) are laid down to restore the architecture. *A,* Bulging due to external pressure and spasm. *B,* Endothelial damage in inflammation, an area of intimal thickening (*e.g.,* due to atheroma), and corrugation due to adjacent scarring. *C,* Aneurysm and a thickened, rigid valve. (From Hadfield, G.: Annals of the Royal College of Surgeons of England, *6:*219, 1950.)

The Constituents of Blood. An increase in the platelet count, an increase in platelet adhesiveness, and a decrease in the clotting time—events that occur after trauma and bleeding—are sometimes important in inducing thrombosis. Likewise, increased viscosity of the blood due to hemoconcentration or polycythemia also leads to thrombosis. Other factors that may induce thrombosis are hyperlipidemia and administration of the birth control pill. The factors involved are complex and not completely understood.

It should be noted that usually more than one factor is implicated in the cause of thrombosis. For instance, there is regional stasis and a high platelet count after a surgical operation. Atherosclerosis acts both by causing a loss of the endothelium and by inducing eddy current formation.

Arterial Thrombosis

Thrombosis generally occurs in arteries as a complication of damage to the arterial wall; *atherosclerosis* is the most important cause, but *arteritis* also accounts for some cases. In an aneurysmal sac, thrombus deposition is a constant feature, and here stasis and eddy currents are important factors.

Effects of Arterial Thrombosis. Except for the aorta and its very large branches, arterial thrombosis results in the complete blockage of the vessel. The effects of this depend on the local architecture. The following are possibilities.

No Effect. When anastomoses are good, no ill effect is noted. Thus, if the radial artery is blocked, the hand is supplied by the ulnar artery because branches of the two vessels are normally joined together by *anastomotic channels*. These channels enlarge so that a *collateral circulation* develops. Blockage of either artery alone, therefore, leads to no serious aftereffects, provided the other vessel is not diseased.

Functional Disturbances. Blockage of a major vessel may render tissue ischemic only with exercise. In coronary occlusion, which is an example of this blockage, the effect is pain on exercise *(angina pectoris)*. Likewise, occlusion of the mesenteric artery can lead to pain after meals when the intestine exhibits marked peristalsis.

Occlusion of the femoral artery can lead to pain on walking. This is called *intermittent claudication.*

Cellular Degeneration. Ischemia can induce enough hypoxia to cause the specialized cells of an organ to degenerate. This is a patchy affair and leads to atrophy. Often there is *replacement fibrosis (e.g.,* myocardial fibrosis); in the central nervous system, there is *replacement gliosis.*

Infarction. The ischemia may be so severe that the whole area undergoes necrosis. This effect is called *infarction* and is considered later in this chapter.

Venous Thrombosis

Although disease of the vessel walls is uncommon, stasis is particularly evident in the veins, especially those of the legs. Thrombosis with a large element of clotting is therefore common. Two distinct entities can be recognized: phlebothrombosis and thrombophlebitis.

Phlebothrombosis. The most common form of leg vein thrombosis is phlebothrombosis, also called *deep vein thrombosis.* This occurs in patients who are confined to bed, particularly if they are in heart failure or have been subjected to trauma, whether accidental or surgical. If the limb has been injured and immobilized *(e.g.,* a fractured femur), the stage is set for thrombosis, because the major cause of thrombosis is *venous stasis* (Fig. 19–12). A small thrombus forms at one site, perhaps when the vein has been injured by pressure such as that produced by a pillow behind the knee. The flow of blood stops in the vein proximal to the thrombus, and the entire column *clots* (Fig. 19–13). This process can extend, or propagate, up to the iliac vein; as the clot retracts, it has minimal attachment to the vessel wall. The great danger then is embolism, for should the clot become detached, it would travel in the circulation to the right side of the heart and subsequently be ejected into the pulmonary artery. Here it would block either the main pulmonary trunk or one of its major divisions, leading to sudden death or infarction of the lung (see a discussion of this later in the chapter).

Thrombophlebitis. Inflammation of a vein (phlebitis) can occur when there is an adjacent

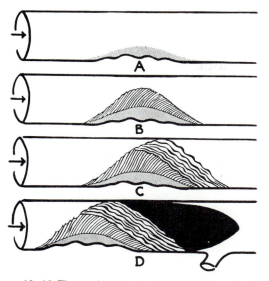

Figure 19–12 The pathogenesis of phlebothrombosis. *A,* An area of intimal damage is covered by a pale platelet thrombus. In the presence of a sluggish stream, this initiates further thrombosis. *B,* Upstanding laminae of platelets with intervening clot constitute the main thrombus. *C,* The lumen is occluded by further thrombosis. *D,* Blood *clot* forms to the next tributary. (From Hadfield, G.: Annals of the Royal College of Surgeons of England, *6:*219, 1950.)

area of infection (*e.g.,* a boil). Thrombosis occurs *(thrombophlebitis)* and is confined to the inflamed area of vein. A propagated clot does not form, and the risk of embolism is slight unless the thrombus itself becomes infected (see Infected Emboli, p. 340).

Thrombophlebitis affecting many veins at different times (called *migrating thrombophlebitis*) is an occasional manifestation of cancer, particularly cancer of the pancreas. The pathogenesis is not understood. The first description of this condition is attributed to Trousseau, a French physician, who observed it in himself and subsequently died of pancreatic cancer.

Local Effects of Venous Thrombosis. In most tissues, because the veins show extensive anastomoses, venous thrombosis produces few obstructive effects. There are some exceptions to this. Obstruction of the superior mesenteric vein leads to intense engorgement of the intestine and edema of the gut wall. This blockage can be so marked that further blood flow through the part becomes impossible, and the intestine undergoes infarction. In the leg, venous obstruction can

lead to some elevation of the venous pressure of the limb, an effect particularly marked if the subject stands for long periods. The result of this is edema of the ankles.

Cardiac Thrombosis

Thrombi may form in any of the chambers of the heart. The constant danger is their detachment and subsequent embolization. A common cause of atrial thrombosis is atrial dilation secondary to mitral stenosis, atrial fibrillation, or heart failure. Ventricular thrombosis is most commonly encountered as a complication of myocardial infarction, either during the acute stage or in an aneurysm that develops subsequently.

Thrombi on the heart valves (called *vegetations*) are a feature of acute rheumatic fever, infective endocarditis, and nonbacterial thrombotic endocarditis (Chapter 20).

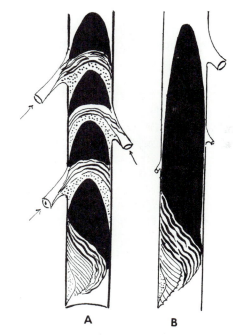

A   B

Figure 19–13 Propagation of clot in phlebothrombosis. *A,* Thrombus formation occurs at each entering tributary. This tends to anchor the clot. *B,* Clotting *en masse* in an extensive length of vein. This occurs when the circulation is very sluggish. The long propagated clot can easily become detached and lead to massive pulmonary embolism. (From Hadfield, G.: Annals of the Royal College of Surgeons of England, *6:*219, 1950.)

Fate of Thrombi

Figure 19–14 summarizes the possible fate of a thrombus. These possibilities are further elaborated in the following.

1. Many thrombi undergo lysis and leave no trace of their previous existence. The fibrinolytic enzyme plasmin is probably important in removing thrombi (see Fig. 19–8).

2. If an occluding thrombus in an artery or vein contains much clot, it retracts sufficiently for blood to pass by, in this way forming a new channel. It becomes endothelialized, and at that point, *recanalization* is said to have occurred. In the pulmonary arteries, a thin web of connective tissue may be all that remains of a previous life-threatening thromboembolism.

3. A thrombus that is not removed may become organized into granulation tissue and subsequent scar tissue.

4. Organized thrombi may become hyalinized and calcified. This response is common in the pelvic veins, and the *phleboliths* so produced may be seen on radiographic examination of the pelvis.

5. Thrombi may be detached to form emboli, a process that is described later in this chapter.

Two important effects of thrombosis are occlusion of the lumen of the vessel involved and detachment from this to form an embolus. Vascular obstruction produces ischemia, which in turn leads to hypoxia.

HYPOXIA

Hypoxia is a state of impaired oxygenation of the tissues. Four types are commonly described:

1. *Hypoxic,* due to a low oxygen tension (PO_2) in the arterial blood; this form of hypoxia is a feature of some types of congenital heart disease and lung disease.

2. *Anemic,* due to an inadequate level of hemoglobin, which carries the oxygen in the blood stream.

3. *Stagnant,* or *ischemic,* due to an inadequate supply of blood to the tissues; this form of hypoxia may be due to a low cardiac output, as in heart failure, or to some local vascular obstruction.

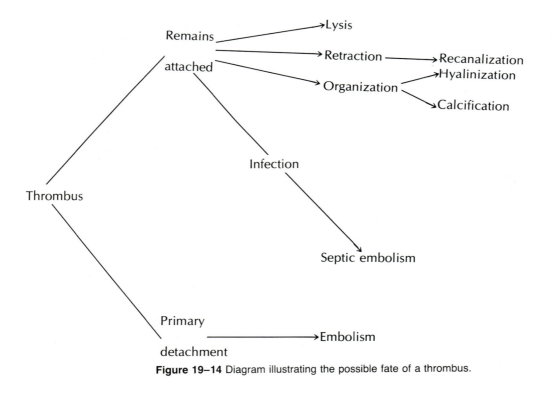

Figure 19–14 Diagram illustrating the possible fate of a thrombus.

4. *Histotoxic,* due to cellular poisoning, which prevents the uptake of oxygen (*e.g.,* cyanide poisoning).

ISCHEMIA

Ischemia is a condition of inadequate blood supply to an area of tissue. It produces harmful effects in three ways.

Hypoxia. A reduced oxygen supply is undoubtedly the most important factor in the production of damage in ischemic tissue. It is particularly important in active cells such as muscle and neurons. On the other hand, it plays no part in the lesions produced by pulmonary arterial obstruction because the alveolar walls derive their oxygen directly from the alveolar gas.

Malnutrition. This is probably a factor of little importance, because the blood contains more nutrients than could be metabolized with the amount of oxygen it contains.

Failure to Remove Waste Products. The accumulation of metabolites is the most probable explanation of pain in ischemic muscles. The presence of waste products or the failure to maintain important electrolyte balances is probably a factor in the pathogenesis of pulmonary infarction.

Causes of Ischemia

General. Ischemia can be caused by an inadequate cardiac output. Not all tissues of the body are equally affected because there is a redistribution of the available blood. The extremities—for instance, the fingertips and toes—tend to be most severely affected; in such cases, the sluggish blood flow leads to peripheral cyanosis. (The term *cyanosis* refers to the blue color of tissues that is produced by the reduced hemoglobin in the vessels.)

Cardiac arrest, such as may occur during the induction of anesthesia or as a result of coronary thrombosis, results in ischemia of all tissues in the body. The effects of this are confined to a single organ, the brain, which is particularly sensitive to hypoxia. If the arrest continues for 15 seconds, consciousness is lost; if the condition lasts for more than 3 minutes, irreparable damage is done. If the patient survives, the neurons degenerate and are replaced by glial tissue. If cardiac arrest lasts for more than 8 minutes, death is inevitable. It follows that *all persons who deal with patients should be capable of diagnosing cardiac arrest (absent heart sounds) and of dealing with it by the maneuvers of external cardiac massage and assisted respiration.*

Local. By far, the most important cause of ischemia is obstruction of the arterial flow. Nevertheless, extensive venous and capillary obstruction can also produce ischemia.

Arterial Obstruction. Most of the causes of obstruction have already been described. In review, they are:

Thrombosis.

Embolism. The effects of an embolus are potentiated by the reflex spasm of the arterial wall and are completed by the rapid development of thrombus over the embolus.

Spasm. See later in this chapter.

Atherosclerosis. See Chapter 21.

Occlusive Pressure from Without. Examples include tourniquets and ill-fitting casts.

Venous Disease. Extensive venous obstruction leads to engorgement of the area drained by the affected veins. This may reach such an intensity that blood flow is impeded and ischemia results.

Capillary Damage. See Chapter 21.

EMBOLISM

An embolus is an abnormal mass of undissolved material that is transported from one part of the circulation to another. The most satisfactory classification is one based on the composition of the embolus.

Types of Emboli

Four distinct types may be recognized: *thrombi* and *clot; gas; fat;* and *tumor;* a fifth category, *miscellaneous emboli,* is also discussed.

Thrombus or Clot Emboli

Pulmonary Embolism. The source of thromboemboli is generally one of the leg veins. If the embolus is large, it produces the syndrome of "massive pulmonary embolism." Either the main pulmonary trunk or many of its branches become plugged, so that the pulmonary circulation is greatly hindered (Fig. 19–15). The output of the right ventricle as well as that of the left ventricle drops precipitously. The effects of this drop are dramatic. The patient experiences sudden dyspnea and chest pain. Loss of consciousness and death may follow. The prevention of massive pulmonary embolism is the prevention of phlebothrombosis. A patient who is confined to bed must be given leg exercises to stimulate the venous circulation. Postoperative physical therapy and early ambulation have done much to reduce this complication of trauma and surgery. Anticoagulant drugs (*e.g.*, heparin) administered before surgery have been somewhat useful.

Small pulmonary emboli produce a different picture. If the subject is otherwise healthy, medium-sized pulmonary arteries can be obstructed without appreciable ill effect. Since the lung derives much of its oxygen from the alveolar gas,

the area beyond a blocked artery does not become hypoxic. Nevertheless, the altered gas tensions in the tissue can lead to bronchospasm, with the result that the area ceases to be ventilated and may collapse. This area can become reinflated within a few hours. The transient radiographic shadows that can be seen after pulmonary embolism may be explained on this basis. At other times, the area becomes edematous; hypoxia is added to ischemia, and necrosis ensues. The end result is infarction of the lung.

The circumstances determining whether infarction will follow pulmonary embolism are not clearly understood, but patients who are in heart failure or who are confined to bed seem to be most prone to this complication.

Systemic Embolism. The embolus usually arises from the heart, either in one of its chambers or from a valve. Thrombi attached to atherosclerotic ulcers in the aorta sometimes embolize distally.

Infected Emboli. If a thrombus contains py-

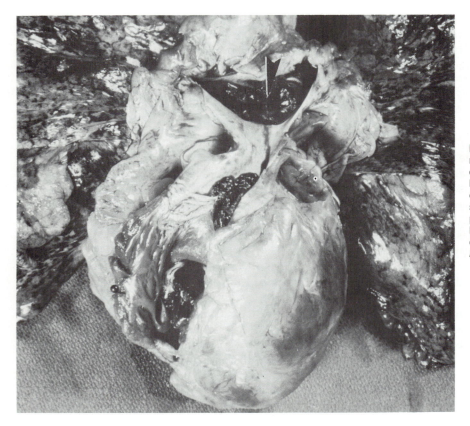

Figure 19–15 Massive pulmonary embolism. The right ventricle and pulmonary trunk have been opened to reveal a large embolus. Part of the embolus is sitting astride the division of the pulmonary trunk and is blocking both pulmonary arteries. This condition is known as a *saddle embolus* and causes sudden death.

ogenic organisms, it tends to break up and produce multiple infected ("septic") emboli. Such a condition, which is called *pyemia*, is a complication of both acute endocarditis and thrombophlebitis in an area of suppurative inflammation (*e.g.*, acute appendicitis). If an infected embolus blocks a vessel supplying tissue that has a poor collateral circulation (*e.g.*, kidney), an infarct is produced and subsequently becomes infected; a *septic infarct* results and soon suppurates. If the tissue has a good blood supply (*e.g.*, liver), no infarction occurs, but a local infection leads to abscess formation—a *pyemic abscess*. Thus, a complication of acute appendicitis is portal pyemia and multiple pyemic abscesses in the liver.

Gas Emboli

Air. Air may accidentally be introduced into a systemic vein during a surgical procedure. During operations on the head and neck, air may be sucked accidentally into the jugular vein and may then pass to the right side of the heart. Small quantities produce no adverse effect, but if a large quantity of air suddenly reaches the right ventricle, it becomes churned into a foamy mass that is compressed during systole but cannot be ejected. The cardiac output drops dramatically and sudden death ensues.

When a needle is introduced into the pleural cavity, as when fluid is aspirated, air may inadvertently be introduced into the pulmonary venous circulation and may reach the left side of the heart. From here it may travel to a coronary or cerebral vessel, occluding it. Even small quantities of air can produce serious, or even fatal, results in this manner.

Air embolism, either pulmonary or systemic, is a serious complication of open-heart surgery. All efforts must be made to exclude air from the circulation at the termination of the operation.

Nitrogen: The Decompression Syndrome. Bubbles of nitrogen appear in the circulation in those who, having been exposed to a high atmospheric pressure, are suddenly decompressed. This occurs in divers and tunnelers if they return to the surface too quickly. It is also seen in pilots if the cabin becomes decompressed at a high altitude. Nitrogen, being soluble in lipids, also appears as bubbles in the central nervous system. This particular effect may result in considerable damage to the spinal cord. The accompanying severe pain, which occurs most often in the joints, gives the condition its colloquial name, "the bends." Permanent damage or death may ensue.

Fat Embolism. Globules of fatty marrow may enter small veins in the area of a fracture of a long bone. With multiple injuries, this embolization can be quite extensive. Usually the emboli are trapped in the lungs and, because of the enormous capacity of the pulmonary vascular bed, can produce little harmful effect. Small areas of collapse can be detected radiographically. Occasionally, fat emboli traverse the pulmonary capillaries and enter the systemic circulation, where they produce the condition known as *systemic fat embolism*. Multiple emboli lodge in the kidneys, causing hematuria; in the brain, leading to severe neurologic changes; and in the skin, causing petechial hemorrhages.

Tumor Emboli. It is probable that all malignant tumors invade the local blood vessels at an early stage of the disease and that isolated malignant cells are a frequent occurrence in the circulation. The majority of these emboli become impacted and are destroyed. A small percentage develop into metastatic deposits. Occasionally, a large mass of tumor invades a major vessel and becomes detached. Thus, in lung cancer, a tongue of tumor can invade a pulmonary vein, become detached, pass into the systemic circulation, and block a large artery such as the femoral artery. The event is uncommon.

Miscellaneous Emboli. A variety of foreign bodies can act as emboli. For example, a portion of polyethylene tube may accidentally become detached and travel to the right side of the heart.

The condition described as *amniotic fluid embolism* is an occasional complication of pregnancy that follows escape of amniotic fluid into the veins of the uterus. It produces a syndrome characterized by shock and a generalized bleeding tendency. Although amniotic fluid does travel to the lungs, the syndrome is attributable not to embolism but rather to the initiation of intravascular clotting and fibrinolysis.

INFARCTION

Infarction is the circumscribed necrosis of tissue due to deprivation of its blood supply. The area of necrosis subsequently becomes organized into scar tissue. The process is as follows.

1. Cells die in the area deprived of its blood supply. Blood, either from anastomotic vessels or from venous backflow, continues to seep into the devitalized area for a short time. Thus, most infarcts contain a great deal of blood in the early stages and are swollen and red in color (Fig. 19–16). The red blood cells entering the affected area escape from the damaged capillaries and lie free in the dead tissue. Infarcts of lax tissue such as the lung and intestine are much more engorged than are those of compact organs such as the kidney and heart. If an infarcted area adjoins a surface, the congested necrotic tissue oozes blood. Hence, with renal infarcts, blood is present in the urine *(hematuria)*, and with infarc-

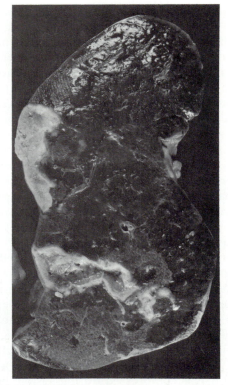

Figure 19–17 Splenic infarction. This section of spleen shows two pale areas of infarction. The specimen is from a patient who died of bacterial endocarditis.

tion of the lung, the sputum is blood-stained *(hemoptysis)*; a small blood-stained pleural effusion may also be detected.

2. The dead tissue undergoes necrosis. In solid organs, the associated swelling of the cells tends to squeeze blood out of the infarct, which then becomes pale (Fig. 19–17). Infarcts of the spleen and kidneys characteristically show this color change and appear as pale, wedge-shaped areas of coagulative necrosis—the apex of such areas being a blocked supplying artery, the base being the capsule of the organ (Figs. 19–16 and 19–17). Infarcts of the heart are also pale, but their shape is more irregular owing to the arrangement of the vascular supply (see Fig. 20–5).

3. Necrotic tissue undergoes progressive autolysis; red blood cells undergo hemolysis. On microscopic examination, the infarct shows a characteristic structured necrosis. The general outline of the cells is visible, but nuclei are either

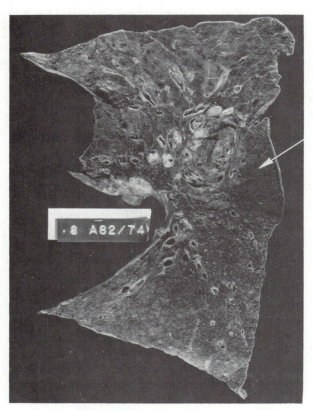

Figure 19–16 Pulmonary infarct. This vertical section through the lung shows an area of hemorrhagic infarction involving the apex of the lower lobe (arrow). Note how the surrounding uninvolved lung has collapsed post mortem; this has left the infarct standing out in relief. The specimen is from a patient who had carcinoma of the lung.

breaking up into fragments or have completely disappeared.

4. At the same time, the surrounding normal tissue shows an acute inflammatory reaction. Hyperemia gives the edge of the infarct a deep red color. Microscopic examination reveals an intense polymorph infiltration. Macrophages subsequently become the predominant cell and play an important part in removing the dead tissue. In pulmonary infarction, the inflammation involves the parietal pleura, and this leads to *pain*, particularly on taking a deep breath. Likewise, splenic infarction may cause pain in the left side of the abdomen.

5. The infarct gradually shrinks and becomes replaced by granulation tissue that subsequently matures to scar tissue. The central portion of a large infarct may remain unorganized for many months and indeed may show dystrophic calcification and never become converted into scar tissue.

Infarcts in particular organs present certain characteristic features. For example, in the lung, the tissue is spongelike, and infarcts in it are always hemorrhagic. In the intestine, the necrotic bowel wall is soon invaded by putrefactive organisms and becomes gangrenous. In the limbs, sudden obstruction leads to infarction, which in turn is associated with infection and leads to *wet gangrene* (Fig. 19–18).

In the central nervous system, on the other hand, the process of infarction is somewhat different, because the necrotic tissue immediately undergoes liquefactive necrosis. The affected area may collapse and eventually be replaced by a glial scar; but if the infarct is large, the end result is the formation of a cyst lined by glial tissue.

VASCULAR SPASM

Although vascular occlusion is generally caused by an organic lesion, there are a number of conditions in which spasm of the vessel wall plays a most important part. Either veins or arteries can be affected by spasm, but it is debatable whether capillaries are capable of independent contraction.

Venous Spasm

Trauma applied directly to the vessel wall can induce intense spasm. This may cause great difficulty during an inexpert venipuncture, *e.g.,* when a transfusion is set up or when blood is withdrawn from a vein. It is the reason the novice has such difficulties in "taking blood."

Generalized venospasm occurs during hypovolemic shock, and it has also been postulated as occurring in heart failure.

Arterial Spasm

Trauma to an artery produces localized spasm; at times, this may be life-saving. There are many cases recorded in which whole limbs have been torn off (avulsed), and yet owing to the spasm of the main artery, the patient has not died of massive bleeding.

The ability of arteries and arterioles to contract can be used to advantage by a surgeon who is faced with severe bleeding during the course of an operation. It is a wise policy to pack the wound and await the onset of spasm rather than make heroic, although blind, efforts with a pair of hemostats. Indeed, *anyone faced with bleeding from a wound should apply local pressure and await vasospasm, rather than panic or apply a tourniquet.*

Although arterial spasm as a response to trauma may be beneficial, it may sometimes be detrimental. Trauma to an artery, *e.g.,* by the close proximity to a bullet path, the jagged ends of a fractured bone, the pressure of a hematoma around a fracture, or the pressure of a plaster cast or tourniquet, may at times produce such persistent widespread spasm that the area involved becomes ischemic and infarcted. Because the process is often painless, the *pulse of a limb beyond an area of damage must always be carefully observed.* Absence of the pulse must be regarded seriously, and every effort should be made to relieve the spasm so that permanent damage will not occur.

Spasm of small arteries and arterioles is a feature of ergot poisoning and Raynaud's phenomenon (Chapter 1). It may lead to gangrene of the toes and fingertips. Widespread arteriolar

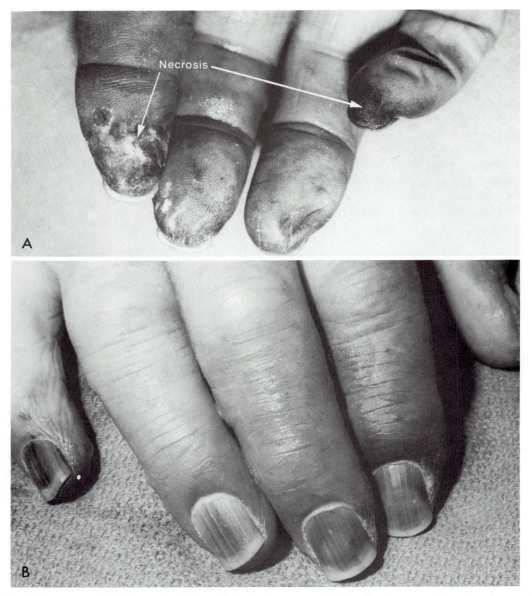

Figure 19–18 Gangrene of the fingertips. This patient died as a result of bleeding from esophageal varices secondary to alcoholic cirrhosis of the liver. He died in shock associated with severe and extensive edema of the subcutaneous tissues, ascites, and pleural effusions. After the insertion of a needle to obtain a sample of arterial blood, the patient developed thrombosis of the right brachial artery and gangrene of the fingertips. There is blue-black discoloration of the tissues and necrosis of the finger pulps *(A).* Acute arterial obstruction associated with pre-existing edema has led to the condition of wet gangrene. The condition would have spread to involve the whole hand and even the arm, but death intervened. See also Figure 19–3.

spasm is a feature of shock and has also been incriminated as a cause of primary hypertension.

Summary

- Normal fluid balance can be upset by deprivation or excess of water or salt. Water excess causes intracellular edema of the brain; water deficiency causes cellular dehydration. Salt and water excess leads to edema, deficiency to circulatory collapse.
- Local edema can be due to the formation of an exudate or a transudate or follow lymphatic obstruction.
- Generalized edema is caused by cardiac failure, the nephrotic syndrome, and starvation.
- Acute hemorrhage is followed by mechanisms designed to maintain the blood pressure and blood volume. If this is not successful, the tissues are underperfused, and shock results. Other causes of shock are trauma, burns, fluid loss, overwhelming infection, and acute heart failure. The metabolic upset that follows entails metabolic acidosis and an acute phase response. Irreversible shock involves secondary changes in lungs, kidney, liver, heart, and other organs; by definition, it ends in death.
- Systemic hypertension may be primary (essential) or secondary (generally to renal disease). Hemorrhage (cerebral), atherosclerosis, arteriolosclerosis, and heart failure are important complications. It may also terminate in a malignant phase.
- Platelets display aggregation and adhesion in response to vascular damage. They form a hemostatic plug in conjunction with fibrin formed as a result of coagulation of blood. Excessive deposition leads to thrombus formation. The properties of vascular endothelium help prevent this. The balance between thromboxane A2 and prostacyclin is also important.
- Thrombosis is precipitated by vascular damage, stasis, and turbulence.
- Phlebothrombosis (deep vein thrombosis) complicates heart failure, immobilization, and trauma. Pulmonary embolism and death are important complications. Thrombophlebitis has no such complications; embolism is rare unless there is infection of the thrombus leading to pyemia.
- The effects of arterial thrombosis depend on the local circulatory arrangements. There may be little effect, local ischemia with functional effects, or infarction. Distal embolism may occur. Some thrombi organize, others undergo lysis.
- Ischemia has many causes. Low cardiac output affects many tissues. Local arterial disease (atherosclerosis, arteritis, thrombosis, embolism, spasm, and pressure from without) is an important cause. Venous and capillary disease are other causes.
- Emboli may consist of thrombus with clot; fat; gas; or tumor.
- Infarction is necrosis due to deprivation of blood supply. In most organs, there is coagulative necrosis; in loose tissues (lung and intestine), the area is stuffed with blood; in solid organs, infarcts soon become pale. In the central nervous system, there is colliquative necrosis.

Selected Readings

Chein, K. R., Pfau, R. G., and Farber, J. L.: Ischemic myocardial cell injury. Am. J. Pathol. *97*:505, 1979.

Colman, R. W., et al. (eds.): Hemostasis and Thrombosis: Basic Principles and Clinical Practice. 2nd ed. Philadelphia, J. B. Lippincott, 1986.

Dinarello, C. A.: Interleukin-1 and the pathogenesis of the acute-phase response. N. Engl. J. Med. *311*:1413, 1984.

Gossling, H. R., and Donohue, T. A.: The fat embolism syndrome. JAMA *241*:2740, 1979.

Handler, C. E.: Cardiogenic shock. Postgrad. Med. J. *61*:705, 1985.

Jaffe, E. A.: Cell biology of endothelial cells. Hum. Pathol. *18*:234, 1987.

Kushner, I.: The phenomenon of the acute phase response. Ann. N.Y. Acad. Sci. *389*:39, 1982.

Mizock, B.: Septic shock: A metabolic perspective. Arch. Intern. Med. *144*:579, 1984.

Price, T. M., et al.: Amniotic fluid embolism. Three case reports with a review of the literature. Obstet. Gynecol. Surv. *40*:462, 1985.

Riede, U. N., et al.: Morphologic development of human shock lung. Pathol. Res. Pract. *165*:269, 1979.

Ryan, N. T.: Metabolic adaptations for energy production during trauma and sepsis. Surg. Clin. North Am. *56*:1073, 1976.

Sharma, G. V. R. K., and Sasahara, A. A.: Diagnosis and treatment of pulmonary embolism. Med. Clin. North Am. *63*:239, 1979.

Young, A. E.: Therapeutic embolism. Br. Med. J. *2*:1144, 1981.

20

Heart

**After studying this chapter, the student
should be able to:**

- Relate the development of the heart to the common
  types of developmental heart disease.
- List the main features of Fallot's tetralogy and of
  coarctation of the aorta.
- Describe the main features of acute rheumatic fever
  and discuss the immediate and long-term effects of
  this disease on the heart.
- Indicate the importance of nonbacterial thrombotic
  endocarditis.
- Contrast acute infective endocarditis with subacute
  infective endocarditis.
- Describe calcific aortic stenosis.
- Discuss the effects of myocardial ischemia and
  describe in detail the clinical and pathologic features
  of myocardial infarction.
- Describe the changes in blood enzyme levels that
  are of value in the clinical diagnosis of acute
  myocardial infarction.
- Define chronic cor pulmonale and indicate the
  mechanisms involved in its evolution.
- List the causes and effects of stenosis and
  regurgitation of each of the four heart valves.
- Describe the pathophysiology and effects of the
  major cardiac dysrhythmias and draw a typical
  electrocardiogram of each type.
- List the cardiac reserves.
- Clarify the causes of heart failure.
- Describe the causes and effects of left ventricular
  failure, right ventricular failure, and congestive heart
  failure.
- Describe what is meant by a cardiomyopathy.
- List the causes of acute cardiac tamponade.
- List the causes of acute pericarditis.

Diseases of the heart are a common cause of
human ill health and death. In the neonatal
period, congenital disease accounts for many
deaths, whereas a heart attack (*myocardial infarction*) is one of the chief causes of death in men

between the ages of 30 and 50 years in the Western world.

Diseases of the heart may affect primarily the pericardium, the myocardium, or the endocardium—in particular, the endocardium that covers the valves. These structures may be attacked separately or in combination. The types and causes of heart disease are therefore many and varied; the effects, however, are few and stereotyped. Since the heart is a pump, it follows that the diseased and failing heart often pumps inefficiently. The consequences of this are circulatory disturbances that together constitute the syndrome of *heart failure*. This complex of disturbances is described later, after individual diseases of the heart have been considered.

DEVELOPMENTAL ANOMALIES

The heart develops early in fetal life, and most of the developmental anomalies are therefore present at birth. This group of diseases is commonly called congenital heart disease, and it is present in about 1 per cent of infants at birth. Without effective treatment, at least 40 per cent of the infants so afflicted die during the first 5 years of life—most, in fact, during the first few months. Many developmental anomalies are known; until recently, however, their recognition was largely a matter of academic interest, particularly to the embryologist. Cardiac surgeons are now able to offer a chance of cure, and interest in congenital heart disease is more than academic. Many techniques have been developed to assist in accurate diagnosis during life. Only a few of the common anomalies are described.

Septal Defects

Because the heart develops from a single tube, a failure in the formation of the septa dividing the left and right chambers is not uncommon. In *atrial septal defects*, some blood passes from the left atrium to the right atrium and from there into the right ventricle and the pulmonary circulation (Fig. 20–1A). The output of the right ventricle is several times greater than normal, but so long as it copes with this additional work,

the patient is not seriously handicapped. This is indeed the most common congenital cardiac anomaly in adults and is not accompanied by cyanosis, as long as the shunt remains from left to right.

Ventricular septal defects are also common (Fig. 20–1B); if small, they cause little functional disturbance. With large defects, the results are serious. There is a large left-to-right shunt that puts a strain on the left ventricle, because in addition to the shunted blood, it must eject an adequate amount of blood into the aorta if life is to be sustained. In time, the left ventricle fails. Furthermore, the right ventricle is subjected to the high pressure of blood coming from the left side so that the pulmonary circulation works at a high pressure. As long as the shunt is from left to right, the patient has no cyanosis. However, in response to the high pressure, the pulmonary vessels become narrowed. The pulmonary resistance increases, and the right ventricular pressure rises even higher. The shunt then changes from left-to-right to right-to-left, and cyanosis ensues. Ventricular septal defects illustrate one of the complexities of treatment in congenital heart disease. If the defect is closed when the patient is young, the child may develop normally and live to old age. If treatment is delayed until the blood flow is from right-to-left because of increased pulmonary resistance, then closure of the defect causes rapid heart failure and death.

Pulmonary Stenosis

An unequal division of the truncus arteriosus may result in the development of a large aorta and a correspondingly small pulmonary artery and valve (pulmonary stenosis) (Fig. 20–1C).

Transposition of the Great Vessels

Owing to a failure of rotation, the aorta can arise from the right ventricle and the pulmonary artery can arise from the left ventricle. If this were the only anomaly, life would not be possible—a complementary defect must also be present. The patient's survival after birth depends on there being some communication, *e.g.,* a septal

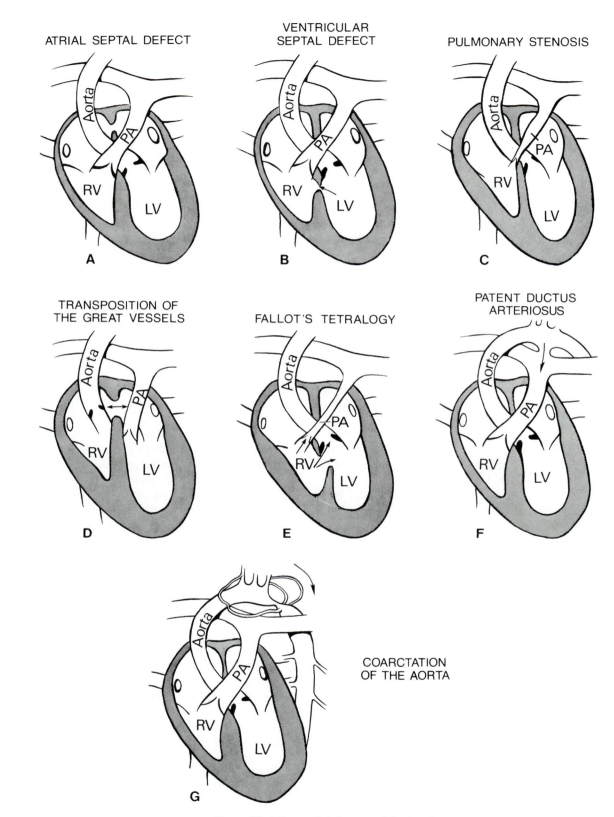

Figure 20–1 Congenital diseases of the heart.

defect, between the two sides of the heart (Fig. 20–1D). Transposition of the great vessels is one of the common fatal anomalies in children under 1 year of age.

Dextrocardia

Occasionally the heart develops as a mirror-image of the normal. If this mirror-imaging involves all organs *(complete situs inversus)*, the patient lives a normal life, since there are no other abnormalities. If only the heart is affected, the results are serious, because other defects are also present.

Multiple Defects

Developmental anomalies are often multiple. Malformations may be found not only in other organs but also in the heart itself. A common combination is the *tetralogy of Fallot* (Fig. 20–1E), which consists of the following: (1) pulmonary stenosis; (2) ventricular septal defect; (3) overriding of the interventricular septum by the aorta, so that blood from both the right and left ventricles enters the aorta; and (4) hypertrophy of the right ventricle—this is compensatory.

Clinical Features of Fallot's Tetralogy

The effects of Fallot's tetralogy illustrate many of the features of developmental heart disease and are considered in some detail in the following paragraphs.

Murmurs. These are often loud and may be heard over the precordium with the aid of a stethoscope. They may even be felt as *thrills*.

Central Cyanosis. Since blood from the right ventricle enters the aorta directly, there is a considerable right-to-left shunt. The arterial blood is not fully oxygenated, and this causes central cyanosis. Patients with Fallot's tetralogy are born as "blue babies." Central cyanosis affects all tissues—skin, mucous membranes, tongue, and the others. Central cyanosis is also found in severe lung disease as well as in direct vascular shunts. It should be contrasted with peripheral cyanosis, which is due to stagnation of the blood in vessels of the skin. Peripheral cyanosis is never seen in the mucous membranes, which have an active blood supply, and this forms a useful clinical point of differentiation.

Polycythemia. This condition (an increase in the total red blood cell mass of the body) is due to hypoxia of the bone marrow.

Clubbing of the Fingers and Toes. This abnormality is generally seen when cyanosis is present and of long duration. The pathogenesis is obscure; it also occurs in other diseases, *e.g.,* chronic suppurative lung diseases, lung cancer, and bacterial endocarditis.

Underdevelopment. Unless the heart defects are corrected, the child shows poor physical development. Early death from infection or heart failure is usual.

Squatting. Patients tend to assume a squatting position after exertion, because this gives them relief from breathlessness.

Hypoxic Spells. A sudden increase in the amount of cyanosis can lead to cerebral hypoxia.

Patent Ductus Arteriosus

In the fetus, blood that reaches the right ventricle bypasses the unexpanded lungs because of the high resistance of the pulmonary circulation. The blood passes from the pulmonary artery into the aorta through the patent ductus arteriosus. After birth, as the pulmonary circulation opens up, the ductus normally becomes obliterated, but occasionally this fails to happen and it remains patent (Fig. 20–1F). The left-to-right shunt that develops puts a strain on the left ventricle, which in due course may fail. In addition, pulmonary hypertension ensues, and this places a burden on the right ventricle. In addition to these hemodynamic effects, a patent ductus arteriosus presents yet another hazard to life. An *infective endarteritis* analogous to bacterial endocarditis may develop at the site of the ductus.

Coarctation of the Aorta*

The process of obliteration that affects the ductus may involve the aorta and may then lead

---

*Although not strictly a disease of the heart, this topic is described here for convenience.

to the formation of a stricture. This generally occurs beyond the subclavian arteries, so that blood reaches the upper half of the body normally by the arch of the aorta and its major branches, but it arrives at the lower half of the body only via collateral vessels (Fig. 20–1G). This condition is important for two reasons: (1) the area of stenosis may become infected, and (2) systemic hypertension may occur in the upper part of the body, leading to left ventricular hypertrophy and failure. Unless it is treated, life is seldom prolonged over the age of 40 years.

The diagnosis of coarctation of the aorta should be suspected if systemic hypertension can be measured in the patient's arms and yet no pulse can be felt in the femoral or other leg vessels.

ACQUIRED HEART DISEASE

Rheumatic Heart Disease

Acute rheumatic fever is a disease of childhood and generally affects those between 5 and 15 years of age. It typically occurs 2 to 3 weeks after a streptococcal sore throat and is currently believed to be due to an immunologic mechanism, but whether the damage is mediated by immune complexes or activation of T cells is unclear. It has been suggested that immune complexes localize in the small blood vessels of the heart and joints and, by activating complement, lead to tissue damage. The reason for the localization of the lesions in rheumatic fever is not known. Patients with rheumatic fever generally have a neutrophil leukocytosis, a raised erythrocyte sedimentation rate, and a high or rising antistreptolysin O titer *(ASO titer)*. Antistreptolysin O is an antibody to streptolysin O, a hemolysin produced by *Streptococcus pyogenes.*

The disease is characterized by *fever,* flitting *pains and swelling of the joints, subcutaneous nodules* (particularly over the bony prominences), and most important, *involvement of the heart.* Since *pericarditis* sometimes occurs, the two roughened surfaces of pericardium cause a characteristic rubbing noise that can be heard with a stethoscope. Some degree of heart failure is common and occasionally is fatal. At necropsy, the heart is dilated, but the myocardium appears surprisingly normal. The characteristic lesion is a chronic inflammatory focus called an Aschoff body, which occurs between muscle bundles. Dilation of the valve annulus can lead to mitral regurgitation, which contributes to heart failure.

The most important lesions of acute rheumatic fever are those of the valves. The valves are swollen, and where the cusps meet, there are depositions of thrombi on the endocardial surface—depositions called *vegetations,* which appear as small nodules along the line of valve closure. The mitral and aortic valves are most commonly affected by this *endocarditis.* Even though most other lesions of acute rheumatic fever undergo resolution, those of the valves do not. They tend to progress to a state of chronic inflammation, and the cusps become thickened, fibrosed, and contracted *(chronic rheumatic endocarditis).* Adjacent cusps adhere to each other, rendering the orifices stenotic. In the mitral valve, this leads to the characteristic fish mouth or buttonhole deformity (Figs. 20–2 and 20–3). The rigid leaflets and thickened chordae tendineae also lead to regurgitation. If the aortic valve is affected, it is also rendered both stenotic and regurgitant.

Not all patients who suffer from an attack of acute rheumatic fever have persistent heart valve damage. Nevertheless, the disease has a tendency to recur, and with each attack, valvular damage increases. Because the disease is precipitated by streptococcal infection, long-term antibiotic therapy is often instituted as a prophylactic measure. In combination with improvements in social conditions, which have reduced the incidence of streptococcal infections, this therapy has considerably reduced the incidence of rheumatic heart disease in North America as compared with 50 years ago.

In those patients unfortunate enough to progress to chronic rheumatic heart disease, mitral stenosis is the most common valvular lesion found. Blood is dammed back in the left atrium, which becomes dilated; its wall becomes hypertrophied. Stasis may lead to the formation of thrombus on the wall of the atrium, particularly if there is atrial fibrillation. Pulmonary venous congestion follows. The effect of this is to make the lungs more rigid, so that breathing is more difficult and requires more effort. This alteration

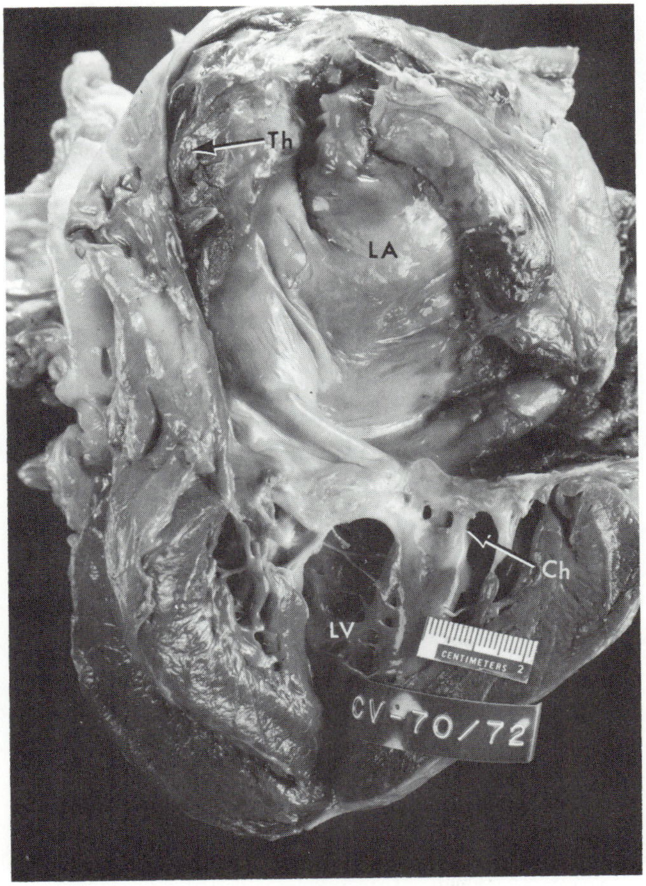

Figure 20–2 Mitral stenosis due to rheumatic disease.
The heart has been opened by an incision passing from
the left atrium (LA) to the apex of the left ventricle (LV).
The left atrium is enormously dilated, and thrombus (Th) is
adherent to its walls. The mitral valve is markedly fibrosed,
and its cusps are fused together; its chordae (Ch) are
greatly thickened and shortened. The left ventricle shows
no abnormality, thereby indicating that the major functional
effect of the valvular lesion was stenosis. (Courtesy of Dr.
M. D. Silver, University of Toronto.)

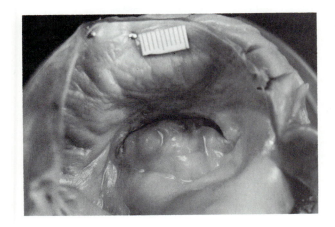

Figure 20–3 Mitral stenosis due to rheumatic disease. The
mitral valve is viewed from the left atrium. Fusion of its cusps
and fibrosis have combined to produce the characteristic rigid
"fish mouth" or "buttonhole" stenotic deformity. (Courtesy of
Dr. M. D. Silver, University of Toronto.)

causes shortness of breath and distress *(dyspnea).* Intra-alveolar bleeding leads to *hemoptysis,* and gradually to brown induration of the lungs (p. 366). In mitral stenosis, the left ventricle is under no strain and is therefore small. However, should there be an additional factor of regurgitation or an aortic valvular lesion, the left ventricle would become enlarged and might subsequently fail. The back-pressure effect on the lungs eventually leads to pulmonary hypertension and right ventricular failure.

In chronic rheumatic heart disease, the valves of the left side are much more frequently affected than are those of the right. Aortic lesions can occur alone or, more commonly, combined with mitral damage.

Nonbacterial Thrombotic Endocarditis

Small warty vegetations along the line of closure of the mitral or aortic valves are a fairly common finding at necropsy. These vegetations are sterile and are of importance in two respects. First, they occasionally become detached and embolize to the brain. About 10 per cent of cerebral embolism has been attributed to this mechanism. Second, the vegetations may form a focus (commonly called a *nidus*) for the development of infective endocarditis. Nonbacterial endocarditis has been called "terminal" or "cachectic" endocarditis, but of necessity, the lesions are encountered most frequently at necropsy. Probably they occur quite frequently. Vegetations on the valves of the right side of the heart are particularly common if a Swan-Ganz or similar catheter has been in place during the period immediately preceding death.

Infective Endocarditis

Case History I

The patient was a 63-year-old man with a 15-year history of essential hypertension and a 5-year history of intermittent claudication. Investigation revealed blockage of the bifurcation of the abdominal aorta. A bypass operation was performed by insertion of an aortoiliac synthetic (Dacron) prosthesis. For the next 4

years, the patient was able to walk without pain; then the claudication returned. Surgery was again performed, and the prosthesis was found to be obstructed by thrombus. The prosthesis was replaced. As a result of the previous surgery, many peritoneal adhesions were present. Unfortunately, the small bowel was accidentally opened during the operation. The tear was sutured, but the fecal contamination led to a postoperative wound infection. In spite of vigorous antibiotic therapy and surgical drainage of abscesses, the patient's condition steadily deteriorated and he died 4 months after the operation. On several occasions during the course of his illness, *Escherichia coli* and *Candida* species had been isolated from the blood.

At necropsy, septic infarcts and pyemic abscesses were found in the brain, myocardium, kidneys and spleen. These were related to endocarditis involving the mitral valve (Fig. 20–4).

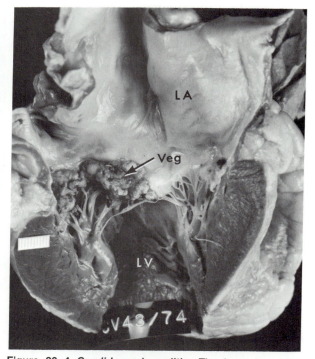

Figure 20–4 *Candida* **endocarditis.** The heart has been opened to show the mitral valve, the left atrium (LA), and the left ventricle (LV). Friable vegetations (Veg) are present on the anterior cusp of the mitral valve. *Candida* was identified in the vegetations both by culture and in histologic sections. The necropsy findings (see Case History I) indicate that this was an example of acute infective endocarditis. Nevertheless, the long clinical course was more suggestive of the subacute variety. Chemotherapy modifies the clinical and pathologic findings; it is more useful to describe endocarditis in terms of the infecting organism rather than as "acute" or "subacute." (Courtesy of Dr. M. D. Silver, University of Toronto.)

Etiology and Pathogenesis. In infective endocarditis, infection of the heart valves is accompanied by inflammation and overlying thrombosis; without effective treatment, it is almost invariably fatal. Depending on the virulence of the infecting organism, the course and pathologic changes vary considerably. If the organism is of low virulence, the illness has a long fluctuating course that by convention is termed *subacute bacterial endocarditis*. With a virulent organism, there is an overwhelming infection that tends to overshadow the cardiac manifestations. This is *acute endocarditis.*

Bacterial endocarditis arises at the site of a pre-existing cardiac anomaly in about 50 per cent of cases. The defect may be a valvular lesion (commonly of rheumatic origin), a congenital lesion (commonly a small septal defect or a patent ductus arteriosus), or at the site of foreign material introduced surgically, such as a patch or a prosthetic valve. Two steps are believed to be involved in the pathogenesis of infective endocarditis: the first is endocardial damage with thrombosis, the second is infection.

The first step in the evolution of infective endocarditis is endothelial damage. Subsequently there is thrombosis and infection. Turbulence is believed to be the cause of endocardial damage, and the distribution of the lesions suggests that this occurs when a high-pressure jet of blood is forced through a small orifice into a low-pressure sink. In mitral valve disease with regurgitation, a jet of blood enters the low-pressure atrium during ventricular systole. Similarly, turbulence occurs when there is aortic stenosis with regurgitation. With a small ventricular septal defect, a jet of blood enters the low-pressure cavity of the right ventricle.

Endocardial damage leads to thrombus formation, and subsequent infection results in endocarditis. Precisely how the organisms reach the thrombus is not known. Possibly there is a chance bacteremia while the thrombus is being formed, or perhaps platelets have specific receptors for certain organisms. Certainly, infection with some organisms is more common than with others. *Streptococcus viridans* was once the most common cause of subacute infective endocarditis but is now less frequent (Fig. 20–4). Other types of streptococci, staphylococci, coliforms, and

other organisms are encountered; indeed, there are few species that have not been encountered. Staphylococci and *Candida* are particularly common in main-line drug addicts, whereas *Staphylococcus epidermidis* and fungi attack heart valve prostheses. In the acute forms of endocarditis, the organism is highly virulent (*e.g., Staphylococcus aureus, Streptococcus pyogenes,* gonococci, pneumococci, and others); a pre-existing valvular lesion is less commonly present than with the more chronic forms of endocarditis.

Because the presence of a valvular or congenital heart lesion predisposes to the development of infective endocarditis, any patient known to have such a lesion should be given adequate antibiotic therapy before being subjected to any procedure (*e.g.,* dental extraction or urinary catheterization) likely to cause bacteremia. The antibiotic is given immediately before the procedure.

Clinical Features. In acute endocarditis, the clinical picture is that of a septicemia with evidence of multiple systemic septic emboli leading to pyemic abscesses or septic infarcts. In the more chronic forms of infective endocarditis (subacute infective endocarditis), the course is quite different. There is a prolonged illness characterized by fatigue, weight loss, intermittent fever, clubbing of the fingers, and signs of valvular disease of the heart. Echocardiography is a useful technique for detecting valvular vegetations. Multiple embolic phenomena are characteristic; the emboli behave as if they were sterile, probably because the patient has considerable immunity and the relatively avirulent organisms in the emboli are killed at the site of impaction. The embolization leads to infarction of spleen, kidney, brain, and elsewhere. Immune-complex vasculitis is responsible for palpable purpura of the skin and the glomerulonephritis that leads to renal failure. The diagnosis of infective endocarditis rests on obtaining a positive blood culture, but because the bacteremia is intermittent, multiple specimens may have to be examined before a positive culture is obtained. The disease is so serious that in a suitable clinical setting, a presumptive diagnosis of the disease warrants the institution of chemotherapy.

Morphologic Features. The aortic valve is affected in about one third of cases, the mitral in a further third; in others, both valves are involved. Involvement of the valves on the right side is uncommon except in intravenous drug addicts.

The affected valves are covered by bulky, red, friable vegetations that are liable to break off and embolize. Because the vegetations are particularly bulky and destructive in acute endocarditis, ulceration of the valve or rupture of one of the affected chordae tendineae is common. Local spread of infection results in a valve annulus or myocardial abscess. The affected valves may show evidence of a pre-existing lesion.

Even if treatment successfully eliminates infection, the affected valves often show gross distortion and calcification. Surgical replacement is then required to prevent heart failure.

Myxomatous Degeneration of Valves

In this form of valvular disease, the dense collagen of the valve leaflets is thinned and replaced by myxomatous tissue. The condition is quite common, and up to 10 per cent of young people, usually women, show evidence of the disease. A few patients have some generalized collagen abnormality, *e.g.*, Marfan's syndrome. The mitral valve is most commonly affected, and the thin ''floppy valve'' can prolapse into the atrium during ventricular systole. Usually the condition is asymptomatic, but some degree of regurgitation can occur. Serious complications include infective endocarditis and rupture of one of the chordae tendineae with marked regurgitation.

Calcific Aortic Stenosis

This condition usually affects elderly men and appears to be a degenerative condition arising in a congenitally abnormal valve. Usually the valve has two cusps rather than the customary three. The aortic valve cusps become calcified and fused together, producing a tight stenosis. The left ventricle is hypertrophied, but in spite of the overaction of this chamber, an inadequate amount of blood is pumped into the aorta. In particular, the blood supply to the coronary vessels is impaired, and these patients are in con-

stant danger of sudden death. Surgical replacement of the diseased valve by a homograft or a plastic prosthesis is therefore indicated.

Ischemic Heart Disease

Two coronary arteries supply the myocardium with blood. These vessels are particularly liable to be affected by atherosclerosis, which causes narrowing of their lumina and subsequent myocardial ischemia.

The incidence of ischemic heart disease steadily increased after 1920, until by 1960 the disease had reached almost epidemic proportion. Tobacco smoking, a sedentary life, gasoline fumes in the air, a diet containing too much saturated animal fat, the stress of modern life, and other factors were all blamed for the increased death rate from myocardial ischemia. Nevertheless, the evidence for any of these factors playing a significant role was not convincing. Quite unexpectedly, since 1965 the incidence of ischemic heart disease in North America has decreased. The reason for this change is not known, for there appears to have been no great change in life style to explain it.

Causes of Myocardial Ischemia and Hypoxia

Myocardial ischemia occurs as an imbalance between myocardial requirements and the availability of blood and oxygen. Coronary artery disease is the most important factor, in particular atherosclerosis. Dissecting aneurysm of the aorta, coronary embolism, polyarteritis nodosa, and other forms of arteritis are occasional causes. When myocardial ischemia occurs in the absence of apparent vascular disease, coronary artery spasm is believed to be the cause in some cases; it has been demonstrated radiographically. Severe hypotension as in shock and aortic stenosis are additional causes. Myocardial hypoxia can also result from increased myocardial metabolic requirements as may occur with sudden violent exercise, prolonged tachycardia, or hyperthyroidism. Reduced availability of oxygen in the blood as in severe anemia may be an additional factor.

Effects of Myocardial Ischemia

Slow occlusion of the coronary arteries leads to increasing ischemia; at first this has no obvious functional effect on the heart, but in due course, angina pectoris can ensue. Patchy destruction of myocardial fibers with replacement fibrosis often accompanies this. On the other hand, sudden complete occlusion commonly causes infarction. However, the correlations are not exact, and it is convenient to describe the four main syndromes associated with myocardial ischemia, without relating them directly to the apparent cause.

Angina Pectoris. Angina pectoris refers to a precordial or retrosternal oppressive pain that sometimes radiates into the neck and down the inner aspect of the left arm. In the common *stable type of angina,* the pain occurs with exercise, particularly in cold weather and after a heavy meal. It can also be precipitated by emotional stress. In *variant angina,* the pain occurs at rest; the ischemia is thought to be due to coronary artery spasm. *Unstable angina,* also called acute coronary insufficiency, describes the sudden onset of angina or the rapid worsening of existing stable angina. It is nearly always associated with severe coronary disease and is likely to be followed by myocardial infarction or death.

The pain in angina is thought to be due to the accumulation of metabolic substances produced by muscle contracting under ischemic conditions. It is not known why only some patients with coronary disease experience angina, whereas others are spared.

Chronic Ischemic Heart Disease. Chronic ischemic heart disease leads to patchy myocardial atrophy with replacement fibrosis and left ventricular failure.

Sudden Cardiac Death. Sudden death may occur without obvious myocardial infarction and is generally due to a sudden cardiac dysrhythmia, usually ventricular fibrillation or heart block due to ischemia of the conducting system. Sudden death is most common during the first 24 hours after the onset of acute ischemia; the value of acute coronary care units is that immediate cardiac massage or defibrillation can save the life of a number of patients. These patients need not necessarily develop subsequent infarction: the acute ischemia may have been transient enough to allow the muscle fibers to survive. It is obvious that the sooner an effective cardiac output is reestablished, the less likely there is to be permanent myocardial or cerebral damage. Hence, it is essential that medical personnel at all levels be trained in the techniques of cardiopulmonary resuscitation.

Myocardial Infarction. Myocardial infarction is the most severe effect of ischemia and is the most common cause of death in Western societies. It is more common in males than in females. In females over the age of 40 years, use of the birth control pill is a factor. Infarction is commonly associated with coronary atherosclerosis either alone or when complicated by thrombosis or hemorrhage into a plaque. The predisposing causes are discussed in the section on atherosclerosis. In some cases, neither coronary artery stenosis nor thrombosis is present, and the ischemia appears to be due to severe hypotension (as occurs in shock) or coronary artery spasm. Blockage by multiple small platelet emboli or thrombi has also been postulated, and their early dissipation can explain why they are not found at necropsy.

Although infarction is caused by ischemia, the pathogenesis is complex. Ischemia may not immediately lead to cell necrosis, but when it is followed by reperfusion of the area, damaging oxygen-derived free radicals are formed and contribute to the necrosis. Experimentally, agents that mop up free radicals limit the damaging effect of myocardial ischemia, and it is to be hoped that in the future this effect can be utilized in the treatment of human disease.

Morphologic Types of Myocardial Infarction. Two patterns of infarction are recognized. In *regional infarction,* a localized area of the left ventricular myocardium undergoes necrosis. A well-developed infarct appears as a firm, yellow area of coagulative necrosis with some surrounding hemorrhage and later inflammation (Figs. 20–5 and 20–6). Thrombosis of the supplying artery is usually present, and the location of the infarct is related to this. Thus, when the anterior descending branch of the left coronary artery is thrombosed, the anterior wall of the left ventricle and interventricular septum are infarcted. If the whole thickness of the ventricular wall is involved (transmural infarction), both pericardium

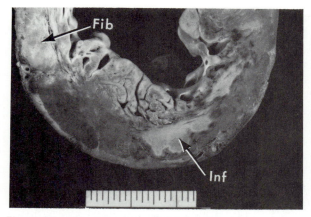

Figure 20–5 Recent myocardial infarction. The specimen shows part of the wall of the left ventricle. The recent infarct (Inf) is pale and has a hemorrhagic border. The lesion is about 10 days old. Fibrosis in other areas (Fib) is the result of a previous heart attack.

and endocardium are affected. In *subendocardial infarction,* a wide zone of myocardium deep to the endocardium is infarcted (Fig. 20–7). This is associated with severe stenosis of all major coronary arteries, but thrombosis is not present.

Clinical Features of Myocardial Infarction. The sudden onset of severe pain in the center of the chest (retrosternal) is characteristic of myocardial infarction. The pain is not relieved by rest or nitroglycerin, and its severity may cause the patient to sweat. Although the typical heart attack is accompanied by severe pain, it is not uncommon for the pain to be relatively mild and atypical. Pain may be situated in the upper abdomen and therefore be mistaken for gastritis. Occasionally, the attack is not accompanied by any pain, and the presence of massive infarction comes as a surprise at necropsy of a patient who died of heart failure for unknown reasons.

Electrocardiographic Changes. Myocardial ischemia and infarction produce changes in the electrocardiogram that are of great diagnostic value (Fig. 20–10D) and from which an idea of the site and extent of the damage can be assessed. Repeated electrocardiograms are of particular value in following the progress of the patient. As with most investigations, the method is not infallible. A patient can die of myocardial infarction and yet have equivocal findings on electrocardiogra-

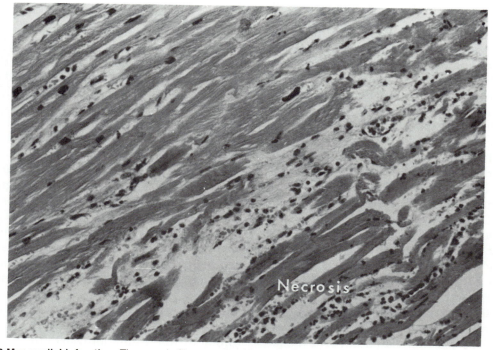

Figure 20–6 Myocardial infarction. The muscle fibers on the right-hand side are shrunken and show intense staining with eosin. Between the fibers is an infiltration by polymorphonuclear leukocytes. A number of red cells are also seen extravasated in the interstitial tissue. Compare these fibers with the normal ones in the upper left part of the picture. This section was taken at necropsy from a man who 8 days previously had sustained an intense crushing pain in the chest and shortly afterward had developed cardiac shock that was not alleviated by treatment (×250).

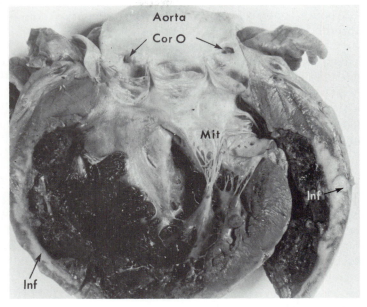

Figure 20–7 Myocardial infarction with extensive mural thrombosis. The dilated left ventricle has been opened, and part of its lateral wall has been swung over to the left. The anterior cusp of the mitral valve (Mit) is clearly shown. Part of the aorta is included in the specimen, and the orifices of the two coronary arteries (Cor O) can be seen immediately above the three cusps of the aortic valve. There is extensive infarction (Inf) of the left ventricular wall immediately adjacent to the endocardium. Attached to the infarcted muscle is a dark mural thrombus. Both coronary arteries were markedly stenosed by atherosclerosis, but no occluding thrombus was present. It is not uncommon to find this pattern of subendocardial infarction in the absence of a thrombosed coronary artery.

phy. Likewise, a patient dying of some disease can have chest pain and electrocardiographic changes "typical" of a myocardial infarct, and yet at necropsy no infarction can be found.

Enzyme Changes in the Diagnosis of Myocardial Infarction. Necrotic heart muscle releases enzymes into the blood stream, and their detection is a useful diagnostic procedure (Chapter 4). The enzyme *creatine phosphokinase (CPK)* is the most specific, and its blood level rises within 6 hours, peaks at 24 hours, and returns to normal by 72 hours. CPK is also present in skeletal muscle, and an intramuscular injection (*e.g.,* of a pain-relieving drug) can cause a considerable rise. The CPK isoenzyme MB is virtually specific for myocardium, but its estimation is expensive and not a routine procedure in most centers. The aspartate aminotransferase level rises in about 12 hours, peaks at 36 hours, and gradually falls by about the fifth day following infarction. The enzyme is also present in liver cells, and very high blood levels suggest liver damage. This could be due to acute congestion and hypoxia secondary to the heart failure precipitated by a myocardial infarction. *Lactic dehydrogenase (LDH),* particularly the isoenzyme LDH-1, predominates in the heart and red blood cells. Its level rises slowly after a myocardial infarct, peaks at 48 hours, and may not return to normal for 1 to 3 weeks. It is evident that the significance of enzyme levels in an isolated sample of blood can be difficult to assess. In the diagnosis of a patient with suspected myocardial infarction, it is advisable to examine samples of blood over a period of several days.

Nuclear Imaging. Technetium-labeled pyrophosphate and diphosphonate accumulate in ischemic or infarcted myocardial fibers, and "hot spots" indicative of damage can be detected by scanning for radioactivity.

Complications of Myocardial Infarction. Three early complications of myocardial infarction should be noted.

Pericarditis. This condition occurs if the infarct involves the pericardial surface.

Mural Thrombosis. This is seen if the infarct involves the endocardium (Fig. 20–7). Portions of this thrombus may break off and embolize to systemic organs (*e.g.,* the brain and the kidneys), thereby producing serious and sometimes fatal results.

Rupture. Occasionally, the necrotic muscle ruptures, causing acute hemopericardium and sudden death. Both this complication and systemic embolism are likely to occur at the end of the first week. Rupture of an infarcted papillary muscle leads to sudden mitral insufficiency, heart failure, and death.

About 70 per cent of patients with coronary thrombosis survive their first attack. The infarct organizes to produce a fibrous scar (Fig. 20–8), which may later bulge and lead to an *aneurysm of the left ventricle.* The aneurysm itself may subsequently rupture, but this is an uncommon event. Usually the patient who has had a myocardial infarct is left with some heart damage, and further episodes of infarction are not uncommon.

In the past, it has been customary to keep patients at rest for several weeks after myocardial infarction. At that time, it was assumed that the heart needed rest for healing to occur. Medical personnel now realize that this rest is unnecessary. It is common practice to keep the patient in bed for 2 weeks only and then to allow increasing exercise. This program of moderate exercise has not increased the death rate and has

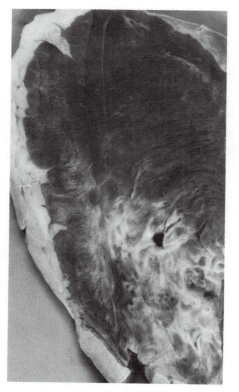

Figure 20–8 Myocardial fibrosis. The specimen is an oblique section through part of the wall of the left ventricle. White fibrous scar tissue has replaced much of the muscle in the lower part of the specimen. This was the end result of an infarct several years before death.

diminished the incidence of complications of bed rest, *e.g.,* pulmonary embolism.

Hypertensive Heart Disease

The presence of systemic hypertension puts a strain on the left ventricle. The muscle fibers enlarge, and this leads to *concentric hypertrophy* of the left ventricle. In due course, often after many years, the left ventricle fails. Attacks of paroxysmal nocturnal dyspnea may occur (Chapter 22). The reason hypertrophic muscle fibers eventually work inefficiently is not known. One explanation is that no new capillaries are formed to provide them with an adequate blood supply. Another factor may be the development of coronary atherosclerosis, which frequently complicates hypertension.

The detection of systemic hypertension is important because effective drug therapy is available and heart failure can be averted.

Cor Pulmonale

Cor pulmonale may be defined as enlargement of the right ventricle secondary to disease or dysfunction of the lungs. The effect on the heart is mediated by *pulmonary hypertension.* The increased pressure in the pulmonary artery is caused by one of three mechanisms. The pulmonary vasculature may be *blocked by material within the lumen* (*e.g.,* thrombus or, rarely, tumor emboli); the vessels may go into *spasm,* an effect generally caused by local tissue hypoxia; finally, the pulmonary vessels may fall victim to *local destructive disease, e.g.,* a type of chronic inflammation such as tuberculosis.

In *acute cor pulmonale,* the right ventricle is acutely dilated and fails owing to an acute obstruction to the pulmonary arterial system. The most common cause is massive pulmonary embolism. A sudden severe attack of bronchial asthma is a less common cause.

In *chronic cor pulmonale,* the right ventricular muscle undergoes hypertrophy secondary to chronic pulmonary hypertension. Causes may be listed:

1. Multiple repeated small pulmonary embolisms.

2. Primary pulmonary vascular disease. Occasional examples of polyarteritis affecting the lung are encountered but are not common. In *idiopathic pulmonary hypertension,* no cause for the small vessel disease can be found.

3. Chronic obstructive lung disease and any other chronic disease that is accompanied by lung destruction, *e.g.,* chronic pulmonary tuberculosis and pneumoconiosis (Chapter 22). Hypoxia adds the effect of vascular spasm to the vascular destruction caused directly by the disease.

4. Impaired pulmonary ventilation from whatever cause, *e.g.,* severe kyphoscoliosis (Chapter 30), muscular paralysis, or obesity (see Pickwickian Syndrome, Chapter 22).

Chronic cor pulmonale is often associated with secondary polycythemia caused by chronic hypoxemia. This increases the viscosity of the blood and adds an additional strain on the already overtaxed right ventricle. Right-sided heart failure eventually ensues.

Valvular Disease of the Heart

The effects of valvular disease are stenosis, regurgitation, or a combination of both. In order to understand the causes of valvular defects, it must be appreciated that although the valve leaflets are the most obvious component of the valves, they are just part of the *valve complex.* In the atrioventricular valves, this complex consists of part of the atrial wall, the annulus, the valve leaflets, the chordae tendineae, the papillary muscles, and the wall of the adjacent ventricle. No papillary muscles are present in the aortic and pulmonary valves, which therefore have a simpler structure.

Valve dysfunction may be acute or chronic. Common causes of acute valve dysfunction are valve leaflet perforation in infective endocarditis, ruptured papillary muscle in myocardial infarction, and rupture of one of the chordae in myxomatous degeneration. In chronic valvular lesions, turbulence around the valve can result in the deposition of small thrombi, which may lyse or become organized. If the thrombus organizes, the valve leaflets become thickened and perhaps eventually calcified; increased turbulence causes further valve damage and dysfunction. This is

the mechanism involved in the development of calcific aortic stenosis associated with a congenital bicuspid valve; also it contributes to the commisural fusion and shortening of the chordae in chronic rheumatic mitral disease.

It is convenient at this point to summarize the valve complex diseases. Details of these are found in other parts of the book.

Mitral Valve Disease. The mitral valve shows structural abnormalities more commonly than does the tricuspid.

Mitral Stenosis. This defect is the most common valvular disease of the heart and is nearly always due to chronic rheumatic endocarditis.

*Mitral Regurgitation.** Some degree of mitral regurgitation is common in chronic rheumatic mitral stenosis. It also occurs in heart failure when dilation of the valve annulus impairs the ability of the annulus to contract and perform a sphincteric function. Calcification of the annulus has a similar effect. The disease is regarded as a degenerative condition and is common in old age. Ischemia of the papillary muscles can affect their function by causing their infarction, rupture, or atrophy with fibrous replacement. Likewise, fibrosis or aneurysmal dilation of the adjacent left ventricular wall can lead to mitral regurgitation by altering the axis of pull of the papillary muscles.

Aortic Valve Disease

Aortic Stenosis. This defect is usually combined with regurgitation in chronic rheumatic heart disease. Congenital stenosis can affect the valve cusps or be due to hypertrophy of the muscle below the valve (subaortic muscular stenosis). Calcific aortic stenosis occurs in old age.

Aortic Regurgitation. There are a number of conditions in which the elastic tissue of the aorta and the aortic valve annulus are so weakened that the annulus becomes dilated. The valve cusps fail to meet, causing severe regurgitation to result. Syphilitic aortitis and medionecrosis of the aorta fall into this group. Syphilitic aortitis is now a rare disease, but a similar type of aortitis with aortic regurgitation is encountered in *rheumatoid arthritis* and *ankylosing spondylitis.* Suffi-

*The terms insufficiency or incompetence are sometimes used to denote regurgitation. Strictly interpreted, however, they could also include stenosis. Regurgitation is more explicit and is used in this book.

cient dilation for causing regurgitation is also seen in hypertension.

Tricuspid Valve Disease. Tricuspid stenosis is generally of rheumatic origin, but it is rare. Tricuspid regurgitation, which is more common than is stenosis, is generally due to dilation of the valve annulus in right-sided heart failure.

Pulmonary Valve Disease. Pulmonary stenosis is nearly always congenital in origin. Sufficient rheumatic endocarditis for causing deformity is rare.

Myocardial Disease

Myocardial ischemia is a common cause of heart failure. Acute infarction, described previously, may precipitate acute heart failure. Repeated infarcts, or gradual coronary occlusion causing fibrosis, may put such a strain on the remaining muscle fibers that failure ultimately occurs.

If one examines the heart muscle from a patient in failure due to hemodynamic conditions, it is disappointing to find that no abnormality can be detected. The muscle fibers may be hypertrophied, but this does not explain why they failed, nor does a biochemical examination elucidate the problem. We have to admit that the heart that fails in hypertension or valvular disease appears normal microscopically, but it does not behave normally. Obviously, our methods of examination are crude and not suited to detecting the lesion involved.

There are a number of diseases in which heart failure occurs as a result of disease that affects the myocardium primarily. These may be divided into two groups, myocarditis and the cardiomyopathies.

Myocarditis

Myocardial damage accompanied by inflammation can be caused by a number of agents. *Toxic myocarditis* is a feature of diphtheria, and the myocarditis of acute rheumatic fever appears to be immunologically mediated. *Infective myocarditis* can be caused by many organisms. In children, acute myocarditis is most often viral; coxsackie A and B viruses have been incriminated most often. Myocarditis can occur in septicemia and pyemia. In South America, trypanosomiasis causes chronic myocarditis (Chagas' disease) and is a common cause of heart failure. Clinically, myocarditis causes chest pain, heart failure, and cardiac dysrhythmia. Embolism can result from mural thrombosis.

Cardiomyopathy

The cardiomyopathies include a group of non-inflammatory diseases that appear to involve primarily the myocardium. Ischemic disease and the effects of valvular disease are excluded. Two groups are described: a primary group in which the cause is unknown and only the heart is involved, and a secondary group in which the heart lesion is part of a systemic disease.

Primary Cardiomyopathy. This group has by definition no known cause, although a previous myocarditis or the effect of some poison has been suspected. The heart may be dilated and flabby, show marked hypertrophy, or exhibit extensive fibrosis.

Secondary Cardiomyopathy (Specific Heart Muscle Disease). The myocardium can be damaged by many agents. These include toxins (*e.g.,* alcohol and doxorubicin used in the treatment of malignant disease), metabolic disturbances (*e.g.,* hemochromatosis, beriberi, and amyloidosis), glycogen storage disease, and infiltration by leukemic or other malignant cells.

Considerable overlap exists between the two types of cardiomyopathy because the primary group is only primary so long as no cause can be identified. Indeed, some authorities now restrict the term "cardiomyopathy" to those conditions of unknown cause and label the secondary group specific heart muscle disease.

Diseases of the Pericardium

The pericardial sac normally contains 30 to 50 ml of fluid, and its smooth lining aids the functions of the heart. An excessive amount of fluid within the pericardial sac occurs under three circumstances.

Hydropericardium. A transudate of low specific gravity may accompany any type of generalized edema, *e.g.,* in heart failure or in the nephrotic syndrome.

Pericardial Effusions due to Pericarditis (see later).

Hemopericardium. Pure blood or blood clot in the pericardium generally results from the rupture of a myocardial infarct or of the outer wall of a dissecting aneurysm of the aorta. Trauma is a third cause and may be inflicted by a stab wound or by the physician's needle when a coronary vessel is inadvertently torn in an attempt to obtain fluid from the pericardial sac.

The effect of excess fluid in the pericardium depends on the quantity of fluid present and the speed with which it accumulates. A slow accumulation of 3000 ml can be tolerated, since the pericardial sac gradually stretches. Rapid accumulation of even 200 ml can lead to *acute cardiac tamponade.* In this, the increased pressure within the pericardial sac hinders venous filling of the atria, and this in turn reduces the cardiac output and coronary blood flow. Hypotension, a state of shock, and finally death can follow rapidly unless the fluid is promptly drained by the insertion of a needle *(pericardiocentesis).*

Acute Pericarditis

Acute serous or serofibrinous pericarditis occurs as a benign condition in young adults. Fever, sudden onset of sharp retrosternal pain that alters with the position of a patient, and a pericardial rub are the main clinical features. Coxsackieviruses and others have been isolated from a few cases, but the majority remain idiopathic.

A sterile pericarditis is a feature of acute rheumatic fever, systemic lupus erythematosus (Chapter 6), and uremia (Chapter 25). It also occurs over an acute myocardial infarct. A typical acute pericarditis may occur weeks or even months after a myocardial infarct. This is called *postmyocardial infarction pericarditis,* or Dressler's syndrome. The pathogenesis is not known, but an autoimmune reaction to damaged tissue has been suggested. Some support for this is the occurrence of a similar acute pericarditis after cardiac surgery. This *postpericardiotomy syndrome*

has been estimated to occur in about 10 per cent of patients who undergo cardiac surgery. It may occur weeks after the surgical event and must be distinguished from a bacterial infection.

Suppurative pericarditis is generally bacterial in origin and is caused by spreading of infection from an adjacent site such as pneumonia or an empyema (see Fig. 5–8). Occasionally, acute suppurative pericarditis occurs as an isolated event, and spread from some inapparent focus of infection via the blood stream is presumed to be the pathogenesis.

The end result of acute pericarditis is generally resolution, perhaps with the formation of a few unimportant fibrous adhesions. Occasionally these adhesions are extensive, and two syndromes are recognized.

Adhesive Mediastinopericarditis

There is massive fibrosis with obliteration of the pericardial sac and adhesion to adjacent structures. This mass of fibrous tissue surrounds the heart, greatly increases the workload of the myocardium, and leads to cardiac hypertrophy and dilation.

Constrictive Pericarditis

Sometimes dense fibrous tissue with foci of calcification surrounds the heart and, by encasing it, impedes venous filling and constricts the venae cavae. The thickened pericardium is not attached to adjacent mediastinal structures, and the heart remains of normal size. In constrictive pericarditis, there is heart failure and prominent venous congestion affecting liver, spleen, and elsewhere. Ascites is a striking feature.

Both adhesive mediastinopericarditis and constrictive pericarditis may be the end result of a suppurative or a tuberculous pericarditis, but often the condition appears to be idiopathic because no evidence of a preceding infection can be found.

Cardiac Dysrhythmias

The term "dysrhythmia" is used to describe any condition in which the heart is beating either too quickly, too slowly, or irregularly. The impulse that initiates cardiac contraction commences in the sinoatrial node in the right atrium, spreads throughout the atria to the atrioventricular node, and then travels down the conducting bundle of His to reach the two ventricles via the two major branches of the bundle of His. This regular spread of electrical impulse can be interrupted in many ways by various pathologic conditions. Only some of the most common disorders are described here (Figs. 20–9 and 20–10).

Ectopic Beats. An ectopic beat arises prematurely from a site other than the sinoatrial node. It may be in the atria, in the atrioventricular node, or in the ventricle (Fig. 20–10C). Distinction between these types can be made only by study of the electrocardiogram. Following the ectopic beat, there is a compensatory pause before the next normal heart beat. This sometimes produces the feeling of the heart "turning over," but apart from this, ectopic beats produce no symptoms. They are common in normal people, but they can also be an indication of myocardial disease. This association with myocardial disease applies particularly to the ventricular ectopic beats, which are encountered in patients with myocardial ischemia and in those who have taken too much digitalis.

Paroxysmal Tachycardia. In this condition, there are attacks of rapid heart action resulting from a regular succession of ectopic beats that last for a few seconds or as long as several days. *Paroxysmal atrial tachycardia* is the most common type and is generally not associated with heart disease. The *ventricular type* is more usually seen in patients with ischemic disease; like ventricular ectopic beats, this condition may precede ventricular fibrillation in patients with myocardial infarction.

Atrial Fibrillation. This is a common and important disorder. It is due to multiple ectopic foci discharging at variable rates in the atria. Rapid fibrillary waves take place rather than normal atrial contraction, and the multiple impulses that reach the atrioventricular node (up to 600 per minute) cannot all be conducted to the ventricles. Approximately 100 to 160 reach the ventricles at a completely irregular rhythm. Because not all ventricular contractions are powerful enough to open the aortic and pulmonary valves, the pulse rate as felt at the wrist is less than that heard at the apex of the heart. Rheumatic heart disease, particularly mitral stenosis, is the most common cause of atrial fibrillation; in older patients, ischemic heart disease, systemic hypertension, and thyrotoxicosis are other important causes.

Atrial fibrillation is generally treated by the administration of digitalis, which acts by impairing conduction in the bundle of His. Fewer impulses reach the ventricles, causing them to

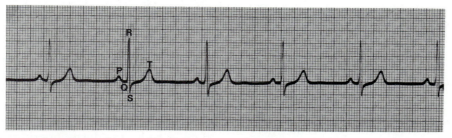

Figure 20–9 The normal electrocardiogram (ECG). The electrocardiogram is a meter that amplifies and records the differences in electrical potential between two points (bipolar leads) on the surface of the body. Originally, three standard leads were used (lead I, left arm–right arm; lead II, left leg–right arm; and lead III, left leg–left arm), but the "unipolar" or V leads are now more commonly used. An exploratory electrode is placed on various parts of the chest wall; for example, VI lead is placed on the fourth right intercostal space near the sternum, and the second electrode is kept at zero potential.

The electrocardiogram is representative of the electrical activity in the heart, and this triggers muscular activity. P, the first wave, represents passage of activity through the atria (depolarization) and triggers atrial systole. The QRS complex represents ventricular excitation corresponding to ventricular systole. The T waves represent ventricular recovery, or repolarization. The Q wave is a small negative deflection and is often absent. With the graph paper used for the standard electrocardiogram, each small square of the abscissa is 1 mm and represents 40 msec. The heart rate can be estimated by counting the number of millimeters between consecutive R waves (or other portion of the complex) and dividing 1500 by this number. In the record shown, the distance between each R wave is 29 or 30 mm, and this corresponds to a heart rate of just over 50 beats per minute. (Courtesy of Dr. R. S. Baigrie, Sunnybrook Health Sciences Centre, North York, Ontario, Canada.)

Figure 20–10 Abnormal electrocardiograms. *A,* Atrial flutter. Normal P waves are absent and are replaced by a flutter wave occurring at approximately 300 per minute. Some impulses reach the ventricles and lead to ventricular complexes. At point A, pressure was applied to the carotid sinus, and this produced reflex vagal activity. The effect of this was to produce a temporary heart block, and for a period there was ventricular standstill.

B, Atrial fibrillation. In this electrocardiogram, no P waves can be seen, and the irregular atrial fibrillation indicates chaotic atrial activity. The ventricles respond in an erratic manner, so that the heart rate in addition to being fast (95 beats per minute) is irregularly irregular.

C, Ectopic ventricular beats. Two ectopic beats are shown in which the QRS complex is abnormal. This abnormality is a reflection of the beats arising within the ventricles themselves and not being a response to normal stimulation from the atria.

D, Myocardial infarction. The outstanding feature of this electrocardiograph is depression of the ST segment. This change was seen shortly after an acute myocardial infarction. In other leads there was ST segment elevation, and analysis of the changes in the standard leads can give a good indication of the site of the infarct.

(Courtesy of Dr. R. S. Baigrie, Sunnybrook Health Sciences Centre, North York, Ontario, Canada.)

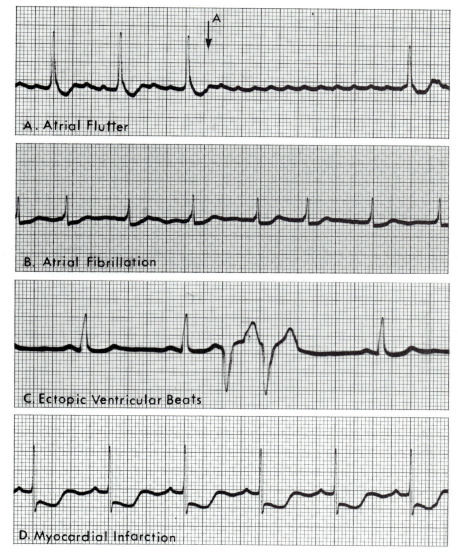

A. Atrial Flutter

B. Atrial Fibrillation

C. Ectopic Ventricular Beats

D. Myocardial Infarction

be slowed, so that each contraction is more effective. The atrial fibrillation is not terminated. Indeed, to try to stop the fibrillation itself may precipitate detachment of a mural thrombus from the atrium.

Atrial Flutter. This form of dysrhythmia is less common than is atrial fibrillation. The atria contract at a rate of about 300 beats per minute, being stimulated by a rapidly firing ectopic pacemaker. Atrioventricular block results in a slower ventricular rate (Fig. 20–10*A*).

Ventricular Fibrillation. This is a most serious condition, and it is generally the immediate pre-

cursor of death in myocardial infarction. Immediate external electrical defibrillation is the most effective treatment if equipment is available.

Heart Block. The term "heart block" is used to describe depression of conduction between the atria and the ventricles. In the early stages, the time required for the impulse to reach the ventricles is merely prolonged, but as the condition progresses, occasional impulses fail to reach the ventricles and a beat is dropped. When conduction is completely blocked, there is *complete heart block;* no impulses from the atria reach the ventricles, which then beat at their own intrinsic rate of about 40 beats per minute. The chief causes of heart block are ischemic heart disease and an overdose of digitalis. When complete heart block occurs suddenly, the ventricles may not start to beat for several minutes, and the patient rapidly loses consciousness and develops convulsions. These episodes are known as *Stokes-Adams attacks*.

Effects of Cardiac Dysrhythmias

Irregular or rapid cardiac contraction may lead to a sensation in the chest that is described as *palpitation*. If the heart rate is either very rapid (*e.g.*, over 160 beats per minute, as in paroxysmal tachycardia and atrial fibrillation) or very low (*e.g.*, below 40 beats per minute, as in complete heart block), the cardiac output is diminished, particularly on exercise. If the heart is otherwise normal, this change in rate may be of no immediate consequence, but if it is superadded to some other heart disease, the results can be serious. Tachycardia increases the heart's requirements for oxygen, and the energy expended is wastefully used by ineffective contractions. Furthermore, during tachycardia, the coronary blood flow is decreased. Most of the coronary blood flow takes place during diastole; with tachycardia, diastole is shortened, and the blood flow is diminished. The heart muscle therefore has an increased need for oxygen at the same time that its supply is reduced. The ischemia that results further impairs myocardial activity and can lead to necrosis, either patchy or massive. Heart failure can therefore be precipitated.

HEART FAILURE

The major contractile element of the heart is the muscular walls of the two ventricles. When the muscle is relaxed *(diastole)*, blood flows into the ventricles; the flow is aided to some extent by atrial contraction. When the ventricular muscle contracts *(systole)*, the atrioventricular valves close, and a volume of blood (the cardiac output) is forced past the pulmonary and aortic valves into the main arteries. At the end of systole, some blood remains in the ventricles; this is called the *residual volume.* Under resting conditions, the venous return to each ventricle is about 5 liters per minute; with exercise, this increases to 25 liters or more. Cardiac output is correspondingly increased by utilizing the three *cardiac reserves* described in the following.

1. The increased filling of the ventricles stretches the heart muscle fibers, causing an increase in the force of the next contraction. This response is known as *Starling's law of the heart*, which states that *the energy of contraction is proportional to the initial length of the cardiac muscle fibers.* In spite of the increased venous return of exercise, the pressure of blood in the atria does not rise under normal circumstances.

2. Increased sympathetic tone causes an increase in the strength of cardiac contraction. This reduces the residual volume and therefore increases the amount of blood ejected with each systole. A change in the force of contraction of the heart without a corresponding change in the initial length of the muscle is termed an *inotropic effect.* The alkaloids of digitalis are used in heart failure because they have an inotropic effect.

3. Increased sympathetic tone also causes an increase in heart rate, *e.g.*, from the normal 70 beats per minute to over double that figure.

The venous return to the right ventricle is the amount of blood draining from all the tissues of the body except the lungs, and this is directly related to the arterial supply to these tissues. The blood supply of a tissue is determined mainly by local self-regulatory mechanisms that are designed to ensure sufficient blood flow to satisfy the activity of the tissue at all times. The venous return, and hence the cardiac output, is governed mainly by extracardiac factors, namely, the metabolic requirements of the body as a whole. By using the reserves described, the normal heart can cope with any normal load placed upon it. When it fails to do this, the result is heart failure, because in the presence of an adequate venous return, it fails to supply the needs to the body. At first the effects of this are seen only during exercise, but as the failure increases, the effects are apparent even at rest. Either the left or the right ventricle may fail separately; more usually the heart fails as a whole. The condition is then called *congestive heart failure.*

Effects of Right Ventricular Failure

Rise in Central Venous Pressure. A failure of the right ventricle to eject all the blood it receives leads to distention of the right atrium by a back-pressure effect. The pressure in the great veins rises, and the jugular veins are seen to be distended with blood when the patient sits up in bed. To some extent this aids heart function, because by stretching the heart muscle, the raised pressure increases the force of contraction. Eventually, however, a point is reached beyond which increased stretching causes a *decrease* in cardiac contraction (Fig. 20–11). Exercise, by increasing the venous return, further reduces the cardiac output and forces the patient to be bedridden. Once this critical point is past, therapeutic bleeding increases the cardiac output by reducing the venous pressure. (This is the basis of the time-honored practice of bleeding as a treatment of heart failure.) A similar effect can be obtained by applying tourniquets to the limbs to obstruct the venous return and to allow pooling of blood in the peripheral vessels. In right-sided heart failure, all the organs of the body are congested because of the increased venous pressure. This effect is particularly evident in the liver, where the center of the lobules is congested and red. Congestion is also apparent in the skin, especially of the face.

Cyanosis. The sluggish circulation allows the blood to become deoxygenated as it passes through the tissues; this response is apparent in the skin as a bluish discoloration known as cyanosis. Cyanosis is evident when the capillary blood contains more than 5 g/dl of reduced hemoglobin. Cyanosis due to stasis is known as *peripheral cyanosis,* and it should be contrasted with the type (central cyanosis) that occurs when venous blood is directly shunted into the systemic arterial system, as in some types of congenital heart disease. Peripheral cyanosis is not necessarily due to heart disease and occurs in other conditions when the circulation is sluggish. It is also seen in shock, whenever there is some local cause of venous obstruction, and when the blood becomes viscous. Stasis in the skin vessels sometimes occurs as a response to cold in people who are otherwise normal. Indeed, it is a common experience to see some degree of cyanosis of the ears, nose, and fingertips on a cold winter's morning.

Polycythemia. An increased red blood cell count occurs as a result of bone marrow hypoxia.

Edema. Edema of the dependent parts is a prominent sign of heart failure. If the patient is up and about, swelling of the ankles is first apparent, whereas if he or she is in bed, swelling of the tissues over the sacrum and external genitalia occurs most often. The pathogenesis of the

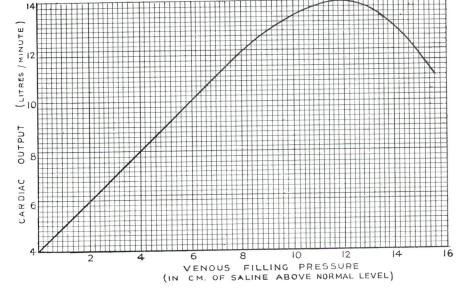

Figure 20–11 Relationship of cardiac output to venous filling pressure (Starling's curve). (From Wood, P.: Diseases of the Heart and Circulation. 2nd ed. London, Eyre and Spottis Wood, 1956.)

edema is complex. In part it is due to the chronic passive venous congestion; this, in itself, is not the complete answer, however. It certainly helps to account for the *location* of the fluid accumulation—be it in the sacral region or legs—but it does not explain *why* the fluid accumulates. In right ventricular failure the output of the heart is inadequate for the needs of the body, and this results in peripheral vasoconstriction, which allows the blood to be most economically distributed. The mechanism is analogous to that which is seen in shock (Chapter 19). The redistribution of blood appears particularly to affect the kidneys and results in a more complete reabsorption of sodium. This causes concurrent water retention and an increase in volume of the extracellular fluids. This increased volume appears as edema. The importance of sodium retention in the pathogenesis of cardiac edema is reflected in treatment. Diuretics that cause excretion of sodium are of great use in treatment of cardiac edema. Likewise, a diet low in salt is frequently prescribed with advantage.

Effects of Left Ventricular Failure

Rise in Pulmonary Venous Pressure. With the onset of left ventricular failure, the left atrial pressure increases, and the atrium together with the pulmonary vessels becomes distended with blood. As in mitral stenosis, dyspnea ensues. The rise in pulmonary venous pressure is extremely serious because of the imminent danger of pulmonary edema. The edema of the lungs may accumulate slowly, but sometimes acute attacks occur, particularly at night. This reaction, which is called *paroxysmal nocturnal dyspnea,* is a life-threatening event. The patient wakes up in the early hours of the morning with a sense of breathlessness and acute oppression of the chest. The patient becomes acutely distressed and coughs up the blood-stained watery sputum that is characteristic of severe acute pulmonary edema. Spasm of the bronchi is often a feature, and the condition resembles bronchial asthma to the extent that it sometimes is called *cardiac asthma.* The pathogenesis of acute paroxysmal dyspnea is only partially understood. It seems to be precipitated by a sudden sympathetic over-

activity. Intense constriction of the peripheral systemic blood vessels drives the blood from the systemic circulation to the pulmonary circuit. The excess blood distends the pulmonary vessels, and there is a transudation of fluid into the alveoli to produce edema. Morphine quiets the patient and has a dramatic ameliorative effect, whereas epinephrine can be fatal. This effect is extremely important to remember, because in bronchial asthma, epinephrine is helpful, whereas morphine is dangerous.

Chronic venous congestion of the lungs results in rupture of some capillaries, and blood-stained sputum (hemoptysis) is produced. Some of the extravasated blood is converted into hemosiderin, and the lungs become brown and slightly fibrotic. This is called brown induration of the lungs, and it is characteristic of long-standing left ventricular failure (and mitral stenosis).

When considering the pathogenesis of heart failure (whether it is left or right), one must remember that the output of both ventricles is the same over any reasonable period of time. In left ventricular failure, the left ventricle is functioning with the aid of increased venous filling pressure, but the right ventricle, on the other hand, is working normally. This leads to a redistribution of blood, more being retained in the pulmonary circuit than is normal. As noted, this produces congestion of the lungs, and ultimately there is a rise in pulmonary arterial pressure. Eventually this causes the right ventricle to fail as well, and congestive heart failure ensues.

Congestive Heart Failure

In congestive heart failure, both ventricles of the heart fail together, and the effects are a combination of those described under the separate headings of left and right ventricular failure (Fig. 20–12). The inadequate output of the left ventricle leads to sympathetic overactivity with resultant peripheral vasoconstriction. In particular, the vessels of the skin tend to be constricted, causing stasis in the skin; this response leads to peripheral cyanosis. The lessened blood supply to the liver leads to atrophy and necrosis of the cells in the center of the classic liver lobules. This change contributes to the appearance of the char-

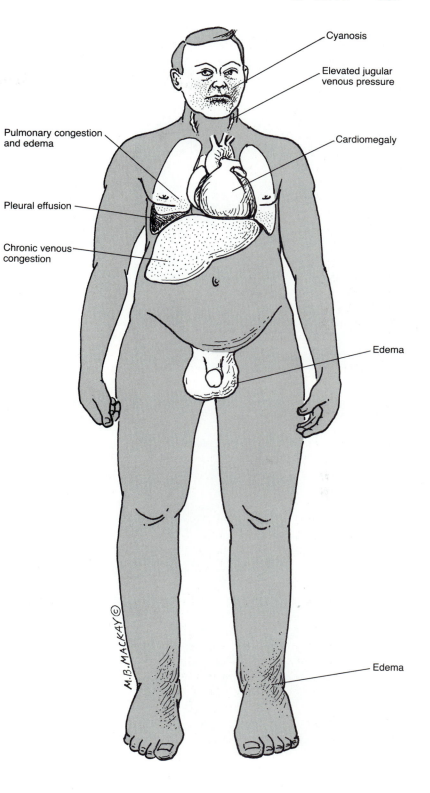

Cyanosis

Elevated jugular
venous pressure

Pulmonary congestion
and edema

Cardiomegaly

Pleural effusion

Chronic venous
congestion

Edema

Edema

**Figure 20–12 Effects of congestive
heart failure.** (Drawn by Margot Mackay,
University of Toronto, Faculty of Medicine, Department of Surgery, Division of
Biomedical Communications, Toronto.)

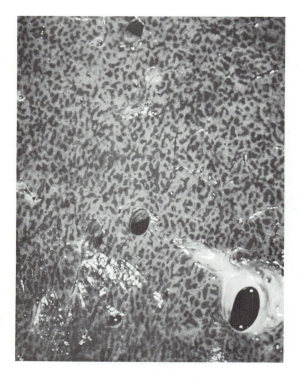

Figure 20–13 The liver in heart failure. This specimen shows the characteristic "nutmeg" appearance of chronic venous congestion in the liver. The dark areas consist of regions where liver cells have undergone necrosis and in which there is intense congestion. They are classically described as the centers of the liver lobules, but in fact they correspond more accurately to the peripheral parts of the liver acinus (see Fig. 24–1). (From Robbins, S. L., and Cottran, R. S.: Pathologic Basis of Disease. 2nd ed. Philadelphia, W. B. Saunders Company, 1979.)

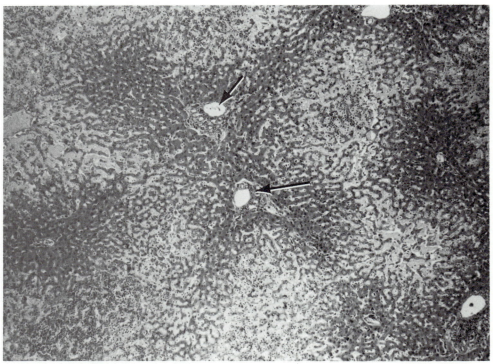

Figure 20–14 The liver in congestive heart failure. Two portal triads are indicated by the arrows; radiating from them are columns of relatively normal liver cells. These are in zone 1 of the Rappaport acinus. The liver cells in zones 2 and 3 have undergone necrosis, and these zones are intensely congested. Correlate this appearance with Figure 20–13 ($\times$60).

acteristic "nutmeg" liver of heart failure (Figs. 20–13 and 20–14). The kidneys respond to the redistribution of blood by salt and water retention, but they show no morphologic evidence of this malfunction. The brain receives an adequate supply of blood until the terminal stages of heart failure. Loss of consciousness tends to be a terminal event.

Causes of Heart Failure

A major cause of heart failure is *myocardial disease* secondary to ischemia (Fig. 20–15). Myocarditis and cardiomyopathy are less common. A heart with a normal myocardium has adequate reserves that enable it to cope with any immediate demand for additional work, but it is not capable of being overburdened for any length of time and eventually fails. Thus, failure may be the result of *overburdening due to a sustained increase in ventricular pressure.* This increase in pressure occurs in systemic and pulmonary hypertension and also in aortic and pulmonary stenosis.

Overburdening due to a sustained increase in cardiac output is another important cause of heart failure. In mitral regurgitation, the left ventricle is forced to eject a large volume of blood, partly back into the left atrium and partly into the aorta. Aortic regurgitation also causes an increase in left ventricular output, because during diastole, blood from the aorta flows back into the left ventricle. With each ventricular systole, a large volume of blood must be ejected so that the effective output

remains normal. In time, both mitral and aortic regurgitation lead to left ventricular failure. Likewise, pulmonary and tricuspid valve regurgitation lead to right ventricular failure.

Another example of overburdening due to an increased cardiac output is seen in a group of diseases in which the resting cardiac output is above normal. This occurs under a variety of conditions. In *anemia,* for example, the tissues require an increased volume of blood to compensate for its low oxygen-carrying power. In *thyrotoxicosis,* the metabolic needs of the tissues are increased. In cases in which a large *fistula* exists between an artery and a vein, the shunt diverts so much blood that the cardiac output must be increased to meet the demands of the rest of the body. There are some common diseases (*e.g., chronic lung disease* and *advanced liver disease*) in which the cardiac output even at rest is high for no very obvious reason. Whenever the resting cardiac output is increased, the heart copes with the load for a while, but it ultimately fails. Even in failure, the output may be above that of the normal resting cardiac output; for this type of condition, the term *high-output failure* is used. Although the cardiac output is raised relative to the normal, it is still insufficient to meet the demands of the body. In the more common type of heart failure, termed *low-output failure,* the cardiac output is less than that of a normal person of similar stature.

Additional factors contributing to heart failure are anxiety, pyrexia, pregnancy, and dysrhythmia. *Anxiety* raises the heart rate and blood

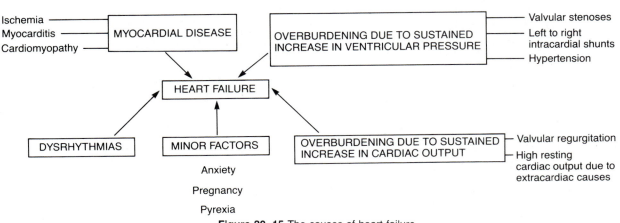

Figure 20–15 The causes of heart failure.

pressure, thereby adding an additional burden to the left ventricle. By raising the metabolic rate, *pyrexia* causes an increase in cardiac output. *Pregnancy* increases the work of the heart as a result of an increased blood volume and the necessity for supplying blood to the fetus. The effects of *dysrhythmia* have been considered earlier in this chapter.

Summary

- Common types of congenital heart disease include septal defects, pulmonary stenosis, transposition of the great vessels, dextrocardia, and Fallot's tetralogy. Central cyanosis, polycythemia, clubbing of the fingers, and underdevelopment are common. Patent ductus arteriosus and coarctation of the aorta are congenital arterial anomalies that have characteristic features.
- Rheumatic heart diseases consist of acute rheumatic fever, which is a pancarditis that follows *Streptococcus pyogenes* infection, and chronic rheumatic valvular disease with predominantly mitral and aortic valvular damage.
- Infective endocarditis often complicates previous valvular damage. Multiple emboli and bacteremia are characteristic.
- Myxomatous degeneration of heart valves is common, but only infrequently does it lead to regurgitation or infective endocarditis.
- Calcific aortic stenosis usually affects elderly men and is a late complication of congenital bicuspid aortic valves.
- Ischemic heart disease is usually caused by coronary atherosclerosis often combined with thrombosis. Arterial spasm and severe hypotension are other causes. The effects include angina pectoris, myocardial fibrosis, myocardial infarction, and sudden death.
- Myocardial infarcts may be regional or subendocardial. Severe pain in the chest is characteristic but may be absent. Blood enzyme studies and electrocardiographic changes assist diagnosis. Pericarditis, mural thrombosis (and embolism), rupture, and heart failure are complications.
- Valvular disease results from an abnormality of the whole valve complex.
- Myocardial disease is commonly due to ischemia, but other causes include myocarditis (toxic, infective, and idiopathic) and a group of cardiomyopathies in which the cause is either unknown or not ischemic or inflammatory.
- Acute pericarditis is commonly viral or bacterial, but noninfective types are known—acute rheumatic fever, collagen vascular disease, and Dressler's syndrome.
- Cardiac dysrhythmias include ectopic beats, paroxysmal tachycardia, various fibrillations, and heart block. Diagnosis is by electrocardiography.
- Heart failure results from myocardial disease; it also occurs when there is chronic overburdening of the

ventricles by sustained increase in ventricular pressure or sustained increase in ventricular output. It may affect predominantly the right or left ventricle. Right-sided failure leads to cyanosis and peripheral edema; left-sided failure causes pulmonary congestion and edema.

Selected Readings

Agarwal, B. L.: Rheumatic heart disease unabated in developing countries. Lancet 2:910, 1981.

Berger, H. J., and Zaret, B. L.: Nuclear cardiology. N. Engl. J. Med. *303*:799 and 855, 1986.

Braunwald, E.: Pathophysiology of heart failure and clinical manifestation of heart failure. *In* Braunwald, E. (ed.): Heart Disease. A Textbook of Cardiovascular Medicine. 3rd ed. Philadelphia, W. B. Saunders Co., 1988.

Conti, C. R.: Coronary-artery spasm and myocardial infarction. N. Engl. J. Med. *309*:238, 1983.

Davies, M. J., and Thomas, A.: Thrombosis and acute coronary-artery lesions in sudden cardiac ischemic death. N. Engl. J. Med. *310*:1137, 1984.

Davies, M. J., Thomas, A. C., Knapman, P. A., et al.: Intracardial platelet aggregation in patients with unstable angina suffering from sudden ischemic cardiac death. Circulation *73*:418, 1986.

Devereux, R. B.: Diagnosis and prognosis of mitral-valve prolapse. N. Engl. J. Med. *320*:1077, 1989.

de Wood, M. A., Spores, J., Notske, R., et al.: Prevalence of total coronary occlusion during the early hours of transmural myocardial infarction. N. Engl. J. Med. *303*:897, 1980.

Friedman, W. F., and Child, J. S.: Congenital heart disease. *In* Wilson, J. D., et al. (eds.): Harrison's Principles of Internal Medicine. 12th ed. New York, McGraw-Hill, 1991, pp. 923–933.

Hampton, J. R.: Falling mortality in coronary heart disease. Br. Med. J. *284*:1505, 1982.

Leading article: Decline in rheumatic fever. Lancet 2:647, 1985.

Leading article: Infective valvulitis in drug addicts. Lancet 2:1180, 1983.

McCord, J. M.: Oxygen-derived free radicals in postischemic tissue injury. N. Engl. J. Med. *312*:159, 1985.

Naylor, W. G., and Elz, J. S.: Reperfusion injury: Laboratory artifact or clinical dilemma. Circulation *74*:215, 1986.

Olsen, E. G. J.: Dilated cardiomyopathy, myocarditis, and the bioptone. Br. Med. J. *283*:90, 1986.

Olsen, E. G. J.: The pathology of the cardiomyopathies. A critical review. Am. Heart J. *98*:385, 1979.

Perloff, J. K.: The Clinical Recognition of Congenital Heart Disease. 3rd ed. Philadelphia, W. B. Saunders Co., 1987.

Scheld, M., and Sande, M.: Endocarditis and intravascular infection. *In* Mandell, G. L., Douglas, R. G., and Bennett, J. E., et al. (eds.): Principles and Practice of Infectious Diseases. 3rd ed. New York, Churchill Livingstone, 1990.

Selzer, A.: Changing aspects of the natural history of valvular aortic stenosis. N. Engl. J. Med. *317*:91, 1987.

Timms, A. D.: Post-myocardial infarction syndrome. Br. Med. J. *289*:636, 1984.

Vaz, D.: Recognizing common cardiac arrhythmias. Am. J. Nurs. *79*:197, 1979.

Woodruff, J. F.: Viral myocarditis: A review. Am. J. Pathol. *101*:425, 1980.

Zabriskie, J. B.: Rheumatic fever: The interplay between host genetics and microbe. Circulation *71*:1077, 1985.

Blood Vessels

**After studying this chapter, the student
should be able to:**

- Describe the three layers of the arterial wall.
- Describe the changes that occur in Mönckeberg's sclerosis.
- List the causes of arteriolosclerosis.
- Describe atherosclerosis with respect to the following:
  - (a) early lesions;
  - (b) late and complicated lesions;
  - (c) vessels affected;
  - (d) risk factors;
  - (e) pathogenesis;
  - (f) complications.
- Classify the inflammatory diseases of arteries.
- List the causes of small vessel obstruction.
- Describe the causes of acute vasculitis.
- Detail the pathologic lesions that can cause peripheral vascular disease of a limb.
- Classify aneurysms according to their cause.
- List the ways in which aneurysms can produce damage.
- Describe the outstanding clinical and pathologic effects of a dissecting aneurysm of the aorta.
- Give an account of the cause and effects of varicose veins of the leg.

Diseases of Arteries

Arterial disease and its complications are responsible for about 40 per cent of all deaths. Arteritis forms a distinct group, but the degenerative diseases (arteriosclerosis) are by far the most important. A knowledge of the structure of arteries is necessary in order to understand their diseases.

Arteries have three coats, as follows:

The Intima. This layer consists of endothelium together with a small quantity of underlying connective tissue—collagen, occasional fibroblasts, and muscle cells.

The Media. The media is the thickest layer and contains elastic fibers and smooth muscle cells, the proportion of each depending on the type of artery.

The Adventitia. This outer coat consists of loose connective tissue and small vessels (the *vasa vasorum*) that penetrate the media and supply it with blood.

ARTERIOSCLEROSIS

Arteriosclerosis, or *hardening of the arteries,* is a term applied to a group of disorders that appear to be degenerative in nature. Three conditions are included.

Mönckeberg's Medial Sclerosis

This disease affects the muscular vessels, particularly those of the lower limbs. The muscle coat becomes replaced by fibrous tissue, which subsequently calcifies and even ossifies. The thickened, pipe-stem arteries produce characteristic radiologic findings. The disease causes no ill effects and is unimportant because the lumen of the affected vessels is not appreciably narrowed.

Arteriolosclerosis

This condition involves *widespread thickening of the walls of small arteries and arterioles. It is an invariable accompaniment of systemic hypertension.* In benign hypertension, the muscle coat shows hypertrophy, but the most striking change is fibrous thickening of the intima *(hyaline arteriolosclerosis).* The changes are most marked in the kidney, and the resultant ischemia leads to patchy degeneration followed by scarring. This is the pathogenesis of benign *nephrosclerosis* (Fig. 21–5).

Similar changes with intimal thickening of small vessels may occur as a localized event; such changes are not related to hypertension. It is found in the small vessels of the ovaries in postmenopausal women, where it is a component of the aging process. It is common in mature scar tissue, is found in areas of chronic inflammation (*e.g.*, in the base of a chronic peptic ulcer), and is particularly marked in the fibrosis induced by ionizing radiation. Under these conditions, the name *endarteritis obliterans* is applied.

In *malignant hypertension,* the size of the arteriolar lumen is greatly reduced by concentric proliferation of smooth muscle cells of the vessel wall; this produces an onionskin appearance. This is termed *hyperplastic arteriolosclerosis* (Fig. 21–1). There may also be necrosis of the arteriolar walls. These changes of malignant hypertension

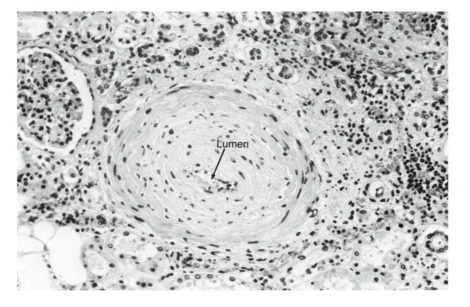

Figure 21–1 Malignant nephrosclerosis. The lumen of the arteriole shown in the center of the field shows concentric proliferation of smooth muscle cells to produce an onionskin appearance. The lumen of the vessel is greatly reduced in size. The changes are characteristic of malignant arteriolosclerosis. (From Walter, J. B.: Pathology of Human Disease. Philadelphia, Lea & Febiger, 1989.)

Lumen

are particularly marked in the kidneys and form the basis for *malignant nephrosclerosis.*

Atherosclerosis

This is the most important component of arteriosclerosis because it is the most common killing disease of all highly advanced communities; its lesions are present to some extent in every adult member of such societies. The disease characteristically affects the aorta and its large elastic branches, such as the common iliac arteries. The abdominal aorta is more severely affected than is the thoracic portion. The lesions are often more advanced at points of bifurcation or around the osteum where a branch (*e.g.,* a lumbar artery) originates. These are points of hemodynamic stress where turbulence is to be expected. Of the medium-sized muscular arteries, the coronary and cerebral arteries are the most commonly and severely involved. This is particularly unfortunate, because the tissues supplied by these vessels are vital to life. Indeed, it is the involvement of these arteries that accounts for the lethal effects of atherosclerosis.

Types of Lesion

The disease may be considered as consisting of two basic types of lesions: *fatty streaks in the intima* and *fibrofatty plaques.* Additional *complicated lesions* occur in advanced disease.

Fatty Streaks in the Intima. Yellow intimal streaks are a common necropsy finding in the aorta of humans from infancy onward (Fig. 21–2). The term *atheroma* is commonly applied to these lesions. The appearances are due to an accumulation of lipid containing foam cells in the subendothelial layer. Some of the cells are smooth muscle cells, but most are macrophages derived from monocytes in the blood. In due course, the cells break down to release their fatty contents into the tunica intima. Perhaps some resolve while others, *e.g.,* in the coronary arteries, progress. When fatty streaks occur in a small artery, they do not produce appreciable narrowing.

Fibrofatty Atherosclerotic Plaques. This is the common type of lesion found in virtually all

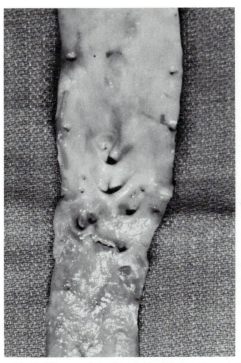

Figure 21–2 Atherosclerosis of the aorta. The abdominal aorta has been opened from behind to expose the intimal surface. The early lesions (atheroma) are the bright, stippled areas and streaks that are seen in the lower part of the specimen. In the fresh state, the lesions were bright yellow in color.

adults. The lesions consist of intimal plaques containing a central mass of fatty, yellow, porridge-like material (the Greek *athere* means porridge). The material contains much cholesterol and its esters. The lesions are associated with dense fibrous tissue that tends to form a cap, thereby giving the plaque a white, pearly appearance when viewed from the lumen (Fig. 21–3). The term *atherosclerosis* is applied to these lesions in contrast to *atheroma* for the fatty streaks. Nevertheless, the two terms are often used interchangeably.

Advanced and Complicated Lesions. Four further changes may be seen in the plaques as they progress.

Hemorrhage. Proliferation of vessels from the vasa vasorum produces increased vascularity in the tissues surrounding the atherosclerotic plaques. Rupture of one of these vessels leads to bleeding into the plaque. In a small vessel such as a coronary artery, this bleeding can produce acute total obstruction.

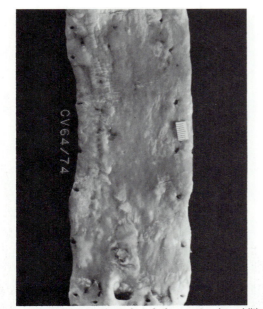

Figure 21–3 Atherosclerosis of the aorta. In addition to yellow streaks, the intimal surface shows raised plaques of fibrous tissue overlying the atheromatous material.

Thrombosis. Turbulence of blood flow around the plaque can lead to superadded thrombosis (Fig. 21–4). The vessel is then lined by shaggy, ragged thrombus.

Ulceration. Sometimes the fibrous covering of the plaque becomes detached so that there is ulceration followed by thrombosis.

Calcification. The fatty material of the atherosclerotic plaque frequently undergoes dystrophic calcification. The vessel wall becomes rigid and on pressure breaks like an eggshell.

Effects of Atherosclerosis

Gradual obstruction to the lumen, thrombosis sometimes with distal embolism, and weakening of the vessel wall causing dilation are the major effects.

Gradual Obstruction. Atherosclerosis of medium-sized arteries, such as the coronary or cerebral arteries, produces intimal thickening and progressive occlusion of the lumen. This leads to ischemia of the area supplied.

Thrombosis. In medium-sized vessels, throm-

bosis can cause sudden complete occlusion and infarction of the area supplied. In a large vessel such as the aorta, the lumen is not appreciably narrowed, but thrombus and atheromatous material can become detached and embolize distally. Occasionally, these emboli are large and can cause serious effects, *e.g.*, renal or cerebral infarction. Usually, however, such emboli are small and inapparent clinically. Nevertheless, the steady occlusion of many small vessels is a contributing factor in peripheral ischemic disease of the lower leg as well as in the progressive renal ischemic disease that often accompanies atherosclerosis.

Dilation and Aneurysm Formation. The presence of an atherosclerotic plaque causes atrophy of the adjacent media. The wall consequently weakens, and the artery involved may show either a diffuse enlargement, termed *ectasia*, or a localized dilation, termed an *aneurysm* (Fig. 21–5). These effects are seen most often in the aorta, in which the atherosclerosis is most severe. The lesions of atherosclerosis tend to be more advanced toward the more caudal regions of the aorta, and it is therefore in the abdominal portion

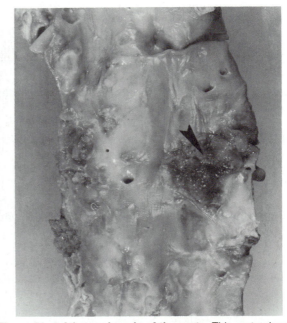

Figure 21–4 Atherosclerosis of the aorta. This aorta shows severe atherosclerosis with complicated lesions. The arrow points to an area of ulceration that is covered by thrombus.

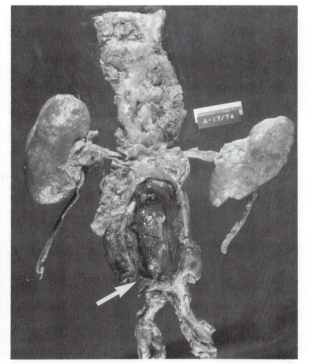

Figure 21–5 Atheromatous aneurysm of the aorta. The aorta shows severe atherosclerosis. An aneurysm situated below the level of the origin of the renal arteries is filled with thrombus but has ruptured (arrow). The kidneys are reduced in size, and their surfaces are granular. This change is due to benign nephrosclerosis combined with the effect of many small atheromatous emboli in the renal arterioles.

that aneurysm formation is most common. The aneurysm is generally below the origin of the renal arteries, which is fortunate, because surgical replacement by a plastic prosthesis is technically possible.

An aneurysm that begins to leak generally causes pain, and this is liable to be followed shortly by complete rupture with exsanguination and death.

Case History I

The patient was a 71-year-old man who had had a 15-year history of hypertension. Five years before the examination, he had been investigated for a possible aortic aneurysm. The findings were equivocal, however, and no treatment was advised. One year before his present admission, he had noted the onset of angina pectoris and intermittent claudication. The angina was easily relieved by nitroglycerin tablets.

The patient's present complaint was that of pain in the abdomen. His blood pressure was 220/115 mm Hg, and the blood urea nitrogen was 18 mmol/L (normal 3 to 6.5 mmol/L). A diagnosis of myocardial infarct was considered, but it was not confirmed by the electrocardiogram. The pain subsided for a few days but suddenly recurred with increased severity and was accompanied by signs of shock. The patient died before treatment for internal bleeding could be undertaken.

Necropsy revealed a ruptured aortic aneurysm, which is shown in Figure 21–5. There was extensive bleeding into the retroperitoneal tissues and into the peritoneum. The heart was enlarged (weight 850 g, compared with 300 g in a normal heart) owing to marked left ventricular hypertrophy. The coronary vessels showed severe atherosclerosis with narrowing.

Etiology of Atherosclerosis

Atherosclerosis is present to some extent in all adult members of the population, yet its precise cause is not known. The subject is discussed under the two headings of risk factors and pathogenesis.

Risk Factors. The most important risk factors that predispose to severe atherosclerosis, particularly as it affects the coronary arteries, are tobacco smoking, hypertension, a family history of atherosclerotic-related diseases, the presence or a family history of hyperlipidemia, and diabetes mellitus or a family history of this disease. Elevated low-density lipoproteins (LDL) are atherogenic and are found in both acquired and familial hypercholesterolemia. On the other hand, an elevated high-density lipoprotein (HDL) level is protective. Obesity itself is not a risk factor except insofar as it is associated with hypertension and diabetes mellitus. The evidence that physical exercise is protective is not convincing. Hormonal factors play some part because the lesions of atherosclerosis tend to progress steadily in males, whereas females are protected during their reproductive life. After the menopause, the lesions progress.

Pathogenesis. The present concept (*the response to injury theory*) is that damage to the endothelium is important in the initiation and development of atherosclerosis. The normal endothelium inhibits thrombosis and regulates the transfer of macromolecules into the vessel wall. The nature of its glycocalyx and the production of prostaglandin I2 (prostacyclin) probably play an important role.

Injury could be caused by hemodynamic stresses, associated vascular disease (*e.g.*, vasculitis), hypertension, smoking, or hyperlipidemia. After injury to the endothelium, monocytes and lipoproteins can enter the intima and lead to the formation of fatty streaks. Intimal damage also leads to the deposition of platelets and the formation of a thrombus.

It is now realized that smooth muscle cells play a very important role in the formation of the atherosclerotic plaque. Normally these cells are not present in the intima, but under the influence of a variety of chemotactic factors, they migrate from the media into the intima, proliferate, and differentiate into a cell that produces collagen, elastin, and the glycosaminoglycans of ground substance. The factors involved are platelet-derived growth factor, which is released from platelets undergoing the release reaction, endothelial cell–derived growth factor, and macrophage-derived growth factor. Furthermore, the connective tissue components formed by the smooth muscle cells are not normal. The elastin tends to bind calcium, and the glycosaminoglycans can bind certain lipoproteins. The smooth muscle cells themselves have LDL receptors and can take up lipid to become a type of foam cell. An interesting discovery, with use of the X chromosome as a marker (see the Lyon hypothesis, Chapter 3), is that the cells of each atherosclerotic plaque are monoclonal as if each were a separate "tumor." The significance of this observation is not known.

It is evident that the pathogenesis of atherosclerosis is complex. A wide array of agents appear to damage the vascular endothelium and set in motion the lipid accumulation, platelet deposition, and smooth muscle migration and proliferation that contribute to the formation of the plaques.

The only effective treatment of atherosclerotic lesions is surgical, and the only way to prevent the lesions from developing is to avoid known risk factors, namely, refrain from smoking and adopt dietary or other measures to avoid developing a lipoprotein profile that is known to be atherogenic. The possibility of using long-term, low-dosage drugs that affect platelets (such as aspirin) is under investigation, and the results appear promising at least so far as coronary disease is concerned.

INFLAMMATORY DISEASES OF ARTERIES

Acute Infective Arteritis

Arteritis may occur in pyogenic infections, and if the vessel wall undergoes necrosis, severe hemorrhage can result. A good example of this is the fatal hemorrhage from the lingual artery that sometimes ends the life of a patient with an ulcerating carcinoma of the tongue. Neoplastic invasion plays its part, but the major weakening effect is the result of infection. Similarly, destruction of an artery at the base of a gastric ulcer is a common cause of bleeding. Fortunately, in many chronic inflammatory lesions, the artery responds by proliferation of its intimal lining so that the lumen becomes steadily occluded (*endarteritis obliterans*) and bleeding is restricted.

Syphilitic Arteritis

An arteritis may occur in tertiary syphilis, and it nearly always affects the aorta. A chronic inflammatory reaction is combined with destruction of the elastic coat and its replacement by fibrous tissue; the vessel becomes thickened, and at the same time is weakened. Either it dilates diffusely or an aneurysm (either fusiform or saccular) is formed. The thoracic part of the aorta is most severely affected; in the past, syphilis was the common cause of thoracic aortic aneurysms (Fig. 21–6). Today the disease is rare, and atheroma accounts for the majority of aortic aneurysms. Dilation of the arch of the aorta and the aortic ring leads to separation of the aortic cusps so that in diastole they fail to meet and *aortic regurgitation* results. Syphilitic arteritis can also affect the cerebral vessels but, like syphilitic aortitis, is rarely encountered today.

Rheumatoid Aortitis

Rheumatoid aortitis, which is very similar to the aortitis of tertiary syphilis, is occasionally

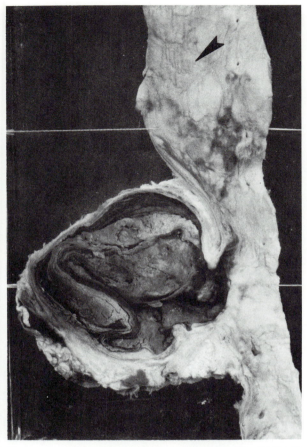

Figure 21–6 Syphilitic aneurysm of the aorta. The specimen shows part of the descending thoracic aorta from which a saccular aneurysm arises. Note the laminated thrombus in the aneurysmal sac and the wrinkled appearance of the aortic wall (arrow). This appearance is characteristic of the syphilitic aortitis of tertiary syphilis. (Specimen from the Boyd Museum, University of Toronto.)

encountered in rheumatoid arthritis. It also leads to aortic insufficiency.

Idiopathic Inflammatory Conditions

There are a number of diseases in which inflammation of the arterial wall leads to thrombosis.

Thromboangiitis Obliterans (Buerger's Disease)

This disease occurs predominantly in young men who are heavy cigarette smokers and affects the arteries and veins of the legs. Thrombosis leads to ischemia and intermittent claudication; ultimately, gangrene of the toes sets in. The arms and viscera are affected less frequently.

Giant-Cell Arteritis

Giant-cell arteritis is a disease of elderly people. The affected artery shows thrombosis and a chronic inflammatory granulomatous reaction with many giant cells forming around disrupted elastic fibers. Since the disease commonly affects the temporal artery, it is also called *temporal arteritis*. It is characterized by pain in the region of the artery and is important because it can affect the ophthalmic artery and lead to blindness.

Polyarteritis nodosa is described in Chapter 6.

SPASM

Arterial spasm may be severe and prolonged enough to cause ischemia of the part supplied. An important example is the spasm that affects an artery involved in an area of trauma, *e.g.*, a fracture. Spasm of the digital arteries as an abnormal response to cold is the cause of the manifestations of Raynaud's syndrome (see also Chapter 1).

ANEURYSMS

An *aneurysm* is a local dilation of an artery or a chamber of the heart and is due to weakening of its walls. It may be saccular or fusiform (Fig. 21–7A).

Causes

Weakening of the wall may be due to any of the following.

Congenital Deficiency. A good example is a berry aneurysm of the circle of Willis (Chapter 33).

Trauma. A tear in the arterial wall can lead to the formation of a hematoma that by becoming incorporated into the vessel wall forms a *false*

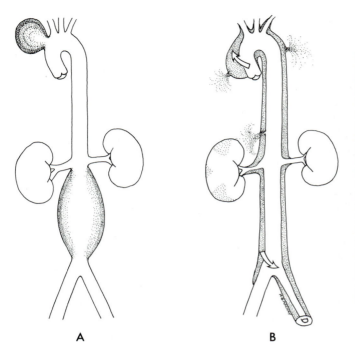

A   B

Figure 21–7 Types of aortic aneurysm. *A*, Two aneurysms are shown. One is saccular and has arisen from the ascending aorta. It is filled with laminated thrombus. Fifty years ago, this type of aneurysm was invariably due to tertiary syphilis; today this form of the disease is so rare that atherosclerosis is the usual cause. The abdominal aorta shows a fusiform aneurysm that is lined by thrombus. This type of aneurysm is usually due to atherosclerosis and invariably affects the aorta below the origins of the renal arteries. *B*, A dissecting aneurysm. Blood has been forced into the media of the aorta and has dissected down to the left common iliac artery. Some branches are obstructed, and the effects of this account for the clinical signs and symptoms. Thus, in the aneurysm illustrated, the left femoral pulse would be weaker than the right, and the ischemia of the right kidney has led to infarction. The false aneurysmal sac may rupture externally at various points or, rarely, may rupture into the aortic lumen (large arrow near the bifurcation of the aorta). (Drawn by Margot Mackay, University of Toronto, Faculty of Medicine, Department of Surgery, Division of Biomedical Communications, Toronto.)

aneurysm. Sometimes an injury can damage not only an artery but also an adjacent vein, thereby establishing a connection. This formation is termed an *arteriovenous aneurysm,* or fistula, and so much blood can be diverted from the peripheral tissues that heart failure ensues.

Inflammation. Syphilitic aortic aneurysm and mycotic aneurysms are examples of infective causes. In polyarteritis nodosa, the inflammation is not directly related to infection.

Degenerative. Atherosclerosis is by far the most common cause of aortic aneurysm.

Effects

An aneurysm can produce its effect in a number of ways.

Pressure. An aneurysm of the thoracic aorta may press on the esophagus and cause difficulty in swallowing, or it may press on the recurrent laryngeal nerve and lead to changes of voice.

Thrombosis. The sac and aneurysm soon become filled by laminated thrombus. This effect is due in part to damage of the endothelial lining, but it is mostly the result of local stasis and turbulence.

Hemorrhage. Rupture of an aneurysm leads to bleeding; for a while, this can be quite trivial because of the plugging effect of the thrombus lining the sac. Nevertheless, when an aneurysm, such as one of the abdominal aorta, has begun to bleed, it is not long before massive hemorrhage follows and the patient dies of exsanguination.

Ischemia. This is due to blockage of the branches of the artery at the site of the aneurysm, an effect produced either by local pressure or by thrombotic occlusion.

DISSECTING ANEURYSM OF THE AORTA

Dissecting aneurysm involves bleeding into the arterial wall rather than the formation of a true aneurysm. The patient suddenly experiences a severe, tearing chest pain that must be distinguished from myocardial infarction. Occasionally there is no pain, and the condition is an unexpected necropsy finding. Untreated, the condition is almost always fatal, but surgical treatment is often successful.

Pathogenesis

The initial event appears to be a tear in the intimal wall of the ascending aorta. Blood is forced into the wall and dissects in the media between its middle and outer thirds. This process extends proximally to the heart and distally so that in due course the whole of the aorta and some of its branches can be involved (Fig. 21–7B). The dissection is usually terminated when the aneurysmal sac ruptures externally. Sudden bleeding into the pericardium, mediastinum, peritoneum, or retroperitoneum causes death. Very rarely, the false aneurysm ruptures internally into the aortic lumen and the patient survives with no treatment. This accounts for the double-barreled aorta that is occasionally found as an unexpected necropsy finding.

The cause of the initial intimal tear is not known but may be related to the presence of hypertension. An alternative but less popular hypothesis is that the initial bleeding into the aortic wall is by rupture of one of the vasa vasorum. The intramural hematoma so formed ruptures into the aortic lumen so that the full force of the arterial blood can tear into the false aneurysm. Regardless of the initial events, the extension of a dissection is aided by the presence of *Erdheim's cystic medionecrosis*, in which loss of elastic fibers is associated with accumulation of mucinous ground substance forming small cystic spaces. The cause of this degeneration is not known, but a similar change is found in Marfan's syndrome.

Effects

The effects of a dissecting aneurysm depend on the extent of the dissection. The accumulation of blood in the aortic wall blocks the lumen of vessels that arise from it. If the dissection extends toward the heart, the coronary arteries are ob-structed, causing myocardial ischemia and perhaps infarction. Likewise, involvement of the arteries supplying the arms leads to weak and unequal pulses at the wrist; the blood pressure measured in the arms is unequal. As the extent of the dissection progresses, the degree of obstruction changes, and there is fluctuation in the limb pulses and blood pressure. Blockage of the intercostal vessels can compromise the blood supply to the spinal cord and result in paraplegia. Involvement of the renal arteries can lead to infarction and renal failure.

PERIPHERAL VASCULAR DISEASE

"Peripheral vascular disease" is an inclusive term used to describe all those conditions in which there is impairment of the blood supply to the limbs. Usually it is the legs that suffer. The following diseases all play their part.

Atherosclerosis. This tends to affect the large vessels such as the iliac and femoral vessels.

Thrombosis. This may be secondary to atherosclerosis.

Embolism. Emboli may be large thromboemboli or small clumps of atheromatous material.

Small Vessel Diseases. Hyaline arteriolosclerosis secondary to hypertension and diabetic microangiopathy are important causes.

Effects of Peripheral Disease

The effects are serious and disabling. The ischemia of the leg leads to atrophy of many structures, including the bones (osteoporosis) and the skin. Trivial injury can lead to chronic, persistent, and extremely painful ulceration. Ischemia of the muscle leads to pain on walking (intermittent claudication) and, ultimately, to pain at rest. Dry gangrene leading to loss of the limb is the all-too-frequent end result.

Diseases of Small Vessels

In consideration of vascular disease, the capillaries and arterioles are usually forgotten. There are, nevertheless, many conditions in which so many vessels in an area are occluded that ische-mia results. Because an additional effect is bleeding, petechial hemorrhages are a common feature of small vessel disease, even though the extent of the occlusion is insufficient to lead to ischemia

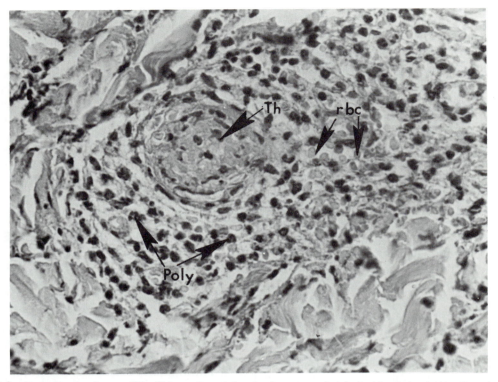

Figure 21–8 Acute gonococcal vasculitis. This section of dermis shows an arteriole that is obstructed by thrombus (Th). The vessel wall has undergone necrosis, and there is a heavy infiltration of polymorphs (Poly). The presence of many red cells (rbc) in the interstitial tissues indicates that the vessel has ruptured. This biopsy was taken from the patient shown in Figure 8–3.

of the total area involved. Some causes of these diseases are briefly described.

Frostbite. The harmful effects of cold on exposed parts are due in large measure to small vessel damage. In mild cases, there is an inflammatory reaction causing large blisters to form; if the damage is severe, the vessels become completely occluded by thrombus, and gangrene occurs.

Occlusion by Red Blood Cells. This response occurs in severe sludging and is a component of shock.

Occlusion by Fibrin. This occurs in disseminated intravascular coagulation (Chapter 18). The kidney is the organ most affected.

Occlusion by Precipitated Cryoglobulins. In cryoglobulinemia, exposure of the extremities to cold leads to vascular occlusion and petechial hemorrhages.

Fat Embolism. See Chapter 19.

Decompression Syndrome. See Chapter 19.

External Pressure. The best example of this is a bedsore. Continual pressure on one area produces such ischemia that necrosis of the skin and underlying tissues occurs. *It is a major duty of health care workers to move nonambulatory patients often enough that no pressure sores develop.*

Occlusion by Antigen-Antibody Interaction. This is a feature of such immune complex phenomena as the Arthus reaction (Chapter 6).

Vasculitis. The term vasculitis is used to describe an inflammatory reaction in the wall of small vessels. Typical lesions occur in the Arthus reaction; the immune complex deposition in the vessel wall causes damage associated with a marked polymorph infiltration and thrombosis (Fig. 21–8). This type III hypersensitivity is thought to occur in many drug reactions as well as in some infections. The petechial hemorrhages seen in the skin in septicemia (*e.g.,* gonococcal septicemia, see Fig. 8–3) and in infective endocarditis are explained on this basis. Internal organs are affected; the kidney appears to be the most vulnerable. In some examples of vasculitis, no cause can be found. The disease then appears to be a component of polyarteritis nodosa (Chapter 6).

Diseases of Veins

Phlebothrombosis and its important complications of embolism and pulmonary infarction are described in Chapter 19. Inflammation of veins (phlebitis) is a common event in any inflammatory process. The overlying thrombosis that accompanies it is not important as a source of embolism because the thrombus is firmly adherent to the wall of the damaged vessel. Only if the thrombus is invaded by pyogenic organisms is embolism a hazard. Under these circumstances, emboli containing bacteria are thrown off and pyemia results (Chapter 19).

VARICOSE VEINS

Elongation and irregular dilation of veins is known as *varicosity*. It is generally assumed that persistent increase in pressure is a cause of this; esophageal varices can certainly be explained in this manner (Chapter 24). Nevertheless, the common condition of varicose veins of the legs is not well understood. There seems to be a familial factor in the incidence of this common disease, and an inherited defect of the venous walls or valves has been postulated. Other suggested causes are the standing for long periods over many years that is required in some occupations and the lack of support for the walls of the veins that is seen in fat people. Because pregnancy seems to initiate varicose vein formation, the disease is more common at an earlier age in women. Once varicose veins have formed, their valves become incompetent, so that on standing, the full hydrostatic pressure of blood is applied to the vessel wall and further dilation ensues. Particularly important is incompetence of valves in the perforating veins that communicate between superficial veins and deep vessels. The extremely sluggish blood flow through the veins can predispose a person to thrombus formation, but embolism from this is extremely rare. The major effect of varicose veins is to produce venous stasis. The increased hydrostatic pressure leads to edema, and the skin exhibits *stasis dermatitis*. Trivial injuries lead to persistent ulcerations that characteristically overlie the medial malleoli. Even though these ulcers can enlarge,

they are not painful. In this respect, they contrast with the ulceration caused by arterial disease (ischemic ulcers).

Two particular circumstances under which venous thrombosis occurs are worthy of special note.

THROMBOPHLEBITIS MIGRANS

Migratory thrombophlebitis is described in Chapter 19.

PAINFUL WHITE LEG (Phlegmasia Alba Dolens)

The painful white leg that is seen in pregnant women in the third trimester—or more often immediately after delivery—is due to ileofemoral venous thrombosis. It is thought that inflammation also involves lymphatics and that this contributes to the formation of such massive edema.

Summary

- Arteriosclerosis includes Mönckeberg's medial sclerosis, arteriolosclerosis, and atherosclerosis.
- Atherosclerosis is the most important lethal disease of humans. Its lesions are fatty streaks, fibrofatty plaques, and complicated lesions with hemorrhage, thrombosis, ulceration, and calcification. The disease leads to gradual and later complete arterial obstruction and aneurysm formation. The precise cause is unknown, but risk factors include tobacco smoking, hypertension, family history, diabetes mellitus, and an atherogenic pattern of plasma lipoproteins. The response to injury theory of its pathogenesis is now favored.
- Arteritis may be infective (*e.g.*, syphilitic), rheumatoid, or idiopathic (Buerger's disease, giant-cell arteritis, and polyarteritis nodosa).
- Aneurysms are associated with congenital abnormality, trauma, arteritis, and atherosclerosis. Dissecting aneurysm of the aorta is associated with medionecrosis of the aortic wall.
- Peripheral vascular disease is caused by atherosclerosis, thrombosis, embolism, and small vessel disease (many types, but particularly associated with hypertension and diabetes mellitus). Intermittent claudication and gangrene are its most important effects.

- Varicose veins of the leg are common and lead to stasis dermatitis and ulceration. A positive family history, standing for long periods, and pregnancy are probable causative factors.

Selected Readings

Benditt, E. R., and Benditt, J. M.: Evidence for a monoclonal origin of human atherosclerotic plaque. Proc. Natl. Acad. Sci. USA 70:1753, 1973.

Botting, R. M.: Regulatory functions of the vascular endothelium. N. Engl. J. Med. 323:27, 1990.

Browse, N. L., and Burnard, K. G.: The cause of venous ulceration. Lancet 2:243, 1982.

Cupps, T. R., and Fauci, A. S.: The vasculitic syndromes. Adv. Intern. Med. 27:315, 1982.

DeSanctis, R. W., et al.: Aortic dissection. N: Engl. J. Med. 317:1060, 1987.

Gajdusek, C., et al.: An endothelial cell–derived growth factor. J. Cell Biol. 85:467, 1980.

Lees, R. S., and Lees, A. M.: High-density lipoproteins and the risk of atherosclerosis. N. Engl. J. Med. 306:1546, 1982.

Pekkanen, J., et al.: Ten-year mortality from cardiovascular disease in relation to cholesterol level among men with and without preexisting cardiovascular disease. N. Engl. J. Med. 322:1700, 1990.

Ross, R.: The pathogenesis of atherosclerosis: An update. N. Engl. J. Med. 314:488, 1986.

Ross, R., Glomset, J., and Harker, L.: Response to injury and atherosclerosis. Am. J. Pathol. 86:675, 1977.

Ross, R., Raines, E. W., and Bowes-Pope, D. F.: The biology of platelet-derived growth factor. Cell 46:155, 1986.

Vane, J. R., Anggard, E. E., and Botting, R. M.: Regulatory functions of the vascular endothelium. N. Engl. J. Med. 323:27, 1990.

Respiratory Tract

**After studying this chapter, the student
should be able to:**

- Define the acinus of the lung.
- Define surfactant and indicate its importance in
  normal lung function and in the pathogenesis of lung
  disease.
- Define respiratory failure and compare the causes
  and effects of ventilatory failure with those of
  impaired alveolar-arterial gas exchange.
- Discuss the causes of dyspnea.
- Describe the defense mechanisms of the lung.
- Give an account of the pathogenesis, clinical
  features, and pathologic findings of lobar
  pneumonia.
- Classify the causes of bronchopneumonia.
- Give an account of the respiratory distress
  syndrome of the newborn.
- Give an account of legionnaires' disease.
- Describe interstitial pneumonia with respect to
  (a) cause and pathogenesis;
  (b) morphologic changes in the lungs;
  (c) end results.
- Describe the common fungal infections of the lung
  and sarcoidosis.
- Define chronic obstructive pulmonary disease
  (COPD) and give an account of chronic bronchitis
  and emphysema with respect to
  (a) definition;
  (b) known causes;
  (c) clinical effects.

- Describe the outstanding features of
  (a) intrinsic asthma;
  (b) extrinsic asthma;
  (c) extrinsic allergic alveolitis.
- Describe the causes of pulmonary edema.
- Describe the causes and effects of bronchial obstruction.
- Give an account of the sudden infant death syndrome (SIDS), bronchiectasis, and the pneumoconioses.
- Give an account of bronchial carcinoid tumor.
- Describe carcinoma of the lung with respect to the following factors:
  (a) known causes;
  (b) gross appearance and types;
  (c) diagnosis;
  (d) histologic types;
  (e) spread.
- Distinguish between a transudate and an exudate with reference to hydrothorax.
- Define pleuritis, empyema, and pneumothorax. Give common causes of each.

DEVELOPMENT AND STRUCTURE OF THE LUNG

The lung develops from a central outpouching from the primitive foregut. This develops into the trachea, and by repeated branching, the bronchi and bronchioles are formed. These act as conducting tubes, and the last passage to perform only this function is defined as a *terminal bronchiole*. The part of the lung distal to a terminal bronchiole is termed the *acinus* of the lung, and it in turn consists of a number of generations of respiratory bronchioles and alveolar ducts, from the walls of which bud the alveoli, in which gas

exchange takes place (Fig. 22–1). The alveoli are packed together like a mass of soap bubbles and are themselves lined by flattened pneumocytes, of which there are two types. *Type I pneumocytes* are the most abundant and line most of the alveolar surface. *Type II pneumocytes* secrete *surfactant,* a phospholipid, surface-active compound that has the very important function of lowering surface tension at the air-liquid interface in the lung. Hence, surfactant aids inspiration by lessening the work needed to inflate the alveoli, and it also prevents alveoli from collapsing after expiration. It should be noted that the acini of the lung are not visible as entities to the naked eye, but a group of acini together form the lobules, the outline of which is often visible by the fact that carbon is deposited in the septa that separate one lobule from the next.

Normal Function

The function of the respiratory system is to enable gaseous exchange to occur between the blood and the atmosphere. The upper respiratory tract functions as an air conditioner for the lungs, the inspired air being filtered and humidified as it passes through the nose, nasopharynx, larynx, and trachea. Air eventually reaches the alveoli of the lung, where it comes into close contact with blood in the capillaries and where conditions for gaseous exchange are ideal (Fig. 22–2). Oxygen is added to the blood, and the carbon dioxide that is removed is exhaled. The gas in the alveoli is maintained at a fairly constant composition by

COMPONENT PARTS OF ACINUS

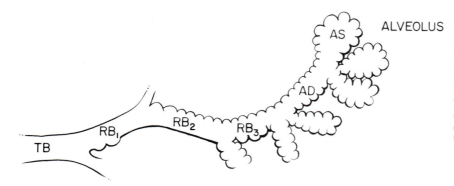

Figure 22–1 This diagrammatic representation of an acinus shows a terminal bronchiole (TB), respiratory bronchioles of the first (RB$_1$), second (RB$_2$), and third (RB$_3$) orders, an alveolar duct (AD), and an alveolar sac (AS). The acinus is the part of the lung distal to a terminal bronchiole. (From Thurlbeck, W. M.: Chronic obstructive lung disease. *In* Sommers, S. C. [Ed.]: Pathology Annual, vol. 3. New York, Appleton-Century-Crofts, 1968.)

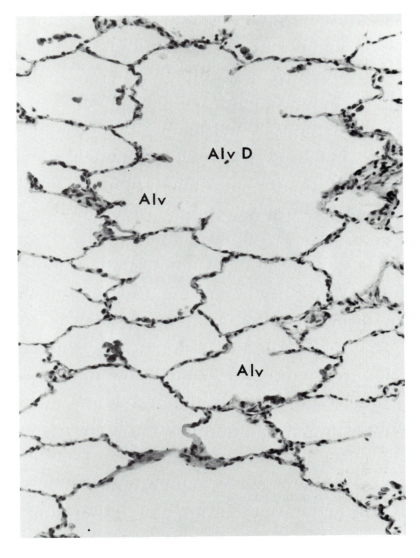

Figure 22–2 Normal lung. This section shows a number of alveoli (Alv) and an alveolar duct (Alv D) from which some of them have arisen. Note how thin the alveolar walls are (×60).

the act of breathing, a process that has two components: *ventilation* and *distribution.*

Ventilation. This is the bellowslike action of the chest, by which fresh air is inspired and stale air is expired. The volume is approximately 7.5 liters per minute in the adult at rest.

Distribution. The inspired air is distributed in such a way in relation to the volume of blood perfusing the lung that the composition of the alveolar gas is maintained at a constant level. The arterial blood, as it leaves the lung, is in equilibrium with the alveolar gas, and it follows that the gaseous tensions of oxygen and carbon

dioxide in the arterial blood are also maintained at this same constant level (Fig. 22–3).

RESPIRATORY FAILURE

If through dysfunction of the lungs there is lack of oxygen or retention of CO_2, the condition is called *respiratory failure.* In the arterial blood under normal conditions, the partial pressure of oxygen, usually written P_{O_2}, is about 100 mm Hg, and the partial pressure of carbon dioxide, written P_{CO_2}, is about 40 mm Hg. In respiratory

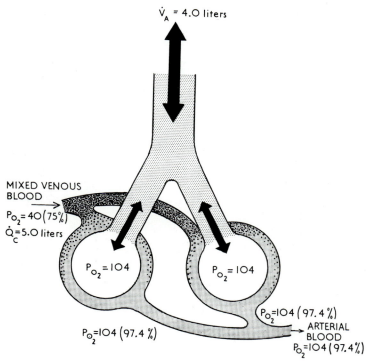

$\dot{V}_A$ = 4.0 liters

MIXED VENOUS BLOOD

P_{O_2} = 40(75%)
$\dot{Q}_C$ = 5.0 liters

P_{O_2} = 104

P_{O_2} = 104

P_{O_2} = 104(97.4%)

P_{O_2} = 104(97.4%)
ARTERIAL BLOOD
P_{O_2} = 104(97.4%)

Figure 22–3 Physiologic relationships within lung. This diagrammatic representation of the lung shows two alveoli with ideal ventilation/blood flow relationships. This relationship is generally written $\dot{V}_A/\dot{Q}_C$, the dot indicating that the volumes of alveolar ventilation (V_A) and capillary blood flow (Q_C) are in unit time. Thus, for the lung as a whole in a normal subject at rest:

$$\frac{\dot{V}_A}{\dot{Q}_e} = \frac{4 \text{ liters per minute}}{5 \text{ liters per minute}} = 0.8$$

In the diagram, the oxygen tensions are in mm Hg, and the figures in parentheses are percentages of the saturation level of oxygen in the blood.

The partial pressure of a gas in a mixture is the contribution that the gas makes toward the total pressure. Thus, for moist air at sea level, the total pressure is about 760 mm Hg. Water vapor contributes about 24 mm Hg, and the remaining 736 mm Hg is contributed by oxygen (about 20 per cent) and nitrogen (about 80 per cent). Hence, the partial pressure of oxygen (P_{O_2}) is 20 per cent of 736 mm Hg or about 147 mm Hg. As fresh air is drawn into the lungs, it mixes with expired gases. Under normal conditions, the gas in the alveoli has an oxygen tension of about 100 mm Hg. (From Walter, J. B., and Israel, M. S.: General Pathology. 6th ed. Edinburgh, Churchill Livingstone, 1987. After Comroe, J. H., et al.: The Lung: Clinical Physiology and Pulmonary Function Tests. 2nd ed. Chicago, Year Book Medical Publishers, 1963.)

failure, the P_{O_2} is under 60 mm Hg *(hypoxemia),* and the P_{CO_2} is over 49 mm Hg *(hypercapnia).*

Types of Respiratory Failure

Two main types can be recognized:

1. *Ventilatory failure,* which is due to an inadequate volume of inspired air available for exchange.

2. *Impaired alveolar-arterial gas exchange,* which is due to failure of distribution or diffusion.

Ventilatory Failure (Hypoxia with Hypercapnia). This condition is caused by the following factors:

1. Airways obstruction, which is considered later in this chapter.

2. Restriction of thoracic movement, such as that resulting from the presence of a pneumothorax or a large pleural effusion.

3. Neuromuscular impairment, such as that found in infantile paralysis.

4. Disturbance of the brain, such as that due to injury or to overdose of a depressant drug *(e.g.,* a barbiturate). Hypoventilation associated with somnolence can occur in obesity (the pickwickian syndrome).

Effects. Since

$$P_{CO_2} \text{ (arterial)} \ \alpha \ \frac{CO_2 \text{ production}}{\text{Alveolar ventilation}}$$

and at rest the CO_2 production is constant, it follows that when alveolar ventilation is reduced, there is an increase in the arterial P_{CO_2} and an arithmetically equivalent decrease in P_{O_2}. Thus, if the P_{CO_2} rises from 40 to 60 mm Hg, then the P_{O_2} falls from 100 to 80 mm Hg. A drop of this magnitude in the P_{O_2} does not greatly affect the amount of oxygen present in arterial blood because hemoglobin has great affinity for oxygen. Desaturation of blood with subsequent cyanosis is a late event in ventilatory failure.

The main effect is a raised arterial P_{CO_2} *(hypercapnia),* and symptoms are related to this response. The pulse is rapid, and the hands are moist and warm. The pupils are small, and the blood pressure is raised. If there is severe CO_2 retention, then confusion, drowsiness, tremors, and coma may ensue. Carbon dioxide is a vasodilator, and severe CO_2 retention causes cerebral edema, which is the explanation of the nervous phenomena and which can be detected clinically by the occurrence of papilledema. Finally, the plasma bicarbonate level is high, and the patient has respiratory acidosis.

Impaired Alveolar-Arterial Gas Exchange (Hypoxia Without Hypercapnia). In this type of respiratory failure, there is a reduction of alveolar-capillary surface available for gas exchange. This reduction may occur as a result of lung destruction, but more commonly it is due to an imbalance in the distribution of perfusion and ventilation. Frequently, these factors are combined; of the two, however, maldistribution is much more important, and it becomes prominent in all progressive lung disease.

Impaired alveolar-arterial gas exchange occurs in emphysema and severe chronic bronchitis, especially postoperatively, when there is mucous plugging of bronchi. It is a feature of pulmonary embolism.

Effects. Oxygen uptake is interfered with, and the venous blood becomes more desaturated during exercise; increasing arterial desaturation also occurs. The patient develops central cyanosis.

Although impaired alveolar-arterial gas exchange leads to a severe interference with O_2 uptake, it interferes little with CO_2 elimination. In the distribution failure group, some alveoli are underventilated relative to alveolar perfusion with blood. This situation is remedied by overventilation of the remaining lung. Overventilation serves to eliminate more CO_2 from the blood, but it cannot compensate for any unequal oxygen uptake because it does not produce an appreciable increase above the normal level in the amount of oxygen taken up by the blood (Fig. 22–4).

DYSPNEA

In a healthy person, the rate and depth of respiration are so regulated that the individual is

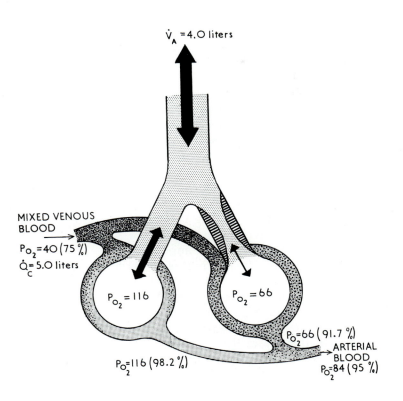

Figure 22–4 Ventilation and perfusion within lung. This diagrammatic representation of the lung shows two alveoli that are unevenly ventilated but uniformly perfused. Note how the overventilation of one alveolus does not compensate for underventilation of the other, with the result that some arterial desaturation occurs and the P_{O_2} is considerably reduced. (From Walter, J. B., and Israel, M. S.: General Pathology. 6th ed. Edinburgh, Churchill Livingstone, 1987. After Comroe, J. H., et al.: The Lung: Clinical Physiology and Pulmonary Function Tests. 2nd ed. Chicago, Year Book Medical Publishers, 1963.)

$\dot{V}_A = 4.0$ liters

MIXED VENOUS BLOOD

$P_{O_2} = 40$ (75 %)
$\dot{Q}_C = 5.0$ liters

$P_{O_2} = 116$

$P_{O_2} = 66$

$P_{O_2} = 66$ (91.7 %)
ARTERIAL BLOOD

$P_{O_2} = 116$ (98.2 %)

$P_{O_2} = 84$ (95 %)

unaware of the movements involved in breathing. *Tachypnea* is an increased rate of respiration. Rapid, shallow breathing occurs when pain restricts respiratory movement, as in pleurisy, or in increasing rigidity of the lungs, as in congestion or fibrosis. Tachypnea is sometimes accompanied by an increase in depth of breathing; the term *hyperpnea* includes both conditions. *Dyspnea* is a state in which the act of breathing causes distress. It occurs under two main circumstances:

1. *When tachypnea or hyperpnea is excessive.*
2. *When the movement of the chest on inspiration is small in comparison with the muscular effort needed to produce it.* This occurs in any disease interfering with the respiratory excursions of the lung, such as fibrosis or congestion. Obstruction to the major air passages—whether due to pulmonary disease like chronic bronchitis or to strangulation—has a similar effect and produces intense dyspnea. Psychological factors also play a part. Thus, the sudden blockage of a tube through which a person is breathing can cause intense dyspnea. However, if the subject is asked to block the tube, the maneuver causes no immediate discomfort.

DEFENSE MECHANISMS OF THE LUNG

Each part of the respiratory tract has its own defense mechanisms. In the upper respiratory tract, not only is the inspired air warmed and humidified, but the mucus-covered ciliated surface of the mucous membrane traps particles just as flies are trapped by flypaper. There is a continuous flow of mucus backward to the nasopharynx, where it is swallowed. Apart from this mechanical role, mucus contains various bactericidal substances, *e.g.,* IgA antibodies, lysozyme, and lactoferrin. The local flora, such as *Streptococcus viridans*, is also important.

The respiratory tract is normally sterile below the larynx. This is a remarkable fact, for each day the respiratory airways and alveoli are exposed to about 10,000 liters of air containing innumerable bacteria as well as particulate inanimate matter.

Particles are deposited on the walls of the various parts of the respiratory passages depending on their size. The momentum of large particles carries them out of the main airstream in areas of turbulence or where there is a sudden change in the direction of flow, *e.g.,* at points of bronchial branching. In this way, most particles larger than 10 μm settle in the nose, whereas most particles larger than 3 μm settle in the upper bronchial tree. Particles smaller than 0.3 μm tend to remain suspended by brownian movement, but those between 0.5 μm and 3.0 μm (this includes bacteria and particles of silica) reach the small bronchi, bronchioles, and respiratory portions of the lung. In the trachea, bronchi, and bronchioles, particles are trapped by the covering of mucus; ciliary action moves the sheet of mucus upward to be swallowed or spat out. This mucociliary escalator is a very efficient decontamination device under normal conditions but is impaired in disease, *e.g.,* in bronchitis, bronchiectasis, and obstruction. Particles that reach the acini are removed by two mechanisms. Those near the bronchioles join the mucociliary stream, but those more distal are engulfed by macrophages and slowly destroyed or removed. Unlike macrophages elsewhere, these cells derive their energy for phagocytosis by aerobic metabolism, and for this reason hypoxia secondary to pulmonary collapse or edema predisposes the affected areas to infection.

CONGENITAL ABNORMALITIES OF THE LUNG

Congenital abnormalities range from very rare conditions such as complete absence of both lungs (agensis) that is incompatible with life to minor abnormalities that can be considered variations of the normal. Sometimes there is a malformation in which the affected part of the lung is not connected to the normal bronchial or arterial system. The presence of an abnormal mass or cyst in the lung always raises the possibility of a developmental abnormality.

RESPIRATORY DISTRESS SYNDROME OF THE NEWBORN

The respiratory distress syndrome of the newborn is a clinical state that may have one of many causes, both extrapulmonary (*e.g.,* heart failure) and pulmonary; by far the most important cause is *hyaline membrane disease,* which is responsible for approximately 30 per cent of all neonatal deaths in North America.

Clinical Features. Respiratory distress generally occurs within 1 hour of birth and is invariably present by 6 hours. It is characterized by rapid grunting respiration, cyanosis, and obvious retraction of the intercostal muscles on inspiration. The overall mortality is about 50 per cent.

Predisposing Factors. The respiratory distress syndrome is more common in infants delivered by cesarean section, in infants subjected to perinatal asphyxia, and in those whose mothers have diabetes mellitus. However, by far the most important predisposing factor is prematurity, and the more premature the infant is, the more likely is the syndrome to be fatal.

Pathogenesis and Morphology. Fetal adaptation from intrauterine life to breathing air depends on orderly and unimpaired lung development. The type II pneumocytes first develop at about 24 weeks' gestation; at this time, surfactant also begins to appear. A deficiency in surfactant activity at birth is the main direct cause of the syndrome. As would be expected, this is most likely to occur in premature infants. The infant who lacks surfactant has difficulty in expanding the lungs because the work of inflating the alveoli is increased. Characteristically, at death the lungs are airless and dark red and have a liverlike consistency. On microscopic examination, the developing alveoli are collapsed, and the larger air passages are dilated and lined by a pink eosinophilic hyaline membrane similar to that seen in adult hyaline membrane disease (see Fig. 22–8).

Prediction and Treatment. Treatment is at present mainly supportive, but the possibility that hyaline membrane disease might occur can be predicted by examining the amniotic fluid. The amniotic sphingomyelin content remains constant throughout gestation, whereas amniotic lecithin levels reflect the development and function of type II pneumocytes. Hence, the ratio of lecithin to sphingomyelin is a good indicator of fetal lung development. If the ratio is greater than 2, it indicates that there is adequate surfactant and that hyaline membrane disease is un-

likely to develop. If the ratio is less than 1.5, significant surfactant deficiency exists, and hyaline membrane disease should be anticipated. The administration of glucocorticoids to the mother induces the formation of surfactant by the fetus, and this therapy has met with some success. Another approach is to instill surfactant down an endotracheal tube in an affected infant.

PNEUMONIA

Pneumonia is defined as an inflammation in the alveolar parenchyma of the lung.

Causes

The following causes may be listed.

Infection. This is generally bacterial, mycoplasmal, or viral.

Physicochemical. The agent may be inhaled (toxic gases, irritant particles, or irritant fluids such as gastric juice), or it may reach the lung via the blood stream (*e.g.,* bleomycin, an anticancer agent). Ionizing radiations form a separate variety of damaging agents.

Types

Two patterns of reaction may be found.

Pneumonia with Exudation into Air Spaces. The unqualified term *pneumonia* is commonly used to refer to this type. Inflammatory exudate fills the alveoli, which are thereby rendered airless and solid. This is called *consolidation,* and a portion of lung obtained at necropsy showing this will sink when placed in a beaker of water.

Pneumonia with Interstitial Exudate. The terms *interstitial pneumonia* and *pneumonitis* are commonly applied to this type.

Pneumonia with Exudation into Alveolar Spaces

This type of pneumonia is invariably caused by a bacterial agent. The clinical presentation is extremely variable, depending on the properties of the causative organism, the amount of lung affected, and the state of the host's defenses. The clinical course can be greatly modified by antibiotic therapy, and indeed many patients who formerly were admitted to the hospital can now be managed at home by their family practitioners. Nevertheless, it has been estimated that pneumonia accounts for approximately 10 per cent of admissions to the hospital in the United States.

Two patterns of reaction are evident in pneumonia, the difference between them being related mainly to the virulence of the causative organism. Highly virulent organisms, usually pneumococci, affect a whole lobe rapidly and cause *lobar pneumonia*. Organisms of lesser virulence initially cause a bronchiolitis; subsequent spread of infection to involve the distal pulmonary acini produces the more common *bronchopneumonia*.

Lobar Pneumonia

Healthy individuals are often affected by this disease, but an underlying debilitating disease, particularly chronic alcoholism, predisposes one to it. The infecting organism is invariably a highly virulent pneumococcus that is acquired by inhalation from another victim or a convalescent carrier. The disease has a sudden onset and is accompanied by rigors, fever, and pain in the chest. The organisms that reach the lung produce a rapidly spreading inflammatory edema that soon implicates a whole lobe or, at times, several lobes (Fig. 22–5).

During the initial stage of the disease, there is a septicemia and sometimes the pneumococci become localized not only in the lungs but also in the meninges, peritoneum, joints, and elsewhere. During the first few days of illness, the patient is desperately ill and may die; the lobe of lung affected is *congested* and shows *inflammatory edema*. It is teeming with pneumococci.

In the next stage, the lung shows complete consolidation and has a solid appearance that has been likened to that of a liver. Hence, it is sometimes called *hepatization*. The alveoli are filled with typical inflammatory exudate, with fibrin and polymorphs abounding.

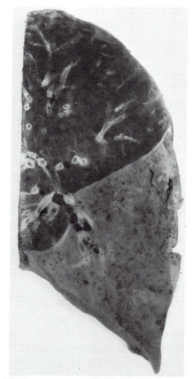

Figure 22–5 Lobar pneumonia. The lower lobe is completely consolidated, whereas the upper lobe is unaffected. Note the sharp division between the two lobes. (From Walter, J. B., and Israel, M. S.: General Pathology. 6th ed. Edinburgh, Churchill Livingstone, 1987. Reproduced by kind permission of the President and Council of the Royal College of Surgeons of England. Hunterian Museum specimen R30.2.)

The last stage of the disease is that of *resolution*. Macrophages replace the polymorphs, the inflammatory exudate is removed, and the lung returns to normal. This is an excellent example of complete resolution after acute inflammation.

During the acute stage of lobar pneumonia, the overlying pleura shows acute inflammation *(pleurisy)* and is covered with a fibrinous exudate. This exudate is responsible for the creaking *pleural rub*, which may be heard with a stethoscope, and for the severe pain that occurs on inspiration.

Clinical Course. After the acute onset, the patient remains seriously ill for 7 to 10 days with high fever. Death may occur during this stage. As suddenly as the disease started, it terminates. Sweating occurs, the temperature drops, and there is a sense of well-being. This is termed the *crisis*. In practice, these stages are rarely seen today, because antibiotics rapidly terminate the course of the disease.

Complications. Lung abscess, pulmonary fibrosis, and empyema may occur but are uncommon, even in the untreated patient.

Bronchopneumonia

Bronchopneumonia, unlike lobar pneumonia, is characterized by discrete foci of inflammation around terminal bronchioles. Patches of consolidation are scattered throughout several lobes of the lung, and the condition is usually bilateral (Fig. 22–6). The wildfire spread seen in lobar pneumonia is not present. The many varieties of

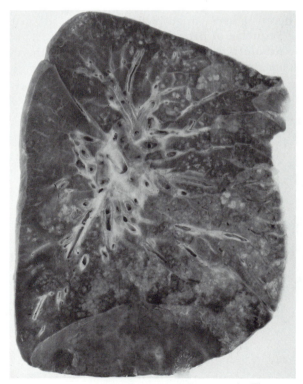

Figure 22–6 Staphylococcal bronchopneumonia. There are many discrete foci of consolidation scattered throughout the lung. Compare this with Figure 22–5, which shows lobar pneumonia. (From Walter, J. B., and Israel, M. S.: General Pathology. 6th ed. Edinburgh, Churchill Livingstone, 1987. Reproduced by kind permission of the President and Council of the Royal College of Surgeons of England. Hunterian Museum specimen R29.3.)

bronchopneumonia are best considered under two headings: *endogenous bronchopneumonia* and *exogenous bronchopneumonia*.

Endogenous Bronchopneumonia

This type of bronchopneumonia is due to infection by commensal organisms normally resident in the upper respiratory passages. These include pneumococci, staphylococci, *Haemophilus influenzae*, *Pseudomonas aeruginosa*, and the coliforms. *They cause infection whenever the defense mechanisms of the host are impaired.* The antagonists are therefore a weakly virulent endogenous organism and an enfeebled host.

Causes. The conditions leading to endogenous bronchopneumonia may be classified as either general or local factors.

General Factors

Extremes of Age. Bronchopneumonia is most common in infancy and old age.

General Debilitating Illness. It is a common terminal event in cancer, cerebrovascular accidents, and uremia.

Impaired Immune Response. It may occur with agammaglobulinemia or agranulocytosis or as a complication of glucocorticoid therapy.

Local Factors. Any local condition interfering with ciliary action and the upward movement of mucus is liable to be followed by bronchopneumonia. Possible causes are listed.

Pre-existing Acute Upper Respiratory Disease. Bronchopneumonia often complicates influenza, measles, and whooping cough. In these infections, the ciliated bronchial epithelium is shed, and organisms that gain access to the lung cannot be removed.

Local Obstruction. The trapped secretions form an admirable medium for bacterial growth, and bronchopneumonia is localized to the segment distal to the obstruction. Foreign bodies and tumors of the bronchi are good examples.

Chronic Bronchitis and Bronchiectasis. These are important predisposing causes of bronchopneumonia. Two factors are involved. First, the ciliated epithelium may be replaced by goblet cells or squamous cells, thereby impeding the upward flow of mucus. Second, the mucus itself is often of viscid consistency, and it cannot easily be removed. An excessive secretion of mucus accompanies the chronic venous congestion of heart failure because of the additional fluid contributed by transudation.

Pulmonary Edema. In edematous lung tissue, the alveolar macrophages are unable to perform their normal protective function. Bronchopneumonia is a common terminal event in congestive heart failure and indeed is a common sequel to edema from whatever cause. The basal edema that occurs in debilitated, bedridden patients, in those who are unconscious, and in those who have just undergone surgery often progresses to pneumonia; this is called *hypostatic pneumonia.* Good nursing and physical therapy can do much to prevent this complication.

Bronchopneumonia is of much longer duration than is lobar pneumonia. If the primary condition is incurable, the pneumonia is merely a welcome terminal event, and obviously little attempt is made at healing. Even in the childhood bronchopneumonias that follow measles and whooping cough, a prolonged course is the rule. The course of the disease is often punctuated by relapses and remissions, depending on whether the organism or the host is gaining the upper hand. Both the onset and the termination of the disease are gradual.

Lesions of Bronchopneumonia. The disease is usually basal, posterior in distribution, and bilateral (Fig. 22–6). If an area of bronchopneumonia is examined microscopically, it is found to consist of acutely inflamed bronchioles full of pus (Fig. 22–7). Some of the surrounding alveoli contain edema fluid in which there are macrophages and polymorphs, whereas others contain a dense, fibrinous exudate in which there are innumerable polymorphs. Some are collapsed as the result of the absorption of air distal to the blocked bronchioles, whereas neighboring alveoli are empty and distended because of compensatory dilation. In contrast to lobar pneumonia, in which all alveoli in a lobe are at about the same stage of the inflammatory process, in bronchopneumonia there is a very varied picture.

Sequelae of Bronchopneumonia

Resolution. This is much less frequent than in lobar pneumonia.

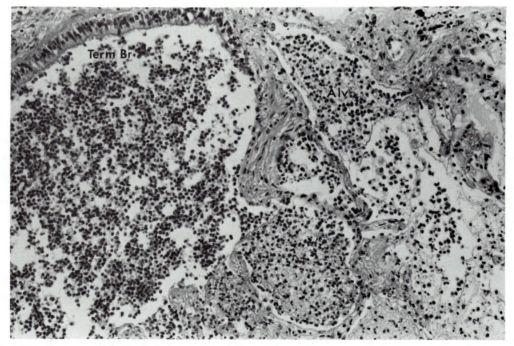

Figure 22–7 Bronchopneumonia. Part of a terminal bronchiole (Term Br) is shown with its lining of ciliated columnar epithelium. The bronchiole contains a mass of inflammatory cells, the majority of which are polymorphs. Alveoli (Alv) adjacent to the bronchiole also contain inflammatory exudate with polymorphs and fibrin. An alveolus further away from the bronchiole contains merely edema fluid.

Progressive Fibrosis of the Lung. This is correspondingly more frequent. The fibrosis is due to organization of the inflammatory exudate in the alveoli. In addition, there is often a continuance of the inflammatory process, so that more and more lung tissue is destroyed and converted into fibrous tissue. This is, of course, the condition of chronic inflammation, and bronchopneumonia often becomes chronic. In due course the infection spreads, and the muscle and elastic tissue of the adjacent bronchi are destroyed and replaced by granulation tissue. Consequently there is widening of the lumina, and eventually the dilation becomes extensive. This is the pathogenesis of *bronchiectasis,* which is both a sequel of bronchopneumonia and a predisposing cause of further attacks (see Fig. 22–19).

Suppuration. Abscess formation is not uncommon, particularly when the host's resistance is exceptionally poor and the causal organism is *Staphylococcus aureus.*

Exogenous Bronchopneumonia

When inhaled, a variety of virulent organisms may lead to severe bronchopneumonia. The host may be either healthy or enfeebled as a result of a previous disease. Examples of virulent organisms causing exogenous bronchopneumonia are listed.

Staphylococcus aureus. The bronchopneumonia may come as a result of hospital cross-infection.

Streptococcus pyogenes. Bronchopneumonia from this source was particularly common in the 1918 influenza pandemic.

Legionella pneumophila. Legionnaires' disease first attracted widespread attention when an outbreak occurred among delegates to a state convention of the American Legion in Philadelphia in July 1976. The incubation period was about 5 days. The main features of the disease were fever; myalgia; a spreading type of pneumonia, sometimes with cavitation; pleural effusion; chest pain; dyspnea; vomiting and diarrhea; renal failure; thrombocytopenia with purpuric rashes; and occasionally encephalopathy. This epidemic had a mortality of about 15 per cent, and although it appeared to be due to an infection (probably airborne), no causative organism could at first be identified. Intensive study finally isolated a previously unrecognized bacterium named *Legionella pneumophila.* Although the organism cannot be visualized in tissues by conventional staining, special silver impregnation and immunofluorescent techniques can demonstrate it. Also, it can now be grown on special media *in vitro.*

In retrospect, it has become apparent that other outbreaks of this disease had occurred previously (*e.g.,* "Pontiac fever" in 1968), and outbreaks of the disease have now been reported from many parts of the world. The diagnosis of the disease is most easily substantiated by obtaining a titer of antibodies of at least 1 in 128 or obtaining a fourfold increase in the titer of antibodies during convalescence. There are at least six distinct serotypes of *L. pneumophila* including a group termed atypical *Legionella*-like organisms.

Interstitial Pneumonia (Alveolitis)

Interstitial pneumonia is a type of lung inflammation in which the inflammatory exudate is confined predominantly to the interstitial tissues of the acinus. Because the main area involved is the alveolar walls, the term *alveolitis* is commonly used. Unless otherwise stated, when either term is used, it is assumed that the condition referred to is diffuse.

Interstitial pneumonia may be acute or chronic and has a variety of clinicopathologic presentations. In some instances, the cause is known; but in the majority of cases, neither cause nor pathogenesis is understood. It is convenient first to describe the various morphologic changes that are found and then to relate these to known causes and mechanisms.

Interstitial pneumonia appears to be initiated by damage to the alveolar lining cells (particularly the type I pneumocytes) and also to the alveolar vascular endothelial cells. Acute and chronic variants of interstitial pneumonia are recognized.

Acute Interstitial Pneumonia (Acute Alveolitis)

Damage to the vascular walls leads to the formation of an exudate in the interstitium of the lung, *i.e.,* in the alveolar walls, in the interlobar septae, in the connective tissue sheaths around blood vessels and bronchioles, and beneath the pleura.

The exudate consists of fluid and a variable number of mononuclear blood cells. Although this exudate is initially interstitial, damage to the type I pneumocytes and their subsequent loss allows a protein-rich fluid to exude into the alveoli and alveolar ducts. The air spaces are still ventilated, and the plasma proteins, fibrin, and cellular debris are thrown onto the air space walls, where they coagulate to form an *eosinophilic hyaline membrane* (Fig. 22–8). The morphologic term for this condition is *alveolitis with hyaline membrane formation.*

Acute interstital pneumonia may terminate in death or complete recovery, or it may progress to one of the chronic forms of interstitial pneumonia. An important example of acute interstitial pneumonitis, adult respiratory distress syndrome, is encountered after severe trauma.

Adult Respiratory Distress Syndrome. It is well recognized that severe trauma is often followed by pulmonary complications that closely resemble acute interstitial pneumonia (acute alveolitis) due to medical causes. This state has been called the *shock lung syndrome,* but the term *adult respiratory distress syndrome* is now more commonly used. It follows complicated surgery, such as that involving cardiopulmonary bypass procedures; trauma of any sort, particularly if associated with shock; burns; narcotic overdose; inhalation of irritants such as smoke in a fire; hemorrhagic pancreatitis; and severe sepsis. The common denominator among these very diverse events is not known, but the initial lesion appears to be an increased permeability of the alveolar capillaries to plasma proteins such that interstitial edema develops. Initially this leads to reflex tachycardia and hyperventilation due to stimulation of interstitial pressure stretch receptors. Respiratory alkalosis results. The lung becomes stiff, and this combined with peribronchiolar

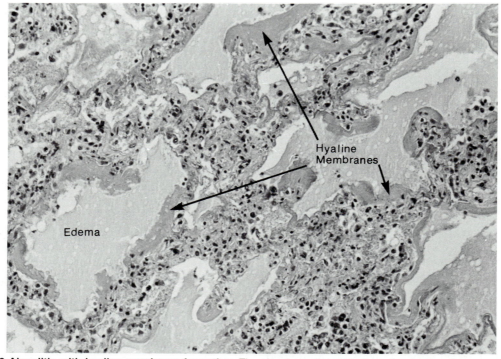

Figure 22–8 Alveolitis with hyaline membrane formation. The alveolar walls are thickened owing to edema, congestion, and a sparse infiltration by inflammatory cells that are mostly mononuclear. A striking feature is the lining of the airway spaces by an eosinophilic hyaline membrane. The alveoli and alveolar ducts are also filled by a pale-staining material, and in this section they are virtually airless. The material is coagulated edema fluid ($\times$120).

edema reduces alveolar ventilation so that some degree of hypoxemia results. The cause of the altered vascular permeability is not known and indeed probably varies under different circumstances. It may be the direct effect of inhaled irritants or hypoxia or the effect of a circulating toxin. A factor that has gained prominence recently is the *toxic effect of oxygen*. Prolonged breathing of gas containing over 50 per cent oxygen can cause this syndrome. After the formation of interstitial edema in the lung, there appears to be damage to the type I pneumocytes so that a similar fluid with high protein content accumulates in the alveoli. Alveolar hypoventilation increases, and arterial PO_2 decreases even more. If the patient dies in this acute stage, the lungs are heavy, plum-colored, wet, and bulging. Collapse of the lung is not a feature.

If the changes are insufficient to cause death, further changes occur in the lung. In those air spaces still ventilated, the alveolar fluid of high protein content is thrown into the alveolar walls and condenses to form a fibrin-rich hyaline membrane. This is particularly well seen in the alveolar ducts, and the picture is that of the *adult hyaline membrane disease* (Fig. 22–8). The type II pneumocytes proliferate, and some are desquamated into the alveoli, which become filled with cells, including macrophages, giving the picture of desquamative alveolitis. The type II pneumocytes eventually differentiate to replace the lost type I pneumocytes. In many cases, after about 2 weeks, both interstitial and intra-alveolar fibrosis occur; the picture of chronic interstitial pneumonitis is mimicked, and the lung is converted into a mass of fibrous tissue containing dilated spaces lined by bronchiolar epithelium, giving a honeycomb appearance *(honeycomb lung)*. These later complications of the acute respiratory insufficiency syndrome that lead to death 2 to 6 weeks after the initial insult have become more common since the establishment of aggressive pulmonary intensive care units that commenced around 1963. Positive-pressure ventilatory support methods can force gas into fluid-filled air spaces and lead to hyaline membrane formation. The excessive use of oxygen leads to the additional effect of oxygen toxicity, and indeed some authorities feel that this is the most important factor in the pathogenesis of the condition. Thus, by prolong-

ing life, the modern pulmonary intensive care unit has made more obvious and more common the late results of the acute pulmonary complications of severe injury.

Viral Pneumonitis. Acute upper respiratory tract viral infections can be complicated by acute interstitial pneumonia. The most important causes are the viruses of measles and influenza; other causes of pneumonitis include echoviruses, adenoviruses, respiratory syncytial virus, cytomegalovirus, and the viruses of chickenpox and herpes simplex. Cytomegalovirus pneumonitis is most common in children under the age of 4 years but has recently come to the fore as a common opportunistic infection at all ages. It is especially common in subjects with AIDS.

Acute Mycoplasmal Pneumonitis. This common disease is described in Chapter 9.

Pneumocystis Pneumonia. Pneumonia caused by infection with *Pneumocystis carinii* was originally described as a type of interstitial pneumonia in malnourished children but is now an important and common type of severe pneumonia in patients with AIDS (see Chapter 6).

Chronic Interstitial Pneumonia

This condition remains a major problem in chest medicine. In a few cases, a potentially removable extrinsic cause can be identified, but there remains a large group of patients in whom irreparable lung damage ultimately leads to pulmonary fibrosis and death. The disease may progress rapidly to a fatal termination within a few months, but more often the onset is insidious with progressive dyspnea and relatively little by way of other symptoms; often there is neither fever nor cough. The chest radiograph shows subtle interstitial changes. The rigidity and the swelling of the alveolar walls render the lungs stiff, so that ineffective alveolar ventilation in relation to arterial profusion increases the alveolar-arterial oxygen pressure difference. The mean survival time is about 4 years from diagnosis. Two main patterns of reaction can be recognized.*

---

*Other types have also been described but are uncommon and are not discussed here.

Desquamative Alveolitis. This is also called *desquamative interstitial pneumonia.* The distinguishing feature of this type is the filling of alveoli by mononuclear cells that were originally regarded as desquamated pneumocytes. It is now thought that these cells are macrophages.

Fibrosing Alveolitis. This is also called *usual interstitial pneumonia* because it accounts for over 80 per cent of the cases. Alveolar fibrin is organized, and the alveolar walls show fibrosis together with a sparse mononuclear cell infiltrate. Alveoli are lined by prominent type II pneumocytes (Fig. 22–9).

Etiology and Pathogenesis of Interstitial Pneumonia

A number of agents or circumstances have been incriminated as the cause of interstitial pneumonia.

1. *Infectious agents.* Many types of viruses cause acute interstitial pneumonia, as described previously.

2. *Pneumoconioses*, particularly asbestosis.

3. *Collagen vascular diseases*, particularly systemic sclerosis and rheumatoid arthritis.

4. *Ionizing radiation*, generally as a result of treatment of an adjacent carcinoma, *e.g.*, of breast, esophagus, or lung.

5. *Chemical agents.* Paraquat, a widely used herbicide, if ingested or absorbed is an important cause of acute alveolar damage. The damaging effect of inhaling high oxygen concentrations has been noted previously. Some drugs can also cause alveolar damage, in particular bleomycin, cyclophosphamide, methotrexate, busulfan, and chlorambucil, all drugs used in the treatment of malignant disease.

6. *Severe trauma.* This has certain distinctive features and is described under the heading Adult Respiratory Distress Syndrome.

In spite of this impressive list, it must be confessed that in over 50 per cent of cases of acute and chronic alveolitis, no cause can be identified. The term *cryptogenic fibrosing alveolitis* is used to cover our ignorance with respect to the chronic cases of unknown etiology. In some patients, IgG deposits have been demonstrated in the alveolar walls, and the damage is presum-

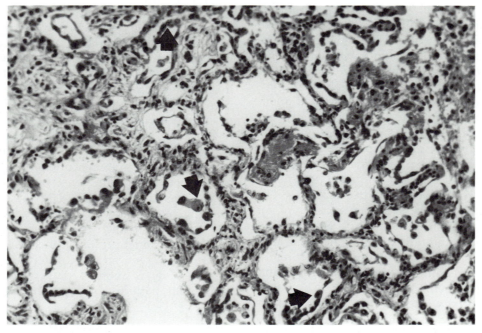

Figure 22–9 Fibrosing alveolitis. The alveolar walls are thickened by fibrous tissue and a mononuclear inflammatory infiltrate. Enlarged type II pneumocytes are seen lining the alveoli, and some of them have become detached from the alveolar walls.

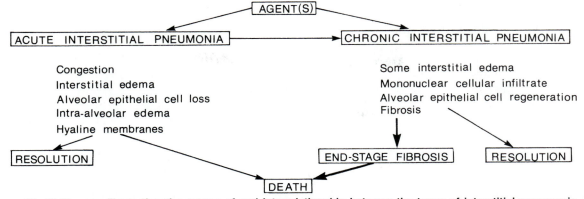

Figure 22–10 Diagram illustrating the course of and interrelationship between the types of interstitial pneumonia. It is suggested that acute interstitial pneumonia may undergo resolution, cause death, or progress to a chronic state. Chronic interstitial pneumonia may or may not be preceded by an acute pneumonia. The histologic "types" of chronic interstitial pneumonia depend on the type and extent of the cellular exudate, combined with the magnitude of the epithelial regeneration and the extent of the fibrosis. Resolution is still possible, but more often there is progressive fibrosis that ends in death.

ably immunologically mediated. Desquamative alveolitis tends to respond to glucocorticoid therapy and has a better prognosis than do the fibrosing types. This raises the important question of the relationship between the various types of alveolitis. It would be logical to assume that the desquamative type progresses to fibrosing alveolitis and ultimately terminates in pulmonary fibrosis. At present there is much contradictory evidence on this point, and future research may clarify the issue.

For the time being, it seems logical to regard the interstitial pneumonias as reaction patterns to many diverse agents. In some cases, several etiologic factors may be involved, and the reaction may well be determined as much by the host's response as by the nature of the agent concerned. The possible relationship between the types of interstitial pneumonia is indicated in Figure 22–10.

It should be noted in passing that it is in this area of chronic lung disease that open lung biopsy has been found to be of considerable value in determining the nature of the lesion and predicting the prognosis.

TUBERCULOSIS AND FUNGAL INFECTIONS OF THE LUNG

Tuberculosis of the lung is described in Chapter 8. In certain parts of the world, fungal infec-

tions are of importance and closely resemble tuberculosis in being acquired by inhalation and producing a pulmonary lesion of granulomatous type that generally heals but may occasionally be followed by widespread dissemination of the organism.

Fungal Infections

Cryptococcosis. The causative organism, *Cryptococcus neoformans,* is a yeast of worldwide distribution. The primary lung lesion is usually small, heals by fibrosis, and passes unnoticed. Occasionally, the organism spreads widely and has an affinity for the central nervous system, where it causes *meningitis.* This widespread dissemination is particularly common in patients with T-cell deficiency.

Histoplasmosis. The causative organism, a dimorphic fungus named *Histoplasma capsulatum,* has a worldwide distribution; infection, however, is particularly common in the Mississippi Valley of the United States, and skin tests indicate that up to 90 per cent of the population have been infected. The organism is found in the soil and is particularly abundant in soil contaminated with bird droppings, *e.g.,* in chicken houses. Once again, the primary lesion is in the lung, and the disease closely resembles tuberculosis (Fig. 22–11). Unless the initial infection has been

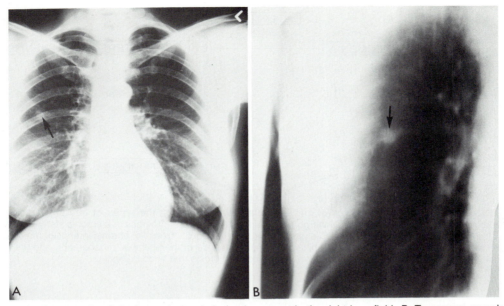

Figure 22–11 Histoplasmosis of the lung. *A,* A coin lesion is present in the right lung field. *B,* Tomogram reveals the shadow with greater definition. (Radiographs courtesy of Dr. D. E. Sanders, Department of Radiology, Toronto General, Division of the Toronto Hospital, Toronto.)

heavy, the disease is generally asymptomatic. Healing usually occurs with calcification. Occasionally the lung lesion cavitates, and metastatic lesions occur elsewhere. Even more rarely, the fungi invade the blood stream in a massive way and cause a generalized infection. An extract of the organism is used in the *histoplasmin test* (analogous to the tuberculin reaction) and is positive in infected individuals.

Case History I

In 1953, at the age of 25 years, the patient, an Englishwoman, developed a flulike illness that was accompanied by pain in the chest on taking a deep breath. Pleurisy complicating "virus pneumonia" was diagnosed initially, but markedly enlarged hilar lymph nodes and normal lung fields were revealed by a chest radiograph. The diagnosis was changed to primary tuberculosis, but since the patient produced no sputum, the diagnosis was never proved; nevertheless, her tuberculin test was initially negative and became strongly positive. This Mantoux conversion was taken as good evidence of a tuberculous infection. Three months of rest in a sanatorium was ordered. The patient made a rapid recovery, married, and had two children without recurrence of the lung infection. She emigrated to North America in 1965.

In 1971, at the age of 43, the patient developed another "flulike" illness (see radiograph, Fig. 22–11).

A "coin lesion" was noted in the right lung field (Fig. 22–11*A*), and a tomogram (Fig. 22–11*B*) revealed the shadow with greater definition. Although the patient was a nonsmoker, a diagnosis of lung cancer was considered. However, a radiograph taken two years previously showed a lesion of similar size to be present. A cancerous lesion probably would have enlarged during this period. Nevertheless, it was decided that this was insufficient evidence on which to exclude such a serious disease. A needle biopsy was performed under local anesthesia, and necrotic tissue was obtained. Neither organisms nor tumor cells could be identified in this. A histoplasmin test proved to be strongly positive. Histoplasmosis is much more common in North America than in England, and the presence of a lung lesion with a strongly positive histoplasmin test in a recent immigrant was regarded as presumptive evidence of primary histoplasmosis. No treatment was given, and the patient remains well to this day.

This case illustrates four points:

1. Persistent lung infections in young people should always raise the possibility of tuberculous infection.

2. The development of hypersensitivity to an organism or its products during the course of a disease is good evidence of infection by that organism, provided the clinical features are consistent with such a diagnosis.

3. A lung lesion in a person over the age of 40 years should be regarded as cancerous until proved otherwise.

4. A knowledge of the geographic incidence of disease can help in arriving at a correct diagnosis.

Coccidioidomycosis. This disease is caused by *Coccidioides immitis*, a dimorphic fungus that is common in the dry desert regions of California, Arizona, and Argentina. In these places, the majority of the inhabitants acquire a primary infection of the lung, but as with other diseases of this type, the lesion soon heals and is either asymptomatic or else causes a mild influenza-like illness known locally as "valley fever" or "desert fever." Occasionally, the disease is progressive, and the destructive lung lesions closely resemble tuberculosis. Rarely, the organism invades the blood, and infection of many organs may subsequently occur.

North American Blastomycosis. This is caused by infection with the yeast *Blastomyces dermatitidis*. The primary lesion is usually in the lung (Fig. 22–12) but may be cutaneous. Widespread dissemination occasionally occurs and tends to involve the bones, skin, and lung.

SARCOIDOSIS

Sarcoidosis is a disease of unknown etiology characterized histologically by the formation of noncaseating tuberculoid follicles. The lung is commonly affected, and the disease is considered here; however, other organs may also be affected, including the skin (erythema nodosum is common), the uveal tract, the spleen, the liver, and the bones particularly of the fingers. The disease is common in northern European communities, particularly in Scandinavia; in North America, it is most common in blacks.

The characteristic of sarcoidosis is the formation of discrete noncaseating follicles, resembling those of early tuberculosis, composed of plump

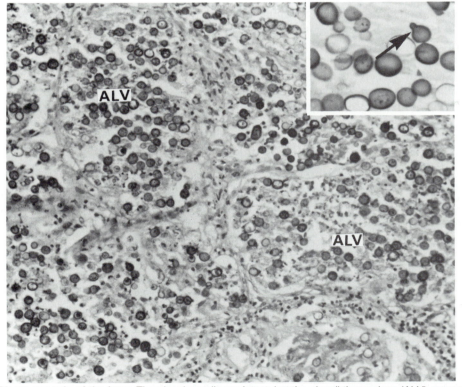

Figure 22–12 Blastomycosis of the lung. The alveolar walls are intact, but the alveoli themselves (ALV) are consolidated, being airless and filled with inflammatory exudate containing amorphous fibrinous material, disintegrating polymorphs, and large numbers of fungi (×250). The inset is from the same case, but the section has been stained by a silver impregnation method. The budding form of the fungus, marked by the arrow, is typical (×600).

epithelioid cells, in which Langhans type giant cells may be found (Fig. 22–13). There may be a few lymphocytes surrounding the tubercles, but they are by no means as plentiful as in tuberculosis.

The initial lesion in the lung is an interstitial alveolitis with an interstitial infiltration of lymphocytes and macrophages; later the characteristic granulomas develop. The hilar nodes are commonly involved, and hilar lymphadenopathy is sometimes the major and only radiologic evidence of sarcoidosis. In the later stages of the disease, the lesions heal with fibrosis and hyalinization. Chronic interstitial fibrosis possibly with honeycombing is the end result.

A common finding is a polyclonal hypergammaglobulinemia accompanied by the presence of circulating immune complexes. The patients have a depressed delayed type hypersensitivity reaction to all common antigens, *e.g.,* tuberculin and lepromin. This state of anergy is not accompanied by significant depression of cell-mediated immunity. The significance of these findings is not understood because no cause for the disease has been found. A curious reaction to some antigen (pine pollen, dust, or metals) or infection with some atypical mycobacterium has been suggested but never substantiated.

Sarcoidosis is sometimes accompanied by hypercalcemia; this is attributed to the hydroxylase content of the epithelioid cells. The enzyme converts vitamin D to an active form.

CHRONIC OBSTRUCTIVE PULMONARY DISEASE (COPD)

Chronic obstructive pulmonary disease (COPD), also called chronic obstructive lung disease (COLD), chronic airflow obstruction, and chronic nonspecific lung disease, is a clinical syndrome that comprises those conditions that are accompanied by *chronic or recurrent reduction in expiratory airflow within the lung.* The traditional teaching is that most cases of COPD are due to chronic bronchitis, pulmonary emphysema, or bronchial asthma. Chronic bronchitis and pulmonary emphysema often occur in the same individual and have many features in common, including a strong etiologic association with cigarette smoking and the associated presence of *small airways disease.* Bronchial asthma has significant differences from these three conditions and is described separately.

Types of COPD

The triad of chronic bronchitis, emphysema, and small airways disease composes the syn-

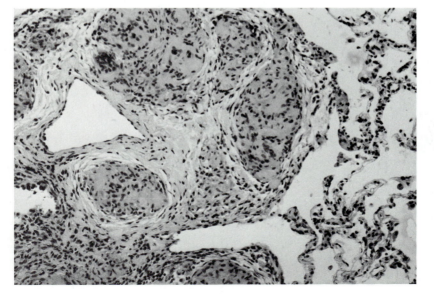

Figure 22–13 Sarcoidosis of the lung. The interstitial tissues of the lung show well-defined noncaseating tuberculoid granulomas, each consisting of a mass of epithelioid cells and occasional giant cells.

drome of COPD. They are described separately, but frequently they occur together.

Chronic Bronchitis

Chronic bronchitis is defined in clinical terms and is present in any patient who has persistent cough with sputum production occurring on most days for at least 3 months of the year for at least 2 successive years. Sputum production due to localized bronchopulmonary disease is excluded from this definition. At first, the expectoration in chronic bronchitis is intermittent and worse on rising in the morning; eventually it becomes continuous. Chronic inflammation of the bronchi is not a constant feature, and Laennec's term bronchial catarrh is particularly apt.

The most constant morphologic change in chronic bronchitis is an increased mass of mucous glands, reflected by an increase in the thickness of the bronchial mucosa. The surface epithelium of the bronchi shows metaplasia with replacement of ciliated cells by mucus-secreting goblet cells. Nevertheless, the mucus contributed by these cells is trivial compared with that produced by the large mucosal glands.

Etiology. The major cause of chronic bronchitis is the inhalation of irritant chemicals. Atmospheric pollution contributes to this, but by far *the most important cause is cigarette smoking.* Heavy smokers have up to ten times the incidence of chronic bronchitis as compared with nonsmokers. In the initial stages the sputum is mucoid, but periodically there are exacerbations of the disease due to infection—the sputum increases in amount and becomes purulent, and features of airway obstruction increase. Specific viral infections may produce similar exacerbations, but more frequently the culprit is a bacterial infection, often by one of the normal commensal inhabitants of the upper respiratory tract. *Haemophilus influenzae* and the pneumococci are particularly common causes. Bronchopneumonia may follow and indeed can be a terminal event of this disease.

Symptoms. Persistent cough with the production of mucoid or mucopurulent sputum is the outstanding symptom. Dyspnea, cyanosis, and right-sided heart failure develop later and are probably associated with the development of small airways disease.

Pulmonary Emphysema

Pulmonary emphysema is best defined as a condition in which there is an abnormal permanent increase in size of the air spaces distal to the terminal bronchioles accompanied by destructive changes of the alveolar walls. The definition is therefore a morphologic one, and two types can be recognized.

Centriacinar Emphysema (Centrilobular Emphysema). In this type of emphysema, the central parts of the acini, *i.e.,* those formed by respiratory bronchioles, are most severely affected (Fig. 22–14). Hence, the enlarged spaces that are formed by the destructive process are readily visible in the center of the lobules of the lung and are surrounded by relatively unaffected areas in which the alveolar ducts and peripheral alveoli reside (Figs. 22–15 and 22–16). Centrilobular emphysema tends to affect the upper parts of the lung fields more severely than the bases; as the disease advances, there can be extensive destruction of all areas of lung with the production of large bullae, *i.e.,* spaces over 1 cm in diameter.

Panacinar Emphysema (Panlobular Emphysema). In this type of emphysema, the destructive process in the alveolar walls involves the acinus uniformly (Fig. 22–17). Hence, the process is more diffuse. This disease, in contrast to centrilobular emphysema, tends to affect the bases of the lungs rather than the upper fields.

Etiology of Pulmonary Emphysema. Elastic fibers form an important component of the alveolar walls, and their destruction leads to emphysema. This can be shown experimentally by allowing animals to inhale an aerosol of neutrophil elastase or the proteolytic enzyme papain. So important is the elastic tissue to the integrity of the lung that there are normally potent anti-elastase enzymes in lung tissue. The most important of these is *alpha*$_1$-antitrypsin, which is manufactured in the liver and reaches the lung via the blood stream. Patients who have a genetic defect causing a reduced or absent alpha$_1$-antitrypsin activity tend to develop emphysema of the panacinar type. These observations have

CENTRILOBULAR EMPHYSEMA

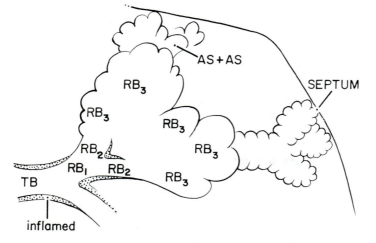

Figure 22–14 Centriacinar (centrilobular) emphysema. The respiratory bronchioles are selectively and dominantly involved. AS, alveolar sac; TB, terminal bronchiole; RB_1, RB_2, RB_3, respiratory bronchioles of the first, second, and third orders. (From Thurlbeck, W.M.: Chronic obstructive lung disease. *In* Sommers, S. C. [Ed.]: Pathology Annual, vol. 3. New York, Appleton-Century-Crofts, 1968.)

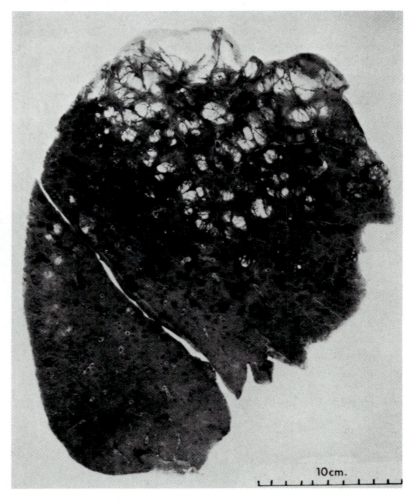

Figure 22–15 Centriacinar pulmonary emphysema. This thin section of whole lung shows severe destructive emphysema. The lesions are so severe in the upper parts of the lung that light can be transmitted through the slice where there are bullae. (From Heard, B. E.: Pathology of Chronic Bronchitis and Emphysema. New York, Churchill Livingstone, 1969.)

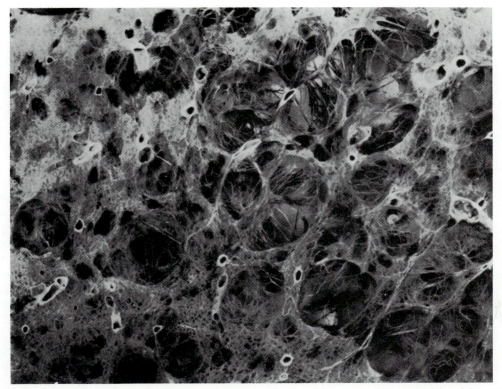

Figure 22–16 Centriacinar pulmonary emphysema. Higher magnification of the center of the upper lobe of the specimen shown in Figure 22–15. (From Heard, B.E.: Pathology of Chronic Bronchitis and Emphysema. New York, Churchill Livingstone, 1969.)

PANLOBULAR EMPHYSEMA

Figure 22–17 Panacinar (panlobular) emphysema. The enlargement and destruction of air spaces involves the acinus more or less uniformly. A, alveolus; AD, alveolar duct; AS, alveolar sac; RB₁, RB₂, RB₃, respiratory bronchioles of the first, second, and third orders; TB, terminal bronchiole. (From Thurlbeck, W.M.: Chronic obstructive lung disease. *In* Sommers, S.C. [Ed.]: Pathology Annual, vol. 3. New York, Appleton-Century-Crofts, 1968.)

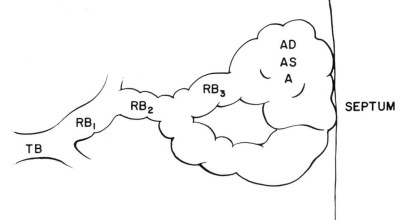

given rise to the concept that *elastase-antielastase imbalance* could be a major factor in the pathogenesis of emphysema.

Inhaled pollutants, particularly tobacco smoke, cause an inflammation that results in the accumulation of neutrophils in the lung and the release of elastase; lung destruction follows. These changes are most pronounced in the proximal portion of the respiratory unit, thereby resulting in respiratory bronchiolitis and centrilobular emphysema. The upper parts of the lung are the best-ventilated areas, and it is here that the emphysema is most advanced.

On the other hand, if the main determinant in causing an elastase-antielastase imbalance is a low level of circulating alpha$_1$-antitrypsin, the effects of elastin destruction are more widespread, and the end result is panlobular emphysema.

It is now accepted that tobacco smoking and inhalation of other pollutants is a major factor in the cause of emphysema. Many mechanisms are involved. Inhibition of ciliary action leads to mucus retention. The irritant smoke can contribute to bronchiolitis and small airways obstruction. Inhalation of smoke leads to an increased number of polymorphs in the alveoli by a direct irritant effect. In addition, macrophages accumulate; these cells, when irritated by tobacco smoke, release a neutrophil chemotactic factor. They also release an elastase that is not inhibited by alpha$_1$-antitrypsin. Furthermore, the level of alpha$_1$-antitrypsin activity is reduced by smoking. One cause of this is its destruction by macrophage elastase. The activity of the enzyme is also inhibited by oxidants in the smoke and by the action of free radicals released by stimulated neutrophils and macrophages. Hence, even a normal level of alpha$_1$-antitrypsin can be inadequate for preventing the development of emphysema in the presence of inhaled pollutants, especially tobacco smoke.

Small Airways Disease

Because of the large total cross-sectional area of the small air passages (less than 2 mm in diameter), they normally offer little obstruction to the flow of air. Nevertheless, in COPD, small airways obstruction can be demonstrated; the bronchioles show goblet cell metaplasia with mucus plugging and inflammatory change with fibrosis in the walls of the airway. Smooth muscle hypertrophy and spasm contribute to the obstruction. Atmospheric pollutants, particularly tobacco smoke, appear to be the main causative factors.

Airways Obstruction

Obstruction of the airways and therefore also to airflow can be demonstrated by a variety of techniques. The simplest is to ask the patient to take a deep inspiration and follow it by a maximum expiration. The total amount of gas expired is termed the forced expiratory volume (FEV), and by suitable measurement, the amount of gas expired in one second (FEV$_1$) can be measured. A decrease in FEV$_1$ indicates airflow obstruction and is therefore a feature of COPD.

In the past, it has generally been considered that airflow obstruction in COPD resulted either from bronchial narrowing in chronic bronchitis or a loss of elastic recoil in emphysema. Although there is some truth in these concepts, it is now felt that chronic bronchitis alone does not produce appreciable obstruction and that small airways disease and emphysema are more important. Usually they occur together in the same patient. As noted, the small airways can be obstructed by mucus in the lumen or by inflammatory disease in the wall, possibly with fibrosis. Furthermore, the loss of elastic tissue in emphysema can allow the small airways to collapse by loss of radial support. Although it is possible to define and describe chronic bronchitis, emphysema, and small airways disease separately, in practice they often occur together and indeed seem to share many etiologic factors.

Classic Clinicopathologic Syndromes of COPD

Two types of this clinical syndrome can be recognized.

Type A—Pink Puffers. Typically the patient is middle-aged and complains of increasing shortness of breath and negligible cough with little sputum. On examination, the chest appears to be overexpanded, and the chest radiograph may exhibit hypertranslucency. The effect of the emphysema is to reduce the total area available for blood-gas interchange, so that the patient must breath more rapidly in order to maintain the blood gases at normal levels. These patients therefore develop progressive, unrelenting dyspnea and yet remain pink. Hence, the term "pink puffers" is applied.

Type B—Blue Bloaters. Typically this patient presents at an earlier age with chronic bronchitis and increasing shortness of breath. Chest auscultation reveals scattered rales due to mucous plugging of some bronchi. Pathologically, there is chronic bronchitis and small airways disease. In spite of airways obstruction there is little dyspnea, and some areas of lung are hypoventilated. This unequal distribution of ventilation in relation to blood supply causes desaturation of the arterial blood, and the patient is therefore cyanosed. The hypoxemia stimulates the bone marrow, so that secondary polycythemia results. The low alveolar P_{O_2} causes vasoconstriction, and this leads to pulmonary hypertension, itself a forerunner of chronic cor pulmonale and heart failure. The poor ventilation of the lungs results in carbon dioxide retention, so that the P_{CO_2} rises. This causes peripheral vasodilation and accentuates the cyanosis of the skin.

Patients with chronic bronchitis, having a raised arterial P_{CO_2} and lowered P_{O_2}, often tolerate these abnormal blood gas tensions remarkably well, and any sudden change can lead to serious consequences. Thus, if the hypoxemia (low P_{O_2}) is relieved by oxygen therapy, ventilation can become so depressed that CO_2 retention with coma ensues. Alternatively, vigorous artificial ventilation can relieve the hypercapnia to the extent that the low arterial P_{CO_2} causes vasoconstriction and cerebral ischemia.

The administration of general anesthetics to chronic bronchitics is particularly hazardous because any further increase in mucus production or spasm of the bronchi is liable to precipitate respiratory failure.

Patients with this syndrome can often be tided over acute attacks with antibiotics and other treatment. They therefore differ from the pink puffers, who progress relentlessly and are resistant to treatment.

Although two types of clinical syndrome have been described, these must be regarded as the two ends of a clinical spectrum, and patients will be encountered who have features intermediate between type A and type B.

BRONCHIAL ASTHMA

Asthma is a condition of widespread narrowing of the bronchial airways that *changes in severity over short periods of time,* either spontaneously or under treatment, and is not due to cardiovascular disease. It is characterized by *paroxysms of wheezing and dyspnea.* The bronchial obstruction is caused partly by spasm of the bronchial muscle and partly by the presence of viscid mucus (Fig. 22–18). Rarely an attack fails to remit, and the patient dies *(status asthmaticus).*

Case History II

The patient was a 28-year-old woman who had a long history of bronchial asthma. She had an acute

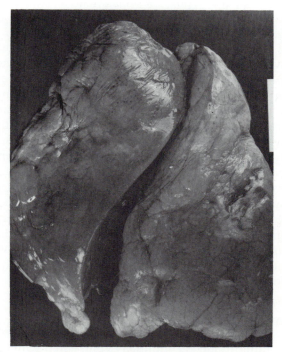

Figure 22–18 Bronchial asthma. The lung is greatly overinflated because the bronchi are plugged with thick, tenacious mucus. See Case History II for clinical details.

attack that became progressively more severe as dyspnea and cyanosis developed. Despite vigorous resuscitation attempts, she had a cardiac arrest and died 9 hours after the onset of the attack. On opening of the chest at necropsy, the lungs were found to be greatly overinflated (Fig. 22–18). The bronchi were plugged by thick, tenacious mucus. During life some air could enter the lungs during inspiration because on inspiration the bronchi dilate. However, the patient could not expel air so easily on expiration, and the lungs became overinflated.

Many examples of asthma (usually termed *extrinsic asthma*) have a hereditary basis, and the disease is one manifestation of atopy. Attacks are brought on by the inhalation of an antigen to which the subject is sensitive. This sensitivity can be detected by skin tests. A small quantity of antigen is scratched into the skin; if the patient is sensitive, there is an immediate response with a wheal and flare. This is an example of a type I hypersensitivity reaction and is mediated by IgE.

Some types of asthma (often termed *intrinsic asthma*) appear to be related to respiratory infections, and other types are triggered by taking aspirin by mouth or by the inhalation of chemicals. The chemicals are usually of industrial origin, such as epoxy resins, plastics, and other chemical dusts and gases. This group may be termed *industrial asthma*.

An uncommon type of asthma is associated with pulmonary infiltrates and blood eosinophilia. In this group, there is combined type I and type III hypersensitivity, and probably many types of this syndrome exist. Some may be manifestations of parasitic infections in which the worms are migrating through the lungs. Another type is due to colonization of bronchi or lung cavities by the fungus *Aspergillus fumigatus*. It is evident that bronchial asthma is a condition in which the bronchi are unduly sensitive to a variety of agents derived from either some immunologic reaction or a physical stimulus. Examples of the physical stimulus are asthmatic attacks in response to exercise, cold, or psychological stress.

ALLERGIC LUNG DISEASE

Lung tissue is continually confronted with airborne antigens, and it is not surprising that allergic disease is common. Many of the types of bronchial asthma discussed in the preceding sec-

tion fall under this heading. In addition, there is a group of interesting diseases termed *extrinsic allergic alveolitis*. Clinically, patients experience sudden onset of fever, headache, dyspnea, and cough coming on 4 to 6 hours after exposure to fine particles of organic material to which the patient is sensitive. It is believed that sensitizing IgG antibodies are involved, and this is an example of type III hypersensitivity occurring in the alveoli. Many known external antigens are described. Perhaps best known is the antigen derived from fungal spores in moldy hay. Breathing in dust containing these spores causes *farmer's lung*. Likewise, inhalation of antigens from maple bark, pigeon excreta, or mushrooms produces a similar picture (*e.g., bird fancier's lung*).

PULMONARY EDEMA

The systolic pressure in the pulmonary artery is 15 to 25 mm Hg; being much lower than that in the systemic vessels, it follows that there is less tendency to edema formation (see Fig. 5–1).

The osmotic effect of the plasma proteins is relatively unopposed; in the initial stages, edema fluid accumulates in the interstitial tissues of the lung. It is drained away by the lymphatic vessels, but when this defense mechanism becomes overloaded, the fluid passes into the alveolar spaces and the lung becomes solid. There are two factors that tend to ensure that pulmonary edema persists and even spreads:

1. The loose nature of the lung prevents any immediate appreciable rise in tissue tension, a fact that in most tissues limits the extent of edema formation.

2. When the lungs have become edematous, the alveoli become filled with fluid, ventilation ceases, the vessel walls become hypoxic, and their permeability to protein increases. It follows that in all examples of pulmonary edema, the fluid has a high protein content. Therefore, it is more difficult to distinguish between transudates and exudates in the lungs than in other tissues.

Causes of Pulmonary Edema

Acute Inflammation. Edema occurs in the early stages of pneumonia; it is particularly marked in acute lobar pneumonia. It was a prominent feature in the bronchopneumonia that complicated the influenza of the 1918 pandemic. The lungs were described as showing acute hemorrhagic edema rather than bronchopneumonia of the classic type. Such a picture is also encountered in poisoning with certain gases, *e.g.*, phosgene, chlorine, and nitrogen peroxide. Acute pulmonary edema also follows the inhalation of gastric juice, such as may occur if a patient vomits during the inexpert administration of a general anesthetic.

Heart Failure. Acute pulmonary edema is a frequent complication of left ventricular failure and mitral stenosis. Although increased pulmonary venous pressure is the usual explanation offered for this complication, it is unlikely that this is the major cause of pulmonary edema in heart failure. More important is the effect of a *redistribution of the blood volume;* attacks of acute pulmonary edema *(cardiac asthma)* occur quite suddenly (sometimes at night), and they are probably initiated by peripheral vasoconstriction. The amount of blood in the peripheral circulation is thus diminished, and the excess volume is displaced into the pulmonary circulation, in which it appears as edema fluid. Support for this contention is the observation that acute pulmonary edema is a well-known hazard of epinephrine administration. This drug causes peripheral vasoconstriction. It must never be given to patients with acute pulmonary edema of cardiac origin. In bronchial asthma, this drug is beneficial, but in cardiac asthma, it can be lethal.

The terms *cardiac asthma* and *paroxysmal nocturnal dyspnea* are often applied to these attacks of acute pulmonary edema. The patient wakes up gasping for breath, with a sense of oppression in the chest, and sits up, but the dyspnea increases. Mounting restlessness drives the patient out of bed to seek the fresh air at the window. The sense of suffocation becomes intense, and with it there is profound distress. The skin has an ashen color because of the vasoconstriction combined with cyanosis, and there is also profuse sweating. The patient may cough up copious blood-stained sputum owing to a rapidly spreading pulmonary edema. In severe cases, death ensues.

Overloading the Circulation. If an excessive volume of fluid is administered intravenously, some of the excess is accommodated in the great veins, but the remainder is diverted to the pulmonary circulation and leads to edema formation. It is obvious that patients already in heart failure are particularly prone to this complication (Chapter 18).

Cerebral Damage. Acute pulmonary edema sometimes complicates damage to the brain, *e.g.*, trauma or cerebral hemorrhage. The most likely explanation is that increased sympathetic nervous impulses from the brain lead to peripheral vasoconstriction and cause diversion of the circulating fluid to the lungs, as described before.

BRONCHIAL OBSTRUCTION

Causes

The common causes of bronchial obstruction are (1) *tenacious mucus*, which is not expelled from the respiratory passages, as in asthma; (2) *chronic bronchitis*; (3) *inhaled foreign bodies*, such as fragments of teeth or peas; and (4) *tumors*, usually carcinoma.

Effects

The effects of obstruction depend on whether the obstruction is partial or complete.

Partial Obstruction. The partial obstruction of a bronchus impedes the ventilation of the lung distal to the obstruction. It therefore follows that the blood perfusing that part of the lung is inadequately oxygenated and that, in effect, a quantity of venous blood is shunted directly into the pulmonary veins and from there to the left side of the heart. Because the blood leaving the lungs is normally fully saturated with oxygen, it follows that no amount of overventilation of the unaffected lung can compensate for this shunt effect (Fig. 22–4). The arterial P_{O_2} is therefore lowered *(hypoxemia)*. A very important example of partial obstruction of the bronchi occurs in chronic bronchitis, especially after a surgical operation requiring general anesthesia.

Widespread partial bronchial obstruction leads to overinflation of the lungs in asthma (see Fig. 22–18).

Infection commonly follows persistent bronchial obstruction. Organisms that are inhaled into the affected lung segment become trapped in the mucus, their expulsion is impaired, and bronchopneumonia follows. The infection also involves the bronchial walls; chronic infection will destroy the muscular and cartilaginous components of the walls so that they are weakened and dilation ensues *(bronchiectasis).* This effect is frequently seen distal to the obstruction caused by a carcinoma or a foreign body.

Complete Obstruction. Where there is complete obstruction of a large bronchus, the lung distal to it shows a progressive absorption of its gas content until it becomes completely airless or collapses *(i.e., a collapsed* lung). A plug of mucus sometimes causes this postoperative complication. Physical therapists can help prevent this by encouraging the patient to breathe deeply and bring up sputum.

SUDDEN INFANT DEATH SYNDROME

Also known as cot or crib death, the sudden infant death syndrome occurs in approximately 0.5 per cent of all live births. The infant, generally under the age of 1 year, is found dead, apparently having died quietly while asleep. Extensive investigations have failed to find any consistent abnormality or to indicate the cause. Immaturity of the respiratory system leading to periods of apnea and inapparent respiratory infections have been suggested as the most likely factors, but the cause of these tragic deaths remains a mystery.

BRONCHIECTASIS

Bronchiectasis is a condition in which bronchi are abnormally and permanently dilated. Weakening of the bronchial wall, generally as a result of infection, and increased traction of surrounding structures are the major factors whereby this comes about. When there is collapse of lung tissue around the bronchi, the inspiratory efforts are transmitted directly to the bronchial walls, and dilation ensues. Fibrosis of the lung has a similar effect, and contracture of the scar tissue is an additional factor.

It follows that bronchiectasis is commonly found distal to a bronchial obstruction because collapse, chronic bronchopneumonia, and fibrosis ensue. Bronchiectasis invariably complicates cystic fibrosis in patients who survive into adult life (Fig. 22–19). It is also found in areas of fibrosis such as those of chronic fibroid tuberculosis. Bronchopneumonia in childhood is an important cause of bronchiectasis in later life; if the pneumonic episodes are forgotten, the condition is liable to be labeled idiopathic.

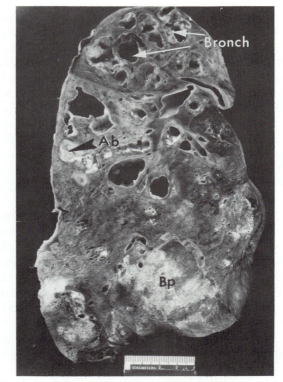

Figure 22–19 Bronchiectasis with repeated lung infection. Since the age of 7 years, this patient had had repeated attacks of pneumonia. When he was 24 years of age, a diagnosis of cystic fibrosis was made. He was treated with vitamins and pancreatic enzymes by mouth but continued to be plagued by repeated lung infections. The terminal event was an overwhelming infection with *Pseudomonas aeruginosa.* The patient died at the age of 32 years. The specimen shows the effects of repeated bronchopneumonia. Toward the base of the lung there are several areas of bronchopneumonia (Bp), and the discrete areas of consolidation have fused together to become confluent. Nevertheless, the appearances are not those of lobar pneumonia. In another area, the pneumonia has progressed to abscess formation (Ab). Toward the upper part of the lung, there is tremendous dilation of bronchi, and the appearances are typical of advanced bronchiectasis (Bronch). Much of the intervening lung has been destroyed.

In preantibiotic days, bronchiectasis was characterized by chronic cough with the production of copious, foul-smelling sputum. Complications such as lung abscess, empyema, bronchopleural fistula, and pyemic spread particularly to the brain were all common. So also was clubbing of the fingers and amyloid disease. Fortunately, antibiotic therapy and surgery have rendered this scenario a thing of the past.

LUNG ABSCESS

Many of the causes of lung abscess have already been encountered; they include the following:

1. Aspiration of infected material. This may occur in unconscious patients (coma, alcoholism, or during surgery) and may complicate oral surgery and dental procedures. Aspiration of gastric juice with its high acid content causes acute pulmonary edema and possibly the later development of abscess.
2. Pneumonia, particularly bronchopneumonia caused by *Staphylococcus aureus.*
3. Bronchiectasis, especially if secondary to an obstruction.
4. Septic embolism.
5. Spread from adjacent foci. Examples include liver abscess, subphrenic abscess, and mediastinitis due to ruptured esophagus or penetrating wounds.
6. Idiopathic. Finally, in some cases, no primary cause can be found.

Inhalation of material tends to cause an abscess in the apical or subapical portion of the lobe, because with the patient in bed, inhaled material readily enters the appropriate bronchi. Furthermore, abscesses are more common on the right side owing to the more vertical course of the right main bronchus. Lung abscesses usually rupture into a bronchus so that their contents are drained and the cavity contains air as well as pus. Regardless of the original causative organism, secondary anaerobic invaders (*e.g.*, *Bacteroides* species) are common. The result is a putrid lung abscess with symptoms, such as foul-smelling sputum, and complications closely resembling those of advanced bronchiectasis.

THE PNEUMOCONIOSES

This group of diseases, produced by the *inhalation of dust,* is mostly occupational in origin. The most important condition is *silicosis,* which occurs in miners and in those whose work entails exposure to silica dust. After the inhalation of this dust, the silica particles are taken up by macrophages and, being toxic, kill these cells. Fibrogenic factors that stimulate the formation of collagen are liberated. The particles themselves are once again phagocytosed by macrophages, and the process is repeated many times. Hence, numerous *silicotic nodules* of dense fibrous tissue are formed that are readily demonstrable on a radiograph (Figs. 22–20 and 22–21). Silicosis predisposes one to pulmonary tuberculosis.

Asbestosis is another important pneumoconiosis. It affects workers who fabricate asbestos fibers; it does not affect the miners who quarry it. Asbestosis is characterized by a diffuse interstitial fibrosis and the formation of pleural plaques of fibrous tissue. The disease is important in predisposing the subject to *cancer of the lung* and to *mesothelioma of the pleura.* It has been estimated that subjects with asbestosis have a tenfold likelihood of developing cancer of the lung. If in addition they smoke cigarettes, the incidence is about 90 times the normal. Asbestos is widely used as an insulating fire-resistant material and in car brake linings, so that many city dwellers are bound to inhale the fibers. Their presence in the lung does not alone constitute asbestosis, but how great a health hazard they constitute is not known.

Anthracosis, which is due to the inhalation of carbon, is the most common of the dust diseases because to some extent it affects all city dwellers. The disease often severely affects coal miners, but since carbon induces little inflammatory reaction or fibrosis, the miners experience no ill effects unless the carbon accumulations are massive. Usually this occurs in association with tuberculosis or silicosis.

Coal miner's pneumoconiosis results from inhalation of coal dust with a low silica content. In its common mild form, there is little fibrosis and virtually no effect on lung function. However, after 10 to 20 years of heavy exposure, *progressive massive fibrosis* may develop. The lungs become

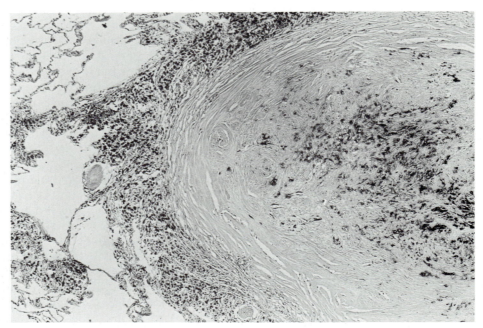

Figure 22–20 Silicosis. The silicotic nodule in the lung shows the characteristic concentric laminated appearance caused by successive waves of fibrosis induced by silica particles. The particles themselves cannot be seen in this picture. The black pigment in the center of the nodule and in macrophages in adjacent alveoli is carbon. (From Walter, J. B.: Pathology of Human Disease. Philadelphia, Lea & Febiger, 1989.)

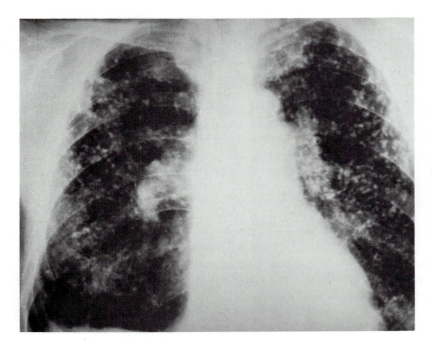

Figure 22–21 Silicosis. This radiograph shows numerous silicotic nodules scattered throughout the lung fields. The bases are relatively spared, and in this respect silicosis resembles the other pneumoconioses. Asbestosis is the only major exception to this rule because the large, heavy asbestos fibers tend to gravitate to the bases of the lungs. (Courtesy of Dr. D. E. Sanders, Department of Radiology, Toronto General, Division of the Toronto Hospital, Toronto.)

converted into solid masses of black fibrous tissue, the disease is progressive, and death is inevitable. Possibly silicosis and tuberculosis are the additional factors that lead to the development of this severe variant.

PULMONARY NEOPLASMS

The vast majority of lung tumors are epithelial in origin.

Bronchial Carcinoid Tumor

The bronchial carcinoid is of APUD cell origin (Chapter 29) and is of intermediate malignancy since it invades locally, is of slow growth, and rarely metastasizes. Hence, lobectomy or pneumonectomy is usually curative. The tumor generally arises in the wall of a large bronchus and causes partial, and finally complete, obstruction. Distal *bronchopneumonia* and bronchiectasis, often with hemoptysis, are frequent (Fig. 22–22).

True benign tumors of the bronchi (adenomas) are rare; it should be noted that the term "adenoma of the bronchus" has often been used in the past to describe the carcinoid tumors, a practice that should be abandoned.

Carcinoma of the Lung

In North America, cancer of the lung now ranks as the most common lethal cancer in males. The incidence in females is steadily increasing and indeed it has overtaken cancer of the breast, which until recently has been in the lead.

Etiology and Pathogenesis

Inhaled carcinogens in tobacco smoke and industrial fumes are believed to be the major cause.

Tobacco Smoking. By far the most important cause of cancer of the lung is tobacco smoking. Reports based on statistical evidence by the Royal College of Physicians and of the Surgeon General of the United States have all incriminated cigarette smoking as the major factor in the cause of

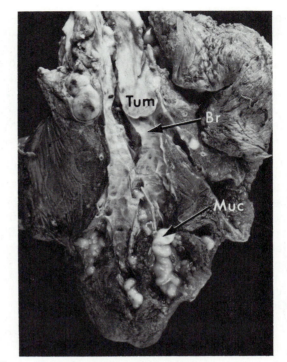

Figure 22–22 Carcinoid tumor of bronchus. This patient developed a patch of bronchopneumonia that did not clear completely with chemotherapy. Bronchoscopy revealed a tumor obstructing the bronchus in the lower lobe. Biopsy showed a carcinoid tumor. A lobectomy was performed, and the patient made a satisfactory recovery. The specimen shows a tumor (Tum) growing into and obstructing a bronchus (Br). Distal to the tumor, the bronchus is widely dilated and contains thick mucopurulent material (Muc). Bronchiectasis distal to an obstructing tumor is characteristic.

lung cancer, particularly the squamous-cell and small-cell types. Compared with the nonsmoker, the average smoker has a tenfold increased risk of developing lung cancer; for heavy smokers, the risk is twice that figure. For those smokers who have kicked the habit, there is some comfort; after 10 years of abstinence, their death rate from cancer is similar to that of nonsmokers. Nevertheless, nonsmokers are probably at some risk because they inhale other people's smoke.

The bronchial epithelium of smokers shows loss of ciliated cells, basal-cell hyperplasia, and cellular atypia. The severity of the changes is related to the amount smoked, and they are thought to progress to carcinoma *in situ* and ultimately to invasive tumor.

Industrial Hazards. A high incidence of lung cancer has been noted in certain industries. In the Schneeberg mines, the cause was probably inhalation of radon. Other industries associated with an increased incidence of lung cancer include those involving uranium ore, nickel ore, chromates, arsenic, and beryllium. Asbestos is a well-recognized carcinogen, and workers exposed to it have a ten times greater risk of developing lung cancer. The incidence is even higher (about 100 times) if the worker is a heavy smoker.

Air pollution in urban districts is another factor, but its importance is difficult to assess because other factors—particularly industrial exposure to carcinogens and cigarette consumption—must be taken into account. It seems that the carcinogenic effect of air pollution is relatively small.

Gross Appearance

Two common types of tumor may be recognized.

Peripheral Lung Cancers. These tumors presumably arise in one of the small bronchi or bronchioles and appear as fairly discrete tumor masses in the lung parenchyma. Symptoms are often absent until the pleura and chest wall are invaded or until distant metastases appear.

Central Lung Cancers. These tumors arise in one of the major bronchi and therefore cause early obstruction with resulting collapse, bronchopneumonia, and bronchiectasis (Fig. 22–23). Frequently, the patient presents with fever and symptoms of pneumonia. Hemoptysis is common, the bleeding being either from the ulcerated tumor itself or, more often, from the inflamed, dilated bronchi beyond.

Diagnosis

Hemoptysis, recurrent or "unresolved" pneumonia, or a persistent shadow on the radiograph should always lead to thorough investigation, particularly if the patient is a smoker (Fig. 22–24). Sputum examination

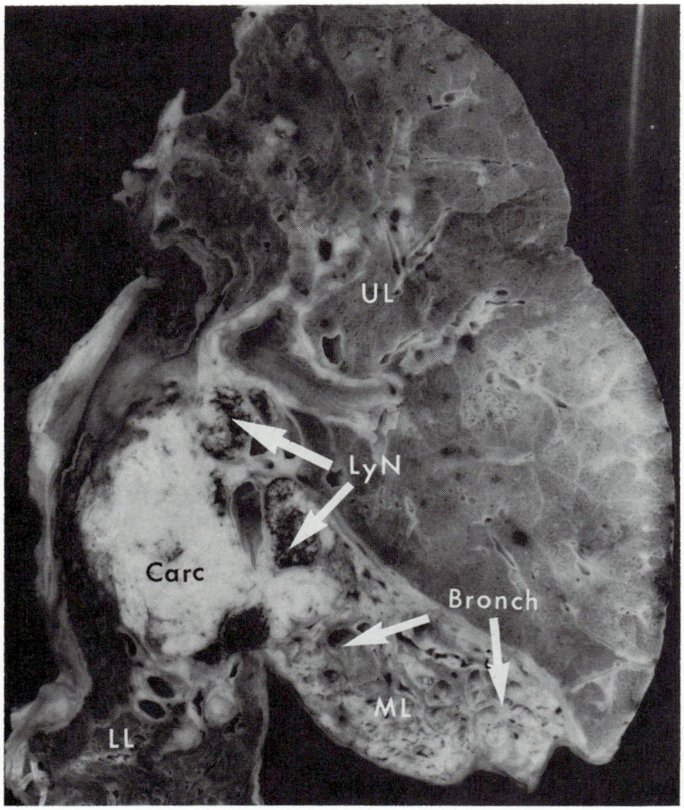

Figure 22–23 Carcinoma of the lung. This section through the lung shows a large carcinomatous mass (Carc) in which an obstructed bronchus is embedded. The main effect of this is seen in the middle lobe (ML), where much of the lung substance has been destroyed and replaced by fibrous tissue. Bronchiectasis (Bronch) is well developed. Tumor is seen to be extending into the lower lobe (LL), but the upper lobe (UL) is unaffected. Several hilar lymph nodes (LyN) are invaded by growth and have fused with the main tumor to form one large mass. The black material in the lymph nodes is carbon. This degree of anthracosis is common in city dwellers.

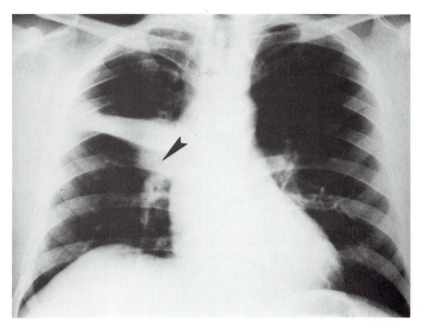

Figure 22–24 Carcinoma of the lung. This radiograph shows a hilar mass (arrow) that is produced by a tumor. The linear shadow extending outward toward the chest wall is due to secondary changes, namely, collapse, infection, and bronchiectasis. This portion of the lung might well appear like the middle lobe in Figure 22–23. (Courtesy of Dr. D. E. Sanders, Department of Radiology, Toronto General, Division of the Toronto Hospital, Toronto.)

may reveal malignant cells. The tumor may be seen and biopsied at the time of *bronchoscopy.* Even if the tumor is beyond the range of the bronchoscope, mucus or pus may be aspirated from individual bronchi. The finding of malignant cells in a specimen will then localize the tumor. *Mediastinoscopy* is a useful procedure in which the mediastinum is examined with an instrument that is inserted through a small incision in the neck. Enlarged lymph nodes may be detected and biopsied. This investigation also gives the surgeon an indication of whether the tumor is operable. If these investigations are negative, thoracotomy and direct biopsy may be necessary, since a policy of "wait and see" is rarely justifiable.

Spread

Lung cancer spreads by all the classic routes.

Local Spread. This can involve lung parenchyma, pleura, bronchi, arteries, and veins.

Lymphatic Spread. The hilar and mediastinal nodes can be involved. This usually occurs early and is most marked with the small-cell anaplastic tumors. Supraclavicular and other lymph nodes are involved as the disease progresses.

Blood-Borne Metastases. Secondary tumors are common in the *liver, bones, adrenals,* and *brain.* Even the spleen and bowel (organs not commonly the site of metastases from other tumors) may be involved. It is the frequency of distant spread that makes the prognosis so poor (Fig. 22–25).

Histologic Types

Although arising from a mucus-secreting epithelium, cancers of the lung are remarkable for their histologic variations.

Squamous-Cell Carcinoma. This resembles squamous-cell carcinoma arising elsewhere microscopically, except that well-differentiated examples are not common. The tumor arises from bronchial or bronchiolar epithelium. Before the development of invasive tumor, the epithelium shows increasing atypia (dysplasia), with the dysplastic cells taking on some features of keratinizing squamous cells. Ultimately the *in situ* carcinoma becomes invasive in a manner reminiscent of that encountered in the cervix uteri. These tumors may be either central or peripheral, and they have the most favorable prognosis.

Adenocarcinoma. These tumors are almost al-

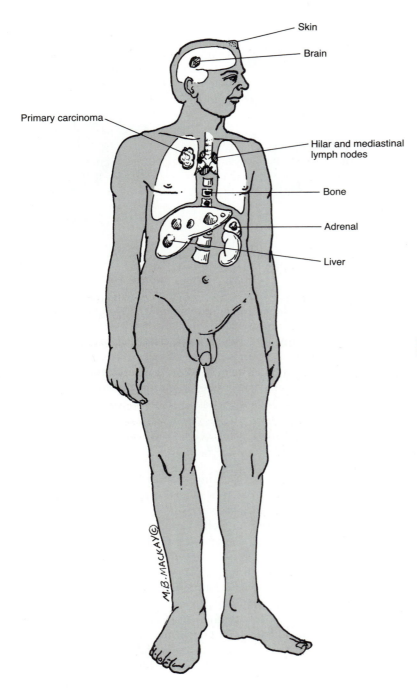

Skin

Brain

Primary carcinoma

Hilar and mediastinal
lymph nodes

Bone

Adrenal

Liver

**Figure 22–25 Common sites of metastases
in carcinoma of the lung.**

ways peripheral and tend to be more frequent in females. Areas of squamous metaplasia are common.

Anaplastic Carcinoma. These tumors show little or no differentiation; two variants are recognized.

Small-Cell, or Oat-Cell, Carcinoma. Small-cell carcinoma of the lung appears to be a distinct tumor, which is probably derived from neurosecretory cells of the bronchial mucosa. In this respect, it shares a common origin with the carcinoid tumor. The tumor is composed of small, darkly staining cells, which may form small rosettes and may be round or oat-shaped (Fig. 22–26). Frequently the tumors are large, and their origin is difficult to determine. They metastasize early and widely. An enormous mediastinal mass may be produced that can impede the heart's action by directly invading the pericardium and myocardium and by compressing the great vessels. Although the tumors are very radiosensitive, the prognosis is extremely bad.

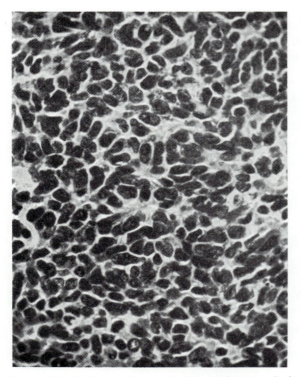

Figure 22–26 Small-cell anaplastic carcinoma of the lung. The tumor cells are small, are fusiform in shape, and have prominent, darkly staining nuclei. Their shape has given rise to the alternative name of oat-cell carcinoma (×500).

Paraneoplastic Syndromes

There are a number of characteristic syndromes associated with carcinoma of the lung. Some of these syndromes are due to the secretion by the tumor of hormones or hormone-like substances, *e.g.,* Cushing's syndrome (adrenocorticotropic hormone), hyponatremia (antidiuretic hormone), hypercalcemia (parathyroid hormone), hypocalcemia (calcitonin), and gynecomastia (gonadotropin). In other syndromes, the pathogenesis is not known. Clubbing of the fingers is common and, if combined with bone and joint changes (hypertrophic pulmonary osteoarthropathy), can closely mimic rheumatoid arthritis. Other syndromes include peripheral neuropathy, myopathy, dermatomyositis, and leukemoid reactions.

Prognosis

The symptoms of lung cancer are often vague, and by the time a diagnosis is made, the disease is so far advanced that only 20 to 30 per cent of cases are suitable for surgical resection. Even with these, only 10 per cent survive over 5 years. The prognosis is better with early squamous-cell carcinoma, but with small-cell carcinoma, the results are so poor that resection is usually contraindicated. With this disease, there is little doubt that prevention is easier than cure. Public appreciation of the dangers of smoking is slowly increasing, but the vested interests of governments and the tobacco industry continue to ensure that carcinoma of the lung and COPD will remain major problems well into the next century.

THE PLEURA

The pleural cavities are normally potential spaces situated between the visceral and parietal pleura, each lined by flattened mesothelial cells. An accumulation of fluid in the pleural space is termed a hydrothorax, or pleural effusion. There are two types, which are described in the following.

Transudate. The fluid has a low protein content and few cells. The common causes are congestive heart failure and the nephrotic syndrome.

Exudate. An exudate is formed as a result of inflammation or neoplastic involvement of the pleura. The protein content approximates that of plasma; inflammatory or neoplastic cells are present in the fluid.

Pleurisy

Inflammation of the pleura (pleurisy or pleuritis) is usually secondary to underlying inflammatory or neoplastic lung disease. This may be apparent, as in acute lobar pneumonia or in a large area of infarction, or it may be inapparent, as in the pleurisy that accompanies a small tuberculous lesion. Occasionally, the cause of pleurisy is to be found below the diaphragm, *e.g.,* a subphrenic abscess.

Fibrinous Pleurisy. "Dry pleurisy" is associated with an audible friction rub and can be extremely painful, particularly when the affected person takes a deep breath. Organization of the exudate leads to the formation of fibrous pleural adhesions.

Serous or Serofibrinous Pleurisy. "Pleurisy with effusion" can lead to the accumulation of so much fluid that the affected lung is collapsed. Persistent pleural effusion should always be adequately investigated. Fluid can be withdrawn through a needle and sent for bacteriologic and cytologic examination. Tuberculosis and carcinoma (primary or metastatic) are two causes that must be considered.

Empyema

The presence of pus in the pleural cavity is termed an empyema. It is generally formed as an extension of infection from a contiguous structure, *e.g.,* a lung abscess or subphrenic abscess (Fig. 22–27).

Pneumothorax

The presence of air in the pleural cavity is termed a pneumothorax. It may arise suddenly in an apparently healthy person (spontaneous pneumothorax), and it is usually due to rupture of a small subpleural emphysematous bulla. The onset is sudden, with severe pain in one side of

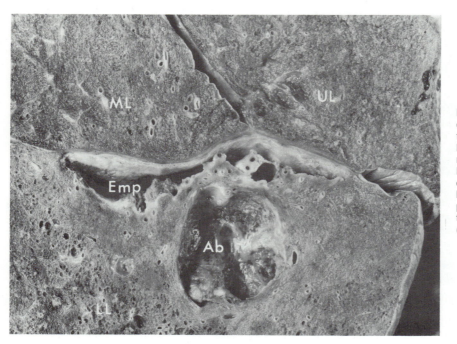

Figure 22–27 Empyema and chronic lung abscess. This section of lung shows the meeting point between the upper lobe (UL), the middle lobe (ML), and the lower lobe (LL). The lower lobe shows a chronic lung abscess (Ab); infection has evidently spread through the pleura, involving the pleural cavity to form a localized empyema (Emp).

the chest. Dyspnea and cyanosis follow, and their severity depends on the amount of air that escapes into the pleural cavity. The condition tends to recur.

Neoplasms of the Pleura

The common primary tumor of the pleura is the mesothelioma. Occasional benign examples are encountered, but the most common type is malignant. This *malignant mesothelioma,* which is related to asbestosis, forms an encasing mass around the lung.

Metastatic tumors, particularly from carcinoma of the lung and breast, are frequent in the pleura.

Summary

- Respiratory failure can result from ventilatory failure or impaired alveolar-arterial gas exchange.
- The lung has a variety of defense mechanisms. The mucociliary escalator and macrophages remove organisms, whereas IgA and other agents in mucus destroy them.
- Hyaline membrane disease is the most important cause of the respiratory distress syndrome.
- Pneumonia is of two main types. The type with exudation into the air sacs is invariably of bacterial origin; pneumonia with interstitial exudate (interstitial pneumonia or alveolitis) is often idiopathic or of viral origin.
- Lobar pneumonia generally affects one lobe and is pneumococcal; bronchopneumonia is usually bilateral and caused by bacteria of lesser virulence.
- Acute interstitial pneumonia or alveolitis with hyaline membrane formation has many causes; one of the most important and severe examples follows severe trauma and is called the adult respiratory distress syndrome.
- The primary lesions of tuberculosis, cryptococcosis, histoplasmosis, coccidioidomycosis, and North American blastomycosis are generally in the lung.
- Sarcoidosis is a noncaseating granulomatous disease of unknown cause that affects many organs, commonly the lung, skin, and eye.
- Chronic obstructive pulmonary disease (COPD) comprises chronic bronchitis, emphysema, and small airways disease.
- Chronic bronchitis is characterized by excess sputum production; the most important cause is cigarette smoking.
- Pulmonary emphysema can be centriacinar or panacinar. Upset in the elastase-antielastase balance is an important pathogenetic mechanism.
- Bronchial asthma can be extrinsic or intrinsic. It is related to type I hypersensitivity and contrasts with extrinsic allergic lung disease, such as farmer's lung, which is a type III reaction.
- Widespread pulmonary edema is commonly due to redistribution of blood volume and occurs in heart failure, overloading of the circulation, and cerebral damage.
- Sudden infant death syndrome occurs in infants under the age of 1 year. The cause is unknown.
- In bronchiectasis, the bronchi are permanently dilated. Pulmonary collapse, chronic interstitial pneumonia, and bronchopneumonia with fibrosis are common causes.
- The pneumoconioses are caused by the inhalation of dust. Silicosis, which causes extensive fibrosis, is the most important; it also predisposes to tuberculosis. Mesothelioma of the pleura is a complication of asbestosis.
- Carcinoma of the lung is the most common lethal type of cancer in many populations. Cigarette smoking is the major cause. The prognosis depends on the stage of the tumor and its histologic type, with squamous-cell carcinoma having the best prognosis, small-cell carcinoma the worst. Paraneoplastic syndromes are common. Widespread metastases—lymph nodes, liver, brain, and bone—are the rule.
- Bronchial carcinoid tumor is of intermediate malignancy.

Selected Readings

Barnes, P. J.: Pathogenesis of asthma: A review. J. R. Soc. Med. 76:593, 1982.

Crystal, R. G., Bitterman, P. B., Rennard, S. I., et al.: Interstitial lung disease of unknown origin: Disorders characterized by chronic inflammation of the lower respiratory tract. N. Engl. J. Med. 310:154 and 235, 1985.

Edelstein, P. H., et al.: Legionnaires' disease: A review. Chest 85:114, 1984.

Fletcher, C. M., and Pride, N. B.: Definition of emphysema, chronic bronchitis, asthma and airflow obstruction: 25 years on from the Ciba Symposium. Thorax 39:81, 1984.

Kelly, D. H., and Shannon, D. C.: Sudden infant death syndrome and near sudden infant death syndrome: A review of the literature, 1964 to 1982. Pediatr. Clin. North Am. 29:1241, 1982.

Kerdel, F. A., and Moschella, S. L.: Sarcoidosis. An updated review. J. Am. Acad. Dermatol. 11:1, 1984.

Leading article: Adult respiratory distress syndrome. Lancet 1:301, 1986.

McGowan, S. E., and Hunninghake, G. W.: Neutrophils and emphysema. N. Engl. J. Med. 321:968, 1989.

Milner, A. D., and Ruggins, N.: Sudden infant death syndrome. Br. Med. J. 298:689, 1989.

Mossman, B. T., and Gee, J. B. L.: Asbestos-related diseases. N. Engl. J. Med. 320:1721, 1989.

Rinaldo, J. E., and Rogers, R. M.: Adult respiratory-distress syndrome. N. Engl. J. Med. 315:579, 1986.

Spencer, H.: Pathology of the Lung. 4th ed. Vols. 1 and 2. New York, Pergamon Press, 1985.

Thurlbeck, W. M.: The pathobiology and epidemiology of human emphysema. J. Toxicol. Environ. Health 13:323, 1984.

Thurlbeck, W. M. (ed.): Pathology of the Lung. New York, Thieme Medical Publishers, 1988.

23

Alimentary Tract

**After studying this chapter, the student
should be able to:**
• Describe the mechanism of swallowing.
• Define dysphagia, classify its causes, and give a
  brief account of each.

418

- List the causes of ulceration in the mouth and describe aphthous ulceration in detail.
- Describe the types of white lesions (leukoplakia) sometimes found in the mouth.
- State the clinical features, differential diagnosis, and complications of acute streptococcal sore throat.
- Compare and contrast carcinoma of the lips, carcinoma of the tongue, and carcinoma of the pharynx.
- Describe the pathogenesis and complications of dental caries.
- Give an account of the pathogenesis and complications of periodontitis.
- Describe the types and complications of hiatus hernia.
- Outline the main features of carcinoma of the esophagus with respect to the following:
  (a) known predisposing causes;
  (b) site of occurrence;
  (c) symptoms;
  (d) prognosis.
- Give two examples of acute sialoadenitis.
- Describe the main features of pleomorphic salivary gland tumors.
- List the factors that stimulate the secretion of gastric juice.
- Describe chronic peptic ulceration with respect to symptoms, site of occurrence, pathogenesis, and complications.
- Give an account of acute gastroduodenal ulcers and their complications.
- Describe carcinoma of the stomach and indicate its prognosis.
- List the complications of partial or complete gastrectomy and indicate how each is brought about.
- Classify the mechanisms involved in the production of diarrhea.
- List the causes of acute gastroenterocolitis.
- Describe the effects of infection with
  (a) *Escherichia coli*;
  (b) *Vibrio cholerae*;
  (c) Salmonella;
  (d) Shigella.
- Describe the manifestations of ischemic bowel disease.

- Describe the lesions and complications of Crohn's disease.
- List the features of the carcinoid syndrome.
- Classify the causes and effects of the malabsorption syndrome.
- Describe the lesions, effects, and complications of
  (a) idiopathic ulcerative colitis;
  (b) diverticular disease of the colon;
  (c) ischemic colitis.
- Outline the incidence and pathologic effects of carcinoma of the colon.
- Describe acute appendicitis with respect to incidence, pathologic findings, clinical features, and complications.
- Outline the causes of peritonitis.
- Distinguish a volvulus from an intussusception.
- List the common sites for a hernia and describe the complications.
- Distinguish between the mechanical and the nonmechanical types of intestinal obstruction. Describe the main causes and effects of each.
- Outline the common causes of an "acute abdomen."

The alimentary tract is usually regarded as being within the body, but it is, in fact, a long tube exposed at each end to the exterior. Its contents, ranging from food in the mouth to feces in the rectum, are never within the body proper. This is an ideal arrangement because within the lumen, the chemical changes necessary for the digestion of food can occur under conditions that could not be tolerated inside the body itself. One effect of this arrangement is that many liters of digestive fluids are poured into the alimentary tract each day. Most of this is reabsorbed, but it can readily be appreciated that if much escapes to the exterior, the volume of fluid lost could reach alarming proportions. Diarrhea and vomiting are indeed potent causes of water and electrolyte loss.

The Mouth and Pharynx

In the mouth, food is masticated and mixed with saliva. By virtue of its mucus content, saliva performs a lubricating action in addition to initiating carbohydrate digestion by the enzyme ptyalin.

Swallowing (*deglutition*) is triggered by the vol-untary contraction of the pharyngeal and buccal muscles. By raising the larynx and tongue, the process of swallowing throws the bolus of food against the posterior pharyngeal wall. Thereafter, an involuntary wave of peristalsis sweeps the bolus down the muscular eosophagus, and as the cardiac sphincter relaxes, the bolus enters the stomach. Difficulty in swallowing (*dysphagia*) is described later in this chapter.

The mucosa of the mouth is keratinized (like epidermis) over the hard palate and the attached gingiva. In these areas, it is adherent to the periosteum of the underlying bone to form a *mucoperiosteum*. Elsewhere, the mucosa is mobile, and the epithelium is not keratinized, for it lacks the outer horny layer. This distinction is important in explaining the distribution of herpetic and aphthous ulcers in the mouth (see later).

LESIONS OF THE ORAL MUCOSA

The oral mucosa shares many diseases with the skin. In *lichen planus** a white lacy appearance of the buccal mucosa is characteristic and may be the first or, indeed, the only manifestation of the disease. Likewise, *pemphigus vulgaris* may first appear in the mouth. Bullous pemphigoid also affects the mouth, but less frequently than does pemphigus. The severe ulcerations of the oral mucous membranes seen in the *Stevens-Johnson syndrome* are described in Chapter 31.

The rash of some acute systemic *viral infections* affects the mucosa, where it is called the *enanthem*, before becoming clinically apparent on the skin, where it is called the *exanthem*. Thus, the vesicles of chickenpox may first appear on the palate. The *Koplik's spots* of measles, which occur during the prodromal stage of the disease, are reliable forerunners of the skin rash that appears within a day or two. Koplik's spots are minute white ulcers with an erythematous base and can be described as resembling small grains of salt, each having a red halo.

The primary infection with herpes simplex virus can occur in the mouth, particularly in children. There is acute inflammation of the oral mucosa (including the hard palate) and the gingivae. This acute *gingivostomatitis* is vesicular, but the blisters soon ulcerate, and the disease is characterized by multiple shallow and painful ulcers. The patient feels unwell and may have a

---

*Lichen planus is a generalized papulosquamous skin disease of unknown cause. The characteristic lesions are flat-topped, violaceous papules, which are extremely itchy.

fever. Healing occurs within about 2 weeks, and recurrent oral ulceration is not a complication (Chapter 9).

The common *aphthous ulcers*, or canker sores, are not due to a viral infection. They have been estimated to affect between 20 and 50 per cent of the population and are invariably recurrent. Sometimes a single ulcer is present, but often several appear either at the same time or shortly after one another. The ulcers affect the mobile oral mucosa (*i.e.*, tongue and inside of lips and cheeks) but not the hard palate or attached gingivae, where the epithelium is keratinized. They are very painful, shallow ulcers covered by necrotic slough and are surrounded by a bright erythematous zone. Healing generally occurs within a week or two, but in a few patients, the lesions enlarge and persist. These may be accompanied by similar ulcerations of the genital mucosa and by recurrent uveitis (*Behçet's syndrome*). It is evident that an examination of the oral cavity can provide essential clues in the diagnosis of other diseases; such a procedure should never be neglected.

Leukoplakia

This term is applied by some authorities to any white patch of the oral mucosa. It includes the following entities.

Simple Keratoses. Keratinization of the mobile mucosa or hyperkeratosis of the hard palate or attached gingivae is generally due to the irritation of smoking or chronic trauma, such as that produced by persistent biting of the buccal mucosa or by the rubbing of an ill-fitting denture. The oral epithelium closely resembles the epidermis of skin microscopically. A lesion of this type is not precancerous.

Lichen Planus. The lesions of lichen planus show some tendency to become malignant, but this is less of a threat than with dysplastic leukoplakia.

Dysplasia of the Oral Epithelium. The lesions appear as white patches that microscopically show dysplasia, either mild or sufficiently severe to warrant the term carcinoma in situ. It is this type of "leukoplakia" that is premalignant and must be regarded seriously. Obviously, any persistent white patch of the oral mucosa should be biopsied to determine its nature and malignant potentiality.

Acute Streptococcal Sore Throat

This is an acute infection of the tonsils and adjacent pharynx by *Streptococcus pyogenes*. The onset is sudden, and the sore throat is accompanied by fever, leukocytosis, and malaise. The tonsils and adjacent pharynx are swollen and red, and a white inflammatory exudate is seen on the surface. The regional lymph nodes are enlarged and tender (*acute nonsuppurative lymphadenitis*). If the strain of streptococcus produces abundant erythrogenic exotoxin, and if the patient has no immunity to this toxin, the sore throat is shortly followed by an erythematous skin rash. At that stage, the disease is called *scarlet fever*.

Streptococcal sore throat is an important disease because in a number of patients it is followed by *acute glomerulonephritis* or *acute rheumatic fever*, conditions that are considered elsewhere in this book.

It should not be assumed that every sore throat, even if accompanied by tonsillar exudate, is due to the streptococcus. Viral infections, for instance those caused by adenovirus or the Estein-Barr virus (of infectious mononucleosis) can have a very similar clinical appearance, although their onset is generally more insidious. In the past, it was essential to consider diphtheria in the differential diagnosis; now, however, the disease is extremely uncommon in the Western world. The diagnosis of diphteria is confirmed by obtaining a positive culture from a throat swab. Likewise, the diagnosis of acute gonorrheal pharyngitis is confirmed by culture.

Neoplasms

Benign tumors (*e.g.*, papilloma and fibroma) of the oral cavity are not uncommon; they are usually small and unimportant and are not considered further. The important tumor is carcinoma, which varies in character according to its site of origin.

Carcinoma of the Lips. Squamous-cell carcinoma of the lips nearly always affects the lower lip and is more common in men than in women. Predisposing causes are pipe and cigarette smoking, often combined with exposure to sunlight. The tumor usually starts as a nonhealing crack in the lower lip to one side of the midline. Provided treatment is undertaken reasonably early, the prognosis for this tumor is good because the growth is well differentiated and lymph node metastases are late in appearing (see Fig. 12–6).

Carcinoma of the Tongue. This is the most frequent intraoral malignant tumor. Although it is more common in men, the tumor also affects women, particularly in association with the Plummer-Vinson syndrome, described later in this chapter. Cancer of the tongue appears as a nodule that soon ulcerates. Any nonhealing ulcer of the tongue, particularly if its edges are indurated, must be biopsied. Even with early treatment, cancer of the tongue has a less favorable prognosis than does cancer of the lips. Approximately 60 per cent of patients live for 5 years after surgery or radiotherapy. If lymph node metastases are already present, the figure is reduced to about 30 per cent.

Squamous-cell carcinoma can occur in other parts of the mouth and oral pharynx. The floor of the mouth is a common site, and it is therefore very important that this area be inspected when a routine examination is carried out. Too often the dorsal surface of the tongue is scrutinized with care, but the carcinoma in the floor of the mouth goes unnoticed. Squamous-cell carcinoma of the pharynx is often poorly differentiated and highly malignant. Even though the primary tumor is quite small, the lesion first manifests itself as enlargement of cervical lymph nodes due to metastasis. The prognosis is poor.

THE TEETH

Caries

Dental caries, commonly known as tooth decay or "cavities," is the most common affliction of mankind. Although it has been recognized since prehistoric times, the precise cause is not known.

It is principally a disease of childhood, adolescence, and young adult life, affecting deciduous and permanent teeth alike. Tooth decay is particularly frequent in the Western world, where it is presumed to be due to dietary factors. Poor oral hygiene and a diet containing much refined carbohydrate appear to be the major factors.

Caries usually starts in pits, fissures, and other areas, such as the cervical parts of the tooth that are not self-cleansing. Bacterial colonies growing on the tooth surface (and forming *dental plaque*) combine with food debris to form a suitable focus for further bacterial growth. Organisms enter the small fissures in the enamel of the teeth and ferment the carbohydrate, leading to the production of acid. This process steadily erodes the calcific material of the enamel and later of the dentine so that a deep cavity appears; this cavity is often much larger than would be suspected from an examination of the external appearance of the fissure. When a cavity has formed, infection can spread to involve the pulp (*pulpitis*). Pulpitis can be acute and extremely painful; chronic pulpitis, on the other hand, can lead to the formation of a chronic apical abcess that is often remarkably silent clinically. It is believed that the abscess can act as a focus (or *nidus*) of infection and can lead to periodic episodes of bacteremia. This mechanism is an important factor in the pathogenesis of bacterial endocarditis.

Although dental caries appears to be related to infection, no one particular organism has been incriminated, since the bacteria that have been isolated from lesions are those constituting the normal flora of the mouth.

Periodontitis

Inflammation of the periodontium (*periodontitis*) is a widespread disease affecting many children and almost the total adult world population. It causes halitosis and is second to caries as a cause of tooth loss. A knowledge of the normal anatomy of the periodontium is essential for a proper understanding of the disease (Figs. 23–1 to 23–3).

Unless meticulous dental hygiene is practiced, colonies of bacteria become attached to the surface of the teeth and form *dental plaque*. If this is allowed to remain, it calcifies to form *dental calculus* ("tartar"). Food debris, plaque, and calculus in the region of the gingival crevice predispose the gingiva to inflammation. This *gingivitis* is the first stage in the pathogenesis of periodontitis. With this condition, the gingivae become red and swollen and tend to bleed, particularly after the teeth have been brushed. The inflammation leads to resorption of the alveolar bone (Figs. 23–3C, 23–4, and 23–5). The fibers of the periodontal membrane are also destroyed. Although the precise mechanism of this destruction is not understood, the process does lead to the formation of a pocket between the gingiva and the cementum of the tooth. Further accumulation of calculus and debris helps perpetuate the inflammation, and the pocket deepens. At the same time, gingival epithelium migrates into the pocket, and the process extends as more and more of the alveolar bone is destroyed. The teeth become loose and rock, even when they are subjected to normal forces during eating. The excessive movement further damages the attachments that remain, and loss of the teeth—one by one—is merely a matter of time.

THE ESOPHAGUS

The esophagus, or gullet, is a muscular tube through which food is propelled to the stomach by peristalsis. Although there is some debate about the existence of an anatomic sphincter at its lower end (the cardiac sphincter), from a functional point of view there is little doubt that a working sphincter exists, because the contents of the stomach do not readily re-enter the esophagus. This phenomenon can be attested to by witnessing the gyrations of the acrobat and by noting that the bat (which has a structurally similar esophagus) can spend half its life upside down with no ill effect.

Esophageal Webs

Folds or webs of the esophageal mucosa are quite frequently demonstrated by radiologists, but their significance as a cause of dysphagia is debatable. Often the lesions cannot be detected

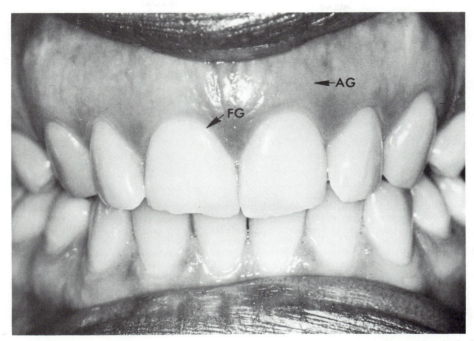

Figure 23–1 Normal gingiva. This photograph of the anterior part of the mouth shows a normal, healthy gingival condition. The free gingiva (FG) is not attached to the underlying enamel but is separated from it by the gingival crevice. The attached gingiva (AG) is firmly adherent to the underlying alveolar bone. (Courtesy of H.D. Glenwright, M.D.S., and the Department of Clinical Illustration, University of Birmingham, Birmingham, England.)

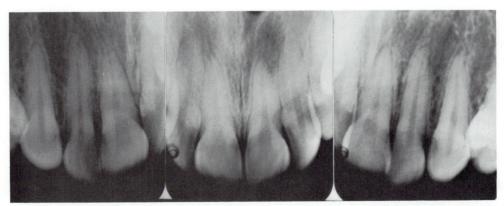

Figure 23–2 Radiograph of a normal mouth. Note how the teeth are deeply embedded in their bony sockets. (Courtesy of H.D. Glenwright, M.D.S., and the Department of Clinical Illustration, University of Birmingham, Birmingham, England.)

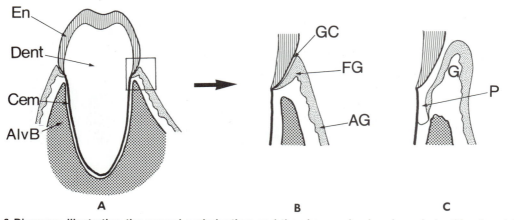

Figure 23–3 Diagrams illustrating the normal periodontium and the changes in chronic periodontitis. *A* and *B* illustrate the normal periodontium, which consists of (1) alveolar bone (AlvB); (2) cementum (Cem); (3) the periodontal membrane, consisting of fibers running between bone and cementum; and (4) the gingiva, including the free gingiva (FG) and the attached gingiva (AG). The gingival crevice (GC) is the space between the free gingiva and the enamel of the tooth (En); Dent, dentine *C*, the changes in chronic periodontitis. There is loss of alveolar bone and the associated periodontal membrane. Extension of the gingival crevice has resulted in the formation of a pocket (P), and this is partially lined by gingival epithelium that has grown in. The gingiva (G) is swollen and inflamed.

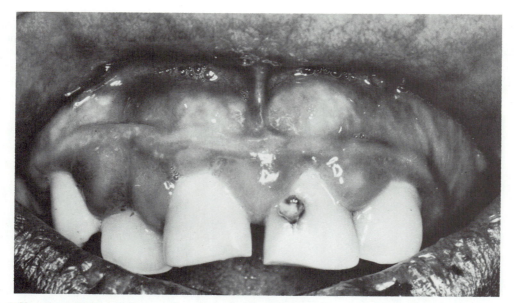

Figure 23–4 Chronic periodontal disease. The gingiva is inflamed, is swollen, and has lost its normal granular surface. The changes are most marked between the teeth. Deep pockets are present. This can be demonstrated clinically by passing a probe between the gingivae and the roots of the teeth. One tooth is obviously carious. (Courtesy of H.D. Glenwright, M.D.S., and the Department of Clinical Illustration, University of Birmingham, Birmingham, England.)

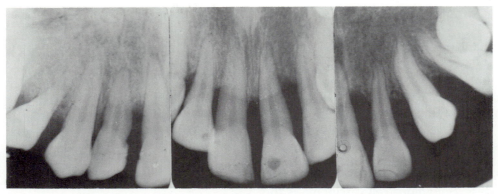

Figure 23–5 Chronic periodontal disease. This radiograph shows marked resorption of the alveolar bone. Some teeth have lost most of their bony support and are loose. They will be shed shortly. (Courtesy of H.D. Glenwright, M.D.S., and the Department of Clinical Illustration, University of Birmingham, Birmingham, England.)

at necropsy. Webs of the upper part of the esophagus are found in the *Plummer-Vinson syndrome*, in which there is the triad of *iron deficiency anemia, dysphagia*, and atrophy of the mucosa covering the tongue (*atrophic glossitis*). The disease is virtually confined to women and is associated with an increased incidence of carcinoma of the oral cavity and upper esophagus.

Hiatus Hernia

The two types of hiatus hernia are illustrated in Figure 23–6. Impaired function of the cardiac sphincter leads to regurgitation of gastric contents; in turn, this leads to an associated esophagitis and peptic ulceration of the lower esopha-

gus. The fibrosis that is associated with the healing of these ulcers can culminate in the formation of a benign stricture.

Esophagitis

Inflammation of the lower esophagus can be due to regurgitation of gastric contents, which causes pain (heartburn). Esophagitis can result from the ingestion of irritating foods, such as hot, spicy meals and strong alcoholic beverages. The deliberate or accidental ingestion of corrosive acids and alkalies (*e.g.*, lye) can lead to severe esophagitis. If the patient survives, marked fibrosis with cicatrization results in an incapacitating stenosis.

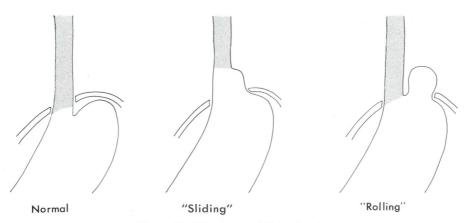

Normal   "Sliding"   "Rolling"

Figure 23–6 The types of hiatus hernia.

Esophageal Varices

An important cause of hematemesis, esophageal varices, is described in Chapter 24.

Neoplasms of the Esophagus

The most important tumor of the esophagus is carcinoma. It is more frequent in males and in those who smoke excessively or who ingest alcohol to excess. Squamous-cell carcinoma is the most common type and generally arises in the lower or middle third of the esophagus. Adenocarcinoma can occur at the lower end of the esophagus and is thought to originate from either esophageal mucous glands or areas of ectopic gastric epithelium. The tumor steadily obstructs the esophagus, causing the patient to experience increasing difficulty in swallowing—at first of solid foods and later of liquids. The onset is insidious; although the tumor tends to invade locally and to metastasize late, by the time the diagnosis has been achieved, resection is difficult because the stomach must be brought up into the chest and anastomosed with the upper esophagus or pharynx, or alternatively a new passage must be reconstructed using a portion of colon or a tube of skin. Often resection of the cancer is impossible. Hence, the prognosis for this tumor is poor. The end stages of this disease are particularly unpleasant because the patient is unable to swallow anything, including saliva. Constant regurgitation from the mouth, inhalation of saliva and food, and starvation combine to terminate the illness. Bronchopneumonia generally intervenes and leads to the patient's death.

Dysphagia

Dysphagia, meaning difficulty in swallowing, is often associated with pain and regurgitation of food. If this causes an inadequate food intake, severe weight loss can occur. The causes of dysphagia, of which there are many, can be considered under three headings, depending on whether the lesion affects predominantly the oropharyngeal mechanism, esophageal peristal-sis, or the lower esophageal sphincter mechanism.

Oropharyngeal Dysphagia

In oropharyngeal dysphagia, there is difficulty in forming the bolus of food in the oral cavity and propelling it from that cavity into the cervical esophagus. It can be caused by painful conditions of the mouth (*e.g.*, acute tonsillitis) or disorders affecting the voluntary muscles of the mouth (*e.g.*, amyloid infiltration of the tongue, or carcinoma), but the common cause is a disorder of the upper esophageal sphincter and the upper intrinsic circular muscle of the esophagus, which fails to relax either at all or in coordination with pharyngeal contraction. Causes include disorders of the central nervous system, of the peripheral nerves, or of the muscles themselves. Local structural abnormalities causing oropharyngeal dysphagia include retropharyngeal abscesses, carcinoma, local scarring, and the Plummer-Vinson syndrome in which esophageal webs may be present.

Aspirated material causes coughing and nasal regurgitation of food after attempts to swallow, particularly liquids. Repeated attacks of pulmonary infection are common and followed by fibrosis.

Dysphagia Due to Disorders of Esophageal Peristalsis

Carcinoma is the serious structural cause of dysphagia. A benign tumor, stricture, and pressure from without (*e.g.* an aortic aneurysm) are occasional causes. Functional motor disturbances leading to dysphagia include the following conditions.

Achalasia of the Cardia. This condition is characterized by degeneration of the ganglion cells of the lower esophagus, which results in disturbed peristalsis and a failure of relaxation of the cardiac sphincter. The patients are generally middle-aged and experience a sensation of food sticking at the level of the lower end of the sternum. Carcinoma of the esophagus develops in about 5 to 10 per cent of patients. A condition very similar to achalasia occurs in Chagas' disease, a form of trypanosomiasis, in which other organs can also be affected (*e.g.*, the heart).

Symptomatic, Idiopathic Esophageal Spasm. This condition usually occurs over the age of 50 years and is characterized by colic that produces substernal pain severe enough to make clinical diagnosis from myocardial infarction difficult. The pain may be precipitated by emotional stress, by the ingestion of hot or cold fluids, or by reflux.

Disordered peristalsis may also occur in diseases of the central nervous system, the peripheral nerves, and the muscles themselves. Fibrosis in systemic sclerosis is an occasional cause.

Disorders of the Lower Esophageal Sphincter Mechanism

In normal individuals, particularly in childhood and pregnancy, it is not uncommon for there to be some disorder of the functional lower esophageal sphincter such that there is a mild degree of gastroesophageal reflux. Reflux is also associated with hiatus hernia.

THE SALIVARY GLANDS

The three pairs of major salivary glands (parotid, submaxillary, and sublingual) can be afflicted by many diseases. With the exception of certain inflammations and one tumor, however, they are uncommon.

Inflammation (Sialoadenitis)

Mumps. A painful swelling at the angle of the jaw is often the first indication of *mumps*, which is due to inflammation of the parotid gland (*acute nonsuppurative parotitis*). The disease is caused by a myxovirus, has a long incubation period (18 to 21 days), and becomes bilateral in about two thirds of cases. Fever and mild malaise accompany the parotitis, and resolution occurs within 1 week. The most common complication of the disease in adult men is an acute orchitis (Chapter 26). Acute pancreatitis, meningitis, and encephalitis are occasionally encountered.

Acute Suppurative Sialoadenitis. This condition is characterized by sudden swelling of the parotid gland, followed by abscess formation. Such an inflammation is encountered in patients who are either dehydrated or in shock and whose level of consciousness is decreased. Poor oral hygiene and a decreased flow of saliva combine to aid the migration of bacteria from the mouth, up the excretory duct, and finally to the parotid gland. It is to prevent this complication that careful cleansing of the mouth is an important component of the nursing care of severely ill patients.

Chronic Sialoadenitis. Recurrent attacks of acute sialoadenitis and chronic inflammation are generally encountered in a submaxillary gland and often related to obstruction of the duct by a stone (sialolithiasis).

Sjögren's Syndrome. Sjögren's syndrome consists of the combination of dry mouth (xerostomia), dry eyes (keratoconjunctivitis sicca), and chronic arthritis. It is predominantly a disease of women over the age of 40 years. Hypergammaglobulinemia and numerous autoantibodies are usually present in the blood, and the syndrome is sometimes associated with systemic lupus erythematosus or other collagen vascular disease.

Neoplasms of the Salivary Glands

The most common tumors of the salivary glands are of epithelial origin, and although any of the salivary glands can be involved, the parotid is the most commonly affected.

Pleomorphic Adenoma. The common tumor of the salivary gland is a pleomorphic tumor of the parotid. This tumor grows slowly to produce a painless mass in front of the external ear. On microscopic examination, it consists of two elements. There are obvious epithelial components showing glandular differentiation with tubule formation (Fig. 23–7). Also, there are less cellular areas consisting of scattered cells with a background of material that may resemble extravasated mucus, myxomatous tissue (*myxoid areas*), or hyaline cartilage matrix (*chondroid areas*). On the supposition that the myxoid or cartilaginous

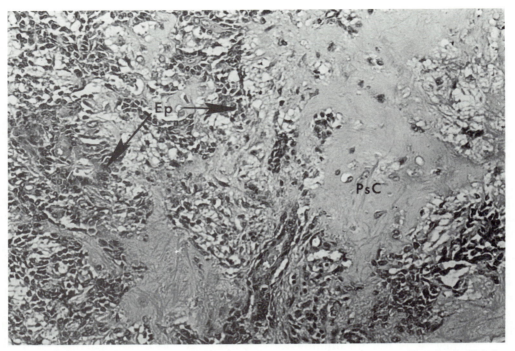

Figure 23–7 Pleomorphic salivary gland tumor. The tumor shows many clumps of obvious epithelial cells (Ep). In some areas, mucin has accumulated in the stroma to produce a pseudocartilaginous appearance (PsC) (×300).

areas are of connective tissue (mesenchymal) origin, the tumor has been called a "mixed parotid tumor," since it appears to contain epithelial and connective tissue neoplastic elements. The current belief is that the tumor is purely epithelial, with the secreting epithelial cells producing the glandular elements of the tumor, and the myoepithelial cells* forming the myxoid or pseudocartilaginous areas. Pleomorphic adenoma is the current name for the tumor, but "mixed salivary gland tumor" is commonly used in conversation.

Although the tumor may appear to be encapsulated, small outgrowths are present. It is from these that growth recurs after a simple enucleation of the tumor. The current treatment is to excise not only the tumor but also the surrounding parotid gland. The recurrence rate is low, and the prognosis is good. Unfortunately, the

facial nerve travels through this gland, and damage to the nerve sometimes follows.

Pleomorphic salivary gland adenoma is regarded as a benign tumor, although occasional examples show local invasion and even metastasis indicating a tumor of intermediate malignancy. On the other hand, if the tumor suddenly enlarges, invades locally, and metastasizes, an obvious adenocarcinoma is found to have arisen within the adenoma.

Pleomorphic tumors occur in the other salivary glands but are much less common than those in the parotid gland.

Warthin's Tumor. This benign tumor is also known as adenolymphoma or papillary cystadenoma lymphomatosum. It constitutes about 10 per cent of all parotid tumors. On microscopic examination, it is a well-differentiated tumor with glandular spaces, many of which contain papillary projections. An outstanding feature is an abundant lymphoid stroma that includes germinal centers—from this characteristic it derives its curious name.

---

*Many glands have two epithelial components. The inner secreting cells are either cubical or columnar, in contrast to the outer flattened myoepithelial cells, which by their contraction help express secretions from the gland.

The Stomach

In the stomach, the masticated food is softened, moistened, lubricated, and partially digested by the gastric juice. The food is kneaded by strong muscular contractions into a semiliquid mass called *chyme*, which passes steadily into the duodenum. The gastric juice has four major active components: (1) *Mucus*, which has a lubricating action, (2) *Intrinsic factor*, which is necessary for the absorption of vitamin B_{12}, (3) *pepsin*, which commences protein digestion, and (4) *Hydrochloric acid*, which has an important bactericidal action and also provides the correct pH for the action of pepsin. Its presence is important in the pathogenesis of one of the common disabling human afflictions—peptic ulceration.

GASTRITIS

Acute Gastritis

Acute gastritis affecting the whole stomach is usually caused by some local irritant such as alcohol, heavy smoking, or ingestion of aspirin. It may be infective in origin and be a component of gastroenteritis.

Another type of acute gastritis accompanies severe shock and may therefore be a complication of burns and severe injury including major surgery. Focal ischemia due to vascular changes mediated by vagal activity has been postulated but never proved. This type of acute gastritis tends to affect one or more relatively discrete areas of the mucosa.

The mucosa in acute gastritis is inflamed, red, and swollen. If the changes are severe, hemorrhage, causing hematemesis and melena, can be severe. The condition is called *acute hemorrhagic gastritis* or *acute hemorrhagic erosive gastritis* if multiple gastric erosions are present. The term erosion is used if the gastric epithelium only is lost; if the whole mucosa is lost, the term ulcer is applied. Indeed, acute stress ulcers may also be present (see later).

Chronic Gastritis

The term chronic gastritis is best used to describe conditions in which the gastric mucosa shows histologic evidence of chronic inflammation. Two types are recognized.

Chronic Fundal Gastritis (Type A). Chronic fundal gastritis is present in pernicious anemia and is associated with autoantibodies against parietal cells and antibodies that prevent the absorption of vitamin B_{12}. The acid-secreting part of the stomach *i.e.,* the fundus and the body, are affected, and the gastric mucosal cells show cellular atypia. The condition is precancerous, and patients with severe changes have a tenfold chance of developing gastric cancer.

Chronic Antral Gastritis (Type B). As its name implies, this type of chronic gastritis affects the antrum and tends to spare the acid-producing areas. It may accompany chronic peptic ulceration; without convincing evidence, it has been attributed to chronic alcoholism, aspirin intake, and biliary reflux.

Acute Gastric Ulcers (Stress Ulcers)

Acute ulcers, commonly called erosions, may be caused by any of the factors noted as a cause of acute gastritis. In practice, acute stress is the usual cause. Acute stress ulcers involve any part of the stomach or first part of the duodenum (Fig. 23–8). They are round, are generally under 1 cm in diameter, and usually heal rapidly with minimal scarring. Occasionally an ulcer erodes a large vessel and gives rise to a severe hemorrhage. The ulcer may perforate into the peritoneal cavity, causing peritonitis.

CHRONIC PEPTIC ULCERS

Peptic ulceration occurs in any non–acid-secreting mucosa that comes into contact with gastric juice. Therefore, it is seen in the pyloric antrum of the stomach, along the lesser curvature of the stomach, in the first and second parts of

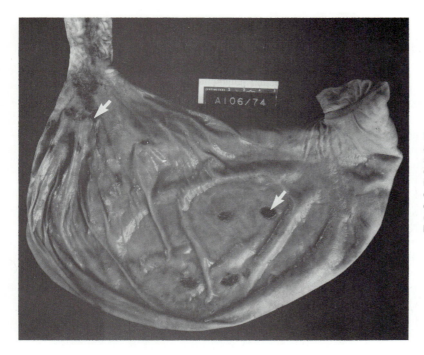

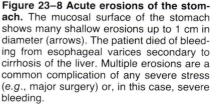

Figure 23–8 Acute erosions of the stomach. The mucosal surface of the stomach shows many shallow erosions up to 1 cm in diameter (arrows). The patient died of bleeding from esophageal varices secondary to cirrhosis of the liver. Multiple erosions are a common complication of any severe stress (*e.g.*, major surgery) or, in this case, severe bleeding.

the duodenum, at the lower end of the esophagus, and at the site of a gastroenterostomy (stomal ulcer). The duodenum is the most common site of peptic ulcer, but its incidence has declined over the last 50 years. Ulcers are more common in males than in females.

Chronic peptic ulcers are usually solitary and present a characteristic appearance (Fig. 23–9). Not only is the mucosa lost, but also the underlying muscle layers are often destroyed, thereby producing a deep round or oval, punched-out ulcer with straight edges. For reasons that are not yet known, regeneration of the mucosal epithelium is inhibited, and chronic inflammation ensues. The floor of the ulcer consists of inflamed vascular granulation tissue covered by necrotic material that forms a slough. Bleeding is common, therefore. Deeper in the base of the ulcer, the granulation tissue matures to form dense scar tissue that ultimately replaces the muscular walls.

Clinical Features. Pain in the epigastrium is common and is related to gastric acidity and muscle spasm. With a duodenal ulcer, the pain comes on 1½ to 3 hours after a meal and frequently is severe enough to awaken the patient at night. It is usually relieved by eating food or,

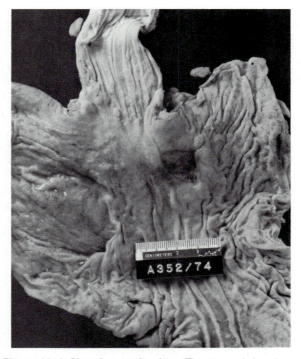

Figure 23–9 Chronic gastric ulcer. The stomach has been opened along its greater curvature to show the mucosal surface. There is a typical chronic peptic ulcer on the lesser curvature about 2 cm from the cardioesophageal junction. Note the folds of mucosa (rugae) that are normal.

in particular, by the administration of alkali. With gastric ulcers, the occurrence of pain is more erratic, and it may not be relieved by food or alkali. Indeed, eating may actually make the pain worse. It should be stressed that peptic ulceration can be present in the absence of any symptoms (see Case History I).

Case History I

The patient was a 65-year-old woman who was diagnosed as having a tumor involving the cerebellum and adjacent medulla oblongata. At surgery, complete removal of the tumor was not possible, but a biopsy was performed and showed an uncommon tumor called a hemangioendothelioma. The patient never fully regained consciousness and died 13 days later. There was a past history of duodenal ulcer, but details were not available because the patient was too ill to give a good history. At necropsy, a large perforated duodenal ulcer was found (see Fig. 23–10 and 23–11). This was associated with peritonitis and a subphrenic abscess. This case illustrates how trauma can precipitate the perforation of a peptic ulcer. In a seriously ill patient, the perforation can be silent, and a subphrenic abscess can develop and be missed clinically.

Complications

Hemorrhage. Repeated bleeding is a common cause of iron deficiency anemia. Sometimes the ulcer penetrates adjacent structures, particularly the pancreas, and a large artery is eroded. When this occurs, there is massive hematemesis and melena (altered blood in the feces, with the stool appearing black and tarry).

Penetration and Perforation. When the ulcer penetrates the peritoneal surface, it produces a localized fibrinous inflammation that may cause adjacent structures to adhere to it. In this way, a chronic duodenal ulcer may penetrate into the substance of the pancreas. If adhesions do not form, the ulcer may perforate, and the gastric or duodenal contents may then be poured into the peritoneal cavity (Figs. 23–10 and 23–11). The patient immediately experiences severe pain, and generalized peritonitis soon develops.

Cicatrization. As an ulcer heals, scar tissue tends to cicatrize and cause stenosis. Pyloric ulcers are particularly susceptible to this complication; the resulting *pyloric stenosis* causes per-

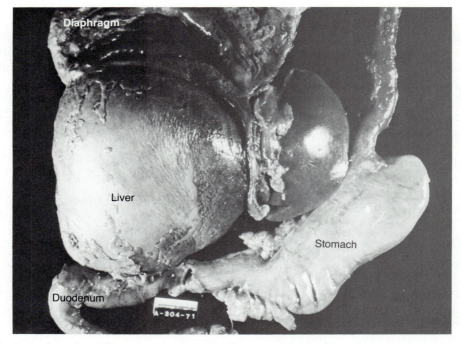

Figure 23–10 Perforated duodenal ulcer. A perforation of the first part of the duodenum is associated with adjacent peritonitis. The upper surface of the liver is coated by a purulent exudate. An accumulation of pus was found between the liver and the diaphragm, constituting a subphrenic abscess. See Case History I for clinical details. (Courtesy of Dr. J.B. Cullen, Toronto General Division of the Toronto Hospital, Toronto.)

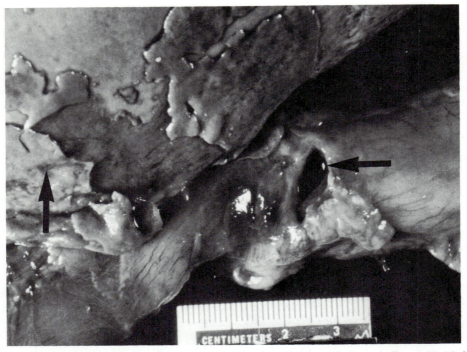

Figure 23–11 Perforated duodenal ulcer. This is a close-up of the ulcer (right arrow) shown in Figure 23–10. Note the loosely adherent purulent exudate on the surface of the liver (left arrow). (Courtesy of Dr. J.B. Cullen, Toronto General Division of the Toronto Hospital, Toronto).

sistent severe vomiting. This can lead to dehydration, starvation, and metabolic alkalosis resulting from loss of acid gastric juices.

Etiology and Pathogenesis. Although the pathogenesis of chronic peptic ulceration is poorly understood, it is evident that one essential factor is the presence of gastric juice containing hydrochloric acid and pepsin. Before the pathogenesis of this condition is studied, it is appropriate to review the mechanism involved in gastric secretion.

Acid gastric secretion is directly stimulated by four factors:

1. *Acetylcholine*, which is released at vagal nerve endings.

2. *Gastrin*, a group of polypeptide hormones produced in the antral pyloric glands. Local stimulating factors (such as digested protein in the gastric chyme) and vagal stimulation lead to gastrin release. A gastrinlike hormone is also released from the duodenum.

3. *Histamine*. The precise role of this powerful stimulant is not known, but it may be the final mediator for cholinergic and gastrin stimulation. The stimulating action of histamine on gastric secretion is due to the effect of the drug on H_2 receptors.

4. *Polypeptide hormones*, a variety of which are released from the small intestine. Some of these stimulate gastric secretion, but others inhibit.

Traditionally, three phases of gastric secretion are described:

1. *Cephalic phase.* The sight and taste of food stimulate gastric secretion. Emotions such as anger have a similar effect. Vagal overactivity is the probable mechanism.

2. *Gastric phase.* Distention of the stomach and an alkaline content are stimulating.

3. *Intestinal phase.* This is both stimulatory (*e.g.*, peptides in the duodenal lumen) and inhibitory (acid and fatty material in the intestinal lumen).

The non–acid-secreting mucosa, bathed in gastric juice, has a defense mechanism that prevents it from being digested and damaged. Two defenses have been proposed:

1. The covering layer of mucus forming a protective blanket. This is currently not regarded as being of great importance.

2. The *mucosal barrier* formed by the integrity of the epithelial cells and the tight junctions between adjacent cells. This provides a barrier to the diffusion of hydrogen ions from the lumen into the tissues.

The medical treatment of peptic ulcers has been based on efforts to inhibit gastric secretion of hydrochloric acid and pepsin. They include avoidance of worry by giving the patient mental and physical rest; use of antihistamine drugs, especially cimetidine, an H_2-blocking agent; use of anticholinergic drugs, which block the action of acetylcholine; frequent small meals to avoid gastric distention; and the administration of antacids, including milk.

These measures are often helpful, but it is evident from the many treatment failures that factors other than abnormal gastric secretion are involved in the pathogenesis of peptic ulcer.

Bile acids, tobacco products, ethanol, and other irritants may damage the mucosal barrier by a direct irritant effect. The administration of glucocorticoids (*e.g.*, prednisone) inhibits the mitotic rate of epithelial cells, and this may interrupt the replacement of cells normally shed from the surface. Aspirin and other nonsteroid analgesic drugs have a similar effect. Possibly infection with the fastidious organism *Campylobacter pyloridis* plays a part, but its role is unknown. However produced, a break in the mucosa exposes the submucosal tissues to the destructive effects of gastric juice.

That hypersecretion of gastric juice is not of overriding importance in the genesis of peptic ulceration is indicated by the observation that most patients with gastric ulcers have normal or even low gastric activity. It has been suggested, therefore, that an abnormality of the pyloric sphincter function is important. A sudden influx of alkaline, bile-containing duodenal contents could damage the non–acid-secreting pyloric mucosa. Once the mucosa is damaged, acid gastric juice could continue the destructive action. Likewise, it is possible that acid gastric contents could

suddenly be allowed to enter the duodenum and damage its mucosa. This is consistent with the observation that most patients with duodenal ulcers have high gastric acidity and a rapid gastric emptying time. Also, duodenal ulcers are usually confined to the first and second part of the organ proximal to the entrance of the pancreatic duct, from which pours alkaline bile and pancreatic secretion.

It must be admitted, therefore, that the precise etiology of peptic ulceration is not known, but it seems that mucosal damage and exposure to gastric juice can combine in some individuals and lead to chronic ulceration. What factors upset the balance between the mucosal defense on the one hand and the destructive actions of gastric juice on the other remain to be determined. Genetic factors play some role in this mechanism, for duodenal ulcers are most common in those of blood group O, whereas stomach ulcers (and also gastric carcinoma) are more common in those of blood group A.

Surgical Treatment. When medical treatment fails, a variety of surgical procedures may be practiced. These include sections of the vagi (vagotomy) and operations on the pylorus and antrum (pyloroplasty and antrectomy). Another procedure is partial gastrectomy with anastomosis of the remaining stomach to the jejunum. The results of surgical treatment are sometimes satisfactory, but a number of complications must be expected. Recurrent ulceration can occur and may involve the small intestine adjacent to the enterostomy (*stomal ulcer*).

Effects of Gastrectomy. The gastric juice is not essential for digestion, apart from the secretion of intrinsic factor and its vital role in the absorption of vitamin B_{12}. Nevertheless, even partial gastric resection leads to a degree of malabsorption, because the stomach provides a place of temporary arrest that allows food to be admitted into the intestine in a slow, controlled manner. After gastrectomy, there is more hurried passage of chyme through the intestine so that digestion is rendered less complete. Furthermore, the disinfectant activity of hydrochloric acid is lost, and the bacterial flora of the intestine is changed. This may be accentuated by various blind loops created by the surgeon. The overall effect of these changes is to impair digestion of protein and fat

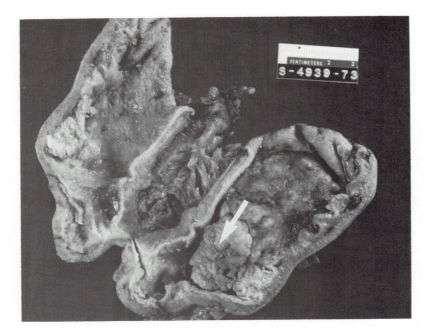

Figure 23–12 Carcinoma of the stomach. The stomach has been bisected, and both halves are shown. The wall is thickened, partly by tumor invasion and partly by muscular hypertrophy that the tumor has caused. The mucosa is obviously invaded, and a polypoid mass of growth is present (arrow). This is shown more clearly in Figure 23–13.

Figure 23–13 Carcinoma of the stomach. Note the cauliflower-like mass of tumor. This is the same case as depicted in Figure 23–12. On microscopic examinations, the tumor was a poorly differentiated adenocarcinoma.

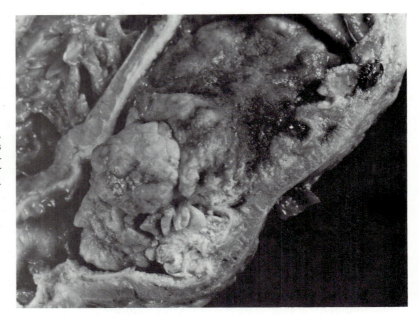

so that considerable weight loss can ensue. Furthermore, an iron deficiency anemia is common. Two specific effects of gastrectomy should also be noted.

The Dumping Syndrome. This occurs shortly after each meal; there is a feeling of epigastric distention and pain, accompanied by pallor, sweating, dizziness, and possibly collapse. The cause is thought to be related to the rapid entrance into the jejunum of the hypertonic chyme from the stomach. Fluid is drawn into the lumen of the bowel, and this leads to intestinal distention. Of greater importance is the passage of fluid into the intestinal lumen with a resultant sudden fall in plasma volume.

Hypoglycemic Attacks. These attacks occur 2½ to 3 hours after a meal and consist of sweating, tremor, tachycardia, and faintness. After a meal, there is rapid absorption of glucose from the bowel so that initially there is a high blood sugar level. This stimulates insulin secretion, which is of such magnitude that the initial hyperglycemia is followed by a phase of hypoglycemia. The symptoms of this syndrome are therefore similar to those of insulin overdose.

CARCINOMA OF THE STOMACH

Gastric carcinoma is not uncommon in northern European communities, but its incidence is now lower than that of colonic carcinoma. It is a common tumor in the Japanese, and in European communities it is more frequent in the lower social echelons than in the social elite. The tumor appears either as a fungating, cauliflower type of growth (Figs. 23–12 and 23–13) or as a typical malignant ulceration. In some instances, the tumor cells invade the stomach wall so diffusely that no definite mass exists. Instead, the entire stomach wall is diffusely thickened by tumor cells and by the dense fibrous stroma that develops in response to them. This formation is called a diffuse infiltrating carcinoma of the stomach, or *linitis plastica.*

The symptoms of carcinoma of the stomach are often vague; they include indigestion, pain not relieved by food or alkalis, and weight loss. Bleeding that causes an obscure anemia is common. Blood may be present in altered form in the vomitus ("coffee-ground vomit"), and melena may occur.

On histological examination, cancer of the stomach is a poorly differentiated adenocarcinoma. The prognosis is extremely poor, and even with early excision, few patients survive for more than 5 years. Metastasis is to the regional lymph nodes and by blood spread to the liver and elsewhere.

The Small Intestine

The small intestine consists of the duodenum, the jejunum, and the ileum and, in all, is about 6 meters long. The chyme that leaves the stomach is acted upon by bile, the pancreatic enzymes, and the intestinal secretion (*succus entericus*). The last contains few enzymes; the most important of these is *enterokinase*, which converts trypsinogen to trypsin, a conversion that is an essential step in the activation of pancreatic enzymes. The function of the small intestine is therefore the final breakdown of fat, carbohydrate, and protein as well as the absorption of the products formed. The complex structure of the mucosa with its numerous villi is well adapted to this function (Fig. 23–14A). Likewise, the microvilli of each luminal cell are designed for absorption of the products of digestion. The glycocalyx (see Fig. 2–4) is thought to contain enzymes, including the important disaccharidases. These are responsible for splitting disaccharides (*e.g.*, sucrose and lactose) into monosaccharides (*e.g.*, fructose and glucose); in this form, these sugars can be absorbed.

About 8 liters of fluid enters the duodenum each day, but only 1 to 1.5 liters leaves the ileum to enter the colon; 100 to 200 ml is passed in the feces. The driving force for the absorption of this large volume of water is mainly the osmotic

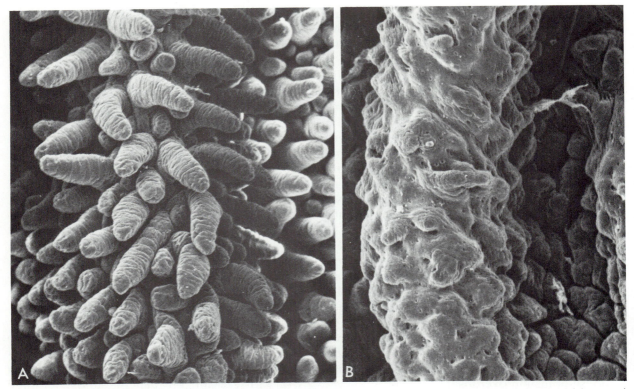

Figure 23–14 Scanning electron micrographs of small intestine. Both specimens are from the small intestine. *A* is normal and shows slender, fingerlike villi; compare this with Figure 2–2. *B* is from an animal infected with a transmissible gastroenteritis virus, which produces an illness similar to human rotavirus enteritis. Note that the mucosa is flattened owing to partial villous atrophy. The loss of villi is complete over the folds. Surface openings of crypts appear as pits on the irregular surface (×40). (Courtesy of Dr. E. Cutz, Hospital for Sick Children, Toronto. From Shepherd, R.W., Butler, D.G., Gall, D.G., and Hamilton, J.R.: The mucosal lesion in viral enteritis: extent and dynamics of the epithelial response to virus invasion in transmissible gastroenteritis of piglets. Gastroenterology, 76:770–777, 1979. Reprinted by Courtesy of Marcel Dekker Inc.)

pressure gradient that follows the active absorption of solutes (*i.e.*, the products of digestion of food). In particular, the absorption of glucose and amino acids induces a flow of water and sodium in the same direction. This is termed *solvent drag.* This phenomenon has been used to great advantage in the treatment of cholera. Even though there is a tremendous outpouring of fluid and electrolytes in the "rice water" stools of this disease, the administration of suitable solutions of glucose and electrolytes *by mouth* is effective treatment. Intravenous therapy is therefore not obligatory in the treatment of cholera, an observation that can save thousands of lives in the event of an epidemic involving an underprivileged area of the world in which intravenous equipment is not available on a mass scale

Electrolyte absorption in the ileum and colon

involves specific transport mechanisms. An important component of this involves cyclic AMP (see later). Before the disorders of intestinal absorption are described, it is convenient to summarize the mechanisms involved in the production of diarrhea.

PATHOGENSIS OF DIARRHEA

Osmotic Diarrhea. The presence within the lumen of the gut of unabsorbed solutes results in water retention within the lumen. This is the mechanism by which sodium and magnesium sulfates act as purgatives. It is also a factor in the diarrhea that accompanies defects of intestinal absorption, *e.g.*, celiac disease.

Defective Permeability. Decreased permeability of diseased bowel to water has been demonstrated in the small intestine in celiac disease and in the colon in chronic inflammatory disease. This is also a contributing mechanism to the diarrhea of many other intestinal diseases.

Inflammation and Ulceration of the Mucosa. An outpouring of inflammatory exudate, often with blood and mucus, causes diarrhea. This is seen in typhoid fever when there is ulceration of the ileum and in the various forms of colitis. Rectal involvement leads to straining at stool, which is termed *tenesmus.*

Intestinal Secretory Diarrhea. Cholera toxin stimulates adenyl cyclase and leads to the formation of cyclic AMP (Chapter 2). This induces such an outpouring of salt and water into the small intestine that the colon is unable to absorb the load, and a severe watery diarrhea results. A similar mechanism is believed to explain the diarrhea caused by enterotoxigenic *Escherichia coli, Staphylococcus aureus*, and *Shigella dysenteriae.*

Endogenous agents may also increase intestinal secretion, possibly by activating the adenyl cyclase–cyclic AMP mechanism. Thus, vasoactive intestinal peptides produced by certain tumors of the islets of Langerhans of the pancreas produce cyclic AMP and are associated with a cholera-like diarrhea. 5-Hydroxytryptamine produced by carcinoid tumors also causes diarrhea, but the precise mechanism is not known.

Increased Intestinal Motility. This is an ill-defined mechanism and has not as yet been well documented.

From this account of the functions of the small intestine, it is evident that any derangement caused by disease can easily be accompanied either by malabsorption or by the loss of large quantities of fluid and electrolytes.

ACUTE IMFLAMMATION OF THE INTESTINE

Many agents cause acute inflammation of the small intestine (*acute enteritis*). Often this is accompanied by gastritis (*acute gastroenteritis*) or colitis (*acute enterocolitis*). It is convenient, therefore, to consider this group of intestinal diseases as a whole.

Etiology

Many causes of gastroenteritis and enterocolitis can be recognized. These include (1) chemicals, (2) preformed bacterial toxins, (3) bacterial infections, and (4) viral infections. In addition, some cases of intestinal inflammation are classified as idiopathic.

Chemicals. Poisoning may be deliberate (*e.g.*, by ingestion of inorganic arsenic) or accidental (*e.g.*, by ingestion of poisonous mushrooms and spoiled potatoes).

Bacterial Toxins. *Staphylococcus aureus* or *Clostridium perfringens* allowed to grow in food such as a meat pie produces toxins that cause acute gastroenteritis when ingested.

Bacterial Infection. A large number of different species of bacteria cause diarrhea by acting on the intestine in various ways.

Pathogenesis of Bacterial Diarrhea. Three mechanisms are involved.

Local Toxin Production. Vibrio cholerae, enterotoxigenic *E. coli, S. aureus*, and some strains of *Clostridium* and *Salmonella* adhere to the small intestinal mucosa and elaborate a toxin that causes an intestinal secretory type of diarrhea. With some toxins, there is activation of adenyl cyclase as described previously. With other toxins, the mechanism is unknown. The intestinal mucosa is not invaded, and there is no true infection as this term is strictly defined.

Invasion of the Intestinal Mucosa. Pathogens invade the mucosa of the colon, damage it, and cause an acute inflammation. This results in frequent small-volume bloody motions. Infections with *E. coli, Vibrio parahaemolyticus, Campylobacter jejuni, C. coli, Shigella, Yersinia enterocolitica*, and some species of *Salmonella* fall into this group.

Damage After Widespread Bacterial Invasion. The pathogens invade the mucosa but damage it days later after a preliminary phase of bacterial multiplication in some other tissue followed by septicemia. Typhoid fever is a typical example and is described in Chapter 7.

Specific Types of Bacterial Infection
Escherichia coli Infections. Although most strains of *E. coli* are normal, harmless inhabitants of the bowel, there are some recognized strains that cause enterocolitis.

Enteropathic E. coli causes serious infantile diarrhea (cholera infantum). The organisms cause a great outpouring of fluid into the intestine by an unknown mechanism.

Enterohemorrhagic E. coli causes a hemorrhagic colitis similar to shigellosis.

Enterotoxigenic E. coli produces a toxin that activates adenyl cyclase and produces a choleraic type of diarrhea. These strains are a common cause of traveler's diarrhea.

Enteroinvasive E. coli invades the colonic mucosa and causes a dysentery-like illness.

Cholera. Cholera, which is caused by *Vibrio cholerae*, has been responsible in the past for several pandemics that have originated in the Bengal basin. The disease is characterized by the sudden onset of intense vomiting and watery diarrhea, which rapidly leads to dehydration and hypovolemic shock, followed in about one third of the cases by death within 2 or 3 days. With efficient treatment by fluid and electrolyte administration, the mortality can be reduced to under 1 per cent. At a time when the disease appeared to be declining in the world, a new strain became prominent (the *El Tor* type); this appeared to have originated in Indonesia in 1961. It subsequently spread to involve large areas of the Far East, India, and Africa.

Cholera is acquired by ingesting the organisms in food or water contaminated by human excreta. The organism produces a secretory type of diarrhea by the action of its toxin on the intestinal wall; there is neither tissue invasion nor a true enteritis.

Salmonella Infections (Salmonellosis). Over 2000 serotypes of *Salmonella* are responsible for human infection. The enteric fever organisms—*typhi* and *paratyphi A, B,* and *C*—are exclusively human pathogens, and the disease that they cause has been described in Chapter 7. The remainder of the salmonellae are predominantly parasites of animals and cause food poisoning in humans. Common types are *S. typhimurium, S. hadar, S.virchow,* and *S. enteritidis.* Infection occurs by eating undercooked infected poultry or meat, or by contamination of other food by raw meat or poultry or by human carrier. The incubation period is 12 to 24 hours; the disease is characterized by an abrupt onset of diarrhea, abdominal pain, and vomiting. The stools may be watery

(due to a toxin-induced enteropathy), or they may contain blood and mucus (due to an invasive colitis). Recovery generally occurs within a few days, and a convalescent carrier state lasting several weeks is common.

Campylobacter Infections (Campylobacteriosis). Infection with *Campylobacter* produces a type of food poisoning similar to that caused by *Salmonella.* Animals generally provide the source of infection, and transmission is via milk or water.

Shigellosis (Bacillary Dysentery). After an incubation period of 1 to 4 days, there is an abrupt onset of fever, abdominal pain, and watery diarrhea. This phase lasts 1 to 3 days and is associated with colonization of the jejunum and a secretory type of diarrhea similar to that described in cholera. With some strains of *Shigella,* there then ensues a prolonged second phase of *colitis* as the stool volume decreases but the mucus and blood content increase. Tenesmus is often severe. This type of diarrhea is the classic feature of dysentery (the bloody flux of Hippocrates); untreated, it can last for weeks and lead to great debility and weight loss. As with other types of dysentery, it occurs in epidemic form and often occurs in custodial institutions, particularly those that care for the mentally retarded.

Bacillary dysentery is characterized pathologically by colitis with ulceration and inflammation of the mucosa.

Other bacterial causes of gastroenteritis include infection by *Y. enterocolitica, V. parahaemolyticus,* and others. Differentiation among these various types of infection is largely a bacteriologic problem.

Viral Infections. Many viruses are known to cause diarrhea. The rotaviruses are a cause of gastroenteritis in children under 6 years old; indeed, under 2 years of age, they are the most common cause (Fig 23–14B).

The *winter vomiting disease* is probably viral in origin, and various virus particles have been demonstrated in the feces of affected individuals. The disease is not uncommon and has a sudden onset of severe vomiting and diarrhea after an incubation period of 24 to 48 hours. Fever, vomiting, abdominal pain, and diarrhea generally last 2 to 3 days and are followed by complete recovery.

Pseudomembranous Colitis

This form of acute colitis causing severe diarrhea can occur postoperatively or in debilitated patients but is usually encountered as a complication of antibiotic therapy (usually with clindamycin or lincomycin). For this reason, it is also called antibiotic-associated pseudomembranous colitis. Early recognition and treatment are important because the condition can be fatal. The colitis is caused by the toxin of *Clostridium difficile*, a normal bowel commensal that can, under certain conditions, proliferate and produce toxin. The colon shows superficial mucosal necrosis, and in severe cases, an extensive pseudomembrane resembling the pseudomembrane of severe *Shigella* dysentery is formed (Fig. 23–15).

Other Clinical Types of Gastroenteritis

Traveler's Diarrhea. It is a common experience to develop acute gastroenteritis when traveling in hot climates, particularly in countries with inadequate sanitation. Colloquial terms such as "Delhi belly" and "Montezuma's revenge" bear witness to the widespread nature of the problem. The irritant effects of local exotic foods are now discounted as a cause, and epidemiology suggests an infective cause. Enterotoxigenic *E. coli* and *Campylobacter* are probably the most common causes. Other causes include infection by *Shigella*, *Salmonella*, and *Giardia*. Often no cause can be recognized. In up to 30 percent of cases, no cause can be found.

Acute Infantile Gastroenteritis. In developing countries, acute gastroenteritis is an important cause of infant mortality and morbidity; even in the Western world, it is among the ten leading causes of death in children under 5 years of age. The disease is less common in breast-fed infants, partly because they are protected by IgA in the milk, and partly because there is less chance of contamination of the food. Rotavirus infection is

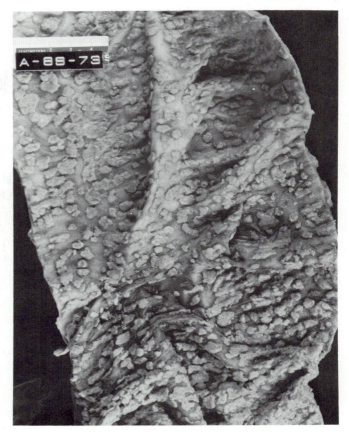

Figure 23–15 Pseudomembranous colitis. The colon has been opened to show necrosis of the mucosa. In some areas there is ulceration; between these denuded areas, necrotic mucosa is loosely attached as isolated islets of pseudomembrane. (Courtesy of Dr. J.B. Cullen, Toronto General Division of the Toronto Hospital, Toronto.)

the most common cause, but *E. coli, Yersinia, Campylobacter, Shigella, Salmonella, Giardia,* and *Strongyloides* are other causes.

Food Poisoning. Food poisoning is used to describe a wide range of conditions with presenting symptoms of diarrhea and vomiting due to gastroenteritis that develop up to 48 hours after the consumption of food or drink. It is customary to exclude the enteric fevers (typhoid), dysentery, and cholera. The causes include the infections described previously, the effects of ingested preformed bacterial toxin, chemical poisons, and probably some examples of food allergies.

ISCHEMIC BOWEL DISEASE

Although massive infarction of the bowel has been recognized for many years, the existence of less dramatic, more subtle lesions due to ischemia has not attracted attention until comparatively recently.

Causes. Ischemia of the bowel can result from the following causes.

Arterial Occlusion. Atherosclerosis, with or without thrombosis, and embolism are common causes. Dissecting aneurysm of the aorta and polyarteritis are less frequently encountered causes.

Venous Occlusion. Thrombosis of the mesenteric vein may arise as a complication of abdominal surgery, cirrhosis of the liver with portal hypertension, or ingestion of birth control pills.

Nonocclusive Underperfusion. This may be due to hypotension complicating shock.

Effects. The effects of ischemia depend on its degree and duration. Mild cases lead to edema, hemorrhage in the bowel wall, and superficial mucosal necrosis. Such effects cause no permanent damage, and healing occurs with minimal scarring. In more severe cases, necrosis involves the whole mucosa and perhaps the submucosa. Such a lesion may heal, but with scarring that may lead to stricture formation. The most severe cases cause full-thickness necrosis of the bowel wall, resulting in the classic picture of infarction. The wall becomes gangrenous and ruptures, leading to peritonitis, shock, and death unless emergency surgery intervenes.

Examples of Ischemic Bowel Disease. Sudden complete vascular occlusion generally leads to infarction of the whole thickness of the gut wall. Examples include mesenteric artery thrombosis or embolism, mesenteric vein thrombosis, volvulus, and a strangulated hernia.

Gradual occlusion of the superior mesenteric artery due to atherosclerosis may cause *intestinal angina,* a syndrome in which abdominal pain occurs shortly after meals owing to the increased peristalsis, which accentuates the effects of the pre-existing ischemia. Diarrhea, weight loss, and a frank malabsorption syndrome can ensue. The condition may terminate in bowel infarction.

Nonocclusive ischemia is generally a feature of shock and is therefore a complication of major trauma and surgery. Underperfusion of the bowel is accentuated by any pre-existing organic arterial occlusion such as atherosclerosis. Older patients are therefore at greater risk than are the young. Any part of the bowel can be affected, and the type of lesion and the extent of the damage vary from case to case. There may be scattered areas of superficial mucosal hemorrhage and ulceration, which may heal or lead to scarring if the patient survives the primary disease. In severe cases, there is widespread hemorrhage and extensive mucosal loss. If the colon is affected, the appearance closely resembles acute ulcerative colitis (described later). Clinically, abdominal pain, cramps, and bloody diarrhea are added to the patient's other problems.

CROHN'S DISEASE (REGIONAL ENTERITIS)

Crohn's disease is a chronic inflammatory disease that can affect any part of the bowel but is usually most obvious in the lower small intestine (see Case History II).

Ulceration is characteristic of Crohn's disease. The ulcers vary in size from minute (aphthoid ulcers) to larger lesions that extend into the bowel wall as narrow fissures. The inflammation therefore involves the whole wall of the bowel and is described as being *transmural;* with lesions in the colon, this characteristic distinguishes it from ulcerative colitis. In some cases, noncaseating tuberculoid granulomas are present not only in the bowel wall but also in the regional lymph nodes. Fibrosis associated with the inflammation and the formation of strictures is another characteristic. The submucosa of the affected bowel is markedly edematous; the appearance of raised mounds of mucosa, separated from each other by intercommunicating fissures and crevices, is described as "cobblestoning" (Fig. 23–16).

With the classic type of the disease affecting the terminal ileum, the bowel is thickened, rigid, and inflexible such that it has been likened to a pipe or rubber hose. The lesions of the small intestine are well demarcated and separated from each other by apparently normal areas of mucosa (*skip lesions*). The adjacent mesentery is thickened in the areas of the lesions, and its fat "creeps" over the gut so that the bowel becomes buried in fat (Fig. 23–17). Involvement of the peritoneal surface leads to local peritonitis and the formation of adhesions between the abdominal organs (Fig. 23–17).

Sinuses and fistulas develop so that communication is established between adjacent loops of intestine, the colon, the bladder, and the skin surface. Anal lesions, with ulceration, fissures, and fistulas, may occur at some time during the course of Crohn's disease and may indeed be the presenting symptom.

Involvement of the colon (*granulomatous colitis*)

in Crohn's disease either alone or with the small intestine is now recognized as being common. Distinction from ulcerative colitis is sometimes difficult or impossible; indeed, most experts accept that the two diseases cannot be distinguished in a number of cases, probably 10 percent. Hence, there is a tendency to group them together as *nonspecific inflammatory bowel disease*.

The clinical features of Crohn's disease include abdominal pain, diarrhea, fever, and weight loss. When the colon is affected, bleeding, perianal abscesses, and fistula are characteristic. The malabsorption syndrome can develop; because the terminal ileum is often affected, vitamin B_{12} absorption is particularly affected. As might be expected, intestinal obstruction and fecal fistulas involving the bladder and the skin surface add to the patient's problems.

The cause of this disease, which tends to affect young adults, is still unknown. Treatment by resection of the affected bowel is sometimes successful, but recurrence in other areas is quite common. The course is therefore protracted and presents great problems to both patient and attendants.

CASE HISTORY II

The patient was a 30-year-old male who was admitted to a hospital with a complaint of abdominal pain

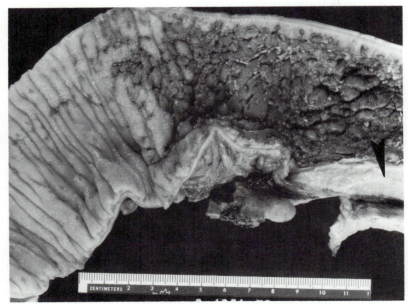

Figure 23–16 Crohn's disease of the small intestine. The mucosa of the affected area is thickened and presents a hyperemic cobblestone appearance. Note the thickening of the intestinal wall (arrow) and the sharp line of demarcation between the diseased bowel and the normal intestine.

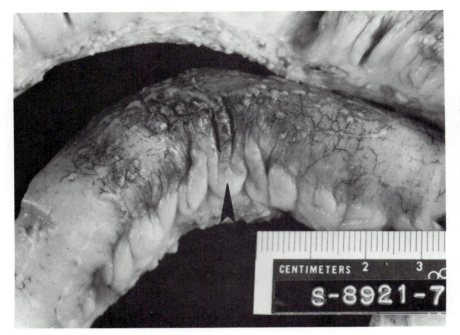

Figure 23–17 Crohn's disease of the small intestine. This portion of the small intestine shows hyperemia and thickening of the peritoneal surface. Focal white areas of inflammation are present, and this loop of intestine has become adherent to adjacent structures. The fat at the mesenteric border (arrow) is prominent and is "creeping" over the gut wall. (See Case History II for additional clinical details.)

and frequency of stool discharge for 1 year. The pain, which was colicky in nature, began between 1 and 2 hours after meals. It was relieved by having a bowel movement, which showed stools that were bulky, light brown, and foul-smelling. They floated in the toilet bowl because of their fat and gas content. Pathologic examination of the feces showed the presence of pus cells, blood, and an increased amount of fat. A barium meal showed narrowing and irregularity of the bowel wall involving two or three loops of ileum. Such findings were suggestive of Crohn's disease. Since the patient was thought to have signs of subacute intestinal obstruction, a laparotomy was performed. About 50 cm of small gut was resected. The disease started about 20 cm from the ileocecal junction and extended upward. Two skip areas were noted between the lesions. The sigmoid colon also showed thickening, which was interpreted as Crohn's disease, but since there was no sign of obstruction, the colon was not resected. The postoperative course was uneventful. Part of the resected specimen is shown in Figure 23–17. Postoperatively, the patient continued to have three or four bowel movements daily, but he felt reasonably well in spite of the occasional passage of blood. It was felt that his Crohn's disease was still present but stable.

TUBERCULOSIS OF THE INTESTINE

This disease is now extremely uncommon.

DIVERTICULA OF THE SMALL INTESTINE

About 3 percent of the population have a Meckel's diverticulum caused by persistence of the vitellointestinal duct. It arises from the antimesenteric border of the small intestine about 3 feet (90 cm) from the ileocecal valve and is about 3 inches (7.5 cm) long. In some cases, the lining mucosa contains ectopic acid-secreting gastric mucosa, and this leads to its major complications—peptic ulceration with hemorrhage or perforation. Furthermore, adhesions can lead to volvulus formation.

NEOPLASMS OF THE SMALL INTESTINE

Small leiomyomas are not uncommon but rarely produce symptoms; carcinomas are rare. The most frequently encountered malignant tumor is the *carcinoid*. This tumor is characterized by the development of a considerable stromal reaction that causes a stricture to develop. The tumor grows slowly, but it ultimately metastasizes to lymph nodes and liver. These metastases sometimes lead to the *carcinoid syndrome*—diarrhea, valvular lesions of the right side of the heart, asthmatic attacks, and periodic flushing of the face. The pathogenesis of this syndrome is not clear, but the release of 5-hydroxytryptamine by the tumor, the activation of plasma kinin, and the deposition of platelets on the heart valves are all involved. Carcinoid tumors also occur in other parts of the intestine—the appendix, in particular; in the appendix the tumor is usually small and does not spread.

MALABSORPTION

An abnormality of the function of the small intestine can lead to failure in the absorption of nutrients owing to a derangement of digestion or defective absorption. Three classes of disorder may be recognized.

1. The defect may be specific for a particular food component; this is usually associated with an enzyme defect, *e.g.*, lactase deficiency causes lactose intolerance. It is a common condition in adults; its prevalence shows a definite racial variation, being most common in Orientals. The individual experiences no trouble during infancy or childhood but later, as lactase production wanes, experiences intolerance to milk, which the patient soon eliminates from the diet in order to avoid symptoms.

2. There may be a lack of a major digestive fluid, *e.g.*, gastric juice after total gastrectomy, pancreatic juice in pancreatic disease, and bile in bile duct obstruction.

3. There may be gross abnormality of the small intestine itself such that many processes are affected. The short bowel syndrome, the blind loop syndrome, and intrinsic disease of the intestine itself, such as celiac disease, are examples.

In the last two groups, there is defective absorption of protein, carbohydrate, and fat; fat absorption is often the most severely affected. In addition, there may be defective absorption of vitamins and minerals. The clinical state is that of the *general malabsorption syndrome.*

The Short Bowel Syndrome. Extensive resection of the small intestine leads to malabsorption because there is loss of absorptive area. Abdominal gunshot wounds, recurrent Crohn's disease, and massive infarction are common causes.

The Blind Loop Syndrome. Fistulas between adjacent loops of bowel and blind loops caused by surgical procedures sometimes lead to a malabsorption syndrome. The precise mechanism is not clearly understood, but it is believed to be related to an upset in the intestinal bacterial flora. The bacteria may directly damage the bowel mucosa, or they may impair digestion by deconjugating bile salts. The free bile acids so formed are absorbed; hence, there is deficiency of bile salts in the intestinal lumen, and fat absorption is impaired.

Celiac Disease. Celiac disease commonly presents in childhood but may first be recognized in adults. Diarrhea, steatorrhea with bulky offensive stools, and evidence of malabsorption are the main clinical features. The technique of peroral intestinal biopsy has proved to be of great value in diagnosis. The specimen obtained can be examined under the dissecting microscope and scanning electron microscope; the characteristic feature of celiac disease is atrophy of the intestinal villi (Fig. 23–18). The intestinal lesions and symptoms can be relieved by a diet low in gluten, a protein contained in flour. For this reason, the disease has been called *gluten-sensitive enteropathy*, but since not all patients are relieved by a gluten-free diet, the name is not entirely appropriate. There is a marked familial incidence, the condition probably being inherited as an autosomal dominant trait with incomplete penetrance. There is little doubt that the lesions are produced by ingested gluten components of flour, but the mechanism is not understood. Gluten or one of its breakdown products may be directly toxic to the mucosa, or possibly the damage is immunologically mediated.

Other causes of malabsorption include *cystic fibrosis* (described in Chapter 24) and tropical sprue. *Tropical sprue* is encountered in the Far East, in some islands in the Mediterranean, but not in Africa. It is not related to gluten sensitivity but, for reasons that are not clear, often responds to oral antibiotics. Macrocytic anemia due to folic acid deficiency is an outstanding feature in addition to the chronic diarrhea and emaciation.

Effects of Malabsorption. The lack of absorption produces some effects that are similar to

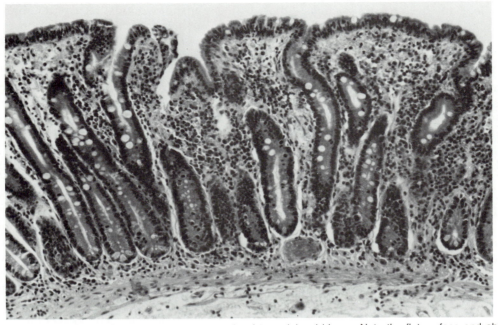

Figure 23–18 Gluten-induced enteropathy. This is a section from a jejunal biopsy. Note the flat surface and absence of villi (compare this with the normal intestine illustrated in Ch.2). The lamina propria is heavily infiltrated with lymphocytes and plasma cells. Under the scanning electron microscope, the appearance would resemble that demonstrated in Figure 23–14*B* ($\times$250).

those of starvation, *e.g.*, the effects that follow the dysphagia of esophageal cancer. Thus, there is a loss of weight and generalized body atrophy.

Fat absorption is usually severely affected; therefore, much fat—some of it undigested—is passed in the feces, which are pale and bulky. Excess fat in the stools is termed *steatorrhea*. There is often poor carbohydrate absorption, and the excess carbohydrate is fermented by bacteria in the bowel. The resulting gas causes the stools to be frothy and offensive.

In addition to the generalized wasting, there are the effects of specific dietary deficiencies (*e.g.*, deficiencies of the vitamin B complex, the fat-soluble vitamins A and D, and calcium). Calcium is poorly absorbed because it is bound by the fatty acids in the bowel. This results in a negative calcium balance with mild hypocalcemia and a tendency to develop tetany. A deficiency of vitamin D aggravates matters, causing osteomalacia to develop (Chapter 30). A deficiency of vitamin K leads to a low plasma prothrombin and a bleeding tendency (Chapter 18). Dermatitis, peripheral neuropathy, and inflammation of the tongue (glossitis) may all be found and may be attributable to vitamin deficiencies. A failure to absorb iron, vitamin B_{12}, and folic acid leads to severe anemia. The effects of malabsorption from the small intestine are both widespread and serious, and their occurrence is a reflection of the importance of this part of the digestive tract.

The Colon

The colon has two main functions: (1) absorbing water and electrolytes, and (2) providing a convenient receptacle for feces so that they may be discharged at the individual's convenience. Acute inflammation of the colon results in a derangement of its functions, and the diarrhea that results causes great inconvenience as well as a considerable loss of water and electrolytes. Infection of the colon leading to ulceration and causing diarrhea with pus, mucus, and blood in the feces is called *dysentery*. *Bacillary dysentery* has been described earlier in this chapter, and *amebic dysentery* is discussed in Chapter 10.

Ischemic colitis has been described earlier in this chapter, and *uremic colitis* is noted in Chapter 25.

CONGENITAL ABNORMALITIES

Hirschsprung's disease and anal atresia, or imperforate anus, are described.

Hirschsprung's Disease (Megacolon)

Megacolon of the congenital type is caused by a failure of the ganglion to develop in a segment of the rectum and sigmoid colon. This leads to obstruction because the aganglionic segment fails to relax. As a result, the colon proximally becomes hypertrophied and enormously dilated as the infant fails to pass feces for weeks or even months.

Anal Atresia

In simple imperforate anus, a thin diaphragm separates the endodermal rectum from the ectodermal anus. If the atresia is more complete, involving the anal canal and lower rectum, the malformation is then complex, and the colon may communicate with the bladder or, in the female, the vagina.

ANGIODYSPLASIA

The presence of ectatic small blood vessels in the mucosa and submucosa of the cecum or ascending colon constitutes angiodysplasia. The lesions are usually small and can be easily missed at laparotomy or on colonoscopy. They can be demonstrated by selective mesenteric arteriography. Angiodysplasia is an important cause of hemorrhage, either recurrent, leading to iron deficiency, or severe. The condition is usually found in elderly patients and is presumably degenerative in nature.

IDIOPATHIC ULCERATIVE COLITIS

Now the most common cause of serious bowel disease in North America, idiopathic ulcerative colitis affects all age groups and often starts in young adult life.

The disease generally commences with an acute attack of colicky abdominal pain accompanied by diarrhea and the passage of blood, mucus, and pus in the feces. Fever and malaise are also present. The acute attack generally subsides and is followed by chronic ulcerative colitis with recurrent exacerbation of symptoms. Pain, diarrhea, and the passage of blood, mucus, and pus are intermittent.

The disease generally affects the rectum and distal colon most severely; in the acute phase, it is characterized by intense hyperemia of the mucosa. On proctoscopy, the mucosa bleeds at the slightest touch. In due course, mucosal ulcers develop, and these tend to undermine the mucous membrane so that tags or pseudopolyps are formed. The ulcers are covered by a slough. Deep to this is an inflammatory reaction from which the blood and pus are derived.

In chronic ulcerative colitis, the disease tends to remain confined to the mucosa. Because the muscle coat itself and the peritoneal surface of the colon are not generally affected, adhesions do not form between adjacent viscera and there is usually no perforation or fistula formation. In this respect, the disease differs markedly from Crohn's disease, which can also affect the colon.

Ulcerative colitis generally pursues a chronic intermittent course, producing misery to the patient and leading to anemia, general debility, and loss of weight. A further complication is the development of carcinoma. It has been estimated that about one third of the patients who suffer from the disease for more than 12 years develop cancer. For this reason, and because of the symptoms of the disease, total colectomy is sometimes performed, and the patient is left with a permanent ileostomy. The ileum is brought to the surface of the anterior abdominal wall, a permanent opening is created, and a suitable container is attached.

Ulcerative colitis is occasionally very acute, either at its inception or at some stage in its development. The colon becomes acutely congested, its muscle becomes atonic, and the bowel dilates enormously. This type of disease follows a fulminating course; generally, the transverse colon is involved, and the patient becomes extremely ill. Multiple perforations develop, and the patient dies of toxemia associated with peritonitis. This variant of ulcerative colitis is called *acute toxic megacolon.*

DIVERTICULAR DISEASE OF THE COLON

The current Western diet, which contains inadequate cellulose (roughage), is believed by some authorities to be responsible for the high frequency of colonic diverticula. This disease is most frequent in the distal part of the colon, particularly the sigmoid part. Apart from the presence of numerous diverticula, the most striking change is muscular hypertrophy and shortening of the colon, presumably due to the muscular overactivity that is necessary to propel the small, hard feces. The diverticula themselves consist of outpouches of the mucosa that penetrate weak points in the muscular coat (Figs. 23–19 and 23–20). Often they are covered by merely a thin layer of peritoneum. Sometimes the orifices of the diverticula become obstructed by fecal material, and inflammation ensues. Overlying peritonitis develops, with the formation of adhe-

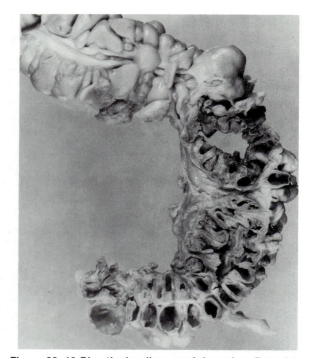

Figure 23–19 Diverticular disease of the colon. Part of the descending and sigmoid colon has been opened. Numerous diverticula are present. There is no evidence of inflammation, and the condition can be labeled *diverticulosis.*

sions, pericolic abscesses, and fistulas. The condition is then called *diverticulitis.* Sometimes a mass of chronic inflammatory tissue forming in the bowel wall is sufficient to cause obstruction and to simulate carcinoma. Occasionally, diverticular disease can cause massive bleeding, which is life-threatening.

NEOPLASMS OF THE LARGE INTESTINE

Adenoma

Adenomas are common and sometimes multiple (Fig. 23–21). They tend to become pedunculated and bleed. Malignant change can occur, but it is not inevitable. Nevertheless, in the hereditary condition of *familial polyposis coli,* there are so many tumors that one invariably becomes malignant and the patient dies of carcinoma.

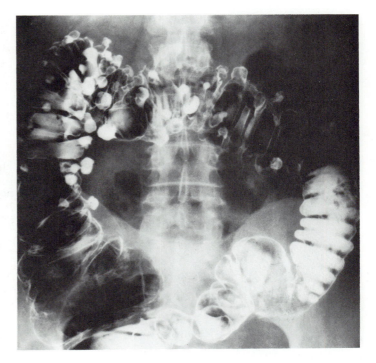

Figure 23–20 Diverticular disease of the colon. This radiograph after a barium enema shows numerous diverticula that are outlined by radiopaque barium. (Courtesy of Dr. D.E. Sanders, Department of Radiology, Toronto General Division of the Toronto Hospital, Toronto.)

Carcinoma

The large bowel ranks with the lung and the breast as the most common site of fatal malignant disease in Europeans. It has a low incidence in Japan. It is more common in populations of high socioeconomic standards and less common in economically deprived areas. These differences in incidence are thought to be environmental and not genetic, since Japanese emigrants gradually acquire the incidence of the inhabitants of their new country. Diet is believed to play an important part; a high intake of animal fat and protein and a low intake of fiber predispose to the disease.

Apart from the high incidence in familial polyposis coli, genetic factors are of importance; it has been estimated that the relations of a patient with colon cancer have a fourfold increased chance of developing colorectal cancer, compared with the remainder of the population. There is an increased incidence of colorectal cancer in chronic inflammatory bowel disease, particularly chronic ulcerative colitis.

A number of tumor markers can be identified in the blood; *carcinoembryonic antigen* is the best documented, and its level in the serum is related to the bulk of tumor present. Thus, the test is of little value in diagnosis because it is positive in late cases but likely to be negative at the early, curable stage. However, reappearance of carcinoembryonic antigen in the blood after surgery is indicative of tumor recurrence or metastases.

Cancer of the colon is usually a well-differentiated adenocarcinoma (see Figs. 12–11 and 12–12). The rectum and sigmoid colon are the sites most frequently involved. Initially the tumor produces a polypoid growth protruding into the lumen, but it generally soon breaks down to produce a typical carcinomatous ulcer (Fig. 23–22). The tumor tends to encircle the gut, and the fibrous stromal reaction that accompanies it produces a stricture (Figs. 23–23 and 23–24). This obstruction produces constipation, but overgrowth of organisms above this soon liquefies the feces so that diarrhea follows. *Alternate constipation and diarrhea are characteristic of partial intestinal obstruction.* When this is combined with

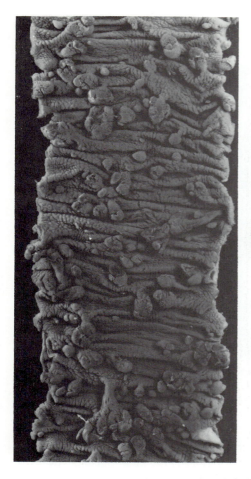

Figure 23–21 Familial polyposis coli. The mucosal surface of the colon shows numerous adenomas, many of which are pedunculated and therefore may be labeled polyps. (Specimen from the Boyd Museum, University of Toronto.)

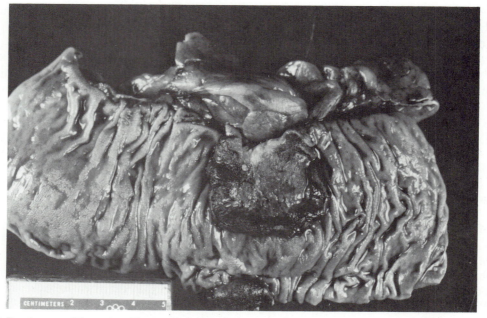

Figure 23–22 Carcinoma of the colon. The specimen shows a typical ulcerating carcinoma. It has a rolled edge where tumor is actively extending.

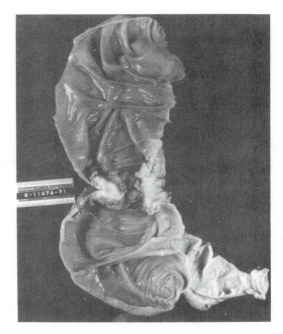

Figure 23–23 Carcinoma of the colon. This surgically removed colon has been distended with 10 per cent formalin solution before being opened. Note how the carcinoma encircles the gut and has produced stenosis.

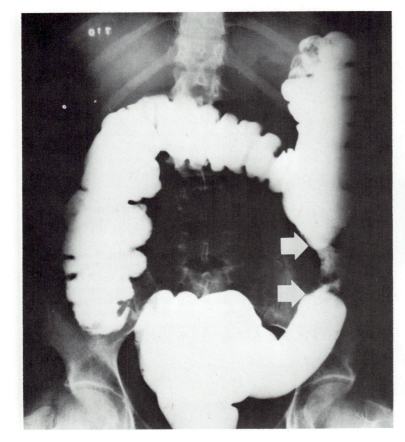

Figure 23–24 Carcinoma of the colon. This radiograph after a barium enema shows obvious obstruction in the descending colon. The lesion proved to be a carcinoma similar to that depicted in Figure 23–23. (Courtesy of Dr. D.E. Sanders, Department of Radiology, Toronto General Division of the Toronto Hospital, Toronto.)

the passage of blood and mucus in the stools, the diagnosis of carcinoma is almost certain. The tumor invades locally, metastasizes to the regional lymph nodes, and finally invades the blood stream to cause metastases in the liver and, later, elsewhere. Growth is often relatively slow, so the prognosis after resection is good if the tumor is detected in the early stages of development and correspondingly poor if the tumor is detected in the later stages.

The Appendix

The importance of the appendix as a site of intra-abdominal mischief is not proportional to its size or apparent uselessness. The organ is a hollow cul-de-sac opening into the cecum, and it is seldom more than 7 cm in length. Its major disease is acute inflammation.

ACUTE APPENDICITIS

Incidence. Acute appendicitis is common in persons living in highly civilized societies but spares the inhabitants of poor and undeveloped areas of the world. The reason for this is not precisely known, but it is presumed to be related to diet; a low-roughage/high-meat diet apparently predisposes to the disease. Appendicitis is rare in children under 2 years of age and has its maximum incidence in young adults between the ages of 20 and 30 years.

Pathology and Pathogenesis. No specific infective agent can be isolated from an acutely inflamed appendix; the organisms present are those normally found in the feces—in particular, *Escherichia coli*. The inflamed organ is red and swollen (Fig. 23–25); its peritoneal coat is dulled by a fibrinous exudate, and the mucosa is ulcerated. Often found blocking the lumen is a hard mass of feces (called a *fecalith*), which may play some part in initiating the disease.

Complications. Acute appendicitis may resolve spontaneously, but often the wall undergoes necrosis, becomes gangrenous, and *perforates*. Pus and fecal material pour into the peritoneal cavity. This material may become walled off by adhesions to produce a *localized*

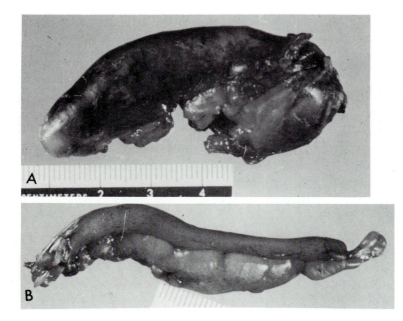

Figure 23–25 Acute appendicitis. The appendix in *A* shows acute inflammation. The organ is turgid and deeply congested. The mottled appearance seen in some areas is due to underlying suppuration. This appendix would almost certainly have ruptured had it not been removed. Specimen *B* is a normal slender appendix for comparison; the presence of fat in the mesentery is normal. (Courtesy of Dr. J.B. Cullen, Toronto General Division of the Toronto Hospital, Toronto.)

abscess, but often *generalized peritonitis* ensues, and the outlook is poor. It is impossible to predict the course of an individual case, and early removal of the appendix (appendectomy) is the treatment of choice in all cases. If the patient is seen later in the course of the disease when a localized abscess mass is present, it is best to allow the inflammation to subside and to treat the person surgically at a later date. Suppurative thrombophlebitis with portal pyemia is an occasional complication.

Symptoms. The inflamed turgid appendix causes *pain* that is referred to the midline of the abdomen at about the level of the umbilicus. *Nausea* and sometimes *vomiting* follow. As the parietal peritoneum becomes inflamed, the periumbilical pain shifts to the right iliac fossa, and local tenderness can be detected.

If each case of acute appendicitis had this typical history, the disease would present no diagnostic problems. Unfortunately, atypical cases are common, particularly in the very young

and the very old, and even the most astute physician can be mistaken and misled. In view of the seriousness of perforation, it is a wise policy to operate if there is a reasonable suspicion of acute appendicitis. Inevitably, some unnecessary operations will be performed and normal appendices will be removed, but the operative mortality is very low. The alternative policy is to risk allowing an acute appendicitis to rupture and to go undetected. In such cases, the mortality is high.

MUCOCELE OF THE APPENDIX

After an attack of appendicitis, the lumen becomes blocked, and the appendix distally becomes distended with mucus. A similar appearance can occur as a result of a low-grade carcinoma of the mucosa; in this type of mucocele, the organ may rupture and lead to pseudomyxoma peritonei (Chapter 27).

Diseases of the Abdominal Cavity As a Whole

The abdominal cavity is lined by a layer of flattened cells that are sometimes classified as epithelial but are actually *modified connective tissue fibroblasts*. After surgical procedures that have left raw areas of peritoneum, the exposed connective tissues rapidly differentiate into new peritoneal cells; hence, it is unnecessary to attempt to cover these raw areas. To cover them is detrimental, because the required sutures lead to inflammation and the formation of adhesions.

ASCITES

The presence of excess fluid in the peritoneal cavity is called ascites. Depending on the nature of the fluid, three types are recognized.

Ascites Due to a Transudate

The fluid has a low protein content and a specific gravity of less than 1.010. Portal hyper-

tension, the nephrotic syndrome, and cardiac failure are common causes.

Ascites Due to an Exudate

An inflammatory exudate occurs in peritonitis (considered later). If the fluid is blood-stained, multiple peritoneal seedings of metastatic carcinoma should be suspected.

Chylous Ascites

In this uncommon type of ascites, the peritoneal cavity is filled with chyle, a milky fluid containing finely emulsified fat globules. Obstruction of the thoracic duct or the mesenteric lymphatic vessels by tumor is the common cause.

INTRAPERITONEAL HEMORRHAGE

Free blood is a feature of trauma with laceration of viscera (*e.g.,* liver or spleen), ruptured tubal pregnancy, ruptured corpus luteum, or ruptured aortic aneurysm, to mention but a few examples.

PERITONITIS

Peritonitis may be caused by chemical irritants or bacterial infection. Either may be localized or generalized.

Sterile Peritonitis

Bile is highly irritant and causes an acute peritonitis if it escapes into the peritoneum. Rupture of an acutely inflamed gallbladder or rupture of the common bile duct after a surgical procedure involving the biliary tract is a common cause. Peritonitis in acute pancreatitis is described in Chapter 24.

Bacterial Peritonitis

The common source of infection is from the intestinal contents; therefore, the causative organisms are *E. coli* and other gram-negative rods, *enterococci, anaerobic streptococci, Bacteroides species,* and occasionally *C. perfringens.* If collections of pus are not drained and if treatment is ineffective, the disease may become chronic.

Localized Peritonitis. This condition occurs over an inflamed abdominal organ. Examples, which have been described elsewhere in this chapter, include acute appendicitis, Crohn's disease, diverticulitis, and peptic ulceration. Localized pelvic peritonitis in the female is generally secondary to salpingitis, often gonococcal salpingitis. The fibrinous component of the exudate tends to wall-off the inflammation and to localize any infection. Aiding in this process is the *greater omentum,* the fibrovascular fatty apron that hangs from the stomach. This structure has been called the "policeman of the abdomen," for it tends to wrap itself around any area of inflammation; by becoming inflamed itself, the greater omentum adds its fibrinous exudate to the adhesions that limit the spread of infection.

Generalized Peritonitis. This occasionally occurs as a primary disease without evidence of infection elsewhere. The route of infection is presumed to be either via the blood stream, from a pulmonary infection, or, in young women, via the fallopian tubes. More commonly, generalized peritonitis is the result of rupture of a part of the gastrointestinal tract, *e.g.,* perforated peptic ulcer, appendicitis, toxic megacolon, volvulus, and penetrating injuries to the abdomen.

In generalized peritonitis, the large area of peritoneum forms an admirable absorptive area for toxins; the patient rapidly becomes ill, develops paralytic ileus, and goes into shock. Even if the person is treated and survives, there may be localized pockets of infection that can form peritoneal abscesses. One such site is the pelvis, owing no doubt to the effects of gravity. Another is the space between the diaphragm and the liver; indeed, an abscess in this situation (*subphrenic abscess*) is of great importance and should always be suspected if the patient develops signs of infection (*e.g.,* malaise, fever, leukocytosis) after an abdominal event (*e.g.,* appendicitis, laparotomy) and the site of infection is not apparent. The old adage "pus somewhere, pus under the diaphragm" is all too often forgotten (see Fig. 23–10).

PERITONEAL ADHESIONS

After acute peritonitis, the fibrinous adhesions can organize to fibrous adhesions. Hence, these are not uncommon overlying an appendix or adjacent to a peptic ulcer. Surgery alone can produce adhesions; the irritant talc or starch used as glove powder is an important factor in their production. The gloves used by the surgeon and assistants should be well rinsed before entering the abdomen. Endometriosis as a cause of adhesion formation is described in Chapter 27.

Adhesions can cause intestinal obstruction either directly or as a complication of internal hernia formation. Extensive adhesions (*e.g.,* after pelvic irradiation for carcinoma of the cervix) render subsequent surgery difficult and hazardous, for the bowel can easily be opened inadvertently.

VOLVULUS

Much of the small intestine and parts of the colon are suspended from the abdominal wall by means of a mesentery. The twisting of a loop of bowel about its mesenteric base is called a *volvulus* and is yet another cause of the "acute abdomen." Twisting of the mesentery soon produces venous obstruction, causing the gut to become rapidly congested and edematous. Soon the arterial supply is cut off, and infarction results. Urgent surgical intervention is required for volvulus. Sometimes the twist can be undone, but usually the affected gut must be resected.

INTUSSUSCEPTION

In this condition, a segment of gut becomes telescoped into the gut immediately distal to it. The trapped portion is pulled in by peristaltic motions, so that the segment of gut and its mesentery are steadily advanced toward the anus. The condition is most common in children and appears to arise spontaneously, perhaps being precipitated by an acute enteritis. In adults, intussusception is sometimes caused by a benign tumor that is caught by the peristaltic motions of the gut distal to it. Symptoms of intussusception include intestinal obstruction and the sequelae of infarction of the affected bowel. Passage of blood *per rectum* is characteristic.

HERNIAS

Protrusion of the whole or part of an organ or tissue through an abnormal opening is termed a hernia. The protrusion is commonly through a weak point in the abdominal wall. An outpouching of parietal peritoneum occurs first. This forms the lining of the hernial sac. Into this sac pass various mobile abdominal viscera—omentum, small intestine, and, less commonly, colon, fallopian tube, and ovary.

In the early stages of development, the contents of the hernial sac can be reduced by pressure and returned to the abdomen. The formation of adhesions may later result in the intestinal loops being permanently trapped or *incarcerated*. The hernia cannot then be reduced.

An occasional complication of a hernia is that the venous return from its contents is impaired by twisting or kinking at its neck; venous congestion causes edema, with the swelling further endangering the circulation until the arterial supply is finally cut off and the contents of the sac become infarcted and gangrenous. The hernia is then said to be *strangulated*. A strangulated hernia is a serious condition, because if bowel is involved (as it usually is), it results in intestinal obstruction and is rapidly followed by generalized peritonitis. Immediate surgical treatment is imperative. The detailed anatomy of the various types of hernias is therefore of great importance to the surgeon who is called upon to operate on them.

The most common site for a hernia is the inguinal region. Two types of *inguinal hernia* are encountered. In the *indirect* type, the sac follows the previous path of the descending testis. In the *direct* type, the hernial sac bulges directly through weakened muscles in the inguinal region. Both types of hernia must be distinguished by the surgeon from a *femoral hernia*, which passes through the femoral canal.

Other types of hernia include the *umbilical hernia*, which is usually present at birth and may close spontaneously. In a *ventral hernia*, the bowel herniates through a weak area in a laparotomy scar. Paraesophageal or *hiatus hernias* have been described earlier in this chapter.

The opening of the lesser sac and the various fossae around the duodenum present potential orifices through which loops of bowel can pass to form *internal hernias*. Likewise, a hernia can form in relation to fibrous bands or adhesions.

INTESTINAL OBSTRUCTION

Intestinal obstruction (or *ileus*, as it is sometimes called) is a serious condition because if it is complete and not relieved, it terminates in death. Two types can be recognized.

Mechanical Intestinal Obstruction

There are many causes of intestinal obstruction: strictures, tumors, hernias, volvuli, and intussusceptions are some forms of mechanical obstruction that have already been described. The obstruction may develop gradually, or it may be complete and sudden, resulting in more severe effects. The higher in the intestinal tract the obstruction occurs, the more profound are its effects and the greater is the threat to life.

Features

Pain. The intestine above the obstruction exhibits increased peristalsis; such effects can be heard with the aid of a stethoscope. The obstruction causes pain that is diffuse, poorly localized, and cramping or colicky.

Failure to Pass Feces or Gas per Rectum. Constipation, which becomes complete, is an important feature of intestinal obstruction.

Vomiting. Vomiting is a prominent feature of high intestinal obstruction. The vomitus soon becomes green in color and eventually has a foul, fecal odor.

Abdominal Distention. The gut above the obstruction ultimately becomes distended with fluid and gas, causing abdominal distention. A radiograph taken with the patient in the standing position has a characteristic appearance with many fluid levels. Abdominal distention is a late event if the site of the obstruction is low in the intestinal tract.

Nonmechanical Intestinal Obstruction

In the absence of a mechanical obstruction, a failure of the intestinal muscle to propel the gut contents forward is commonly called *ileus.* (Strictly speaking, "ileus," from the Greek *eilos*, meaning "intestinal colic," can be applied to any type of obstruction.) Three types are recognized.

Adynamic or Paralytic Ileus. Peritonitis is the most important cause of paralytic ileus. To a minor degree it occurs after every abdominal operation, but in such cases it does not last more than 3 days. The fully developed syndrome occurs in acute peritonitis, such as that complicating acute appendicitis or a perforated peptic ulcer. The gut dilates, vomiting occurs, peristalsis is absent, and the abdomen is silent — a silence that leads to the grave. Paralytic ileus sometimes complicates painful conditions, such as renal colic, and it is also a feature of severe hypokalemia.

Ileus due to Vascular Occlusion. Mesenteric arterial occlusion or mesenteric venous thrombosis leads to focal intestinal paralysis and obstruction. Gangrene often follows.

Spastic Ileus. Spasm is an uncommon cause of obstruction. It is occasionally encountered in uremia.

THE ACUTE ABDOMEN

The sudden onset of acute abdominal pain, often combined with vomiting and fever, is commonly referred to as acute abdomen. It is usually caused by peritoneal infection derived from a perforated abdominal organ. The task of diagnosis and treatment, which usually falls to the surgeon, is a subject dealt with in texts of surgery. Only a few of the common causes are listed here: acute appendicitis, acute cholecystitis, perforated peptic ulcer, ulcerative colitis, diverticulitis, mesenteric thrombosis, volvulus, and strangulated hernia. Each of these conditions demands prompt surgical treatment. However, there are a number of other causes for which surgery is not required and, in fact, is often contraindicated. Acute pancreatitis, acute enteritis, basal pneumonia, and acute myocardial infarction are good examples of this group. It is evident that the management of the "acute abdomen" requires great skill and considerable experience.

Summary

- Important lesions of the oral mucosa are mucosal lesions of certain skin diseases (lichen planus, erythema multiforme, pemphigus vulgaris, acute viral enanthems), herpes simplex, aphthous ulcers, and leukoplakia.
- Carcinoma of the lips has a better prognosis than does carcinoma of tongue and oropharynx.
- Caries and periodontal disease are the common causes of loss of teeth.
- Dysphagia has many causes; carcinoma of the esophagus is the most serious.

- Important salivary gland diseases are mumps, suppurative sialoadenitis, Sjögren's syndrome, and tumors.
- Acute gastritis and stress ulcers are complications of severe trauma or stress. Chronic gastritis may accompany pernicious anemia and is precancerous (type A), or it may accompany chronic peptic ulceration (type B).
- Chronic peptic ulcers affect esophagus (often with hiatus hernia), stomach, duodenum, or site of gastroenterostomy. Their etiology is complex; hemorrhage, penetration, perforation, and cicatrization are the chief complications.
- Carcinoma of the stomach is common in Japan; it is now uncommon in the United States and Europe but has a poor prognosis.
- Acute gastroenteritis may be due to chemical irritants, bacterial toxins, or infection by a wide variety of gram-negative bacteria including *E. coli, Vibrio cholerae, Salmonella, Campylobacter,* and *Shigella*. Viruses and unknown causes account for the remainder. When the colon is affected, the diarrhea with pus and blood is termed dysentery.
- Ischemic bowel disease includes intestinal angina, focal damage with scarring and obstruction, and massive infarction.
- Nonspecific inflammatory bowel disease includes Crohn's disease, which can affect any part of the bowel, and chronic ulcerative colitis. Both affect young adults, are of unknown etiology, can have similar symptoms, but differ in the type of bowel lesions.
- Meckel's diverticulum is solitary and causes hemorrhage and perforation.
- Carcinoid tumor of the intestine may lead to the carcinoid syndrome.
- Important causes of the malabsorption syndrome are the short bowel and blind loop syndromes, celiac disease, cystic fibrosis, and tropical sprue. Wasting, steatorrhea, and vitamin deficiencies are important effects.
- Anal atresia and Hirschsprung's disease are important congenital defects.
- Angiodysplasia of the large intestine is an important cause of bleeding per rectum.
- Carcinoma of the colon is one of the most common types of fatal malignant disease. It may evolve from adenoma, especially if there are multiple tumors. Carcinoembryonic antigen is a useful tumor marker.
- Acute appendicitis is an important cause of peritonitis; its cause is not known.
- Ascites may be due to accumulation of a transudate, an exudate (in peritonitis), or chyle.
- Intestinal obstruction may be functional, as in the paralytic ileus that accompanies peritonitis, or mechanical and due to volvulus, intussusception, or strangulated hernia.

Selected Readings

Almy, T. P., and Howell, D. A.: Diverticular disease of the colon. N. Engl. J. Med. *302*:324, 1980.

Field, M., Rao, M. C, and Chang, E. B.: Intestinal electrolyte transport and diarrheal disease. N. Engl. J. Med *321*:800 and 879, 1989.

Gorbach, S. L.: Traveller's diarrhoea. N. Engl. J. Med. *307*:881, 1982.

Kirsner, J. B., and Shorter, R. G.: Recent developments in "nonspecific" inflammatory bowel disease. N. Engl. J. Med. *306*:775 and 837, 1982.

Leading article: Angiodysplasia. Lancet 2:1086, 1981.

Leading article: Evolution of colonic polyps. Br. Med. J. 2:257, 1980.

Leading article: *Campylobacter pylori* becomes *Helicobacter pylori*. Lancet 2:1019, 1989.

Lucas, R. B.: Pathology of Tumours of Oral Tissue. 4th ed. Edinburgh, Churchill Livingstone, 1984.

Morson, B. C., and Dawson, I. M. P.: Gastrointestinal Pathology. 2nd ed. London, Blackwell, 1979.

Shklar, G.: Oral leukoplakia. N. Engl. J. Med. *315*:1544, 1986.

Soll, A. H.: Pathogenesis of peptic ulcer and implications for therapy. N. Engl. J. Med. 322:909, 1990.

Trier, J. S.: Intestinal malabsorption: Differentiation of cause. Hosp. Pract. 23:195, 1988.

Turnberg, L. A.: The pathophysiology of diarrhoea. Clin. Gastroenterol. *8*:551, 1979.

Williams, R. C.: Periodontal disease. N. Engl. J. Med. 322:373, 1990.

24

Liver, Biliary Tract, and Pancreas

**After studying this chapter, the student
should be able to:**

- Describe the structure of the normal liver and
  distinguish between the classic liver lobule and the
  acinus of Rappaport.
- Indicate the circumstances under which infarction of
  the liver may occur.
- Describe the effects of portal hypertension.
- Describe the main pathways of the metabolism of
  bilirubin.
- List the types of jaundice and describe the main
  features of each.
- Relate the effects of hepatocellular failure to the
  normal functions of the liver.
- Define the following terms and indicate the
  circumstances under which the conditions are found:
  (a) zonal hepatic necrosis;
  (b) focal hepatic necrosis;
  (c) bridging hepatic necrosis;
  (d) massive hepatic necrosis.
- Outline the main features of viral hepatitis with
  respect to
  (a) causative agents and mode of infection;
  (b) changes in the liver;
  (c) clinical manifestations;
  (d) prognosis.
- Distinguish among chronic lobular hepatitis, chronic
  persistent hepatitis, and chronic active hepatitis.

- Define cirrhosis of the liver. Discuss the causes, main pathologic lesions, and outstanding clinical features of the following:
  (a) micronodular cirrhosis;
  (b) macronodular cirrhosis;
  (c) biliary cirrhosis.
- Classify the primary tumors of the liver.
- Name the structures that constitute the biliary tract.
- List the common types of gallstones and indicate the factors that cause them.
- List the complications of gallstones.
- Describe the clinical and pathologic features of the following conditions:

(a) chronic cholecystitis;
(b) carcinoma of the gallbladder;
(c) carcinoma of the ampulla of Vater.
- List the secretions of the pancreas.
- Describe the main features of cystic fibrosis as it affects the pancreas, the lung, the liver, and the sweat glands.
- Outline the main features of
  (a) chronic pancreatitis;
  (b) carcinoma of the head of the pancreas;
  (c) carcinoma of the body of the pancreas.

The Liver

The liver is the largest organ in the body and performs many vital functions. Its blood supply is unique; in addition to receiving arterial blood via the hepatic artery, nearly all the venous blood draining the gastrointestinal tract passes to it via the portal vein. It is therefore not surprising that the liver occupies a key position in relation to the digestive tract and that it performs many metabolic functions, particularly in relation to fat, carbohydrate, and protein metabolism. The secretion of bile is another important function of the liver. Bile contains the bile acids, which aid digestion, as well as the end products of hemoglobin catabolism. The size of the liver is therefore well matched by the multiplicity of its functions. In disease, each aspect of liver function can be disturbed either separately or, more commonly, in combination.

THE LIVER IN RELATION TO ITS VASCULAR SUPPLY

The liver has a dual blood supply. Oxygenated blood from the radicles of the hepatic artery as well as blood from the portal vein enters the liver sinusoids; the mixed blood is then collected into tributaries of the hepatic vein. The region supplied by one terminal branch of the hepatic artery has been named an *acinus* by Rappaport (Fig. 24–1). This functional unit differs from the classic hexagonal *liver lobule*, which is pictured as centered on a hepatic venule (Figs. 24–2, 24–6, 24–7, and 24–8). The liver receives much of its oxygen from the hepatic arterial blood; a defi-

ciency of this supply results in necrosis in the peripheral part of Rappaport's acinus (zone 3; see Fig. 24–1). Such a response is seen in heart failure ("nutmeg liver"; see Fig. 20–14). Likewise, extensive necrosis is not uncommon in shock and septicemia. Ischemic necrosis involving the whole of many acini to produce an *infarct* is rare because of the dual blood supply, but it is occasionally encountered after obstruction to the hepatic artery or one of its major branches. Hepatic vein thrombosis (*e.g.*, secondary to invasion by a tumor) is another occasional cause.

The normal portal blood is of low pressure (3 to 13 mm Hg) but of large volume (some 1000 to 1200 ml enter the liver from this source per minute). The portal pressure can be measured in several ways. If a catheter is passed through an arm vein and past the right atrium of the heart and then wedged into one of the tributaries of the hepatic vein, the pressure measured in the catheter gives a good indication of the pressure in the terminal part of the hepatic sinuses. This reading is called the *postsinusoidal pressure*.

If a needle connected to a manometer is passed through the skin into the spleen, the intrasplenic pressure measured is closely related to that of blood in the portal vein itself. This is called the *presinusoidal pressure*. Splenic puncture may usefully be followed by injection of a radiopaque substance, the course of which can be followed by radiography. This is one method of demonstrating esophageal varices, a subject discussed later in this chapter.

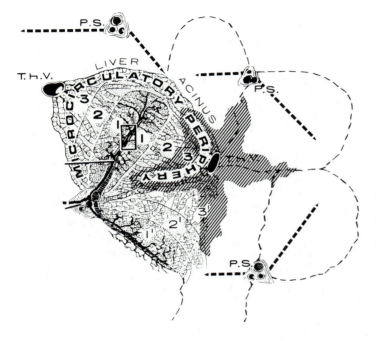

Figure 24–1 The liver acinus. The liver acinus is depicted as an area supplied by a terminal branch of the hepatic artery arising in the portal triad (labeled P.S.). The cells in zone 1 are closest to their blood supply, whereas those in zone 3 are most remote. Note that the acinus contains cells belonging to two adjacent classic hexagonal lobules, which are pictured as being centered on a terminal hepatic venule (T.h.V.). When the blood supply of the liver is impaired (as in congestive heart failure), the cells in zone 3 undergo necrosis first. The damaged area therefore assumes the shape of a sea star (designated by heavy crosshatching). (Courtesy of Dr. A.M. Rappaport. From Rappaport, A.M.: The microcirculatory acinar concept of normal and pathological hepatic structure. Beitrage Pathologie (Stuttgart), *157*:215, 1976.)

Figure 24–2 Normal liver. The cut surface shows the characteristic lobular pattern that is slightly accentuated by congestion. Each lobule has a dark center around a hepatic venule and is surrounded by a pale zone. The arrow points to a small subcapsular cavernous hemangioma.

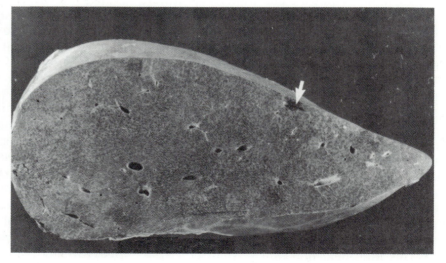

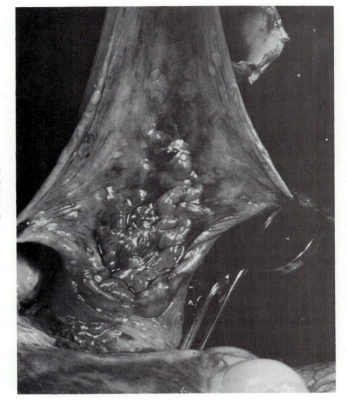

Figure 24–3 Esophageal varices. The esophagus has been opened longitudinally and the lower part held apart to show widely dilated, tortuous varicose veins. Esophageal varices are not usually seen this clearly at necropsy because the vessels collapse. In this instance, the veins were thrombosed.

Portal Hypertension

Obstruction of the blood flow through the liver is a common event in chronic liver disease and leads to portal hypertension. The effects, described in the following sections, are serious.

Development of Portal-Systemic Anastomoses. There are many areas where small tributaries of the portal vein anastomose with those of the systemic circulation. When there is portal hypertension, these anastomoses enlarge and become varicose. Around the colon, such varicosities are of little consequence; but when they are around the lower end of the esophagus, the thin-walled dilated veins project into the esophageal lumen, and the overlying mucosa is liable to ulcerate after the trauma of swallowing food or as a result of esophagitis (Figs. 24–3 and 24–4). Massive bleeding is the result, and a pint or more of blood can be vomited (*hematemesis*).

Portal-Systemic Shunting of Blood. Portal blood destined for the liver is shunted directly into the systemic circulation. Toxic substances from the intestine pass into the systemic circulation and contribute to the neuropsychiatric manifestations described later. Ammonia is believed to be one of these substances. Others are less well defined, but they may be responsible for the fecal odor of the breath noted in patients with chronic liver disease. Organisms from the gut can also gain access to the general circulation and can cause septicemia. Gram-negative endotoxic shock is sometimes seen as a terminal manifestation of liver disease.

The reduction in hepatic blood flow due to shunting can lead to hepatocellular necrosis but usually only as a terminal event when combined with systemic hypotension.

Congestive Splenomegaly. Chronic venous congestion leads to splenic enlargement, an important diagnostic clinical sign of portal hypertension. Occasionally, hypersplenism occurs.

Ascites. This condition is considered later.

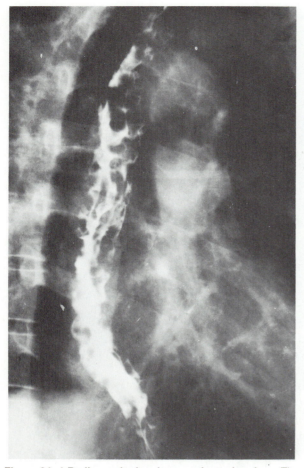

Figure 24–4 Radiograph showing esophageal varices. The patient was given a suspension of barium sulfate to swallow; the radiograph shows the outline of the esophageal lumen. Instead of appearing as a simple tube, the esophagus shows numerous indentations that are due to the bulging veins. The patient had advanced cirrhosis of the liver. (Courtesy of Dr. D.E. Sanders, Department of Radiology, Toronto General Division of the Toronto Hospital, Toronto.)

JAUNDICE

Of all the symptoms of liver disease, jaundice, or *icterus*, is the most immediately apparent. It is due to an excessive amount of bilirubin in the plasma and tissues. Virtually all the tissues of the body become a bright yellow; this coloration is apparent in the skin when the plasma bilirubin level reaches about 50 μmol/L (3 mg/dl). A sign of early jaundice is yellow discoloration of the sclera. This is a particularly useful sign in dark-skinned individuals, in whom jaundice in the skin is less apparent. Jaundice can be understood only in relation to bilirubin metabolism (Fig. 24–5).

When red blood cells are broken down, the porphyrin moiety of the hemoglobin molecule is converted into bilirubin in the cells of the mononuclear phagocyte system. Bilirubin is insoluble in water; after its release from the mononuclear phagocyte cells, it is carried in the blood via attachment to albumin. The liver has three important functions in regard to bilirubin:

1. *The liver extracts bilirubin from the blood.*

2. *The liver conjugates bilirubin with glucuronic acid to form bilirubin diglucuronide.* The level of the conjugating enzyme is low in the newborn but can be increased by giving phenobarbital.

3. *The liver excretes the conjugated bilirubin into the bile.*

Under normal conditions, 15 to 20 per cent of the bilirubin content of bile is derived from sources other than red blood cell destruction. Much of this originates from the bone marrow during the *formation* of hemoglobulin (*ineffective erythropoiesis*). The amount of bilirubin formed in this way may be increased in disease, such as in thalassemia and pernicious anemia, and this increase contributes to jaundice. A small amount of bilirubin results from the metabolism of other porphyrins present in enzymes such as oxidases and cytochromes. Figure 24–5 illustrates the main features of bilirubin metabolism. It should be noted in particular that bilirubin in the intestine is converted into urobilinogen by bacterial action; since some of this urobilinogen is reabsorbed and returned to the liver, there is a very considerable enterohepatic recirculation. A small quantity of urobilinogen is excreted in the urine.

Types of Jaundice

Obstructive Jaundice (Cholestasis). This occurs when there is an obstruction to the passage of conjugated bilirubin from the liver cells to the intestine. Bilirubin diglucuronide is reabsorbed into the blood, and if the obstruction is complete, the patient rapidly becomes deeply jaundiced. The serum bilirubin level may reach 680 μmol/L (40 mg/dl). Since the conjugated bilirubin is soluble in water and is easily excreted by the kidneys, the urine is dark, contrasting with the feces, which are clay-colored. Urobilinogen disappears from the urine.

Two major types of obstructive jaundice are recognized. In *extrahepatic cholestasis*, the bile duct is blocked mechanically. This condition is commonly caused by a gallstone in its lumen or pressure from outside by a carcinoma of the head of the pancreas. In *intrahepatic cholestasis*, the other type of obstructive jaundice, no obvious mechanical cause can be found in the major bile ducts. Instead, it is assumed that the obstruction is in the canaliculi of the liver itself. This condition can occur in a variety of situations. It is seen after the administration of certain drugs, such as chlorpromazine and other phenothiazine derivatives; it is an occasional complication of pregnancy; and it is also seen in the acute fatty alcoholic liver and sometimes during the early stages of acute viral hepatitis.

Other characteristic features of obstructive jaundice should be noted.

Pruritus. Often severe, this condition is probably due to retention of *bile salts*.

Malabsorption. Due to the lack of bile in the intestine, this is a feature of chronic biliary obstruction.

Hypercholesterolemia. This condition is due to increased synthesis by the liver rather than to biliary obstruction. Lipid-laden macrophages accumulate in various organs and may form tumorlike masses termed *xanthomas*. These structures tend to be bright yellow because of their content of carotenoid pigments;* they are most obvious in the skin.

Elevated Plasma Alkaline Phosphatase. This results from an increased production of the enzyme in the liver in response to the obstruction.

Hemolytic Jaundice. An excessive rate of destruction of red blood cells causes an increased rate of bilirubin formation; consequently, the liver is unable to deal with the increased load. Increased erythropoiesis adds to this load by contributing additional bilirubin (Fig. 24–5). The bilirubin in the blood in hemolytic jaundice is unconjugated. It is therefore insoluble in water and is not excreted in the urine. Jaundice of this type is therefore said to be *acholuric*. Increased quantities of bile pigments are excreted in the feces, and the amount of urobilinogen returned to the liver is increased.

Hemolytic jaundice rarely reaches the intensity of that seen in the obstructive variety. An exception to this is that seen in hemolytic disease of the newborn. Because unconjugated bilirubin is relatively soluble in lipids, in severe hemolytic jaundice of infancy, bile pigments pass into the brain tissue and can cause severe damage to the developing central nervous system. This is called *kernicterus*.

Hepatocellular Jaundice. Damage to the liver cells can upset any aspect of their function; there may be a failure of uptake of bilirubin from the blood, a failure in conjugation, or a failure in excretion of bile into the bile canaliculi. This type of jaundice is the most complex. Examples of the most common types are given.

Icterus Neonatorum. A mild degree of jaundice is apparent during the first few days after birth and is due to deficiency of glucuronyl transferase combined with an increased rate of red blood cell destruction that occurs during the neonatal period. This physiologic jaundice is rarely severe but can be more marked in premature infants or if the infant develops a severe bacterial infection. When Rh-hemolytic disease is added, the jaundice can be severe enough to cause kernicterus.

Gilbert's Disease. This disease is characterized by episodes of benign, intermittent jaundice starting in childhood. It is the most common form of unconjugated hyperbilirubinemia. Some cases are familial, and the defect appears to be a reduced glucuronyl transferase activity in the liver cells. The condition is probably not a single entity but rather a heterogeneous group of diseases.

Jaundice Accompanying Liver Cell Damage. Liver cell damage from any cause, *e.g.*, the effects of drugs, alcohol, or viral infection, leads to jaundice. The jaundice is usually of mixed type because there is failure in bilirubin uptake, conjugation, and excretion.

HEPATOCELLULAR FAILURE

The main manifestations of hepatocellular dysfunction are related to the processes of protein

*The carotenoid pigments, or lipochromes, are exogenous lipid-soluble hydrocarbons that constitute the coloring material in beets, carrots, and tomatoes. They give adipose tissue and other lipid material a yellow color. This is particularly well shown in atheromatous plaques, the normal corpus luteum of the ovary, and xanthomas.

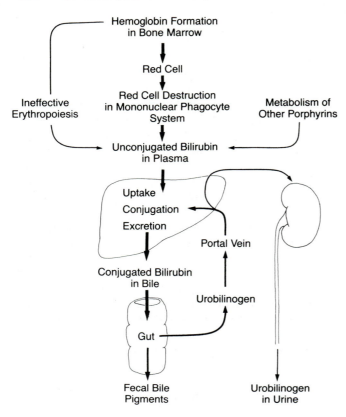

Figure 24–5 Metabolic pathways in the formation and excretion of billrubin.

and carbohydrate metabolism and to detoxification.

Disturbances of Protein Metabolism. The liver is responsible for the synthesis of most of the plasma proteins, with the major exception of the immunoglobulins. Progressive hepatocellular dysfunction is characterized by hypoalbuminemia. This dysfunction contributes to the formation of edema of the dependent parts in addition to being a factor in the production of ascites.

The liver is responsible for the synthesis of most of the clotting factors, the only notable exception being factor VIII, which is made by endothelial cells of the blood vessels. It is hardly surprising, therefore, that liver disease is often accompanied by a tendency to bleed.

The liver is the principal site of deamination of amino acids and is probably the only organ that can convert the ammonia so produced into urea. The other site of ammonia formation is the intestine, where it is formed by bacterial decomposi-

tion of protein. Shunting of this ammonia from the portal blood into the systemic circulation has already been mentioned as a possible cause of cerebral dysfunction.

Disturbances of Carbohydrate Metabolism. After total hepatectomy in an experimental animal, there is profound hypoglycemia. The hepatic reserve is great enough that hypoglycemia is rarely a feature of human disease; occasionally, however, it is seen in acute hepatic necrosis and after an acute episode of alcoholic debauchery. Impaired gluconeogenesis is the mechanism. The impaired glucose tolerance encountered in liver disease is due to portal-systemic shunting.

Failure of Detoxification. The liver is responsible for detoxifying many agents—either by conjugating them with glucuronic or sulfuric acid, or by conjugating them with an amino acid. The conjugated products are then excreted in the bile or in the urine: conjugation of bilirubin is a classic example of this process. Many drugs are treated in a similar way, and the administration of depressant drugs such as barbiturates or morphine may induce a coma in a patient with hepatocellular dysfunction. Likewise, some steroid hormones are conjugated in the liver before their excretion in the urine. The failure to detoxify aldosterone is a possible factor in the formation of ascites. The gynecomastia, testicular atrophy, and loss of body hair sometimes seen in male patients with cirrhosis have been attributed to estrogen excess resulting from inadequate inactivation.

Hepatic Encephalopathy. Patients with chronic liver disease often exhibit steady deterioration in their intellect: forgetfulness and confusion can progress to stupor and finally to coma. Ataxia and a characteristic "flapping" tremor of the outstretched hands are noteworthy accompaniments. The neuropsychiatric manifestations may be chronic, with the patient exhibiting personality changes, mental deterioration, and other neurologic symptoms. On the other hand, the syndrome may be acute and terminate in coma with convulsions.

Animals with a portacaval shunt, or Eck shunt,* can be maintained in a reasonable state of health if given a low-protein diet. If given a large protein meal, they develop coma and die rapidly ("meat intoxication"). It is believed that these manifestations are caused by nitrogenous substances; their precise nature is not known, but ammonia, phenol, octopamine, and gamma-aminobutyric acid (GABA) have all been suggested. Hepatic encephalopathy is seen in patients who have undergone a similar portacaval anastomosis as treatment for cirrhosis of the liver.

Acute encephalopathy is sometimes precipitated by bleeding esophageal varices; the explanation is that a large quantity of protein-containing blood passes into the intestine and amounts to a heavy protein meal. Since bacterial action in the intestine appears to lead to the formation of damaging nitrogenous products, the administration of the antibiotic neomycin is currently recommended. It is also of some value in chronic liver disease with impending encephalopathy.

---

*This is an artificial shunt made surgically between the portal vein and the inferior vena cava. Portal blood tends to flow directly into the vena cave rather than through the liver.

Osteodystrophy. Bone changes, termed hepatic osteodystrophy, having features of osteomalacia, osteoporosis, or a combination of the two, are seen in some cases of terminal liver failure. The pathogenesis of this painful condition is not understood.

Terminal Manifestations of Hepatic Failure. As the patient's condition deteriorates, certain ill-understood events occur. The plasma sodium level falls, probably because of the intracellular deviation of sodium, and not because of excessive excretion, because administration of salt is not beneficial but, in fact, hastens death by producing circulatory overload and widespread edema. A terminal rise in blood urea nitrogen is common and appears to be due to renal failure. This is common in severe hepatic failure, and the combination is known as the *hepatorenal syndrome*. It is debatable whether this is a separate entity. It probably represents renal failure occurring for a variety of reasons in a patient with terminal liver disease.

DEGENERATIVE CONDITIONS OF THE LIVER

The liver cells are very susceptible to the effects of many poisons. Poisonous mushrooms, carbon tetrachloride, chloroform, and many drugs (important among which is the anesthetic agent halothane) can all cause severe liver damage, either by a direct action or by some type of hypersensitivity response. Infections, in particular by the viruses of hepatitis, can also produce liver damage.

The effects of hepatotoxic agents can vary from mild cloudy swelling and fatty change to extensive necrosis. There is a variable inflammatory response, and the terms "hepatic necrosis" and "hepatitis" are often used synonymously.

Hepatic Necrosis

If the liver cells are severely affected, they undergo necrosis. This usually has a *zonal distribution*; that is, the cells of a particular zone in every lobule undergo necrosis. Centrilobular necrosis (affecting Rappaport's zone 3) is the most common (Fig. 24–6). Sometimes the foci of necrosis are erratically distributed: such a response is termed *focal*, or *spotty, necrosis*. It is typical of acute viral hepatitis (Fig. 24–7).

Necrosis may be more widespread and connect central veins to each other and to portal tracts. This is termed *bridging hepatic necrosis* (Fig. 24–7). Causes include hepatitis B infection; non-A, non-B hepatitis; hepatitis due to drugs; and chronic active hepatitis of unknown cause.

Occasionally the necrosis is massive and panlobular. Wide tracts of liver are destroyed. This *massive hepatic necrosis* is a feature of acute fulminant hepatitis. Causes include viral hepatitis and acute poisoning; often no cause can be identified.

The outcome of necrosis depends on the severity of the lesions and whether the cause persists. With *zonal and focal necrosis*, the patient may have no symptoms or may suffer from an acute febrile illness with jaundice and gastrointestinal symptoms and then recover. The necrotic liver cells autolyze and are removed; the sinusoidal structure and reticulin framework of the liver lobules remain intact and there is excellent regeneration as surviving liver cells divide to replace those that are lost so that there is complete restoration of the liver to normal.

Bridging necrosis is a more serious affair, for although recovery is still possible, the process may pursue a chronic course; regeneration occurs

from isolated groups of liver cells that remain. Since the scaffold on which these cells may be arranged has largely been destroyed or has collapsed, irregular nodules termed *regeneration nodules* are formed. The final result is one form of cirrhosis of the liver (*macronodular cirrhosis*) (Fig. 24–7).

With massive necrosis, the patient can die of acute liver failure in the initial phases. In the few patients who recover, remaining liver cells can regenerate quickly before the lobular framework collapses. The liver therefore *returns to normal*. In some cases it is probable that regeneration nodules are formed, and this results in cirrhosis.

Fatty Liver

Fatty change is an important lesion and can be caused by an inappropriate diet. Starvation and overeating both cause fatty change, but an imbalanced diet results in the most severe change (see Kwashiorkor, Chapter 15). It is also common in chronic alcoholism.

If the cause of fatty liver is removed, complete recovery is usual; such recovery is not possible if the condition is due to alcoholism and is allowed to persist indefinitely. Gradually, fibrous tissue forms around Rappaport's acinus. Hepatic cells become isolated as the lobules are split up. Some cells undergo necrosis, whereas others regenerate. This results in a finely nodular cirrhotic liver (Fig. 24–8).

Fatty liver is characteristic of *Reye's syndrome*, an acute, often fatal illness of infants and children up to the age of 15 years that typically follows infection with influenza A or B viruses or chickenpox. The pathogenesis is not known, but an important additional factor is the administration of aspirin; hence, *this drug should not be given to children with influenza or chickenpox*. Cerebral edema causing acute encephalopathy is also characteristic of Reye's syndrome; in patients who survive, there is residual neurologic damage.

Acute fatty liver is a rare complication of the last trimester of *pregnancy*. Typically there is sudden onset of nausea, vomiting, jaundice, and liver failure.

ZONAL NECROSIS

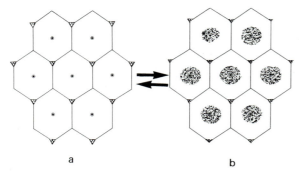

a   b

Figure 24–6 Zonal hepatic necrosis. *A,* The classic liver lobules are represented as hexagons. *B,* The shaded areas depict necrosis, which in this example is centrilobular in distribution. (Drawn by Rasa Skudra, Artlab Two Thousand, Toronto.

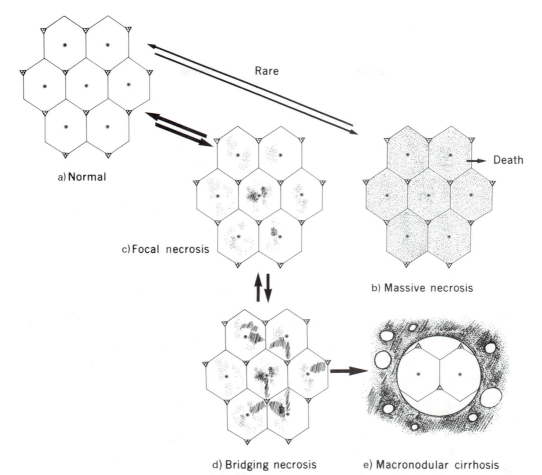

a) Normal

c) Focal necrosis

b) Massive necrosis

Rare

Death

d) Bridging necrosis

e) Macronodular cirrhosis

Figure 24–7 Focal and massive hepatic necrosis. Massive necrosis *(b)* generally results in death from cholemia. Occasionally, the liver cells regenerate so rapidly that the liver structure returns to normal *(a)*. Focal or spotty necrosis *(c)* is typical of viral hepatitis. The areas of necrosis are distributed erratically throughout the liver lobules. Usually recovery is complete, but in some cases, necrosis is more extensive and connects central veins to each other and to portal tracts. This is bridging necrosis *(d)*. Fibrosis often follows, and a macronodular type of cirrhosis develops *(e)*. Note that the regeneration nodules vary greatly in size and that in the large nodules, areas of normal lobular structure remain. (Drawn by Rasa Skudra, Artlab Two Thousand, Toronto.

Drug-Induced Liver Damage

The liver is responsible for detoxifying many drugs; during this process, toxic intermediates can be formed as is described with acetaminophen (Chapter 4). Some drugs produce liver dysfunction to all individuals provided a sufficient dose is given. The dose needed to cause damage varies from one individual to another because of individual susceptibility. Hence, even a "normal" dose of a drug may lead to trouble in the rare individual who is highly susceptible (*e.g.,* the birth control pill; see later).

Drugs in this group include erythromycin estolate (not the base or other salts), acetaminophen, carbon tetrachloride and other halogenated hydrocarbons used in industry, furosemide, and many anticancer drugs, *e.g.,* methotrexate.

Certain steroids such as methyltestosterone and norethandrolone cause cholestatic jaundice apparently by inhibiting the peristalsis of canalicular membranes. Estrogens in large doses have a similar effect and in susceptible women lead to jaundice during pregnancy or after the administration of the birth control pill.

The great majority of adverse reactions to

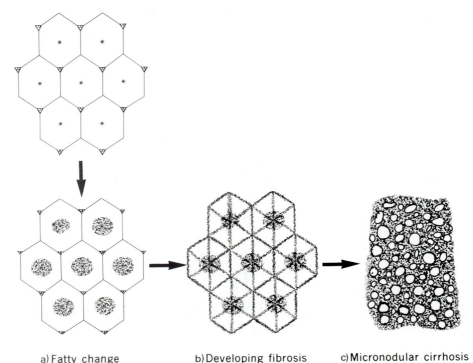

a) Fatty change   b) Developing fibrosis   c) Micronodular cirrhosis

Figure 24–8 Alcoholic liver disease. In the early stages of alcoholic liver disease, fatty changes develop in the centrilobular zones *(a)*. Gradually liver cells undergo necrosis, and fibrous tissue forms around the acini of Rappaport *(b)*. In this way, the lobules are split up, and multiple small regenerative nodules are produced. Micronodular hepatic cirrhosis is the end result *(c)*. (Drawn by Rasa Skudra, Artlab Two Thousand, Toronto.

drugs occur unpredictably. Few individuals are affected and often the damage is immunologically mediated; concurrent fever, arthralgia, and blood eosinophilia point to such a mechanism. Several patterns of reaction are recognized. *Cholestatic hepatitis* is most commonly caused by chlorpromazine, and about 1 per cent of patients on this drug develop an obstructive type of jaundice after one month's therapy regardless of dose. An *acute hepatitic pattern* is the most serious type of drug-induced liver damage; both clinically and pathologically it resembles acute viral hepatitis. Drugs causing this hepatitic reaction include the anesthetic agent halothane, methyldopa, rifampicin, isoniazid, and para-aminosalicylic acid.

VIRAL INFECTIONS OF THE LIVER

Many viruses, *e.g.*, the virus of yellow fever, cytomegalovirus, herpes simplex virus, and the Epstein-Barr virus, can cause hepatitis. However, the term "acute viral hepatitis" is commonly applied to a common acute illness caused by a group of viruses that, although of different structure, produce a similar type of illness.

Acute Viral Hepatitis

At least three types of acute viral hepatitis are known. *Virus A hepatitis* is due to hepatitis A virus (HAV) and has in the past been called infectious or epidemic hepatitis. *Virus B hepatitis* is due to hepatitis B virus (HBV); it is known as serum hepatitis. A third type of illness is due to neither of these agents and is provisionally termed *non-A, non-B viral hepatitis*. It probably includes several separate agents; one of them is hepatitis virus C.

Symptoms of Viral Hepatitis

The onset is usually insidious with mild fatigue, lassitude, and sometimes fever. Nausea, vomiting, and diarrhea are not uncommon, and an aversion to both food and cigarette smoking is a curious but common symptom. Such a vague illness may be the only manifestation of hepatitis (*acute nonicteric viral hepatitis*), but in more severe cases, jaundice appears (*acute icteric viral hepatitis*). Occasionally the jaundice may be severe and of the obstructive type, thereby mimicking obstructive jaundice of extrahepatic type, *e.g.*, due to a stone (*acute cholestatic viral hepatitis*). Recovery is the usual end result, but it may take 3 to 4 months or even longer.

Hepatitis B tends to have a more insidious onset than does hepatitis A. During the early stages, evidence of immune complex disease can occur—fever, arthralgia, and erythematous or urticarial skin eruptions. Hepatitis B tends to be more severe; in a few cases, the disease progresses either to massive hepatic necrosis ending in death (*acute fulminant hepatitis*) or to a chronic form of liver disease (*chronic hepatitis*) that may culminate in *cirrhosis* or finally *carcinoma*.

Etiology, Epidemiology, and Course of Viral Hepatitis

The three types of hepatitis are described separately.

Viral Hepatitis A. Viral hepatitis A is caused by HAV, a small RNA picornavirus 25 to 28 nm in size. The virus is present in the stools for about 5 days in patients who are incubating hepatitis, but with the onset of the clinical disease, the virus rapidly disappears.

Hepatitis A has an incubation period of 2 to 6 weeks and commonly occurs in institutions like schools and military camp. It is contracted by the ingestion of food or water contaminated with feces (fecal-oral route). The disease is generally mild, and recovery is complete in virtually 100 per cent of cases. Subclinical hepatitis A infection in childhood is common in North America as witnessed by the fact that 60 per cent of the population have anti-HAV antibodies. The anti-

bodies are protective, and such individuals have lifelong immunity to the disease.

Viral Hepatitis B. Viral hepatitis B is caused by HBV, which is a double-shelled 42-nm DNA-containing virus. The virus is complex and has a central core (the Dane particle) and an outer coat, both of which are antigenic. The virus is present in the blood of patients with hepatitis and in carriers.

Antigens of HBV

Hepatitis B Surface Antigen (HBsAg). This antigen was first called *Australian antigen* because it was originally found in the blood of an Australian aborigine. It is a component of the surface of the virus particle, but since it is produced in great excess in infected individuals, it is also present free both in liver cells and in the blood. In the blood, two forms are detectable electron microscopically. One is a 22-nm spherical particle and the other is a long tubular form about 20-nm in diameter and of variable length (Figs. 24–9 and 24–10).

Hepatitis B Core Antigen (HBcAg). This can be demonstrated only after disruption of the outer shell of the virus. It is not demonstrable in the blood but may be found in the nuclei of the liver of infected patients. The core also contains a second "e" antigen (HBeAg), and the presence of this antigen in the blood is associated with infectivity.

Antibodies to these various antigens may be found in the blood, and present evidence suggests that whereas anti-HBcAg provides no immunity, anti-HBsAg provides good protection. Effective vaccines have been developed. The first (Hepatavax-B) consisted of the 22-nm HBsAg particles purified from the blood of carriers and inactivated. By utilization of the techniques of recombinant DNA technology, this has now been replaced by HBsAg antigen made by yeast cells into which the appropriate gene has been spliced (Engerix-B). About 15 per cent of the North American population have anti-HBsAg and are presumably immune to infection, having recovered from a subclinical attack of the disease. Hepatitis B is transmitted predominantly by the parenteral route, by blood transfusion, by the use of blood products, or by the contaminated needles or syringes of intravenous drug abusers. Needle-stick accidents are a harzard to health

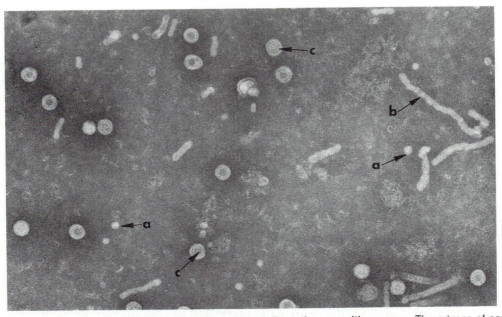

Figure 24–9 Hepatitis B; negative-stained preparation of Australia antigen–positive serum. Three types of particle can be seen: spherical particles 20 nm in diameter (a); elongated tubular filaments up to 230 nm in length, 20 nm in diameter (b); and Dane particles, 42 nm in diameter and having a double shell (c) (×119,700). (Courtesy of Micheline Fauvel, Laboratoire de Santé Publigue du Québec.)

workers. Since the body secretions are also known to contain the virus, infection by close contact, such as kissing and sexual intercourse, may be a means of contracting the disease. HVB infection is particularly prevalent in male homosexuals. Those whose work entails close contact with human blood are also at risk— laboratory technicians and the staff of renal dialysis units. Vertical transmission from infected mother to infant also occurs during the perinatal period, either during delivery via blood and secretions or during the immediate postnatal period.

The incubation period of hepatitis B ranges from 6 weeks to 6 months. The disease cannot be distinguished clinically from hepatitis A, although it tends to be more severe. The mortality is 1 to 2 per cent. About 90 per cent of patients recover completely and the remaining 10 per cent develop chronic hepatitis. A carrier state develops in 5 to 10 per cent of infected persons, and they may or may not have evidence of continuing liver damage. Approximately 0.1 per cent of North Americans are carriers, but in some parts of the world, *e.g.*, Southeast Asia, the carrier rate

is approximately 15 per cent of the population and in some areas even up to 30 per cent.

Viral Hepatitis Non-A, Non-B. It was anticipated that the testing and elimination of all HBsAg-positive persons as blood donors would virtually eliminate the hazard of acquiring hepatitis by transfusion, but this has not been the case; 90 per cent of post-transfusion hepatitis is due to a virus that is neither HAV nor HBV and has been provisionally labeled non-A, non-B. This is probably not a single entity but a group of separate viruses. Complex DNA technology has indicated the presence of one agent, termed hepatitis virus C.

The Delta Virus. The delta virus is a defective RNA virus, the core of which is encapsulated by the surface antigen of hepatitis virus B. It can survive only in patients infected with HBV, and its presence contributes to the development of fulminant hepatitis, severe progressive chronic active hepatitis, and cirrhosis. The infection is endemic in Mediterranean countries and Venezuela but is becoming more common in nonendemic areas such as northern Europe and the United States.

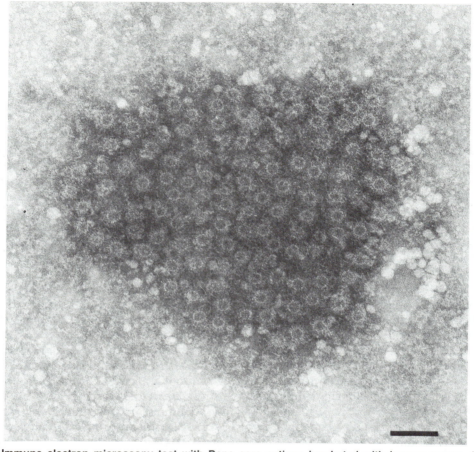

Figure 24–10 Immune electron microscopy test with Dane core antigen incubated with human serum. A concentrated sample of Dane particles was treated with a detergent (polysorbate 80) in order to disrupt the outer coat and release the internal component. This Dane core measures 27 nm in diameter. The suspension of particles was incubated with serum from a patient who had recovered from an attack of virus B hepatitis. An anticore antibody causes the core particles to adhere to each other and form immune complexes. This method can be used to detect anti-HBcAg (bar represents 100 nm)($\times$119, 700). (From Fauvel, M., Babiuk, L., Sheaff, E.T., and Spence, L: Preparation of a Dane core (hepatitis B) antigen from human plasma. Canadian Journal of Microbiology, *21*:905–910, 1975.)

Morphology of the Liver in Viral Hepatitis

The liver shows focal necrosis throughout the lobules. The loss of liver cells, often called *liver cell dropout*, causes interruption in the pattern of the plates of liver cells so that the normal orderly lobular appearance is difficult to make out. This *disarray of the lobules* is highly characteristic of viral hepatitis. Side by side with the degenerative changes and necrosis there is a lymphocytic infiltrate and evidence of liver cell regeneration in the form of mitotic figures, binucleate cells, and variation in size and shape of the hepatocytes. Sometimes recovery is delayed and may take 3 or 4 months or even longer. A liver biopsy performed during this period may show continuing focal hepatic necrosis (*chronic lobular hepatitis*) or merely a lymphocytic infiltrate in the portal triads (*chronic persistent hepatitis*). In either event the prognosis is excellent, and the distinction between these two types of chronic hepatitis is made on the biopsy findings. It is of academic interest only.

In severe cases of hepatitis, the necrosis is more extensive and confluent, thereby joining portal triads to central veins. This is termed *bridging necrosis* (previously called subacute hepatic necrosis). Recovery is still possible, but in some subjects the process continues. It may end fatally or progress more slowly to chronic active hepatitis and cirrhosis. Rarely in acute hepatitis the necrosis is massive and affects the whole of many lobules. This is the pathology of acute fulminant hepatitis.

The pathogenesis of viral hepatitis is not understood. The liver damage appears to be due not to the direct presence of the virus in the cells but to an immunologic reaction, possibly to the liver cell membrane altered by the presence of viral antigen. Hepatitis B antigens can be detected in the liver, but there is an inverse relationship between the amount of virus demonstrable and the severity of the disease; for instance, a great excess of HBsAg is seen in the cytoplasm in carriers who have minimal or no disease. These cells have characteristic groundglass cytoplasm.

OTHER INFECTIONS OF THE LIVER

Blood-borne infections can be complicated by hepatic involvement, *e.g.*, miliary tuberculosis, leptospirosis, secondary and tertiary syphilis, and pyemia. Liver involvement in schistosomiasis, hydatid disease, and amebiasis is particularly important where these diseases are endemic.

Infection may reach the liver via the biliary tree. Ascending cholangitis, sometimes with abscess formation, is a complication of obstruction, commonly a stone, to the outflow of bile from the liver.

CHRONIC HEPATITIS

Chronic hepatitis is defined as chronic inflammation of the liver continuing without improvement for at least 6 months. Needle biopsy of the liver must be done to establish the diagnosis and prognosis. In practice, the term "chronic hepatitis" is not used to describe alcoholic hepatitis, cholangitis, and any inflammatory lesion of obvious infective nature. *Chronic lobular hepatitis* and *chronic persistent hepatitis* have been described

previously and are found in patients with delayed recovery from an attack of acute hepatitis. Chronic active hepatitis is a serious condition and is described in more detail.

Chronic Active Hepatitis

Chronic hepatitis is a clinicopathologic entity that can have a number of different causes. In addition to an infiltrate of lymphocytes and plasma cells in the portal tracts, there is necrosis of the adjacent liver cells. This process is called *piecemeal necrosis*. The formation of fibrous tissue is stimulated, and the steady destruction of liver cells with replacement fibrosis frequently results in cirrhosis.

The first recognized type of chronic active hepatitis usually affects young women and is accompanied by the presence of a variety of autoantibodies in the blood. Antibodies that react with smooth muscle are present in most cases, and both antinuclear and rheumatoid factors are usually present in the blood. For this reason, the disease was initially called "lupoid hepatitis," although there is no evidence that it is related to lupus erythematosus. The clinicopathologic syndrome of chronic active hepatitis has now been extended to include other groups of patients. This heterogeneous group includes cases related to drug toxicity, alpha$_1$-antitrypsin deficiency, or chronic infection with HVB.

CIRRHOSIS OF THE LIVER

The term "cirrhosis" (from Greek *kirrhos*, orange yellow + *nosos*, disease) was introduced by Laennec, who was impressed by the tawny color of the liver in this condition, but this is due merely to fatty change of the liver cells. The important structural features of cirrhosis are the *destruction of the liver parenchyma* and its *replacement by fibrous tissue*, thereby disrupting the normal lobular architecture. There is also active regeneration of the liver cells occurring at the same time as this fibrous reparative process. The *formation of regenerative nodules* is the third essential component of cirrhosis.

Cirrhosis is best regarded as an end-stage condition resulting from liver damage due to any cause: poisons, alcohol, inadequate diet, infection, genetic error, and others. Unfortunately, an etiologic classification of cirrhosis is unsatisfactory, because the cause is unknown in many cases (*crytogenic cirrhosis*). For purposes of disease classification, the condition is categorized by descriptions that are based on the gross appearance of the liver. If the nodules are small and of uniform size, the term *micronodular cirrhosis* is applied (Fig. 24–11). This condition commonly, but not always, is due to alcohol abuse. It contrasts with *macronodular cirrhosis*, in which the nodules are of varying size, many of them being large and containing areas of normal lobular structure. Broad bands of fibrous tissue surround the nodules (Fig. 24–12). In the past this type of cirrhosis has been called postnecrotic or posthepatitic cirrhosis, misleading terms because it rarely follows an overt attack of hepatitis or hepatic necrosis. The most common cause is chronic active hepatitis. In practice, there is no sharp line of demarcation between these two types of cirrhosis; many cases fall into a mixed group, and the macronodular type can evolve from micronodular cirrhosis (Figs. 24–13 and 24–14).

Symptoms of Cirrhosis. Cirrhosis is commonly asymptomatic until some complication makes the condition obvious. The appearance of jaundice, edema of the ankles, or progressive abdominal enlargement may bring the disease to the attention of the patient. Increasing weakness, loss of weight, loss of body hair, and testicular atrophy are all features that may appear. Commonly the first symptom is massive hematemesis, and this is followed by the rapid development of hepatocellular failure with coma and death.

Case History I

The patient was a 62-year-old woman with a long history of chronic alcoholism. Six days before admission to a hospital, she noticed black tarry stools (melena). A few days later, she vomited about pint of blood. On admission, her blood pressure was 95/60 mm Hg, and she was in a state of shock. Her abdomen was distended because of ascites, and her spleen could not be felt. Jaundice was not evident. Laboratory investigations at this time revealed the following:

Serum bilirubin: 29 µmol/L (normal less than 20 µmol/ L)
Serum proteins:
    Albumin: 18 g/L (normal 40 to 50 g/L)
    Globulin: 39 g/L (normal 25 to 35 g/L)
    Total: 57 g/L (normal 65 to 80 g/L)
Serum potassium: 2.5 mmol (normal 3.2 to 4.7 mmol/L
Hemoglobin: 109 g/L, red blood cells normochromic and normocytic

The hypokalemia was attributed to previous diuretic therapy. Gastroscopy revealed bleeding esophageal varices, but in spite of transfusion and other supportive treatment, the blood pressure continued to fall, and the patient became more and more confused. She

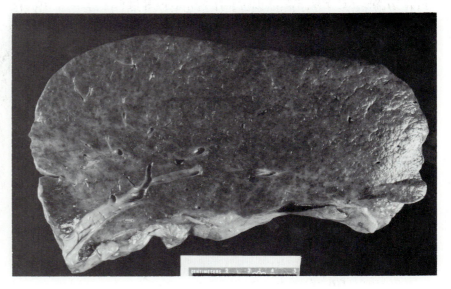

Figure 24–11 Micronodular cirrhosis of the liver. The cut surface of the specimen shows complete loss of the normal lobular pattern (compare with Fig. 24–2). The liver parenchyma now consists of poorly delineated regeneration nodules that are best seen where light is reflected from the surface of the right-hand side of the picture. In some areas, extensive fibrosis appears as obvious gray-white tissue. The specimen is from a patient who died of bleeding esophageal varices and who exhibited little clinical evidence of hepatic dysfunction until shortly before death. For a more complete description, see Case History I.

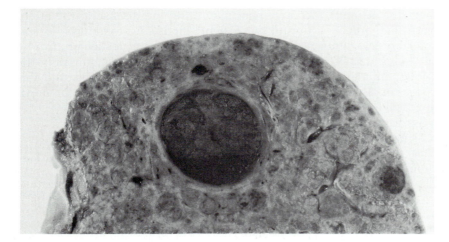

Figure 24–12 Macronodular cirrhosis of the liver. There is replacement of the liver by regeneration nodules that vary greatly in size. The two large hemorrhagic nodules consist of hepatoma.

vomited a small quantity of blood on several occasions but showed no obvious dramatic hemorrhage. Terminally, her urine output diminished, her blood urea nitrogen rose to 32 mmol/L, and the patient suffered a cardiac arrest. She was successfully resuscitated but had a second arrest and was pronounced dead.

Necropsy revealed bilateral pleural effusions and 1500 ml of ascites. There were multiple small acute gastric erosions, and the small hematemeses occurring in the hospital were attributed to them. The kidneys were swollen because of edema, but necrosis was not detectable microscopically (Chapter 25). The cirrhotic liver, which weighed 1900 g (normal, about 1500 g), is shown in Figure 24–11. Esophageal varices were present, but no definite point of bleeding could be iden-

tified; this is often difficult, since the veins are emptied of blood after death.

Ascites is a common manifestation of cirrhosis and has several causes. Hypoalbuminemia and aldosterone excess are contributory factors, but the main cause appears to be obstruction of the flow of blood through the liver. This obstruction is postsinusoidal and results in an increased rate of formation of lymph in the liver. Normally the lymph is drained away by lymphatics into the thoracic duct, but in cirrhosis, the excess of lymph produced oozes or weeps from the liver

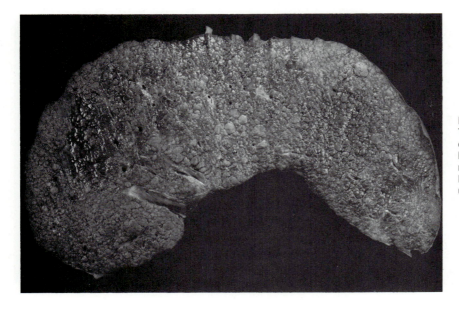

Figure 24–13 Cirrhosis of the liver. The cut surface of the liver shows complete replacement of normal liver by regenerative nodules. Many of the nodules are small, but others are larger. See Figure 24–14 for close-up view.

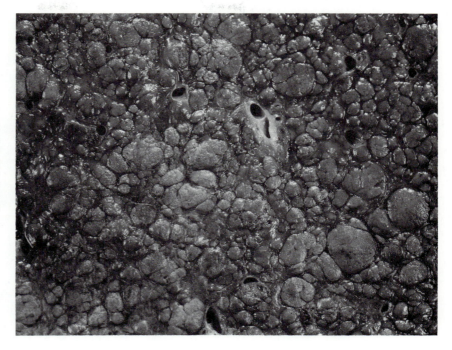

Figure 24–14 Cirrhosis of the liver. This is part of the liver shown in Figure. 24–13. Note the wide variation in the size of the nodules. On microscopic examination, recognizable lobular structures can be identified in the large nodules. This example of cirrhosis may therefore be classified as of mixed type.

and drips into the peritoneal cavity. A second effect of portal hypertension is an increased transudate of fluid from the surface of the viscera drained by the portal vein. This fluid presumably has a low protein content. When it is added to the lymph from the liver, the result is an ascitic fluid having a protein content of 10 to 20 g/L. Most of this protein is albumin. Relief of ascites by removal of the fluid also removes much albumin, often adding to the patient's problems. Also the sudden removal of a large quantity of fluid can lead to hypovolemia and shock.

The other symptoms of terminal cirrhosis—including neuropsychiatric features, coma, and a bleeding tendency—have been described under hepatocellular failure.

Alcohol and the Liver

Alcoholism has long been linked to the development of cirrhosis of the liver; as might be expected, the increasing alcohol consumption associated with affluence has elevated cirrhosis of the liver to a leading cause of death in North America. The mechanism of liver damage in alcoholism is not settled. It has been attributed to a nutritional deficiency brought about by the preference that alcoholics have for alcohol over normal food. It seems more likely that alcohol has a direct toxic effect on the liver possibly related to a subtle metabolic defect secondary to the conversion of alcohol to acetaldehyde with consumption of ATP. About 20 per cent of heavy drinkers develop cirrhosis of the liver, and it is evident that factors other than alcoholism play a part in its pathogenesis. A genetic predisposition is suspected.

The liver of the chronic alcoholic often shows fatty change, and an alcoholic spree may cause an acute fatty liver with cholestatic jaundice. In some subjects, fibrosis occurs around the terminal hepatic (central) veins. This is termed central hyaline sclerosis.

Some alcoholics, particularly spree drinkers, sustain repeated attacks of alcoholic hepatitis. Liver cells, usually in Rappaport's zone 3, undergo necrosis, whereas others become swollen and contain coarse hyaline clumps or skeins of eosinophilic material composed of intermediate filaments and called *alcoholic hyaline or the Mallory body* (Fig. 24–15). Repeated episodes of alcoholic hepatitis with necrosis lead to progressive fibrosis around the terminal hepatic veins

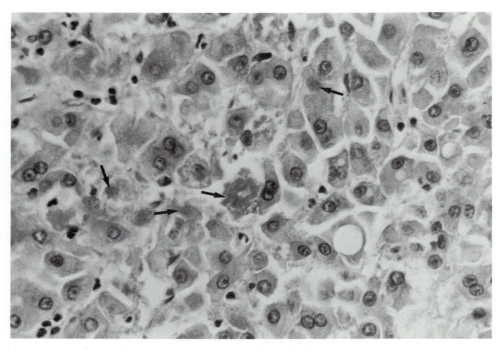

Figure 24–15 Alcoholic hyaline. This section is from a patient with alcoholic hepatitis. Some hepatocytes appear necrotic; they are enlarged and have no nuclei. Irregular clumps of alcoholic hyaline are present in many of the cells (arrows) but are best seen in this section in the necrotic cells. A scattered infiltrate of neutrophils is present.

(*central hyaline sclerosis*); the obstruction so caused can lead to portal hypertension and ascites, even in the absence of cirrhosis. With increasing alcoholic damage, Rappaport's acini are dissected out by fibrous bands that connect the triads with the terminal hepatic veins. The regenerative nodules typical of cirrhosis form isolated groups of liver cells.

Alcoholic Cirrhosis of the Liver

In the initial stages, the liver in alcoholic cirrhosis may be enlarged, particularly if the patient continues drinking and fatty change is marked. As fibrosis increases, the liver becomes small and hard; it has a finely nodular surface of the classic hobnail liver. On section there is uniform appearance of micronodular cirrhosis. Later, extensive fibrosis can produce wide bands of collagenous tissue, and areas may resemble those of postnecrotic cirrhosis. At this stage, the cirrhosis is labeled mixed micro-macronodular type.

Other Types of Cirrhosis

Cirrhosis is a feature of hemochromatosis, Wilson's disease, and alpha₁-antitrypsin deficiency. In hemochromatosis, also called bronzed diabetes, there is a genetic error that leads to abnormal accumulation of hemosiderin in many organs. This causes damage. Involvement of the liver leads to cirrhosis, the myocardium to heart failure, and the islets of Langerhans to diabetes mellitus. In Wilson's disease, there is deposition of copper in liver and central nervous system. Alpha₁-antitrypsin deficiency is described in Chapter 16. Indian childhood cirrhosis encountered in Southeast Asia and the Middle East as well as in India is of unknown etiology but may be related to copper toxicity.

Biliary Cirrhosis. Obstruction to the bile duct, particularly if combined with infection (*cholangitis*), can sometimes lead to such severe liver cell damage that cirrhosis develops. There is, in addition, a *primary form of biliary cirrhosis*. This is most frequently encountered in middle-aged women. Itching is usually the first symptom, and this is followed by the development of obstructive jaundice. The disease has an autoimmune component, for the blood contains IgM antibodies active against bile duct components as well as IgG anti-mitochondrial antibodies. The detection of the latter is a useful diagnostic feature of primary biliary cirrhosis.

NEOPLASMS OF THE LIVER

The finding of one or more *vascular hamartomas* (hemangiomas) of the liver is a common event at necropsy, but apart from the very rare occurrence of intraperitoneal bleeding, these are of no significance during life (Fig. 24–2). *Adenomas* are rare, although recently a number of cases have been reported in women on the birth control pill. The tumors are vascular and clinically can present as a sudden intraperitoneal hemorrhage. This appears to be a rare complication of taking the birth control pill, but since the event has only recently been recognized, its true incidence has yet to be determined.

Carcinoma of the Liver

Cancer of the liver can arise in a normal liver, but it is more often encountered in livers that are already the site of some other disease, most commonly cirrhosis (Figs. 24–12 and 24–16). Nevertheless, many other factors are involved, for although in North America and Europe it has been estimated that between 4 and 10 per cent of patients with cirrhosis eventually develop cancer of the liver, in some parts of Africa and the Orient the figure is closer to 60 per cent. Additional factors that seem to be involved are the ingestion of aflatoxin, an alkaloid derived from a fungus that infects peanuts, in the African diet, and chronic infection with hepatitis B virus.

Two types of primary carcinoma of the liver are recognized.

Hepatoma. This tumor is composed of atypical hepatocytes and usually occurs in patients with cirrhosis. Quite often, portal vein invasion and thrombosis lead to the sudden development of ascites in a patient known to have cirrhosis. Massive hepatomegaly is usually a feature. Tumor cells may contain HBsAg, alpha$_1$-antitrypsin, and alpha$_1$-fetoprotein. Indeed, elevated blood levels of alpha$_1$-fetoprotein are common in patients with hepatocellular carcinoma but are not diagnostic of this tumor since they are also raised, but to a lesser level, in cirrhosis and other nonmalignant hepatic diseases.

Cholangiocarcinoma. About 20 per cent of primary liver tumors are derived from the bile ducts, and histologically they are scirrhous adenocarcinomas. Cirrhosis of the liver is less often a precursor to this type of cancer than it is to hepatoma.

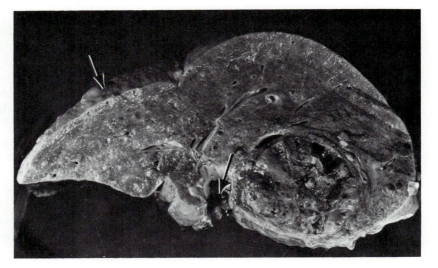

Figure 24–16 Carcinoma of the liver. The specimen shows a large, spherical mass of tumor with several small satellite nodules. The tumor has invaded the inferior vena cava, and there is superimposed thrombosis (arrow at lower center). The remainder of the liver shows the characteristic feature of a micronodular cirrhosis. The nodularity can be seen best on the surface of the liver (arrow at upper left).

The patient had a 13-year history of chronic liver disease and had died following massive bleeding from ruptured esophageal varices. Necropsy revealed tumor invasion of the vena cava and the portal vein. Small pulmonary deposits were the only metastases found. Splenomegaly, ascites, edema of the legs, and testicular atrophy were other findings related to the liver disease.

Secondary Neoplasms of the Liver

It has been estimated that metastatic liver carcinoma is found in about 36 per cent of all cancer patients. It is more common in patients with cancer of the breast, stomach, and colon than in those having primary tumors of other sites. The liver is also a common site for metastatic melanoma.

A raised level of plasma alkaline phosphatase is characteristic of metastatic tumor and is a useful clinical test. Each nodule of tumor obstructs a number of small bile ducts, and the test is positive before there is significant retention of bilirubin. Except as a terminal event, jaundice is not common in tumors of the liver unless there is an associated cirrhosis. This emphasizes the tremendous reserve capacity of the liver and its ability to regenerate.

The Biliary Tract

Bile is formed continuously by the liver and passes down the *intrahepatic bile ducts* to reach the *common bile duct*. This duct empties into the duodenum, and its orifice is guarded by the *sphincter of Oddi*. Immediately above the sphincter there is a dilation called the *ampulla of Vater*. The sphincter of Oddi is normally closed, and bile therefore flows through the *cystic duct* to reach the *gallbladder*, where it is stored and concentrated. When gastric contents—particularly those containing fat—enter the duodenum, the duodenal mucosa secretes a hormone (*cholecystokinin*) that causes the gallbladder to contract and the sphincter of Oddi to relax. Bile then enters the duodenum.

Diseases of the gallbladder are frequent. Inflammation of this organ (*cholecystitis*) ranks with appendicitis as a cause of abdominal pain requiring surgical exploration. The presence of gallstones (*cholelithiasis*) is often associated with inflammation: this topic is discussed first.

CHOLELITHIASIS

Gallstones may be found in any part of the biliary tract, but they are most frequent in the gallbladder. They are more common in women than in men, in a ratio of about four to one. Pregnancy appears to predispose to stone formation, and the typical sufferer is caricatured as being "female, fertile, fat, and forty." Nevertheless, gallstone disease often affects young adults, and any associated with obesity appears to be without foundation.

Types of Gallstones. Gallstones are occasionally composed of pure cholesterol (usually solitary stones) or bile pigments (calcium bilirubinate); most gallstones are *mixed* and consist of cholesterol, bile salts, and calcium salts. Often they are multiple (Figs. 24–17 and 24–18).

Cause of Gallstones. Until recently, *infection* and *stasis* were considered to be the main factors leading to gallstone formation. It is now thought that infection and stasis are the *effects* of cholelithasis, and that the major cause is the *secretion of an abnormal bile by the liver*. The large amount of cholesterol in bile is kept in solution by its being aggregated to form *micelles* having an outer coating of lecithin and bile salts. A deficiency of bile salt formation appears to be the major factor in producing gallstones. Recently, attempts have been made to alter the composition of bile by medical treatment. Chenodeoxycholic acid by mouth appears to lead to the dissolution of cholesterol stones, and there is every hope that in the future the treatment of cholelithiasis will be medical and not surgical.

Complications of Gallstones. The most common complications are obstruction and infection.

Obstruction. A stone may become impacted in the neck of the gallbladder or in the cystic duct. Because bile cannot enter the gallbladder, it becomes distended with mucus (*mucocele*). A stone impacted in the bile duct (*e.g.,* in the ampulla of Vater) causes intermittent obstruction with ob-

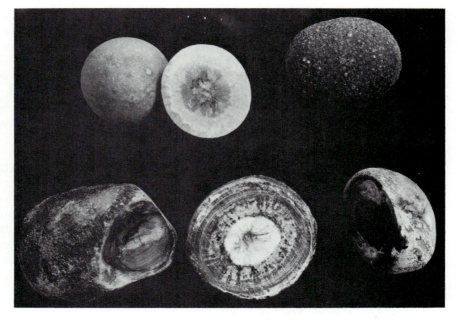

Figure 24–17 Gallstones. The two gallstones shown in the upper part of the picture were solitary stones, each being found in a separate gallbladder. The stones are composed mainly of cholesterol. One of the stones has been bisected to show its internal structure; the appearance of lines radiating from the center is due to crystal of cholesterol. The three faceted stones in the lower part of the picture were found in one gallbladder. One has been cut and shows a pale center of cholesterol. This is surrounded by rings that contain varying amounts of bile pigment. These stones are considered "mixed".

structive jaundice. This condition fluctuates in intensity in contrast to the progressive jaundice of carcinoma.

If a gallstone suddenly obstructs one of the bile passages, distention of the wall causes severe pain that is felt in the midline of the abdomen. The common cause is a stone in the cystic duct. The pain is of sudden onset, persists for some hours with unremitting severity, and then abates as suddenly as it began. This is called *biliary colic*

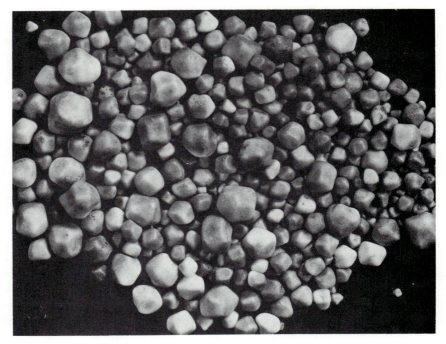

Figure 24–18 Gallstones. One gallbladder contained these small mixed stones. Note how each is faceted as a result of contact with its neighbors during its formation. Several "families" of stones are present.

and differs from intestinal colic, in which crampy pains recur and remit at intervals.

Infection. The presence of stones in the gall-bladder predisposes the patient to the development of cholecystitis. Likewise, a stone in the common bile duct predisposes to infection in the entire intrahepatic biliary system (*ascending cholangitis*). This can be mild and clinically inapparent, or it can cause severe symptoms. Attacks of fever with liver tenderness and jaundice indicate suppurative cholangitis with liver abscess formation.

ACUTE CHOLECYSTITIS

Acute cholecystitis is characterized by the sudden onset of pain, fever, nausea, and vomiting. The pain, accompanied by tenderness, is in the right upper quadrant of the abdomen. Gallstones are present in over 90 per cent of cases, and there is often either a history of a previous attack or other symptoms attributable to the stones.

The cause and pathogenesis of acute cholecystitis are not known. Infection is rarely a cause because in most cases of the disease, organisms are not present in the bile, at least in the early stages. Impaction of a stone is probably an important factor in initiating an attack, and the retained concentrated bile acts as a chemical irritant. Whatever the initiating cause, infection usually follows. Distention of the gallbladder may imperil its blood supply so that infarction occurs.

Many cases of acute cholecystitis subside spontaneously. The mode of treatment is controversial; some surgeons delay operating until absolutely necessary. In some cases the gallbladder ruptures, leading to a severe peritonitis, which is due partly to an irritating effect of bile and partly to organisms that are found in the later stages of an acutely inflamed gallbladder.

CHRONIC CHOLECYSTITIS

Repeated attacks of acute cholecystitis (either mild or severe) combined with stones result in the gallbladder's becoming greatly thickened, shrunken, and functionless. At this stage, the symptoms are vague: flatulence, aversion to fatty foods, indigestion, and ill-defined pain in the upper abdomen.

CARCINOMA OF THE BILIARY TRACT

Carcinoma of the Gallbladder

This tumor is more common in women and the elderly. The prognosis is very poor because local spread to the liver has generally occurred by the time the diagnosis has been made.

Carcinoma of the Ampulla of Vater

This is an occasional cause of obstructive jaundice.

The Pancreas

The pancreas is a dual organ. Its exocrine portion originates from two buds of the primitive gut. The endocrine portion forms the islets of Langerhans, which, despite their small size, are of vital importance because they secrete insulin, glucagon, and other polypeptide hormones.

The pancreas lies on the posterior abdominal wall and pours its exocrine secretions into the duodenum. In about 80 per cent of normal people, the main pancreatic duct and the common bile duct enter into a common chamber (the ampulla of Vater) that opens into the duodenum. The opening is guarded by the sphincter of Oddi. Pancreatic secretions contain the precursors of three important groups of digestive enzymes. The active enzymes are formed in the duodenum. In this way, the pancreas is protected from its own secretions; upset of this mechanism, with activation within the pancreas, is an important factor in acute pancreatitis. The enzymes include (1) *proteolytic enzymes*, including trypsin, chymotrypsin, carboxypeptidases, aminopeptidases, and elastase; trypsin is activated by enterokinase, an enzyme found in the duodenal mucosa, and trypsin so formed activates the other proteolytic enzymes; (2) *lipolytic enzymes*, including lipase, phospholipase A, and cholesterol esterase; and (3) *amylase*, which splits carbohydrate. The reserve capacity of the pancreas is so great that only severe atrophy of the exocrine elements or blockage of its duct leads to upsets in digestion and absorption. In practice, impairment of fat absorption is the most important disorder; steatorrhea and lack of absorption of fat-soluble vitamins are the predominant symptoms of this condition (Chapter 23).

CYSTIC FIBROSIS

This disease, also called fibrocystic disease and mucoviscidosis, is inherited as a mendelian recessive trait. It is one of the most common hereditary diseases of the white population but is rare in blacks and almost unknown in Orientals. The defective gene is on chromosome 7 and is closely linked to a polymorphic marker that can be detected by a specific DNA probe. Carriers can therefore be detected.

Cystic fibrosis is characterized by an abnormality of the exocrine secretory glands and is remarkable for the great variety of its presentations, depending on which glands are affected.

When the pancreas is involved, the gland secretes thick mucus that obstructs the ducts and causes them to dilate. The gland itself atrophies. If the disease develops *in utero*, the absence of pancreatic enzymes together with the abnormal viscid mucus secreted by the intestine itself leads to such viscosity of the intestinal contents (called *meconium*) that intestinal obstruction and even perforation of the gut ensue (*meconium ileus*). In the more common type of cystic fibrosis, the infant or child develops a chronic *malabsorption syndrome*, accompanied by an excessive appetite, failure to gain weight, and often constipation.

When the lung is involved, the thick mucus together with infection produces bronchopneu-

monia, bronchiectasis, and lung abscesses (see Fig. 22–19). Chronic lung disease is a feature of most cases of cystic fibrosis in patients who survive for several years. Hypovitaminosis A and other effects of malabsorption complicate this clinical picture.

Occasionally the liver is affected, and chronic bile duct inflammation leads to a type of *cirrhosis*. Involvement of the cervical mucus leads to *infertility* in most female patients, and likewise most males are *sterile*. It is evident that there is involvement of many exocrine glands and that in some sites this causes symptoms. A remarkable feature of the disease is that the eccrine sweat glands secrete a sweat containing a high concentration of salt. *Chemical examination of sweat for the level of salt is a diagnostic test.*

The fundamental defect in cystic fibrosis is not yet known. The secretion of viscid mucus plays an important role in the pancreatic and lung lesions. It does not explain the abnormal sweat gland function, because sweat contains no mucus.

ACUTE PANCREATITIS

Acute pancreatitis can be mild and can lead to vague abdominal symptoms, but more often it is severe and of sudden onset and presents with intense pain; it is one cause of "acute abdomen."

Areas of pancreas undergo necrosis, and there is an associated acute inflammatory reaction. The pathogenesis is obscure, for although in a few instances the cause is a known infectious agent (*e.g.,* mumps virus), the vast majority of cases are not so related. The disease appears to be due to the sudden release of active pancreatic enzymes, particularly trypsin, within the organ itself. Blood vessels are digested, and in severe cases the whole pancreas is converted into a necrotic, hemorrhagic mass. Released lipases cause necrosis in adjacent peripancreatic fat and omentum; because of their *dystrophic calcification*, these areas of fat necrosis are soon evident as chalky white areas (Fig. 24–19). So rapidly may this calcification occur that the patient actually develops symptoms of hypocalcemia (*e.g.,* tetany). The necrotic pancreatic cells release amylase, which can be detected in the blood. A blood

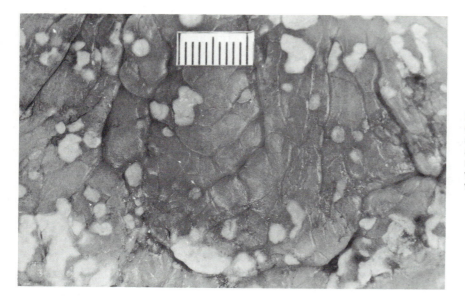

Figure 24–19 Pancreatic fat necrosis. The specimen is from the surface of the greater omentum of a patient who died of acute hemorrhagic pancreatitis. The opaque white areas are foci of fat necrosis with heterotopic calcification.

amylase determination is a useful test for the diagnosis of acute pancreatitis.

Symptoms of acute hemorrhagic pancreatitis are sometimes difficult to distinguish from those of other causes of acute abdominal pain (*e.g.,* perforated peptic ulcer, acute cholecystitis, and acute appendicitis). Laparotomy is often performed because of the difficulty in arriving at a diagnosis; the surgeon is confronted by blood-stained ascitic fluid containing globules of fat. The detection of amylase in the fluid further confirms the diagnosis. Also characteristic is the presence of many foci of fat necrosis with calcification.

Etiology and Pathogenesis. Acute pancreatitis is commonly associated, particularly in women, with gallbladder disease; in males, attacks often occur *after a large meal* or an *alcoholic spree.* Apart from chronic gallbladder disease and alcoholism, other predisposing causes include hyperlipoproteinemia, pregnancy, hypothermia, and hyperparathyroidism.

The cause of the initial damage is believed to be the release and activation of pancreatic enzymes in the parenchyma of the pancreas itself. The enzymes damage cells, leading to necrosis and acute inflammation. The elastic coat of blood vessels is digested by elastase, and bleeding ensues. Trypsin is the key enzyme because not only is it a powerful proteolytic enzyme itself,

but it also activates the other pancreatic enzymes. In addition, it activates prekallikrein and the Hageman factor. Activation of the clotting mechanism and the formation of plasmin and kinins contribute to the severe local hemorrhagic necrotic local reaction associated with profound shock. Many theories have been put forward to explain how the release and activation of the pancreatic enzymes comes about.

Bile Reflux. Obstruction of the common channel that the bile duct shares with the pancreatic duct by a gallstone, pancreatic stone, mucosal edema, or spasm of the sphincter of Oddi could allow bile to regurgitate into the pancreatic ductular system. This once popular theory does not explain all cases because an obstructing stone is rarely found, and pancreatitis can occur in patients who do not have a common channel.

Hypersecretion Theory. The sudden release of secretin after a large meal, particularly one containing alcohol, might cause a sudden secretion of pancreatic juice. If combined with obstruction, such as spasm of the sphincter of Oddi, there might be such a build up of pressure that small pancreatic ducts rupture.

Duodenal Reflux. This theory supposes that duodenal contents containing enterokinase regurgitate into the pancreas and activate its enzymes. A damaged or incompetent sphincter of Oddi (*e.g.,* by alcohol, by trauma, after passage of a stone) might allow duodenal contents to enter the pancreatic duct.

Pancreatic Intracellular Damage. It has been postulated that there is an upset in the mechanism whereby packaged enzymes within the pancreatic acinar cells are excreted; possibly they could be acted upon and activated by lysosomal enzymes within the secreting cells themselves. Drugs (*e.g.*, a thiazide diuretic or alcohol) or a viral infection might produce this effect.

It must be admitted that the precise pathogenesis of acute pancreatitis is not known and indeed may not be the same in all cases.

Course of Acute Pancreatitis. As many as 5 per cent of patients die in shock during the first week. Surgery can contribute to this. Complications in those who survive this period are *abscess* and *pseudocyst formation;* which consists of a loculated accumulation of fluid in the peritoneum adjacent to the pancreas. Such a cyst usually requires surgical drainage. Another cause of pseudocyst formation is direct injury to the pancreas by a blow to the abdomen.

CHRONIC PANCREATITIS

Chronic pancreatitis—like the acute form of the condition—is also associated with gallbladder disease, overindulgence, and alcoholism. The clinical picture is vague; it ranges from no symptoms at all to repeated attacks of mild acute pancreatitis that are not severe enough to warrant surgical intervention. Sometimes the major complaint is one of a constant pain in the back.

In its early stages, chronic pancreatitis leads to no digestive upset. Later, however, signs of malabsorption may appear; in a few cases, impaired glucose tolerance and diabetes mellitus supervene.

An important feature of chronic pancreatitis is that a surgeon may easily mistake the hard, fibrous organ for carcinoma. Even when biopsy or necropsy material is available, the distinction between a fibrosed atrophic pancreas and a scirrhous carcinoma can be very difficult.

CARCINOMA OF THE PANCREAS

Cancer of the pancreas arises from the ducts and is the most important tumor to be consid-

ered. About two thirds of the tumors arise in the head of the pancreas. Obstructive jaundice is often the first sign, and characteristically the obstruction is associated with palpable distention of the gallbladder. Carcinoma of the body or tail of the pancreas produces few symptoms until the growth is large, has invaded local structures, or has metastasized. Loss of appetite, loss of weight, vague back pain, and general malaise with mental depression are the symptoms of this silent killer.

The incidence of cancer of the pancreas is increasing, and the disease is now an important cause of death. Heavy tobacco smoking, a diet high in fats, and industrial exposure to aromatic amines (such as benzidine) have been suggested as possible etiologic factors.

The treatment of carcinoma of the pancreas is extremely unsatisfactory. Occasionally surgical resection is possible, but the inaccessibility of the pancreas and the closeness of important anatomic structures make this disease untreatable in the majority of the cases. Anastomosis of the gallbladder to a loop of intestine relieves the obstructive jaundice with its distressing pruritus.

THE ISLETS OF LANGERHANS

Diseases of the islets are considered in Chapter 16 because their major effects are on glucose metabolism.

Summary

- Portal obstruction results in portal hypertension. It results in portal-systemic shunting of blood, congestive splenomegaly, and ascites. The most common cause is cirrhosis of the liver.
- Jaundice can be obstructive, hemolytic, or of hepatocellular type.
- Hepatocellular failure causes widespread metabolic effects, particularly in relation to protein metabolism and detoxification of drugs. The end result is hepatic encephalopathy.
- Hepatic necrosis can be zonal, massive, or spotty. Bridging necrosis can progress to chronic active hepatitis and cirrhosis.
- Fatty liver is common in starvation and in alcoholics. In the alcoholic form, alcoholic hepatitis and the formation of Mallory's hyaline can develop and progress

to cirrhosis. Reye's syndrome is an acute form of fatty liver that occurs in children.

• Drug-induced liver damage produces many patterns of liver disease; these can resemble obstructive jaundice, acute viral hepatitis, or chronic liver disease.

• Acute viral hepatitis is due to one of the hepatitis viruses. Hepatitis virus A causes a mild disease spread by the oral-fecal route. Hepatitis virus B is transmitted by contaminated blood. It has an appreciable mortality and can lead to chronic hepatitis and ultimately carcinoma. Other hepatitis viruses are the delta virus and hepatitis virus C.

• The most important type of chronic hepatitis is chronic active hepatitis

• Cirrhosis of the liver features destruction of liver cells, fibrosis, and formation of regeneration nodules. It may be micronodular (often alcoholic) or macronodular.

• Primary carcinoma of the liver is either hepatoma (sometimes developing in a cirrhotic liver) or cholangiocarcinoma.

• Gallstones (cholelithiasis) can be asymptomatic but can cause obstruction (with pain and often jaundice) and predispose to ascending cholangitis.

• Acute cholecystitis is a common cause of acute abdominal pain.

• Cystic fibrosis (mucoviscidosis) is an inherited disease with defective secretion of many exocrine glands. It affects the intestine, the lung, and occasionally the liver. The sweat test is used in diagnosis.

• Acute pancreatitis is related to alcoholism and cholecystitis, but the pathogenesis is obscure. It can be mild, or it can be severe and have a 5 per cent mortality.

• Carcinoma of the pancreas is common; it causes pain and ill-defined symptoms unless the bile duct is obstructed, in which case painless jaundice is characteristic.

Selected Readings

Alter, M. J., and Sampliner, R. E.: Hepatitis C. N. Engl. J. Med. *321*:1538, 1989.

Fulginiti, V. A., et al.: Aspirin and Reye's syndrome. Pediatrics *69*:810, 1982.

Leading article: The A to F of viral hepatitis. Lancet 2:1158, 1990.

Lefkowitch, J. H.: The epidemiology and morphology of primary malignant liver tumors. Surg. Clin. North Am. *61*:169, 1981.

Longnecker, D. S.: Pathology and pathogenesis of diseases of the pancreas. Am. J. Pathol. *107*:103, 1982.

Sherlock, S.: Disease of the Liver and Biliary Tract. 8th ed. Oxford, Blackwell, 1989.

Toledo-Pereyra, L.: Pancreas: Principles of Medical and Surgical Practice. New York, Wiley, 1985.

Weisberg, H. F.: Pathogenesis of gallstones. Am. Clin. Lab. Sci. *14*:243, 1984.

Kidneys and Urinary Tract

**After studying this chapter, the student
should be able to:**

- Describe the major functions of the kidney.
- Outline the process of urine formation and indicate
  the relative roles of the various parts of the nephron.
- Define polyuria, polydipsia, nocturia, anuria, and
  retention with overflow.
- Describe the principles underlying the creatinine
  clearance test.
- List the methods that are used to examine urine in
  clinical medicine.
- List the types of casts that are found in urine and
  indicate their significance.
- Describe the important causes and manifestations of
  acute renal failure, chronic renal failure, and the
  nephrotic syndrome.
- List the types of glomerulonephritis and indicate the
  outstanding features of each type.
- Describe the main features and known causes of
  interstitial nephritis.
- Describe the causes and course of acute tubular
  necrosis.
- Discuss the pathogenesis of urinary tract infection
  and describe the clinical features of each of the

following: acute urethritis with cystitis, acute pyelonephritis, and chronic pyelonephritis.
• Describe what is meant by the term "end-stage kidney."
• Compare clear-cell carcinoma of the kidney with carcinoma of the bladder.

• Describe the common causes and effects of urinary tract obstruction.
• Classify the types of urinary calculi and list their effects.

The Kidneys

It is a popular misconception that the only major function performed by the kidneys is the excretion of the waste products of metabolism. In fact, the kidneys have many other functions, particularly in relation to maintaining a fixed internal environment. Unless these other functions are appreciated, the features of renal failure cannot be understood.

FUNCTIONS OF THE KIDNEY

Excretion of Urea and Creatinine. These two substances are the nitrogenous end products of protein metabolism. The normal level of blood urea is usually expressed as the blood urea nitrogen (BUN). The normal BUN is 3.0 to 6.5 mmol/L (8 to 18 mg/dl). The normal level of blood creatinine is 50 to 110 μmol/L (0.6 to 1.2 mg/dl). Renal failure results in a rise in the level of these two nitrogenous substances in the blood; the resultant condition is called *azotemia*, a term derived from *azote*, a name for nitrogen proposed by Lavoisier.

Metabolism and Excretion of Other Substances. Inulin and many drugs are examples.

Regulation of Extracellular Fluids. This is accomplished by controlling the excretion of water and electrolytes, particularly sodium.

Regulation of Acid-Base Balance. The kidney contributes to the maintenance of a stable blood pH by the excretion of hydrogen ions. This excretion takes place mainly in the distal tubule where hydrogen ions are combined either with phosphate or with ammonia. The synthesis of ammonia by the kidney and its conversion into ammonium ions is an important mechanism in acid-base homeostasis.

Regulation of Blood Pressure. The kidney is capable of forming both vasodilator and vasoconstrictor substances, but their role in the regulation of the systemic blood pressure is not understood. The vasodilators are prostaglandins and kinins. The ischemic kidney releases renin, an enzyme that leads to the formation of the powerful vasoconstrictor angiotensin II.

Regulation of Erythropoiesis. Erythropoietin is produced mainly by the kidney and acts as a stimulus to red blood cell production. The precise physiologic role of this process is not understood; it is known, however, that anemia is very common in renal failure. Occasionally, tumors of the kidney result in excessive erythropoietin production, causing polycythemia to ensue.

Vitamin D Metabolism. See Chapter 30.

Mechanism of Urine Formation: Normal and Abnormal

The formation of urine by the normal kidney is described in textbooks of physiology; consequently, only a brief outline of the salient features is presented here.

The glomerular filtrate (approximately 180 liters per day) is derived from blood flowing through the glomerulus and has a similar composition to plasma, except for having a very low protein content. In the proximal convoluted tubule, 80 per cent of the water and virtually all of the protein and glucose are reabsorbed. If the blood glucose level (and therefore the level in the glomerular filtrate) is high—as in diabetes mellitus—the proximal convoluted tubules are unable to reabsorb all the glucose, and this substance passes into the urine (a condition called *glycosuria*). Occasionally, glycosuria occurs in the presence of a normal blood glucose level; this condition, which is known as *renal glycosuria*, is due to defective tubular function.

In many renal diseases, the glomerular vessels become more permeable to protein, and the proximal convoluted tubules are unable to reabsorb the excess protein. The *proteinuria* that results is an important and common finding in renal disease.

Absorption of electrolytes in the proximal tubules is such that the luminal fluid is isotonic with plasma, and the process is therefore called iso-osmotic absorption. Urea passes freely out of the tubules.

In the ascending limb of the loop of Henle, there is considerable transfer of sodium chloride from the lumen to the interstitial fluid of the medulla. Because this part of the renal tubule is impermeable to water, it follows that the modified filtrate within the lumen becomes progressively hypotonic, whereas the interstitial fluid becomes hypertonic.

In the distal tubule, the pH of the filtrate and its electrolyte composition are finally adjusted. When the hypotonic fluid leaves the loop of Henle and enters the distal tubule, it becomes isotonic with plasma once more, since this part of the nephron is fully permeable to water.

Because the filtrate is surrounded by the hypertonic interstitial fluid of the medulla, in its course through the collecting tubules it tends to maintain osmotic equilibrium by transferring some of its water to the interstitial fluid. The filtrate thereby attains the final composition of urine. The permeability of the distal tubule and collecting tubules is regulated by the circulating level of antidiuretic hormone (ADH) released by the posterior lobe of the pituitary. This hormone, by rendering the tubules more permeable to water, aids the transfer of water from the tubules into the interstitial tissue. A high level of ADH, such as occurs during dehydration, results in the production of a highly concentrated urine. In the absence of antidiuretic hormone, such as occurs in *diabetes insipidus*, a large quantity of dilute urine is produced. Normally 1½ to 2 liters of urine is passed daily; if this quantity is exceeded, the condition is termed *polyuria*. Tubules damaged by hypercalcemia or hypokalemia are less responsive to the action of ADH, and this situation also leads to polyuria. Likewise, the regenerating epithelium of the tubules after tubular necrosis is unresponsive to the action of ADH, and again polyuria results.

If the fluid in the tubules contains an excess of an osmotically active substance such as glucose, water absorption is impeded. It follows that in diabetes mellitus, polyuria is a characteristic feature. Since water is lost, thirst is increased, and an excessive quantity of water is drunk (*polydipsia*). A similar situation occurs in chronic renal failure. The blood urea level is high, and the amount of urea in the glomerular filtrate is also raised, hindering water absorption. Polyuria and polydipsia ensue. It is evident that one of the features of the normal kidney is its ability to produce a highly concentrated or a highly dilute urine according to circumstances. As renal function becomes impaired, this ability is lost, and eventually a urine of fixed osmolality is produced.

The continuous production of urine with a specific gravity of about 1.010 regardless of the fluid intake has several important consequences. If the fluid intake is high, then water retention occurs. If the water intake of the body is low, then dehydration results. Finally, the normal ability to produce a concentrated urine during sleep is lost, forcing the patient to get up to pass urine during the night, a feature described as *nocturia*.

Tests of Renal Function

Clearance Values. Inulin is a substance that passes freely from the plasma into the glomerular filtrate and is neither absorbed by the tubules nor secreted by them. The amount of plasma cleared of inulin per minute is equal to the glomerular filtration rate. It is evident that

Filtered inulin = excreted inulin
Filtered inulin = glomerular filtration rate (GFR) × plasma inulin concentration (P)
Excreted inulin = urine inulin concentration (U) × volume of urine (V) in ml/min

Hence

$$GFR \times P = U \times V$$

$$GFR = \frac{U \times V}{P}$$

This forms the basis of a useful clinical test, and the normal value for the glomerular filtration rate is about 120 ml per minute. In practice, the inulin clearance test is difficult to perform, but since creatinine is treated similarly, the *creatinine clearance* is estimated and is a good measure of the glomerular filtration rate. The required measurements are the blood creatinine level, the volume of urine passed over a 1-hour period, and the creatinine content of a sample of this urine. The normal range is 90 to 130 ml per minute. The urea clearance test is also a commonly performed test, but since some urea is reabsorbed by the tubules, the urea clearance is approximately ⅝ of the normal glomerular filtration rate; *i.e.*, the normal range is 60 to 100 ml per minute.

Blood Urea. The BUN is related in part to the protein intake in the diet and in part to renal function. Figure 25–1 shows the relationship between glomerular filtration rate and blood urea. Note that the BUN is an insensitive indicator of renal function and that at least 50 per cent of kidney substance must be destroyed before an appreciable rise in the BUN is seen. The blood creatinine level is related to muscle bulk and not to dietary intake, and the level of blood creatinine is a more useful indication of renal function.

Examination of Urine

Diseases of the kidney and urinary tract are often reflected in abnormalities in the urine and are so common that an examination of the urine (*urinalysis*) is a mandatory procedure with any patient admitted to a hospital or undergoing a routine physical examination. The following methods can be used.

Chemical Examination. Simple tests are available for detecting protein, glucose, hemoglobin, and ketone bodies. If necessary, the amount of protein can be measured; the normal quantity excreted in 24 hours is under 150 mg. Individual proteins can be identified by electroimmunophoresis; for example, Bence Jones protein can be categorized by this method.

Specific Gravity. The normal kidney can concentrate urine such that the specific gravity reaches 1.022 or more after a period of dehydration or an injection of vasopressin. Specific gravity readings are misleading if heavy solutes such as glucose or protein are present in the urine. Under these circumstances, the freezing point method of detecting osmolarity must be used.

The normal kidney can dilute urine after a water load, but tests based on this are unreliable and are not used in practice.

Microscopic Examination. Much can be learned by an examination of the centrifuged deposit from a sample of *fresh* urine. A scanty number of red blood cells, polymorphs, and epithelial cells are normally present. An excess of red blood cells indicates bleeding. The presence of these cells can usefully distinguish between *hematuria*, which is the presence of red blood cells in the urine, and *hemoglobinuria*, which is the existence of free hemoglobin in solution, as in blackwater fever. An increased number of polymorphs indicates inflammation in either the kidney or the urinary tract; generally this condition is due to infection, but it must be

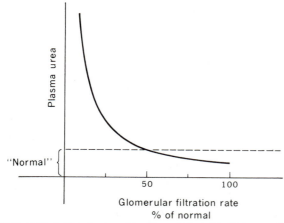

Figure 25–1 Graph showing the relationship between the glomerular filtration rate and the plasma urea concentration. Note that the plasma urea concentration remains within normal limits until the glomerular filtration rate has fallen to less than 50 per cent of normal. (From Epstein, F. H.: Approach to the patient with renal disease. *In* Wintrobe, M. M., et al. [Eds.]: Harrison's Principles of Internal Medicine. 7th ed. New York, McGraw-Hill, 1974. Reproduced with permission of McGraw-Hill, Inc.)

confirmed bacteriologically. If there is no growth on routine media, a search must be made for tubercle bacilli.

Casts are cylindrical structures formed in the renal tubules and composed of a protein that is derived from the tubules themselves (Tamm-Horsfall mucoprotein). *Hyaline casts* are translucent, and a few are sometimes present in the urine of healthy people. An increased number suggests renal disease. More significant are *granular casts*, which have a specked or granular appearance due to an admixture of albumin, immunoglobulin, lipoprotein, or breakdown products of cells. When first formed, the granules are coarse (*coarsely granular casts*), but with intrarenal stasis, the granules break up to produce *finely granular casts*. Ultimately the granules disappear, and highly refractile, brittle, *waxy casts* are formed. The presence of these casts is abnormal and generally indicates tubulointerstitial renal disease. Waxy casts in particular point to severe disease. *Renal tubular epithelial cell casts* contain recognizable tubular cells, and their presence indicates tubular damage. Likewise, *fatty casts* indicate tubular damage, because the fat is derived from the tubular cells. *Red blood cell casts* contain recognizable red blood cells and possibly breakdown products of hemoglobin. The red blood cells are usually derived from damaged glomeruli, but bleeding can also occur in acute renal tubular necrosis. Leukocyte casts indicate acute inflammation, often infective; hence, they are characteristic of pyelonephritis.

Because casts are formed in renal tubules, the diameter of the casts is an indication of the diameter of the tubule in which they are formed. Hence, large, *broad casts* are formed in dilated tubules of severely scarred kidneys, and their presence is of grave significance.

Bacteriologic Examination. Urine normally contains some bacteria that are derived from the anterior urethra, but the organisms are too scanty to be seen on a stained smear of *uncentrifuged* urine. A bacterial count of over 100,000/ml is regarded as abnormal and indicates a renal or urinary tract infection.

CLINICAL EFFECTS OF RENAL DISEASE

The four main syndromes are described next before the complex topics related to individual kidney disease are reviewed. The syndromes are the nephritic syndrome; the nephrotic syndrome; persistent urinary abnormalities; and renal failure, acute and chronic.

The Nephritic Syndrome

The nephritic syndrome is characterized by proteinuria, hematuria that is microscopic or gross with the presence of red blood cell casts, oliguria, diminished glomerular filtration rate, retention of sodium and water, edema, and hypertension. Post-streptococcal proliferative glomerulonephritis is the prototype of this syndrome.

The Nephrotic Syndrome: The Protein-Losing Kidney

The small amount of protein normally in the glomerular filtrate is mostly reabsorbed by the proximal tubules; the urine normally contains less than 0.15 g per 24 hours. There are a number of conditions in which the permeability of the glomerulus is so increased that large amounts of protein, mainly albumin, escape into the glomerular filtrate and are passed in the urine because the capacity of the tubular cells to absorb it is overwhelmed. The cells of the proximal convoluted tubules contain large "hyaline droplets" composed of protein material absorbed from the glomerular filtrate.

A loss of 10 to 20 g of protein per day is not unusual in the nephrotic syndrome. This exceeds the body's capacity to replace it, and the plasma albumin often falls below the level of 10 g/L; this leads to edema. The combination of *severe proteinuria*, *hypoalbuminemia*, and *generalized edema* constitutes the nephrotic syndrome. There is also an increased plasma lipid level, the cause of which may be related to overproduction of lipoproteins but is not well understood.

Renal function is generally good in the nephrotic syndrome; often the glomerular filtration rate is raised in the early stages of the disease. There is, however, an increased susceptibility to infection probably related to the low level of immunoglobulins in the plasma resulting from its loss in the urine. Pneumonia, peritonitis, and other pyogenic infections are very common. Hypertension and uremia do not generally occur unless the cause of the nephrotic syndrome is itself responsible for progressive renal destruction.

Causes of the Nephrotic Syndrome. Common causes include minimal-change disease (particularly in children), membranous nephropathy, diabetic nephropathy, and amyloidosis.

Persistent Urinary Abnormalities in the Absence of Clinical Symptoms

Persistent or recurrent hematuria or proteinuria can occur in the absence of clinical symptoms.

Renal Failure

Renal failure may be of sudden onset (*acute*), or it may develop gradually (*chronic*). If recovery does not occur, the terminal state of *uremia* ensues. Each of these must be examined in some detail.

Acute Renal Failure

Acute renal failure is a common clinical emergency; its causes may be classified as follows.

1. *Prerenal causes.* Acute tubular necrosis resulting from renal hypoperfusion is the most common cause.

2. *Renal causes.* Examples are severe proliferative and crescentic glomerulonephritis; acute pyelonephritis, especially when complicated by papillary necrosis; acute interstitial nephritis; thrombosis, embolism, and vasculitis of renal vessels; malignant nephrosclerosis; and acute intrarenal obstruction (*e.g.*, by myeloma, protein, or uric acid crystals). In children, the most common cause is the hemolytic uremic syndrome.

3. *Postrenal causes.* These include sudden obstruction to the urinary outflow or rupture of the urinary bladder.

Features of Acute Renal Failure. Acute renal failure is characterized by severe oliguria—com-

plete anuria in the worst cases—associated with the retention of nitrogenous substances (*e.g.*, urea and creatinine), potassium, magnesium, phosphate, and other anions in the blood. These substances are mainly derived from the endogenous breakdown of muscle protein, and the changes are aggravated if the patient is given additional protein. Metabolic acidosis is due to the failure of the tubules to excrete hydrogen ions. There is an increase in the volume of the extracellular water, particularly if an inappropriate amount of fluid is given to the patient. A rapidly developing anemia may occur owing in part to increased blood volume secondary to water retention and in part to a hemolytic process that occurs in uremia.

The *causes of death* in acute renal failure are *potassium intoxication* causing cardiac arrest, *overhydration* leading either to water intoxication or else an overexpanded extracellular compartment with pulmonary edema, or concomitant *infection*.

Death follows a clouding of consciousness due apparently to waste products of unidentified nature. There is often a dramatic relief of symptoms after dialysis even before the blood urea and electrolyte levels are corrected.

Chronic Renal Failure

This syndrome is common and its causes are extremely numerous. Frequently it is the *end stage* of many chronic renal diseases, such as glomerulonephritis, chronic pyelonephritis, nephrosclerosis, lupus erythematosus, diabetic nephropathy, extensive renal tuberculosis, and radiation nephritis. Chronic obstruction of the outflow of urine, such as that caused by prostatic enlargement, is a common cause in males.

Effects of Chronic Renal Failure. The effect of chronic renal failure is uremia that is due to a failure of the kidney to regulate the internal environment. The kidneys can neither concentrate nor dilute, and the urine has a fixed specific gravity of 1.010. This leads to nocturia and easy upset in water metabolism.

Uremia is a clinical state produced by renal failure that is associated with retention of nitrogenous substances in the blood. Some of its features can be explained on the basis of known biochemical anomalies. In many instances, we are ignorant of its exact pathogenesis. The features of uremia are enumerated in the following.

General. Weakness, easy fatigue, lethargy, insomnia, and malaise are common.

Cardiovascular Symptoms. Hypertension is common and may lead to heart failure. This contributes to edema both of the tissues in general and of the lung. A terminal sterile fibrinous pericarditis is often seen.

Gastrointestinal Symptoms. Anorexia, nausea, vomiting, hiccup, and diarrhea are frequent. One explanation of these symptoms is that urea present in the gastrointestinal fluids is broken down to ammonia, which is an irritant and causes *gastritis* and *colitis.* Vomiting and diarrhea can precipitate acute renal failure.

Neurologic Manifestations. Mental clouding, inability to concentrate, and lethargy are common in advanced uremia. Convulsions and coma may occur terminally. These symptoms may be due to water intoxication and metabolic acidosis. Muscular twitching has been related to hypocalcemia. A peripheral neuropathy similar to that encountered in diabetes mellitus may occur.

Hematologic Effects. A severe normocytic normochromic anemia, quite unresponsive to treatment, is common in the late stages of renal failure. It is due to diminished production of erythropoietin by the diseased kidney. Defective platelet function is the cause of purpura, another frequent feature of renal failure.

Infection. Advanced renal insufficiency is commonly complicated by infection. Often this is a urinary infection and terminates in septicemia.

Metabolic Acidosis. This condition leads to a sighing respiration.

Renal Osteodystrophy. Retention of phosphate can lead to a lowering of blood calcium and hyperparathyroidism secondary to this. In addition, the metabolism of vitamin D is impaired, and the active 1,25-dihydroxycholecalciferol is formed in inadequate amounts.

Retention of Potassium. Hyperkalemia can lead to sudden death.

CLASSIFICATION OF RENAL DISEASE

The classification of renal disease is based primarily on the light microscopic appearances (morphology) combined with the techniques of electron microscopy and immunopathology. Considerable insight has been obtained on etiology and pathogenesis of many diseases, and investigations have been greatly aided by the availability of fresh kidney obtained by needle biopsy. The following outline is used in the account that follows:

1. Glomerular disease—glomerulonephritis.
2. Tubulointerstitial disease.
3. Renal disease associated with hypertension.
4. Congenital diseases.
5. Cystic disease.
6. Neoplasms.

GLOMERULONEPHRITIS

Glomerulonephritis is a term applied to a group of diseases that are not obviously of infective nature and in which primarily the glomeruli are affected. In most types of glomerulonephritis, the lesions are associated with the deposition of immune complexes in the glomeruli. Glomerulonephritis is a feature of serum sickness and chronic immune complex disease (Chapter 6). In naturally occurring glomerulonephritis, similar immune-complex deposition can occur, and the antigen may be derived from a number of sources. These may be exogenous, such as infections (streptococcal infections, malaria, syphilis, or hepatitis) or drugs. In a number of cases, the antigen is endogenous; glomerulonephritis is a well-known accompaniment of tumors, particularly carcinoma of the lung. In these instances, the renal damage appears to be due to the deposition of circulating immune complexes, but the reason for their deposition in the glomeruli is poorly understood. The kidney appears to be damaged as an "innocent bystander," and the pathogenesis is thought to involve the activation of complement via either the classic or the alternative pathway. In many examples of glomerulonephritis, although immune-complex deposition can be detected, the nature of the antigen is unknown. This applies to the common post-streptococcal glomerulonephritis (Fig. 25–2*A*). In all these examples, it is assumed that the immune complexes are formed in the blood and subse-

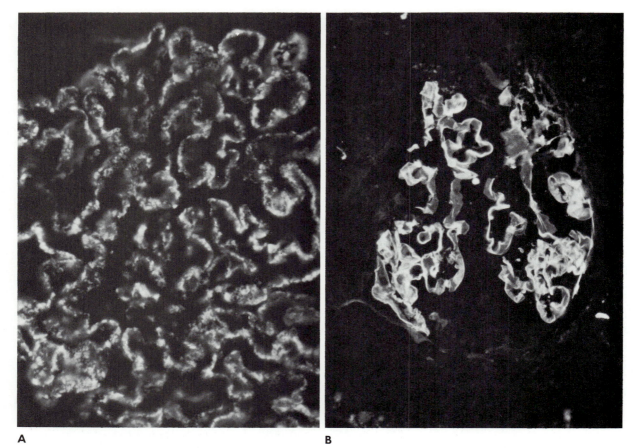

A   B

Figure 25–2 Immunofluorescent patterns in glomerulonephritis. *A*, Part of a glomerulus in acute post-streptococcal glomerulonephritis. Note the granular deposits of IgG in the immune complexes deposited in the basement membrane zone. *B*, Goodpasture's syndrome. There is a uniform linear band of staining along the basement membrane of the vessels in the glomerulus. (Courtesy of Dr. Susan Ritchie, Department of Pathology, Toronto General Division of the Toronto Hospital, Toronto.)

quently filtered off in the glomeruli. Another proposed mechanism is that antibodies form complexes directly with antigens already present in the kidney. The antigen may be part of the normal or slightly altered glomerular structure, and this is believed to be the mechanism in the production of the lesions in Goodpasture's syndrome. In other examples, it is thought that foreign antigens become localized or planted in the kidney and that subsequently antibodies form complexes with them.

Although many classifications of glomerulonephritis have been proposed, none has been found to be entirely satisfactory. The types at present recognized have been delineated on the basis of three parameters, as follows.

Clinical Findings. The clinical features of glomerulonephritis vary enormously. The onset may be acute or insidious. Hematuria is common but may range from insignificant to severe: the red blood cells present in urine may be detectable only by microscopic examination, or the urine may be "smoky" or obviously red. Albuminuria is invariable and if severe leads to the nephrotic syndrome. A patient may recover spontaneously from glomerulonephritis; occasionally the disease is fulminating and leads rapidly to death from renal failure; more often, the damage is progressive, and renal failure occurs after a protracted course of many years. Associated clinical features sometimes suggest the cause of glomerulonephritis. For example, some types are associated with infection by *Streptococcus pyogenes*. For the most part, however, the origin of glomerulonephritis is unknown.

Immunologic Findings. In many types of human glomerulonephritis, deposits of immunoglobulin (IgG or IgA) and complement can be demonstrated by immunofluorescence. The technique used is similar to that illustrated in Figure 31–9. The precise localization of the deposits varies; usually the deposits are granular and are situated in relation to the basement membrane or the mesangium. In a few types—notably the glomerulonephritis of Goodpasture's syndrome— specific antikidney antibodies can be detected in the blood and in the kidney, where they are laid down in a linear manner along the capillary basement membrane zone (Fig. 25–2*B*).

Histopathologic Findings. Light microscopy reveals several types of glomerular change. The glomeruli may appear normal or show the changes described as proliferative, membranous, or crescentic. These are described later. It must be stressed that the changes are purely descriptive. They are merely reaction patterns of the glomerulus to damage and are not specific for any one type of disease.

Electron microscopy has greatly added to our knowledge of the types and causes of glomerulonephritis. Deposits of material (mostly immune complexes and complement) are found in the basement membrane itself or on either side of it. Various patterns and types of deposit have been described, but these details are beyond the scope of this book.

A characteristic electron microscopic finding is extensive effacement ("fusion") of the foot processes of the epithelial cells of the glomerulus (Figs. 25–3 and 25–4). The processes become short and stumpy, so that in places the epithelial cells appear to be directly applied to the basement membrane. This change appears to be an effect of an increased permeability of the glomerular vessels to protein and is therefore present whenever there is proteinuria.

The technique of needle biopsy, by which a core of kidney substance can be safely removed during life, has greatly aided the investigation of glomerulonephritis in patients. The material obtained is particularly suited for immunofluorescence studies and electron microscopy as well as for routine light microscopic examination.

Types of Glomerulonephritis

Minimal-Change Glomerulonephritis. The glomeruli appear normal under light microscopy, but under electron microscopy, fusion of the foot processes of the epithelial cells is revealed.

The majority of the patients are children with the nephrotic syndrome. They respond well to glucocorticoid therapy.

Membranous Glomerulonephritis. On light microscopy, the basement membrane of the glomeruli is shown to be thickened (Fig. 25–5). Eventually this thickening causes obliteration of the vessels, and the glomeruli become functionless. The majority of patients are adults with the nephrotic syndrome. Approximately 30 per cent recover spontaneously, and the remainder continue on with their disease and ultimately die of chronic renal failure. Membranous glomerulonephritis and minimal-change glomerulonephritis at one time were both classified as types of *nephrosis*. Systemic lupus erythematosus can produce an identical histologic picture.

Proliferative Glomerulonephritis. The glomeruli are enlarged and hypercellular because of mesangial proliferation and infiltration by polymorphs (Fig. 25–5). Post-streptococcal glomerulonephritis is the common type of proliferative glomerulonephritis. The illness occurs about 3 weeks after a streptococcal infection; children and young adults are commonly affected, but no age group is exempt. The disease typically starts with a *nephritic syndrome*. There is oliguria, albuminuria, hematuria ("smoky urine"), and periorbital edema that is most obvious on waking in the morning. The edema is due to water and sodium retention by the kidney; occasionally there is a nephrotic syndrome. Recovery is usual in acute glomerulonephritis, particularly in children and in cases occurring during epidemics of streptococcal infection. On the other hand, adults fare less well, and about one third of patients develop progressive renal disease, often with hypertension (Fig. 25–6).

Membranoproliferative Glomerulonephritis (Mesangiocapillary). The glomeruli show a com-

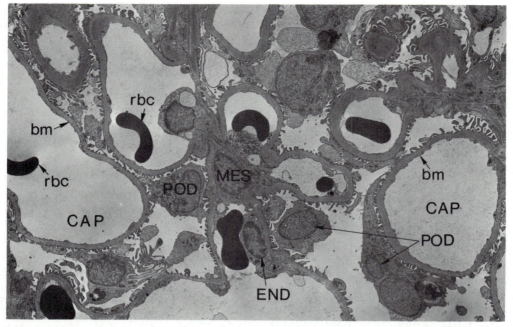

Figure 25–3 Normal kidney. Survey electron micrograph of a portion of a normal human glomerulus. The capillaries (CAP) are lined by attenuated endothelial cells; the nucleus of one of these is labeled END. Red cells are easily identified (rbc). A mesangial cell (MES) is situated between several capillary loops. The capillaries possess a well-marked basement membrane (bm) and are covered by epithelial cells or podocytes (POD) of the visceral layer of Bowman's capsule. These cells are attached to the basement membrane of the capillaries by numerous foot processes or *pedicles* (×3600). (Courtesy of Dr. Susan Ritchie, Department of Pathology, Toronto General Division of the Toronto Hospital, Toronto.)

bination of basement membrane thickening and mesangial proliferation. Several types of membranoproliferative glomerulonephritis are recognized. One type is associated with *Streptococcus viridans* endocarditis; another is associated with a low blood complement level. The location and type of deposits found in immunofluorescent and electron microscopic studies help in delineating these types.

The patients often present clinically with the nephrotic syndrome. The prognosis is poor.

Rapidly Progressive Glomerulonephritis. The glomeruli show proliferative changes and deposits of fibrin. The characteristic lesion, however, is proliferation of the epithelial cells of Bowman's capsule and accumulation of macrophages to produce a *crescent* (Fig. 25–5).

Clinically, rapidly progressive glomerulonephritis is associated with the rapid development of renal failure and consequent death. The disease is occasionally encountered in post-streptococcal glomerulonephritis and in polyarteritis no-

dosa. It is also characteristic of Goodpasture's syndrome, a condition that affects young men and is characterized by pulmonary hemorrhages, hemoptysis, and renal failure. Antibodies are present that react specifically with basement membrane material of the pulmonary and glomerular capillaries.

Focal Glomerulonephritis. Unlike the other types of glomerulonephritis described, this group affects some glomeruli but not others; indeed, it may affect parts of only some glomeruli. The details relating to the various types of focal glomerulonephritis are beyond the scope of this book.

Chronic Glomerulonephritis

Chronic glomerulonephritis is the term used to describe the small, pale, finely granular kidneys that are found in patients with chronic renal disease (Fig. 25–6). Microscopy reveals many

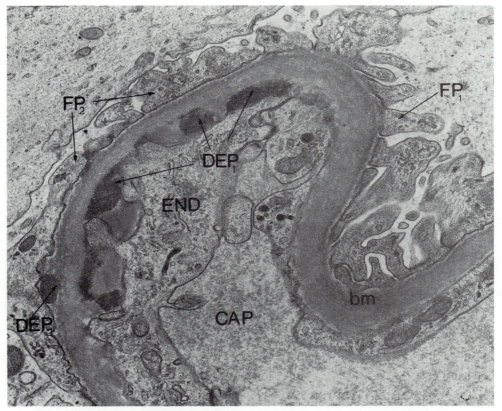

Figure 25–4 Electron micrograph of glomerulus in lupus erythematosus. In some areas, the foot processes (FP₁) of the podocytes appear relatively normal, but elsewhere they are swollen and spread over the basement membrane (bm) of the capillary (FP₂). This change is commonly described as *fusion of the foot processes*. Prominent subendothelial deposits are present (DEP₁). Subepithelial deposits are smaller and less obvious (DEP₂). In this patient, the deposits were shown by immunofluorescence to contain IgG and components of complement (×27,500). (Courtesy of Dr. Y. Bedard, Mount Sinai Hospital, Toronto.)

hyalinized glomeruli, tubular atrophy, interstitial fibrosis, and a scattered lymphocytic infiltrate. The changes are most marked if the patient has been kept alive by dialysis. Retention cysts are common, as are vascular changes associated with the hypertension that is often present. There are usually no early lesions on which to base a diagnosis of a specific renal disease. Indeed, chronic glomerulonephritis is best regarded as the end stage of many types of glomerulonephritis and indistinguishable from the end stage of chronic tubulointerstitial disease.

Summary

The diagnosis of glomerulonephritis is the task of the expert who has access to such sophisti-cated tools as electron microscopy and immuno-fluorescence. Precise diagnosis is of value in giving the prognosis and in suggesting the best treatment available.

GLOMERULAR LESIONS ACCOMPANYING SYSTEMIC DISEASE

Renal changes are common in many systemic diseases; examples include systemic lupus ery-thematosus, amyloidosis, vasculitis, hyperten-sion, and diabetes mellitus. In some cases, the lesions resemble the changes of a primary renal disease; in others, the lesions are distinctive.

Lupus Nephritis. Glomerulonephritis of either a proliferative or a membranous type is common in systemic lupus erythematosus (Fig. 25–4). Im-

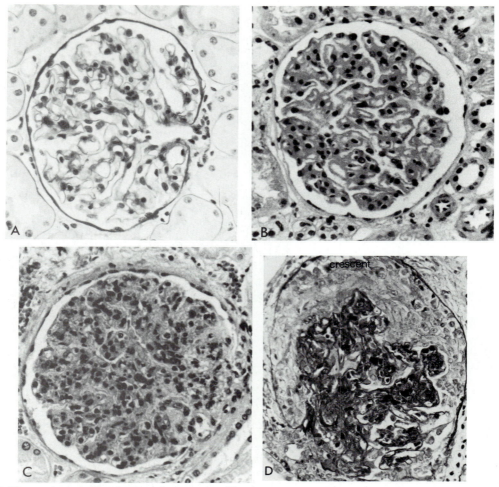

Figure 25–5 Glomerulonephritis. *A*, Normal glomerulus. The basement membrane zones of the parietal layer of Bowman's capsule and of the glomerulus are well shown (PAS stain). *B*, Membranous glomerulonephritis. Note the thickening of the basement membrane of the glomerular capillaries (H & E stain). *C*, Proliferative glomerulonephritis. The glomerulus is enlarged and shows increased cellularity that is due partly to mesangial proliferation and partly to a polymorph infiltration. *D*, Rapidly progressive glomerulonephritis. The glomerular tuft is collapsed, and the deep staining of the basement membrane material is well shown. Proliferation of the epithelial cells of Bowman's capsule has produced a typical crescent (PAS stain). (*A* and *C* courtesy of Dr. Susan Ritchie, Department of Pathology, Toronto General Division of the Toronto Hospital, Toronto.)

mune deposits of DNA–anti-DNA are a prominent feature. Lupus nephritis can cause a nephrotic syndrome and ultimately lead to renal failure.

Nephrosclerosis. Nephrosclerosis is a term used to describe the renal lesions of systemic hypertension. In the *benign type*, the arteriosclerosis causes patchy ischemia. The affected nephrons become atrophic and are ultimately replaced by scar tissue. Hence, the kidneys in benign nephrosclerosis show thinning of the cortex and a granularity of the surface. In malignant hyper-

tension, the arteriolar necrosis causes extensive patchy foci of necrosis (*malignant nephrosclerosis*). Renal failure is a common cause of death (Chapters 19 and 21).

Diabetic Nephropathy. This condition is described in Chapter 16.

DISEASES AFFECTING THE TUBULES

There is a group of conditions in which tubular damage is evident, glomeruli are unaffected, and

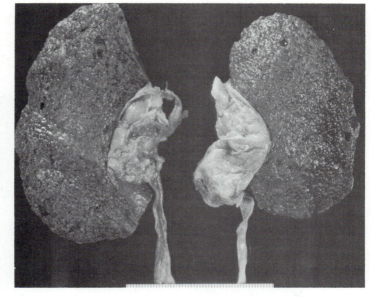

Figure 25–6 Chronic glomerulonephritis. Both kidneys are reduced in size and display a fine granular surface. The patient had developed acute glomerulonephritis after a streptococcal sore throat. Renal failure and systemic hypertension slowly evolved over the next 15 years. Death was due to cerebral hemorrhage. It is not possible to distinguish between the various types of chronic renal disease by a gross examination.

the interstitial tissues are infiltrated by inflammatory cells. The terms *tubulointerstitial disease* and *interstitial nephritis* are used for this group. There is a second type of tubular damage occurring without appreciable interstitial inflammation and sometimes culminating in tubular necrosis. This is *acute tubular necrosis*.

Tubulointerstitial Disease

The most common type of tubulointerstitial disease is caused by infection and is labeled pyelonephritis because the renal pelvis is invariably involved. It is described later. Similar histologic changes in the kidney can be found in the absence of obvious infection and without involvement of the renal pelvis. This is termed *interstitial nephritis*. In some examples the cause is evident, *e.g.*, radiation nephritis, whereas in others the damage is immunologically mediated. Lupus erythematosus and the kidney undergoing graft rejection fall into this group.

Acute Drug-Induced Interstitial Nephritis. A variety of drugs, *e.g.*, methicillin, ampicillin, rifampicin, and thiazide diuretics, can cause this type of interstitial nephritis. The damage is immunologically mediated in most cases, and antitubular basement membrane antibodies may be present. There is tubular damage associated with an inflammatory reaction in the interstitial tissues, the glomeruli being spared until late in the disease. Clinical features include fever, hematuria, and, in severe cases, acute renal failure. Early recognition of the disease is important because complete recovery is the rule if the offending drug is withdrawn.

Chronic Interstitial Nephritis. Poisoning with mercury, lead, and other heavy metals can cause this type of nephritis. Another cause is chronic ingestion of large doses of analgesic drugs. This condition, called *analgesic nephropathy*, is a cause of chronic renal disease particularly in Scandinavia, Australia, and New Zealand. The subjects are usually women who self-administer analgesic drugs (usually phenacetin and aspirin) for a variety of real or imaginary pains, *e.g.*, headache, low back pain, whiplash injury, and fibrositis. Acetaminophen, a metabolite of phenacetin, is thought to be responsible for the condition; it causes cell damage, and the effect is potentiated by ischemia produced by aspirin, which inhibits the formation of prostaglandin—a vasodilator. About 1 g per day for 3 years is needed to produce lesions; often a total of 20 to 30 kg has been consumed.

The characteristic lesion of analgesic nephropathy is *papillary necrosis* (Fig. 25–7). The tips of one or more papillae become necrotic and appear shriveled and black; sometimes the necrotic tips

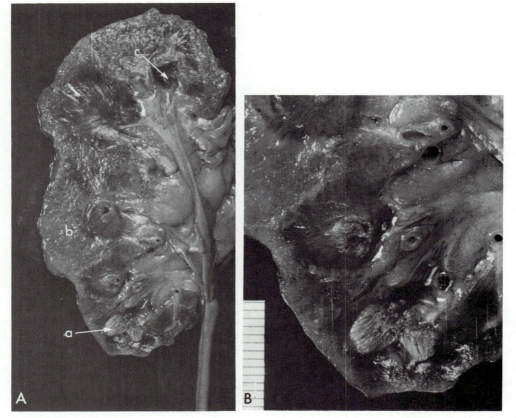

Figure 25–7 Analgesic nephropathy. *A*, The kidney shows several necrotic papillae (seen best at a). Note how the cortex overlying this area is thinned, compared with the more normal cortex (at b). One papilla has become necrotic and has completely disappeared (c). *B*, This close-up shows necrotic papillae. The white flecking is due to dystrophic calcification.

break off and cause renal colic and hematuria. The affected area of kidney shows tubular atrophy with scarring and interstitial infiltration with lymphocytes. As more and more papillae become necrotic, increasing areas of renal parenchyma are destroyed, and this is associated with deterioration of renal function and ultimately uremia.

It is evident that all people involved in administering health care should endeavor to dissuade patients from abusing the many analgesic mixtures that are so prominently advertised on radio and television and in the drug stores.

Acute Tubular Necrosis

Acute tubular necrosis (ATN) is characterized by a sudden drop in urinary output and the steady development of uremia. It is the most common cause of acute renal failure in clinical practice. Biopsy of the kidney sometimes shows tubular necrosis, later followed by signs of regeneration; in other cases, the kidney, although perhaps swollen, appears normal on microscopy even at necropsy. Hence, the term acute tubular necrosis is not strictly accurate but nevertheless is in common use.

Ischemia of the kidney due to underperfusion is the most common cause of ATN; hence, it is a common feature of shock. Not only is the perfusing pressure low, but there is intense vasoconstriction affecting particularly the kidney. ATN is therefore a feature of acute hemorrhage, severe trauma (including surgery), sepsis, burns, and various complications of pregnancy, *e.g.*, abruptio placentae, eclampsia, and septic abortion. The basement membrane of damaged tubules shows areas of disruption; hence, the term for this type is tubulorrhectic ATN.

A less common cause of ATN is poisoning with chemicals or drugs. Heavy metals (*e.g.*, mercuric chloride), organic solvents, and ethylene glycol (used as an antifreeze) are important causes. Certain drugs are also nephrotoxic, *e.g.*, aminoglycosides, nonsteroid analgesic drugs, anesthetic agents, and x-ray contrast media used in arteriography.

An uncommon type of ATN is pigment-induced. It occurs in acute hemolysis, mismatched blood transfusion, and acute rhabdomyolysis.

Clinical Course of ATN. In the initial stages, there is a rise of the BUN followed shortly by a fall in urine output to 400 ml per day or less. Complete anuria is unusual. The urine has a specific gravity of 1.010 and contains granular and cellular casts. During this *oliguric phase*, there is metabolic acidosis and retention of nitrogenous substances (urea and creatinine), potassium, magnesium, phosphate, and other anions. A rapidly developing anemia is also a feature, in part due to an increase in plasma volume and in part due to a hemolytic element that accompanies uremia. The patient may die of potassium intoxication, overhydration causing heart failure or pulmonary edema, infection, or uremia.

In recent years, a *nonoliguric form of ATN* has been recognized. It appears to be associated with vigorous plasma volume–expanding therapy (using saline and mannitol) and the administration of vasodilator drugs that lower the renal vascular resistance.

If the patient survives, the urine output increases and may reach 3 liters per day. The onset of this *diuretic phase* may be gradual or quite sudden. The urine is at first little more than a protein-free plasma filtrate. Loss of water and electrolytes is considerable during this stage, and the patient's life is in jeopardy because of dehydration and electrolyte imbalance. Infection continues to be a hazard.

Specific Defects of Tubular Function

During the flow of the glomerular filtrate down the renal tubules, many substances are absorbed so that the final fluid (urine) is much reduced in volume and changed in composition. Not surprisingly, there are circumstances under which one or more of these functions is impaired. Most of the conditions are rare congenital inherited diseases, but occasionally they occur later in life as a result of disease, *e.g.*, pyelonephritis. Impaired water reabsorption causes *nephrogenic diabetes insipidus*: the kidney fails to respond to antidiuretic hormone. Other syndromes are known in which there is impairment of the absorption of amino acids, glucose, or phosphate.

RENAL AND URINARY TRACT INFECTION: PYELONEPHRITIS

Bacterial infection of the urinary tract is very common and constitutes a major medical problem. The infecting organisms are usually the gram-negative intestinal bacilli, including *Escherichia coli*, *Pseudomonas aeruginosa*, and *Streptococcus faecalis*, as well as *Proteus*, *Klebsiella*, and *Enterobacter* species.

Acute Pyelonephritis

The causative organisms are derived from the patient's own fecal flora. Two routes of infection have been described, and their relative importance has long been debated.

Hematogenous Infection. It is believed that some infection is blood-borne from the colon. Normally, organisms that avoid the clearing action of the mononuclear phagocyte system of the liver pass into the systemic circulation; they escape into the glomerular filtrate and are voided in the urine.

Ascending Infection. It is now thought that the most common route of infection is ascent of organisms from the perineum to the urinary tract. Acute cystitis is more common in females of all ages after the first year of life. It is common in pregnancy. The shortness of the urethra and the ease with which vulval organisms can ascend the urethra is probably the explanation. Direct introduction of organisms into the bladder can complicate catheterization, particularly if it is repeated.

After acute cystitis, ascending infection due to reflux of urine into the ureters can occur. Indeed, vesicoureteric reflux is an important cause of upper urinary tract infections in children; furthermore, intrarenal reflux may further promote the involvement of renal parenchyma by ascending infection.

It is evident that obstruction of the urinary flow is an important predisposing factor to infection. This can be demonstrated experimentally and is in keeping with the observed incidence of infection. Thus, urethral obstruction, such as that due to prostatic enlargement, generally causes bilateral pyelonephritis; whereas if one ureter is obstructed, *e.g.*, by a calculus or a neoplasm, pyelonephritis is usually unilateral. If there has been previous blockage, the hydronephrotic kidney becomes infected to produce a sac of pus, which is known as *pyonephrosis*.

A number of factors predispose to urinary tract infection. It is more common in diabetes mellitus and in patients on glucocorticoid therapy. Furthermore, there may be genetic differences between individuals, so that certain people are more liable to be colonized and infected by certain strains of organisms. Evidence in support of this is the finding that the uroepithelium of some individuals can have receptors for certain strains of *E. coli*. The organisms become adherent to the epithelium, and subsequent invasion is facilitated.

Clinical Features. The clinical features of acute urinary tract infection are those of any severe acute pyogenic infection—rigors, fever, and malaise. Pain is experienced in the loins in pyelonephritis. With cystitis and urethritis, the inflammation leads to urgency of micturition together with pain and burning on passing urine. The acute attack generally subsides rapidly either spontaneously or under treatment with antibiotics.

The urine in acute cystitis and acute pyelonephritis contains numerous pus cells; organisms can usually be seen in a stained smear of urine; hematuria is common.

Lesions in Acute Pyelonephritis. The interstitial tissues show an acute inflammatory reaction that also involves the tubules. Numerous pinpoint cortical abscesses are characteristic, and the pelvis and calyces are intensely inflamed. An occasional complication of acute pyelonephritis, especially common in diabetic subjects and if there is urinary obstruction, is *papillary necrosis*. The lesions are similar to those encountered in analgesic nephropathy.

Chronic Pyelonephritis

Chronic pyelonephritis is generally regarded as a chronic or recurrent infection that leads to chronic inflammation with progressive renal scarring. The disease is characterized by the presence of multiple cortical scars associated with underlying dilated or deformed calyces. The scarring tends to be patchy, and the kidney substance between the areas of scarring may show tubular hypertrophy; hence, the kidney in chronic pyelonephritis is coarsely scarred, and if the disease is bilateral, the involvement is asymmetric. Chronic pyelonephritis is characterized by the presence of multiple cortical scars with the scars overlying dilated or deformed calyces. In the areas of scarring, there is a chronic inflammatory infiltrate and extensive loss of tubules; glomeruli are spared until late in the course of the disease. Systemic hypertension, sometimes of the malignant type, is common in chronic pyelonephritis, and both scarred and nonscarred areas of kidney show secondary changes of nephrosclerosis. The result is a scarred end-stage kidney not distinguishable from other end-stage disease.

The cause of the persistent infection is unknown; some obstruction to the urinary outflow may be present, and if none is obvious, some intrinsic renal damage or the scars of previous infection may cause local obstruction. This type of disease is called *chronic obstructive pyelonephritis*. However, in the majority of cases, no definite obstruction can be demonstrated; it is believed that vesicoureteric and intrarenal reflux play the dominant role, for even without obvious infection, this appears to damage the kidney and lead to chronic pyelonephritis. This type is called *chronic reflux-associated pyelonephritis*.

Clinical Features. The clinical features of chronic pyelonephritis are usually those of progressive renal failure terminating in uremia or are attributable to hypertension and its complications. Occasionally, a specific tubular defect such as one causing aminoaciduria or the nephrotic syndrome occurs.

Other Infections of the Kidney

Tuberculosis of the urinary tract is now an uncommon disease. Routine urine culture is negative, but tuberculosis should be suspected in any case of "sterile pyuria." The kidney can be infected in any generalized infection, *e.g.*, candidiasis.

CONGENITAL DISEASES OF THE KIDNEY

Occasionally one kidney is small (hypoplastic) or completely absent (agenesis). The kidneys may be abnormally placed either at the brim of the pelvis or in the pelvic cavity itself. In *horseshoe kidney*, the two organs are fused together either at their upper or lower poles to produce a horseshoe deformity. These anomalies are of importance to the radiologist or surgeon who is investigating urinary tract disease. Horseshoe kidneys are found in approximately 0.1 per cent of the population. A more frequent malformation is *polycystic kidney*. The common adult type of this condition is inherited as an autosomal dominant trait but does not become manifest until the teens or later. Numerous cysts steadily form, so that ultimately both kidneys become enormous (Fig. 25–8). The cysts communicate with the renal tubules so that bleeding into one of them causes hematuria, in addition to the pain due to the mechanical distention of the cyst wall. Systemic hypertension is common, and eventually renal failure ensues. In the past, such patients rarely lived beyond the age of 50 years, but this gloomy outlook has been changed by the advent of renal transplantation. Berry aneurysms are present in about 15 per cent of cases, and subarachnoid hemorrhage is an additional hazard, especially since there is often high blood pressure (Chapter 33).

NEOPLASMS OF THE KIDNEY

Adenoma. The common benign renal tumor is an adenoma that is usually pinhead-sized and

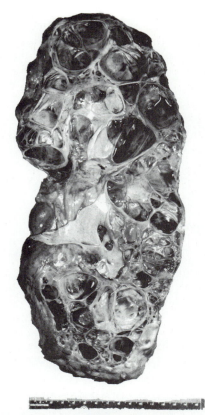

Figure 25–8 Polycystic kidney. The patient was first diagnosed as having polycystic kidneys at the age of 23 years, when he was investigated after an episode of hematuria. He remained in fairly good health until the age of 30, by which time he had developed hypertension and a blood urea nitrogen of 64.3 mmol/L. He complained of a dragging sensation in the abdomen, evidently due to the enormous enlargement of both kidneys. Peritoneal dialysis was carried out, but the patient's condition deteriorated, and he died of uremia at the age of 31. This was in 1963, when renal transplantation was not as readily available as it is today.

The specimen is the left kidney, which has been sectioned to show extensive replacement of renal substance by innumerable cysts ranging in size from microscopic to over 6 cm in diameter. The kidney weighed 4000 g, and its size was recorded as 35 cm × 15 cm × 8 cm.

appears as a yellow-white nodule situated beneath the capsule. Its cells are usually arranged in a papillary cystadenomatous pattern and closely resemble those of a carcinoma.

Carcinoma. This is the malignant counterpart of the adenoma and usually appears as a large, soft mass at one or the other pole (see Case History I and Fig. 25–9). A section shows that it has a variegated appearance, with some areas being white, others yellow or orange; elsewhere

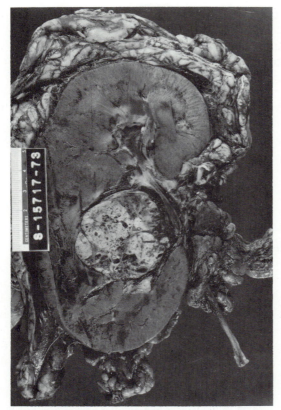

Figure 25–9 Carcinoma of the kidney. The kidney contains a well-circumscribed tumor about 4 cm in diameter. It was yellow in color in the fresh state. Microscopy revealed a clear-cell renal carcinoma. See Case History I for clinical details.

there are foci of bleeding. On microscopic examination, it consists of large spheroidal cells with clear cytoplasm. In well-differentiated tumors, these cells are arranged to form tubules. Although the cells resemble those of the normal renal tubules, it was at one time believed that the tumor arose from ectopic adrenal tissue situated on the surface of the kidney. This belief was the origin of the name *hypernephroma*, a term that is still widely used. It has since been discovered that the tumor arises from renal tubular epithelium; all grades of transition can be found between the anaplastic tumors and the benign adenoma.

The clear appearance of the cells is due to their high content of lipid and glycogen, both of which are lost during routine paraffin wax sectioning. The yellow appearance is due to the carotenoid pigments dissolved in the lipid. Probably the best name for this tumor is *clear-cell carcinoma of the kidney.*

Clinically, carcinoma of the kidney is often silent for a long time. *Painless hematuria and an abdominal mass are the two common presenting features.* Distant and blood-borne metastases are common, with the liver, lungs, and bones being especially involved.

Case History I

In 1967, at the age of 57 years, the patient presented with a complaint of chronic cough. A radiograph showed ill-defined shadows in both upper lung fields; these were interpreted as being produced by fibrosis. Nineteen years previously, a radiograph was reported to have shown similar shadows, and at that time pulmonary tuberculosis had been suspected. The diagnosis had never been proved, and no treatment had been given.

Several samples of sputum and gastric washings were examined for tubercle bacilli without success. A lymph node biopsy taken at mediastinoscopy revealed noncaseating granulomas. No organisms could be identified in the sections. However, shortly after the procedure, a nodule was noted on the left nostril, and a biopsy again revealed a granulomatous reaction; this time, fungi were detected. A repeat biopsy of the nodule was cultured, and *Histoplasma capsulatum* was grown. Amphotericin B therapy was instituted, and the patient's condition improved. Nevertheless, he complained of easy fatigue and periodically had attacks of nausea and vomiting. No cause was found.

Two years later, difficulty in passing urine and nocturia led to a transurethral resection of an enlarged prostate. Histopathologic studies revealed a benign prostate enlargement, but a radiograph revealed a translucent area in the first lumbar vertebral body. In spite of the pathology report, a diagnosis of carcinoma of the prostate with bone metastases was made. Stilbestrol (a synthetic estrogen) therapy was initiated. Several episodes of painless hematuria were attributed to carcinoma of the prostate. Two years later, however, a cystoscopy failed to detect any bladder or prostatic lesion. Further investigations (an intravenous pyelogram and an arteriogram) showed a lesion in the left kidney. A nephrectomy was carried out for carcinoma of the kidney (see Fig. 25–9). Shortly after surgery, the patient collapsed and died in shock.

Autopsy revealed no evidence of carcinoma of the prostate. Both adrenal glands showed almost complete replacement by caseous material due to histoplasmosis (see Fig. 29–3). The lesion in the vertebra also showed histoplasmosis. The upper lobes of both lungs were fibrotic and contained scanty granulomas. This case illustrates several points:

1. Histoplasmosis, like tuberculosis, can become active after remaining dormant for many years.

2. Attacks of vomiting combined with weakness suggest a diagnosis of Addison's disease.

3. Major surgery in a patient with Addison's disease is hazardous unless adequate glucocorticoids are given.

4. In the absence of pathologic proof, it was unwise to make a clinical diagnosis of prostatic cancer. The significance of the attacks of painless hematuria was not appreciated, causing the diagnosis of carcinoma of the kidney to be delayed for over 1 year.

An interesting feature of the tumor is the phenomenon of dormancy. Bone metastases may suddenly erupt many years after the apparently successful removal of the primary growth.

Nephroblastoma, or Wilms' Tumor. The nephroblastoma is a malignant tumor affecting children under the age of 5 years. It is presumed to arise from a primitive nephroblast, a cell that gives rise to both epithelial and connective tissue components of the kidney. The tumor is likewise mixed, having both epithelial and connective tissue elements. Although the tumor is highly malignant, modern treatment has greatly improved the prognosis.

The Lower Urinary Tract

URINARY TRACT OBSTRUCTION (OBSTRUCTIVE UROPATHY)

Ureteric Obstruction. Sudden complete obstruction of one ureter, such as by a calculus, leads to atrophy of the affected kidney and compensatory enlargement of the other. Partial obstruction of a ureter by a stone, tumor, or pressure from an adjacent mass leads to dilation of the ureter above the obstruction (*hydroureter*) and dilation of the pelvis of the affected kidney (*hydronephrosis*).

Urethral Obstruction. The following causes should be noted:

1. Carcinoma of the urethra. This is uncommon.

2. Fibrous stricture. This may follow repeated catheterization or may be an aftereffect of gonococcal urethritis.

3. Carcinoma of the prostate.

4. Benign prostatic enlargement. This is by far the most common and important cause of urethral obstruction and is considered in detail.

Benign Prostatic Enlargement. It has been estimated that between 30 and 50 per cent of men develop some degree of obstruction from this cause after the age of 50 years. Common symptoms are difficulty in starting the act of urination (micturition), a poor stream of urine, and incomplete emptying of the bladder after micturition.

This increase in the residual urine predisposes to *infection*. As the bladder refills, the urge to urinate returns, and there is *frequency of micturition and nocturia*. The bladder dilates, and its muscular wall hypertrophies in response to the increased work needed to expel urine. Its wall becomes trabeculated (see Fig. 26–2). Protrusions of mucosa produce outpouchings, or *diverticula*, which further predispose to urinary stasis and infection.

Sudden urethral obstruction due to benign prostatic enlargement can occur at any time and is presumably due to congestion or infection. The enlarged median lobe of the prostate overlying the urethra can act like a ball valve.

Acute urethral obstruction must be distinguished from anuria. In both conditions, no urine is passed through the urethra; but with obstruction, the bladder becomes painfully enlarged. Ultimately, the increased pressure may force some urine through the urethra. This *retention with overflow* can deceive the unwary attendant into believing that the obstruction has been relieved.

The treatment of acute urinary obstruction requires expert attention. Either a catheter is passed through the urethra or else a needle is inserted into the bladder through the anterior abdominal wall; in either event, the obstruction is relieved. Urine must not be drained too quickly, however, or the sudden reduction in pressure will lead to bleeding. In addition, sudden decompression can cause an equally sudden diuresis, and this can cause hypovolemic shock.

Effect of Urinary Obstruction on the Kidney. Obstruction of the outflow of urine produces a back-pressure effect on the kidney that results in tubular atrophy and ultimately in destruction of renal parenchyma. The pelvis dilates, and hydronephrosis results (Fig. 25–10). Evidence of chronic renal failure, such as a raised BUN, in an elderly person always suggests the likelihood of obstructive uropathy, particularly if the azotemia (excess of nitrogenous substances in the blood) fluctuates in intensity over a period of a few days.

NEUROGENIC BLADDER

When lesions of the spinal cord damage the corticospinal tracts, there is loss of voluntary control of micturition. As the bladder dilates, local reflexes are responsible for automatic evacuation of urine. If the cord lesion is low, or if the nerves to the bladder are directly involved, even this automatic reflex is lost, and the bladder fills and finally overflows. In either event, urinary

stasis—particularly when combined with repeated catheterization—predisposes the patient to urinary tract infection.

Case History II

In 1948, at the age of 44 years, the patient noticed that his urine suddenly became red. Microscopic examination of the urine showed numerous red blood cells; tests for hemoglobin were positive. Cystoscopy revealed numerous "papillomas" in the bladder, and these were *fulgurated* (burned with an electric spark). Because of numerous recurrences, the diagnosis was subsequently changed to papillary carcinoma. During the next 25 years, the bladder tumors were treated on at least 34 occasions. In 1973, when the patient was 69 years of age, a mass was noted in the left side of the abdomen. This was identified as a nonfunctioning kidney and was removed. There were further recurrences of tumor, and in 1975 a partial cystectomy (removal of part of the bladder) was undertaken. A tumor similar to that shown in Figure 25–11 was found.

URETERIC REFLUX

It is not uncommon to find hydroureter and hydronephrosis in the absence of any organic obstructive lesion. In such cases, it is believed

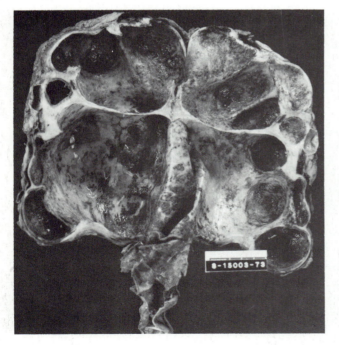

Figure 25–10 Hydronephrosis. The kidney shows dilation of the pelvis and severe damage to the renal parenchyma such that the organ is converted into a bag of fluid. The condition resulted from intermittent ureteric obstruction by a low-grade carcinoma of the bladder. See Case History II for clinical details.

that these are examples of neuromuscular incoordination. Radiographic studies indicate that in some patients, urine passes up the ureter by abnormal peristaltic waves traveling in an upward direction.

NEOPLASMS OF THE URINARY PASSAGES

Apart from carcinoma, tumors of the urinary passages are uncommon.

Carcinoma. Well-differentiated tumors of the transitional epithelium are often multiple and appear as noninvasive papillomatous growths with delicate fronds that give the lesions a resemblance to a sea anemone (Fig. 25–11). On histologic examination, these tumors are papillomatous and appear benign, but unfortunately they tend to recur even after local treatment (see Case History II). In practice, it is wise to regard them

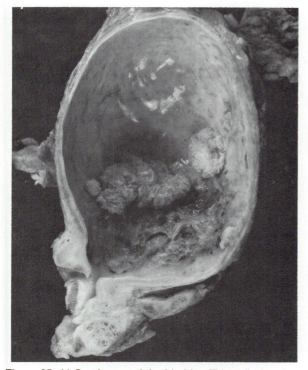

Figure 25–11 Carcinoma of the bladder. This radical cystectomy specimen was inflated with 10 per cent formalin solution before being opened. Numerous papillomatous tumors are seen attached to the bladder lining. Microscopy revealed a papillary transitional-cell carcinoma.

as low-grade carcinomas. Nevertheless, some authorities recognize the entity of benign papilloma of the bladder and attribute recurrence to the formation of new tumors. The less well differentiated transitional-cell tumors are the obvious carcinomas that show invasion of the wall and appear as sessile nodules or papillomatous lesions that break down into indurated malignant ulcers.

On histologic examination, the tumors are transitional-cell carcinomas of varying degrees of differentiation. In some tumors, there are areas of squamous-cell change; not infrequently, tumors are found in which the entire growth is composed of squamous-cell carcinoma. These cases tend to have a poor prognosis. Cancer of the bladder is particularly common in the Middle East and is associated with schistosomiasis. The increased incidence of bladder cancer in aniline dye workers and in those engaged in the rubber industry has been noted in Chapter 12. There is also an increased incidence in those who indulge in heavy cigarette smoking. Users of analgesic mixtures containing phenacetin are at a much higher risk of developing transitional-cell carcinoma of the renal pelvis than are nonusers. Carcinoma may therefore be a late complication of analgesic nephropathy, which is described earlier in this chapter.

URINARY CALCULI

Urinary stones, or calculi, have plagued mankind for centuries; they are particularly common in the hot desert regions of the Middle East. Calculi can be divided into two main groups: primary and secondary.

Primary Calculi. These are presumed to occur because of a high concentration of chemicals in the urine or because of a defective mechanism for keeping these crystalloids in solution. Three common types are known.

Urate Stones. These are smooth, consist of uric acid and urates, and are common in patients who suffer from gout.

Calcium Oxalate Stones. These characteristically have a spiky surface that causes hematuria by damaging the mucosa.

Mixed Calcium Oxalate and Phosphate Stones.

This type of stone occurs in the hypercalcemia that accompanies hyperparathyroidism and prolonged periods of recumbency.

Secondary Calculi. These stones are composed of calcium and magnesium oxalates and phosphates. They are formed around a focus of necrotic tissue, organisms, fibrin, a foreign body, or a primary stone. They are often secondary to infection. The most common type is found in the renal pelvis; as it grows, it assumes the shape of the pelvis and produces a shape that has been likened to that of a staghorn.

Effects of Urinary Calculi

1. Infection. Patients with recurrent urinary tract infection should always be investigated for the possibility of urinary stones.

2. Obstruction. This is frequently intermittent.

3. Hematuria.

4. Pain. A stone formed in the renal pelvis can pass down the ureter and cause severe colicky pain lasting for a time ranging from several minutes to several hours. This *renal colic* is usually accompanied by hematuria.

Summary

- The kidney has many functions other than the excretion of waste products. The kidneys regulate fluid and acid-base balance, blood pressure, erythropoiesis, and vitamin D metabolism.
- Clearance values are a useful test of renal function, as is urine analysis—chemical, microscopic, and bacteriologic.
- Features of renal disease are the nephritic syndrome, the nephrotic syndrome, persistent urinary abnormalities, and renal failure, both acute and chronic.
- Glomerulonephritis is classified on the basis of clinical, immunologic, and histopathologic findings.
- Proliferative glomerulonephritis may be post-streptococcal and causes the nephritic syndrome—oliguria, albuminuria, hematuria, and edema.
- Minimal-change, membranous, and membranoproliferative glomerulonephritis are often associated with the nephrotic syndrome—heavy albuminuria, hypoalbuminemia, hyperlipidemia, and marked edema.
- Chronic glomerulonephritis is an end stage of many diseases.
- Interstitial nephritis, if acute, may be drug-induced (*e.g.*, methicillin). If chronic, analgesic drugs are sometimes causative (analgesic nephropathy); papillary necrosis is a complication.
- Acute tubular necrosis commonly complicates shock, less often infection and poisoning. It has an oliguric phase followed by a diuretic phase if recovery occurs.
- Acute pyelonephritis is generally the result of ascending infection. Vesicoureteric reflux, urinary tract obstruction, diabetes mellitus, and immunosuppression are predisposing factors.
- Chronic pyelonephritis is not obviously of infective origin in many cases. Chronic reflux may be a factor. Uremia and hypertension are complications.
- The dominantly inherited polycystic kidney is associated with berry aneurysm of a cerebral vessel. It causes hypertension, hematuria, and uremia.
- Important malignant tumors are clear-cell carcinoma of the kidney and transitional-cell carcinoma of the urinary passages. Both cause painless hematuria. By contrast, hematuria with urinary calculi is associated with painful colic. Obstruction and infection are other features of calculi.
- Benign prostatic enlargement is the most common cause of urethral obstruction in elderly men. Bladder diverticulum may be associated.

Selected Readings

Brenner, B. M., and Rector, F. C., Jr. (eds.): The Kidney. 4th ed. Philadelphia, W. B. Saunders Co., 1989.

Davidson, A. (ed.): Nephrology. Vol. 1. Philadelphia, W. B. Saunders Co., 1988.

Heptinstall, R. H.: Pathology of the Kidney. 3rd ed. Vols. 1, 2, and 3. Boston, Little, Brown & Co., 1983.

Kaplan, N. K.: Systemic hypertension: Mechanisms and Diagnosis. *In* Braunwald, E. (ed.): Heart Disease. 2nd ed. Philadelphia, W. B. Saunders Co., 1984.

Myers, B. D., and Moran, S. M.: Hemodynamically mediated acute renal failure. N. Engl. J. Med. 314:97, 1986.

Schoolnik, G. K.: How *Escherichia coli* infect the urinary tract. N. Engl. J. Med. 320:804, 1989.

26

Male Reproductive Organs

After studying this chapter, the student should be able to:

• Describe balanoposthitis, phimosis, paraphimosis, condylomata acuminata, and bowenoid papulosis.
• Describe the clinical and pathologic features of benign prostatic enlargement.

• Describe carcinoma of the prostate with regard to the following factors:
  (a) frequency;
  (b) clinical features;
  (c) spread.
• Describe the development of the testis and relate this to the following:
  (a) the occurrence of inguinal hernias;
  (b) the blood supply of the testis;
  (c) the metastatic spread of testicular tumors;
  (d) spermatogenesis.
• Describe cryptorchidism and its complications.
• Give an account of torsion of the testis.
• Classify the common causes of orchitis and epididymo-orchitis.
• Classify the tumors of the testis.

The most important organs of the male genital tract are the testes, where spermatozoa are manufactured. Sperm, together with secretion from the epididymides, pass as seminal fluid to the urethra. The external genitalia comprise the penis and scrotum.

PENIS, URETHRA, AND SCROTUM

The newborn infant should always be carefully examined for congenital defects because they may be the outward evidence of a serious error

505

in sexual development, such as pseudohermaphroditism; or the error may point to other less obvious internal abnormalities. Thus, if the genital folds fail to fuse correctly, the urethra opens on the ventral surface of the shaft of the penis or, if the malformation is severe, in the perineum. The result is *hypospadias*, which may be accompanied by other abnormalities in the urinary tract. A less common malformation is *epispadias*, in which the urethra opens onto the dorsal surface of the penis.

Infections

Gonorrhea, syphilis, and other sexually transmitted diseases are described in Chapter 8. *Balanoposthitis* is the result of smegma retention due to poor personal hygiene, particularly in patients with phimosis or a large redundant prepuce. Bacterial colonization and nonspecific pyogenic infections of the glans and prepuce follow and may cause severe ulceration and subsequent scarring.

Phimosis

If the preputial opening is small, retraction of the prepuce is either difficult or impossible. If the tight foreskin is forcibly retracted, it can act as a constricting ring to cause swelling of the glans so that the prepuce cannot be replaced. This extremely painful condition is called *paraphimosis*; unless relieved, it causes acute urinary obstruction and even ischemic necrosis of the glans penis.

Neoplasms of the Penis

Condylomata Acuminata. Condylomata acuminata are very common warty growths on the glans, prepuce, or shaft of the penis (Fig. 26–1). They are caused by the human papillomavirus (HPV type 6 or 11). Condylomata acuminata are not generally precancerous, but an exception to this is the *giant condyloma*. This lesion generally occurs as a bulky papillomatous growth of the glans penis. A similar lesion can occur on the

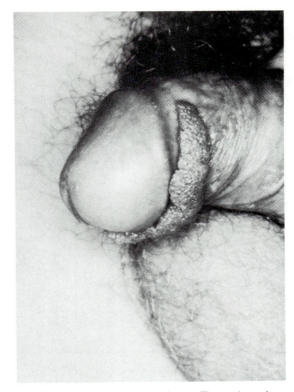

Figure 26–1 Condylomata acuminata. The undersurface of the prepuce shows a confluent mass of papillomas. (Courtesy of Dr. B. K. Fisher, Wellesley Hospital, Toronto. From Walter, J. B.: Pathology of Human Disease. Philadelphia, Lea & Febiger, 1989.)

vulva or in the anal region of both sexes. Histologically similar tumors are found in the oral cavity and have been called *verrucous carcinoma*. These lesions steadily enlarge and invade locally but almost never metastasize.

In Situ **Squamous-Cell Carcinoma.** *In situ* squamous-cell carcinoma can occur in the anogenital region and clinically appear as Bowen's disease. On the glans penis (and also in other mucous membranes such as the mouth), keratinization is often absent and the lesion, termed *erythroplasia of Queyrat*, has a red velvety appearance. A third type of lesion is *bowenoid papulosis*. Clinically, there are multiple raised pigmented lesions resembling skin tags or seborrheic keratoses in the anogenital region. On microscopic examination, they show carcinoma *in situ*, but do not behave as premalignant lesions. They appear to be a curious reaction to the wart virus, probably HPV-16.

Carcinoma of the Penis. Squamous-cell carcinoma of the penis is uncommon in North America and Europe but elsewhere is not uncommon in the uncircumcised, particularly in areas where standards of cleanliness are low. It is almost unknown in those communities that practice ritual circumcision at an early age (*e.g.*, Jews and Muslems). In spite of the exposed position of this tumor, the 5-year survival is about 50 per cent. About one third of cases have metastasized at the time of diagnosis.

Carcinoma of the Scrotum

The description of squamous-cell carcinoma of the scrotum in chimney sweeps by Percival Pott in 1775 was a landmark in the recognition of chemicals as carcinogens. The moist corrugations of the scrotal skin favor retention of industrial carcinogens such as soot, tar, and machine lubricating oils. Preventive measures have greatly reduced the incidence of this tumor.

Extramammary Paget's Disease

An underlying adenocarcinoma may be associated with Paget's disease that occurs on the scrotum and perianal skin.

THE PROSTATE

The prostate gland is situated at the base of the bladder and is traversed by the first part of the male urethra. Its functions are largely unknown, but it contributes its secretions to the seminal ejaculate; its enlargement is a source of considerable annoyance and morbidity in old age.

Prostatitis

Acute prostatitis is generally a complication of urinary tract infection and can be a complication of gonorrhea. It is sometimes precipitated by catheterization and cystoscopy. The changes are similar to those of inflammation in other situations and therefore can terminate in suppuration.

Chronic prostatitis is extremely common as an incidental finding at necropsy. It generally accompanies urinary tract infection and may be associated with numerous calculi within the gland. Chronic prostatitis of clinical significance leads to fibrosis, which may give the gland a firmness that can be mistaken for carcinoma.

Benign Prostatic Enlargement

This is the most common disease of the prostate and is also called *prostatic hypertrophy* or *nodular hyperplasia*. The disease is extremely common in men over 50 years of age, and its incidence increases with age. Consequently, in men over the age of 70 years, about 95 per cent have some degree of involvement. The prostate gland becomes enlarged and nodular. This can be detected clinically by rectal examination. On cross section, cystic nodular areas are found, which can be proved microscopically to be due to foci of glandular hyperplasia. In other areas, there is overgrowth of smooth muscle or fibrous tissue. These elements give the gland a texture that is firm but not usually so hard that it mimics carcinoma. The nodular elements press on local blood vessels, so that focal areas of infarction are not uncommon. Bleeding can occur into these areas, and clinically hematuria is a frequent symptom. The other major effect of prostatic enlargement is distortion of the prostatic urethra and its obstruction (Fig. 26–2). The clinical features and secondary effects of this enlargement on the bladder and kidneys are described elsewhere (Chapter 25).

The cause of benign prostatic enlargement is not known, but it is presumed to be related to hormonal imbalance of old age. A deficiency of androgens or an excess of estrogenic substances has been suggested but not proved.

The treatment of significant benign prostatic enlargement is surgical. Prostatectomy can be performed through an abdominal incision or through the urethra with use of an operating endoscope. Not all patients with prostatic enlargement require treatment. It has been estimated that between 5 and 10 per cent of patients

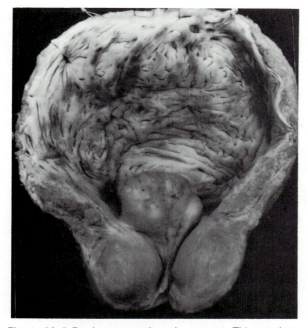

Figure 26–2 Benign prostatic enlargement. This specimen of bladder and prostatic urethra has been opened from the front. The prostate is enlarged, and its nodular median lobe projects into the bladder, acting as a ball valve to obstruct the passage of urine. The bladder wall is thickened. Hypertrophy of muscle bundles is responsible for the ribbed or trabeculated appearance of its lining. (Specimen from the Boyd Museum, Toronto.)

require surgical resection for relief of urinary tract obstruction or infection.

Carcinoma of the Prostate

Carcinoma of the prostate is the second most frequent cause of death from carcinoma in men in the United States. It is common to find small foci of carcinoma in elderly patients dying from other causes, but the significance of these has been disputed. Progressive clinical cancer of the prostate is less common and may present with urinary obstruction or the development of symptoms due to local invasion or metastatic growth. Cancer of the prostate involves such local tissue as seminal vesicle, rectum, and bladder (Fig. 26–3); it also metastasizes to the regional lymph nodes. More significant is the blood-borne metastatic spread; approximately 70 per cent of cases show bone metastases, particularly of the lower

spine. These lesions are noteworthy for being osteosclerotic. Metastatic spread to the liver and lungs is also common.

On microscopic examination, cancer of the prostate is generally a well-differentiated adenocarcinoma, and it tends to excite a considerable scirrhous reaction. A prostate with cancer is stony hard—the salient clinical feature, which can be detected by rectal examination. In any patient suspected of having malignant disease, particularly with metastatic bone spread, a rectal examination is mandatory if the patient is over 50 years of age.

The normal prostatic epithelium secretes acid phosphatase. In carcinoma, particularly if the bulk of tumor and its metastases is great, there is an elevation of the blood level of this enzyme. A test of the level of prostatic acid phosphatase is useful diagnostically, but a normal level does not exclude an early carcinoma.

Prostatic massage can express material through the urethra; malignant cells can be found in this fluid. This method is not completely reliable and has been criticized, since malignant cells appear in the blood after massage, and this could conceivably initiate the formation of metastases.

The most satisfactory method of diagnosis after clinical suspicion is a biopsy, which can generally be performed through the urethra.

The normal prostate is dependent on andro-

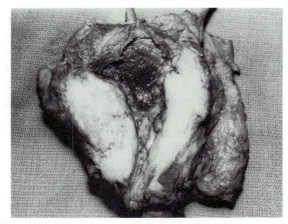

Figure 26–3 Carcinoma of the prostate. The prostate is replaced by firm white tumor that envelops the urethra and extends upward to invade the bladder wall. (From Walter, J. B.: Pathology of Human Disease. Philadelphia, Lea & Febiger, 1989.)

gens, and many carcinomas also are dependent on androgenic hormones. Some degree of hormonal control of cancer of the prostate can be obtained by estrogen (diethylstilbestrol, DES) administration, castration, or a combination of the two. The results are sometimes quite striking; generally, they are of limited duration.

Other types of hormone therapy are also of value. Administration of powerful analogues of gonadotropin-releasing hormone (*e.g.,* leuprolide) produces a brief period of stimulation, followed by a prolonged inhibition of follicle-stimulating hormone and luteinizing hormone release. The serum testosterone level falls to castration levels. Ketoconazole, an antifungal agent, has a similar effect. Administration of antiandrogens (*e.g.,* flutamide) is another approach. The results of these new forms of treatment are being assessed; they appear to be at least as effective as DES but to have fewer side effects.

THE TESTIS AND EPIDIDYMIS

The testes develop from a mass of mesoderm in the posterior abdominal wall. While still retaining their original blood supply, they migrate downward and forward, traversing the anterior abdominal wall through the inguinal canal until they finally come to lie in the scrotum. A process of peritoneum accompanies this descent, forming the tunica vaginalis, which surrounds the testis and its epididymis. The sac usually loses connection with the peritoneal cavity, but the inguinal region remains a point of weakness throughout life and is a common site for the development of a hernia. This is the price that has to be paid for having the male gonads in the scrotum, where the temperature can be maintained at a lower level than is found in the abdomen, from which the testes descended. There is evidence that this cool environment is necessary for the development of sperm (spermatogenesis).

The testis is both an endocrine organ (secreting testosterone) and an exocrine organ (secreting spermatozoa).

The Testis as an Endocrine Organ

The luteinizing hormone of the pituitary gland stimulates the interstitial cells to secrete testosterone, the principal androgen in the circulation. Androgens are vital for male phenotypic sexual differentiation during embryonic life and for sexual maturation at puberty. There are many syndromes related to a failure in the normal formation of androgens by the testis or lack of appropriate hormone receptors on target organs. These *androgen deficiency syndromes* range from severe anatomic defects such as pseudohermaphroditism to subtle changes manifested as infertility in otherwise normal males.

The Testis as an Exocrine Gland

It has been estimated that in involuntarily childless marriages, approximately 50 per cent are due solely or partially to male infertility. The defect may be inadequate production of a normal number of normal spermatozoa or some error in their delivery to the ovum. The details of this complex subject are beyond the scope of this book.

Cryptorchidism

In *cryptorchidism,* one or both testes fail to descend and reach the scrotum. The glands are then situated either within the abdomen or in the inguinal canal. Failure in spermatogenesis results in infertility if both testes are affected. An undescended testis remains immature and is liable to develop a malignant tumor, particularly a seminoma. Unless an undescended testis can be made to descend, by either medical or surgical means, it should be removed, since it remains a permanent hazard.

Torsion of the Testis

During violent exercise or after trauma, the testis can rotate, causing a twist of the spermatic cord and its blood vessels. This rotation causes sudden pain; unless the testis can be untwisted soon (either by manipulation or by open surgery), first the veins and then the arteries become obstructed. The organ becomes intensely congested and subsequently infarcted. Torsion of the testis tends to occur if the testis is abnormally mobile because of a mild developmental defect, which is sometimes bilateral. Hence, after torsion of one testis, the other should be fixed to prevent a similar event from occurring on the other side.

Hydrocele

A collection of clear fluid in the tunica vaginalis, the sac that surrounds the testis, is termed a hydrocele. Transillumination readily distinguishes it from a testicular mass. A hydrocele may accompany any type of generalized edema or form as a complication of epididymo-orchitis or a testicular neoplasm. Often no cause can be found. A *hematocele*, a collection of blood in the tunica vaginalis, generally follows direct trauma.

Infections of the Testis and Epididymis

Acute infections of the epididymis (epididymitis) and testis (orchitis) generally occur secondarily to infection of the urinary tract or prostate. Acute epididymo-orchitis sometimes follows prostatitis and is a well-recognized complication of surgery on the prostate unless the vas deferens and its related lymphatics have been tied previously. Gonococcal epididymo-orchitis is an important complication of this infection. In bacterial infections, the brunt of the damage falls on the epididymis; the testis is affected secondarily. In mumps orchitis, it is the testis that suffers most. It has been estimated that from 20 to 25 per cent of adult males who develop mumps suffer from acute orchitis about 1 week after enlargement of the parotid glands. With resolution of the disease, some testicular atrophy takes place; if this is severe—particularly if it is bilateral—permanent sterility can result. The testis is enclosed in a dense fibrous coat, the tunica albuginea; in acute inflammation, there is a rapid rise in tissue tension. Hence, severe pain is a feature of acute orchitis and epididymo-orchitis.

Tuberculosis of the urinary tract sometimes spreads and affects the epididymis. Years ago, in tertiary syphilis, a testicular gumma was not uncommon, but now this lesion is distinctly rare.

NEOPLASMS OF THE TESTIS

Although rare, neoplasms of the testis are the most common form of cancer to affect males between 15 and 35 years of age.

Germ-Cell Tumors

The majority of the tumors are thought to arise from primitive pluripotential germ cells. As might be expected, they give rise to tumors that vary greatly in their differentiation and prognosis. Four major types, which are described, have been recognized.

Seminoma. This is the most common tumor and occurs in a somewhat older age group than do the others. It consists of uniform cells having clear cytoplasm, and it tends to produce a uniform bulky enlargement of the testis. Local invasion beyond the testis is not evident, but the tumor first metastasizes to the lymph nodes. It should be noted that the lymphatics of the testis follow the blood vessels and terminate in lymph nodes around the aorta. Seminoma of the testis, although malignant, is very responsive to radiotherapy and chemotherapy. Hence, with treatment, it has a good prognosis; a 5-year survival rate of 90 per cent of patients can be expected.

Teratoma. This neoplasm shows a mixed histologic picture, having both epithelial and connective tissue elements. Occasionally, the tumor is well differentiated and cystic, and it resembles the ovarian teratoma. Nevertheless, the vast majority of testicular teratomas are solid and show areas of anaplastic growth, usually of the epithelial element. Teratomas tend to form a discrete nodule in the testis and subsequently invade the capsule. Since there is metastasis to the regional lymph nodes and via the blood stream, the prognosis is worse than that of seminoma. The 5-year mortality of patients with this tumor is approximately 30 to 50 per cent.

Embryonal Carcinoma. This term is used to describe a tumor that microscopically resembles a carcinoma and shows glandular differentiation and considerable pleomorphism. The tumor, which is often quite small, exhibits a more aggressive and lethal behavior than does either seminoma or teratoma. The 5-year survival rate of patients is about 35 per cent.

Choriocarcinoma. This is the least common and most malignant type of testicular tumor. It metastasizes via the blood stream, and the primary growth is often small. In fact, the growth is sometimes of microscopic dimension, so that the patient presents clinically with multiple metastases—the primary tumor being located only at necropsy after a painstaking search. On histologic examinations, the tumor resembles its counterpart in the female.

Combined Tumors. These tumors show a mixture of the types described in the preceding discussion. Their existence supports the concept that these testicular tumors have a common cell type of origin. Further support for this thesis is the production of *chorionic gonadotropins* and *alpha-fetoprotein** by these tumors. As would be expected, this is most marked with choriocarcinoma, but it is also found with some cases of teratoma and embryonal carcinoma. The presence of these substances in the blood can be used as an aid to the diagnosis of testicular tumors as well as to detect the presence of metastases after removal of the primary neoplasm.

Sex Cord and Gonadal Stroma Tumors

The developing testicular stroma forms the Leydig cells (interstitial cells), the Sertoli cells of the sex cords, and the testicular connective tissue. Like their ovarian counterparts, the cells are under the control of pituitary hormones and are responsible for hormone production. It is therefore not surprising that neoplastic lesions, *e.g.*, *Leydig (interstitial) cell tumors* and *Sertoli cell tumors (androblastomas)*, can also produce sex hormones and be associated with a variety of syndromes.

---

*This is a globulin normally found in the blood during early fetal life but absent after birth. Its reappearance in the blood suggests the development of a tumor; liver and testis are the usual primary sites.

Other Tumors of the Testis

Malignant lymphoma may commence in the testis, particularly in the elderly subjects in whom it is the most common type of testicular tumor.

Summary

- Malformations of the external genitalia, such as hypospadias, in which the urethra opens onto the ventral surface of the penis or perineum, are important pointers to other malformations.
- Phimosis, with a small preputial opening, can lead to infection (balanoposthitis) or paraphimosis.
- Condylomata acuminata (venereal warts) are common and rarely become malignant.
- Carcinoma *in situ* of the penis is recognized clinically as Bowen's disease, erythroplasia of Queyrat, or bowenoid papulosis. Invasive carcinoma of the penis rarely occurs in the circumcised.
- Benign prostatic enlargement is the most common disease of the prostate, affecting to some extent most men over 70 years of age. It causes urinary tract obstruction.
- Carcinoma of the prostate is the most common malignant tumor of elderly men. The tumor cells secrete acid phosphatase, causing a raised blood level. The tumor causes obstruction and metastasizes to lymph nodes, bone (especially the lower spine), and elsewhere. Being hormone-dependent, it can be treated by reducing the availability of testosterone.
- Failure of the testis to descend is a cause of infertility and predisposes to malignancy.
- Torsion of the testis is a hazard in athletic males.
- Germ-cell tumors are the most common form of cancer between the ages of 15 and 35 years. They are characterized by secretion of human gonadotropin and alpha-fetoprotein. In order of ascending malignancy, there is seminoma (95 per cent cure rate if treated), teratoma, embryonal carcinoma, and choriocarcinoma (most patients dead in 5 years).
- Some other uncommon testicular tumors secrete male or female hormones.

Selected Readings

Donohue, J. P.: Testis Tumors. Baltimore, Williams & Wilkins, 1983.

Merrin, C. E.: Cancer of the penis. Cancer *45*:1973, 1980.

Peters, M. S., and Perry, H. O.: Bowenoid papules of the penis. J. Urol. *126*:482, 1981.

Wilson, J. D.: The pathogenesis of benign prostatic hyperplasia. Am. J. Med. *68*:745, 1980.

Young, R. H., and Scully, R. E.: Testicular Tumors. New York, Raven Press, 1990.

27

Female Reproductive Organs: Pregnancy and Its Disorders

After studying this chapter, the student should be able to:

- Describe the hormonal changes that are associated with the following:
  - (a) the development of the female secondary sexual characteristics;
  - (b) the menstrual cycle;
  - (c) pregnancy;
  - (d) lactation.
- Describe the common infections of the vulva.
- Describe what is meant by the transformation zone of the cervix uteri.
- Give a general account of carcinoma of the cervix with regard to the following:
  - (a) predisposing causes and etiology;
  - (b) age of onset;
  - (c) mode of development;
  - (d) symptoms.
- Define amenorrhea, menorrhagia, metrorrhagia, and dysmenorrhea. Give at least one cause of each condition.
- Describe the outstanding features of each of the following:
  - (a) uterine fibroids;
  - (b) carcinoma of the endometrium;
  - (c) endometriosis;
  - (d) endometrial hyperplasia.

- Describe the causes and important effects of salpingitis.
- Describe the polycystic ovary syndrome.
- Classify the tumors of the ovary; relate them to corresponding testicular tumors, and indicate which ovarian tumors are the most frequent.
- List the features of toxemia of pregnancy.
- Describe what is meant by "ectopic pregnancy."
- Define spontaneous abortion and give one common cause of this process.
- Classify the causes of bleeding during pregnancy.
- Contrast placenta previa with abruptio placentae.
- Describe the outstanding features of hydatidiform mole and choriocarcinoma.

HORMONAL ASPECTS OF THE FEMALE GENITAL TRACT

The hormones secreted by the ovary play a leading part in regulating the development of the female reproductive system. It is therefore appropriate to describe these before the individual organs and their abnormalities are discussed.

Childhood and Adolescence. During childhood, the ovary secretes small quantities of *estrogen*; this secretion is sufficient to inhibit the hypothalamus. Hence, gonadotropins are not released from the pituitary (Chapter 29). After the age of about 7 years, the hypothalamus becomes less sensitive to estrogen, and its setpoint is raised; this leads to release of gonadotropin (chiefly *follicle-stimulating hormone*) from the adenohypophysis. Ovarian estrogen production is thereby stimulated sufficiently to cause the *development of secondary sexual characteristics*: the breasts and uterus enlarge, and the subcutaneous fat is redistributed to produce the characteristic female contours. Shortly after this, the "cycling" center in the hypothalamus comes into operation, and menstruation commences.* Under the influence of follicle-stimulating hormone, the ovarian follicles enlarge and secrete estrogen. At midcycle, there is a surge of pituitary *luteinizing hormone* that causes ovulation. The follicular cells are converted into the corpus luteum, and *progesterone* is secreted.

---

*The rhythmic cycling center that awakens at puberty is peculiar to the female. It is responsible for the coordinated formation of releasing factors that in turn control the adenohypophysis and ultimately ovarian function. The presence of male hormones in the fetus prevents the development of a cycling center in the male.

Endometrial Changes in the Menstrual Cycle. During the first half of the menstrual cycle, the endometrium (both glands and stroma) undergoes hyperplasia. After ovulation, progesterone causes the glands to form secretion; the endometrium is thus suitably prepared for implantation of the developing fetus. If conception does not occur, the corpus luteum degenerates, and estrogen and progesterone levels decline; the endometrium undergoes necrosis and is passed in the menstrual flow as the cycle starts again.

Pregnancy. The fetal chorionic tissue that forms the placenta secretes *chorionic gonadotropin*,* which maintains the corpus luteum for the duration of pregnancy. In turn, the corpus luteum secretes estrogen and progesterone. These inhibit the hypothalamic-hypophyseal system so that ovulation does not occur. Breast development is induced by the combined effects of placental hormones (estrogen, progesterone, and placental lactogen). During the latter part of pregnancy, pituitary prolactin induces further changes.

Lactation. After delivery, lactation is established under the influence of prolactin. The act of suckling causes release of oxytocin; this helps express the milk by causing contraction of myoepithelial cells.

THE VULVA

Disorders of the vulva may be classified as congenital lesions, infections, noninfectious dermatoses, and neoplasms.

Congenital Lesions

Imperforate hymen is an uncommon malformation that becomes apparent with the onset of menstruation when blood is retained in the vagina (*hematocolpos*) and uterus (*hematometra*). The complex abnormalities associated with the var-

---

*Human chorionic gonadotropin is produced soon after implantation of the fertilized ovum. Its detection in the urine forms the basis for the common pregnancy tests. The test becomes positive at the time of the first missed menstrual period.

ious forms of hermaphroditism are not considered.

Infections

The vulva, being covered by stratified epithelium, is relatively resistant to infection by most common pyogenic organisms. Some organisms, however, can penetrate its keratinizing squamous epithelium, for instance, those causing syphilis, chancroid, and lymphogranuloma venereum; these are described in Chapter 7.

Gonorrhea. The gonococcus does not infect the vulva or vagina in adults. Sometimes there is infection of the urethra and adjacent Bartholin's glands. Acute bartholinitis causes a painful swelling that may progress to abscess formation. The infection can become chronic and if the duct becomes obstructed, a *Bartholin cyst* develops. Infants occasionally develop acute gonococcal vulvovaginitis.

Candidiasis. Candidiasis of the vulva and vagina is common; it is characterized by a thick, white, curdy vaginal discharge and intense itching. Diabetes mellitus, pregnancy, immunosuppression, and the administration of certain drugs (glucocorticosteroids; broad-spectrum antibiotics, *e.g.*, tetracycline for acne; and the birth control pill) predispose to this infection.

Herpes Genitalis. Herpes genitalis is now one of the major sexually transmitted diseases, particularly in teenagers and young women. This has been attributed to the widespread use of the birth control pill and reduction in the use of barrier methods of contraception. Herpesvirus, type 2, is commonly the cause. The vulva, vagina, or cervix can be affected. As with primary herpes elsewhere, there is much local swelling and pain associated with vesicles and shallow ulcers. The virus persists in the sacral dorsal root ganglia, and recurrent vulvar herpetic lesions are common.

Condylomata Acuminata. Condylomata acuminata are caused by infection with human papillomavirus (HPV), usually HPV-6, 11, or 16. The types of virus are numbered according to their DNA composition and can be identified by electron microscopy or immunostaining with specific antibody. However, the most sensitive method is by identifying viral DNA by Southern blot analysis. Condylomata acuminata, also called *venereal warts*, are generally multiple and can involve the anal canal, the perianal skin, and the vulva, the vagina, and the cervix.

Noninfectious Dermatoses Affecting the Vulva

Various skin diseases can also involve the vulva; the following are important: contact dermatitis (either primary irritant or allergic), lichen planus, psoriasis, erythema multiforme, and pemphigus vulgaris.

Vulvar Dystrophy. This term is used to describe a group of conditions specific for the vulva. Two types of lesion, and a third mixed group, are included under this heading.

In *atrophic vulval dystrophy*, also known as *lichen sclerosus*, the vulva develops pale atrophic plaques. Subsequently there is scarring and resorption of the labia. Pruritus is characteristic. The introitus is constricted and intercourse painful.

Hyperplastic vulvar dystrophy is also known as *lichen simplex chronicus*. It is the result of the repeated trauma of scratching secondary to itching.

Vulvar dystrophy with cellular atypia is now grouped under the heading of *vulvar intraepithelial neoplasia* with grades 1 to 3. Grade 3 is carcinoma *in situ*. These lesions are associated with infection by HPV-16 or 18. Precisely how many of these lesions become invasive is not known.

Neoplasms of the Vulva

Condylomas are very common and have already been described. A wide variety of neoplasms, either benign or malignant, can occur, and an adenocarcinoma can be associated with extramammary Paget's disease. Squamous-cell *carcinoma of the vulva* is the most common malignant tumor and is a disease of the postmenopausal age group. The tumor may form a bulky fungating mass or appear as an indurated ulcerating tumor. The overall 5-year survival is about

60 per cent. *Malignant melanoma* is an uncommon tumor.

THE VAGINA

Some infections of the vagina have been included in the section on the vulva. Trichomonal vaginitis is described in Chapter 10.

Nonspecific Vaginitis

A malodorous vaginal discharge not due to trichomoniasis, candidiasis, or gonorrhea is commonly called nonspecific vaginitis. *Gardinella vaginalis* accompanied by anaerobes (*e.g.*, *Bacteroides*) appears to be the cause.

Carcinoma of the Vagina

This is an uncommon tumor and is usually of the squamous-cell type. *Adenocarcinoma* is less common, but the recognition of this tumor in young women whose mothers had taken diethylstilbestrol (DES) during their pregnancy led to the recognition of the carcinogenic properties of this synthetic estrogen.

THE UTERUS

The two müllerian ducts form the fallopian tubes and normally fuse to form a single midline uterus and vagina. If this fusion is incomplete, a variety of malformations can result; thus, there can be a septum dividing the uterine cavity either partially or completely. Such congenital anomalies can produce curious clinical effects such as when a therapeutic abortion with curettage of one half of a septate uterus is followed by continuation of a pregnancy present in the other half.

Diseases of the cervix uteri differ from those of the body of the uterus, and each is described separately.

The Cervix Uteri

The cervix (neck) of the uterus is divided into two parts. The *endocervix* is lined by a columnar, mucus-secreting epithelium and has an underlying layer of vascular tissue that gives it a red color in contrast to the pale appearance of the squamous-covered *exocervix*. The squamous cells' content of glycogen (formed under the influence of cyclic hormonal stimulation) forms the basis of the Schiller iodine test (see later). In some women, the squamocolumnar junction is some distance from the external os, and the exposed red endocervical type mucosa can be seen on vaginal examination. The term congenital "erosion" of the cervix is sometimes applied to this condition. A similar condition, called *eversion or ectropion of the cervix*, follows parturition. It is caused by pouting of endocervical mucosa from the cervix that follows the trauma of childbirth.

The area of exposed columnar endocervical type epithelium tends to be transformed into squamous type epithelium; this is termed the *transformation zone*, the area where squamous epithelium is developing and maturing central to the original squamous-columnar junction. It is a common site for the development of carcinoma.

Abnormalities of Keratinization of the Cervix and Vagina

The epithelium of cervix and vagina is not normally keratinized, but a layer of keratin may form and give the area a white appearance ("leukoplakia"). This can result from mechanical irritation (*e.g.*, wearing a support pessary), or no cause may be apparent. Localized white patches of this type must be distinguished from areas of cellular atypia or neoplasia. It is now appreciated that some lesions on the cervix of this nature are in fact flat warts that lack the typical papillomatous appearance of condylomas. Their relationship to early lesions of cervical intraepithelial neoplasia is not defined (see later).

Cervicitis

Sexually transmitted infections, such as in gonorrhea, syphilis, and genital herpes, can affect the cervix uteri as well as other parts of the genital tract. *Chlamydia trachomatis* is a common cause of mucopurulent cervicitis, the female equivalent of urethritis in men.

Chronic nonspecific cervicitis occurs in women of child-bearing age; it affects the endocervix as well as the exposed endocervical mucosa in an area of ectropion. It causes a troublesome discharge.

Cervical Polyps

Inflammatory folds, or polyps, of endocervical mucosa are very common and can protrude through the external os into the vagina. Ulceration and bleeding, particularly after intercourse, can arouse suspicion of cancer. Polyps do not, however, predispose to malignancy.

Carcinoma of the Cervix

Carcinoma of the cervix is a leading cause of death in some parts of the world but is now less common in North America. Much of this decline can be attributed to Papanicolaou, who introduced and popularized cervical cytologic examination as a means of detecting early precursor lesions. It is now appreciated that the tumor develops slowly through a series of changes, described as dysplasia (atypia), that progress in severity to carcinoma *in situ* and ultimately to invasive cancer. These early lesions can be detected and treated.

Etiology. The highest incidence of carcinoma of the cervix is in women who commenced sexual intercourse at an early age and who have had multiple sexual partners, particularly promiscuous partners. These are the major risk factors and, as might be expected, the disease is common in female prostitutes and rare in virgins. Low socioeconomic class, early marriage, increased parity, and cigarette smoking have been noted as risk factors but are probably related to the major factors. The most likely explanation is that the disease is sexually transmitted, and currently herpes simplex virus and human papillomavirus are suspected.

The incidence of *herpesvirus* (HSV-2) infection is high in patients with cervical intraepithelial neoplasia and invasive carcinoma. Viral nucleic acid can be identified in the tumor, and the virus is oncogenic to cells in culture and to immunosuppressed mice. However, since both carcinoma of the cervix and HSV infection are sexually transmitted, it is to be expected that both would often be found in the same patient. Absolute proof that the virus is directly involved in the neoplasia is lacking.

Human papillomaviruses (HPV-16 and 18, and less often 31) or sequences of their DNA can be identified in 80 to 90 per cent of human tumors. Of significance is the observation that DNA is integrated in the genome of the malignant cells. Virus can also be identified in 10 to 20 per cent of patients without cancer, in either normal or dysplastic tissue. Here the DNA is extrachromosomal. It is apparent that certain types of papillomavirus are involved in the genesis of carcinoma of the cervix, but it is probable that other factors are involved.

Early Lesions of Carcinoma. Cytologic examination of cervical smears has led to the recognition of lesions in which the cervical epithelial cells exhibit abnormalities in nuclear/cytoplasmic ratio, nuclear morphology, and cellular maturation. The lesions are described as *dysplastic*, and the degree of dysplasia can be categorized as *mild*, *moderate*, or *severe* depending on the extent of the atypical epithelial cells within the epithelium. This contrasts with *carcinoma in situ*, in which there is a lack of differentiation and atypia extends full-thickness. The present approach is to regard dysplasia and carcinoma *in situ* as parts of a spectrum of changes termed *cervical intraepithelial neoplasia*. Three grades of cervical intraepithelial neoplasia are defined. Grade 1 corresponds to mild dysplasia, grade 2 to moderate dysplasia, and grade 3 to severe dysplasia and carcinoma *in situ*. The natural tendency, it is thought, is for there to be a progression from a better-differentiated state to a less differentiated state. It seems likely that the more severe the dysplasia, the more likely it is to progress to *in situ* and invasive carcinoma.

The lesions of cervical intraepithelial neoplasia usually occur in the transformation zone of the cervix uteri and may or may not be detectable by the unaided eye. As an aid to their detection, the Schiller test is used. A solution of iodine is applied to the mucosa; normal epithelium stains brown because normal cells contain much glycogen; dysplastic epithelium is unstained. Unfortunately, the test is unreliable. *Colposcopy* is now employed. The examination, which demands the services of a skilled colposcopist, involves the examination of the cervix, vagina, and vulva with use of a stereoscopic microscope. If acetic acid is applied to the mucosa, it dehydrates the epithelial cells so that abnormal areas with nuclear crowding appear white. Such abnormal areas can be biopsied. Removal of a large "cone" of cervical tissue with removal of all the affected area is another approach, but the scarring that results may affect subsequent fertility and delivery. Abnormal areas may be treated by excision, cryotherapy, or laser therapy. It must be emphasized that colposcopy is not a screening test, but is used to investigate patients with abnormal cervical cytologic findings.

It is evident that routine Pap smears of all women who have commenced sexual activity and the investigation of patients with an abnormal smear should detect the early lesions that evolve into carcinoma. Their treatment should virtually eliminate the disease. This requires many highly trained (and highly paid) personnel and compliant patients. Carcinoma of the cervix is still an important cause of death in women because, in practice, women who are at greatest risk are often poor and the least compliant.

The detection and treatment of carcinoma of the cervix involves technical skills and good judgment. There are few other areas in medicine in which collaboration among social workers, technologists, pathologists, and clinical physicians is so necessary to guarantee that their patients receive the best treatment. Overdiagnosis and overtreatment can result in unnecessary surgery that can prevent young women from bearing children. Underdiagnosis and undertreatment, on the other hand, can kill the patient.

Clinical Features. In the past, the peak incidence of carcinoma of the cervix has been between 40 and 60 years of age, but there is now evidence that the disease is occurring in younger women. The dysplastic and preinvasive stage occurs 10 to 15 years earlier. Vaginal bleeding, particularly after intercourse or douching, is the common symptom; with advanced ulcerated, infected lesions, there is a foul vaginal discharge and evidence of invasion of local structures.

Carcinoma of the cervix generally begins in the transformation zone. It may project into the vagina as a fungating mass (*exophytic type*), or it may invade the cervix to produce a nodular, hard mass with overlying ulceration (*endophytic type*). The tumor invades locally to involve bladder, ureters, rectum, vagina, and peritoneum. Lymph node metastases occur relatively late, as do blood-borne metastases. For treatment, radiation and radical surgery both have their advocates, and the results are comparable. About 75 per cent of the tumors are squamous-cell carcinomas; the remainder are mainly adenocarcinomas derived from the endocervix.

The Body of the Uterus

The body of the uterus consists of a powerful muscle (the *myometrium*) and a mucosal lining (the *endometrium*).

The changes that take place in the endometrium during the normal menstrual cycle have already been described. Endometrial abnormalities often cause changes in menstruation; these are described first.

Abnormalities of Menstruation

Some menstrual irregularity occurs in every woman's life. This section deals with only certain facets of this important and complex problem.

Amenorrhea, or absence of menstruation, is normal before the menarche, after the menopause, and during pregnancy and lactation. *Primary amenorrhea* denotes a failure to commence menstruation and is usually due to ovarian disease (*e.g.*, ovarian dysgenesis) or to hypothalamic-pituitary disorders. *Secondary amenorrhea* is usually defined as absence of menstruation for more than 12 months, excluding pregnancy and the menopause. Hormonal imbalance due to detectable disease of the ovaries, hypothalamus, or endocrine glands is an occasional cause, but amenorrhea is also a feature of numerous general illnesses, including mental disturbances such as worry, emotional disappointment, and depression. The mechanism is presumably related to nervous influences on the hypothalamic cycling center.

Menorrhagia, meaning excessive or prolonged blood loss occurring at menstruation, is extremely common. Sometimes it is due to a failure of ovulation. No corpus luteum is formed, and estrogens acting in the absence of progesterone lead to *endometrial hyperplasia*. Curettage performed during the latter half of the menstrual cycle shows *absence of secretory activity*. The procedure of curettage is therefore a useful way of diagnosing this type of anovulatory bleeding.

Metrorrhagia refers to intermenstrual bleeding or such irregularity that no periodicity is present. Sometimes this condition is due to an irregular endometrial response to normal ovarian hormonal influence. Thus, secretory and proliferative areas of endometrium exist side by side.

Abnormalities of menstruation may be symptomatic of local uterine disease—polyps, endometrial hyperplasia, endometriosis, fibroids, or carcinoma. The term *dysfunctional uterine bleeding* is used when no local cause is apparent. Often this is due to *anovulatory cycles*.

If ovulation does not take place, no corpus luteum is formed, and the endometrium is subjected to excessive stimulation by estrogen. This results in abnormal endometrial proliferation, and periodic endometrial breakdown results in bleeding. Anovulatory cycles are most common during the first year after menarche or at about the time of the menopause. In the unfortunate few, normal cycles are never established, and the patient experiences irregular periods and sometimes heavy blood loss. There may be associated obesity, infertility, hirsutism, and polycystic ovarian disease; in most patients with anovulatory cycles, however, no definite cause can be identified, although mental or physical stress and intercurrent illness have been blamed.

Endometrial Hyperplasia

Thickening of the endometrium is a common finding in patients with menorrhagia or metrorrhagia. It may occur in young women and is a feature of the Stein-Leventhal syndrome. Most frequently, however, it is an affliction of women at the time of the menopause. On microscopic examination, there is glandular hyperplasia, indicating that the condition is due to the unopposed action of estrogen. The menstrual cycle is usually anovulatory. The hyperplasia may affect the whole endometrium, or its distribution may be focal.

The hyperplastic endometrium may show focal areas of atrophy microscopically; the atrophic glands show cystic dilation, and the appearance may be described as a "Swiss cheese" pattern. Of greater significance and importance is the presence of *epithelial atypia*. This can vary from slight atypia to carcinoma *in situ*. Hence, endometrial hyperplasia with atypia is considered to be a condition that can evolve into endometrial carcinoma, which, as noted later, is predominantly a disease of postmenopausal women. There is considerable evidence that prolonged exposure to estrogen is a major cause of this. The source may be exogenous in the form of medication given to treat menopausal symptoms, or it may be endogenous from an estrogen-producing tumor of the ovary. Much more frequently, it is produced as a result of some hormonal dysfunction of undetermined cause.

Endometriosis

In endometriosis, ectopic endometrium is present in the pelvic organs (ovaries, uterine ligaments, vagina), in the peritoneal covering of the bladder and uterus, and occasionally elsewhere. The pathogenesis of this remarkable state has been much debated. Endometrial tissue regurgitated through the fallopian tubes during menstruation could become implanted in the pelvic organs. Alternatively, peritoneal cells could undergo metaplasia. The occasional occurrence of endometriosis in the umbilicus—and even in the lung—has raised the possibility of lymphatic or blood-borne spread. The pathogenesis remains a mystery!

Endometriosis is a disease of women during active reproductive life; the endometrial tissue undergoes the same changes as does the uterine endometrium during the menstrual cycle. Bleeding into the affected areas causes pain and often stimulates marked fibrosis. If this is extensive, it can lead to the formation of dense adhesions to the pelvic organs. Chronic pelvic pain, dysmenorrhea, dyspareunia, and pain on defecation or urination are common symptoms. The effects and symptoms of endometriosis are therefore very similar to those of chronic pelvic inflammatory disease.

Adenomyosis (Endometriosis Interna)

This is a common condition in which normal-appearing endometrium invades the myometrium and causes enlargement of the uterus. Menorrhagia is the most common functional effect, but patients may also complain of dysmenorrhea and dyspareunia.

Neoplasms of the Body of the Uterus

Leiomyoma. The leiomyoma is a benign tumor of smooth muscle and usually contains an admixture of fibrous tissue (Fig. 27–1). Hence, it is also called a fibroleiomyoma or "fibroid." Fibroids arise in the myometrium and are generally multiple. They vary in size from those that are scarcely visible to the naked eye to those weighing over 100 pounds! Some fibroids become pedunculated and appear as subserosal or submucosal nodules. Uterine fibroids are the most common tumor to afflict women and are present in about 25 per cent of the adult female population. They may cause symptoms in various ways. Their presence may be associated with menorrhagia and irregular bleeding. Occasionally they cause mechanical difficulties during labor. Fibroids appear to be estrogen-dependent because they diminish in size, degenerate, and even calcify after the menopause.

Carcinoma of the Endometrium. Adenocarcinoma of the endometrium is a disease of postmenopausal women; its peak incidence is between 50 and 60 years of age. It is less common than is carcinoma of the cervix, but the incidence is on the increase, partly because of longer life expectancy. The disease is more frequent among childless women than among multiparous ones. There is considerable evidence that the tumor is related to prolonged exposure to estrogens. These may have been administered for menopausal symptoms or formed in the body. An association with obesity can be explained by the production of estrogens (e.g., from androgens) by adipose tissue.

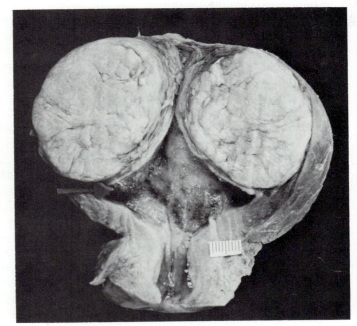

Figure 27–1 Leiomyoma of the uterus. The uterus has been opened to show one large, well-circumscribed tumor. Several smaller fibroids were also present, but they are not visible in this photograph. The tumor was an incidental finding in a patient who died as a consequence of carcinoma of the colon. (Courtesy of Dr. A. Vayalumkal, M.D., Ophthalmologist, Hamilton Civic Hospitals, Hamilton, Ontario.)

Carcinoma of the endometrium is characterized by irregular vaginal bleeding accompanied by leukorrhea. The disease probably begins with the development of endometrial hyperplasia, dysplasia, and carcinoma *in situ*. Nevertheless, this orderly sequence of development is less well documented than are the stages of development of carcinoma of the cervix.

THE FALLOPIAN TUBES

The upper, or cephalic, part of the müllerian duct normally remains separate and forms the fallopian tube. Note that the lumen of the fallopian tubes remains open to the peritoneal cavity, because it is through this opening that the ova reach the lower genital tract.

Inflammatory Disease

Pyogenic infections of the female genital tract tend to spare the vagina and endometrium but attack the fallopian tubes severely. The result is *acute salpingitis*. The fimbriated ends of the tubes become sealed over, and the infection enters a chronic phase. The tubes are distended with pus and assume the shape of retort tubes (*pyosalpinx*). Ultimately the infection subsides, and the tubes remain distended with clear fluid (*hydrosalpinx*). Sometimes the infection is not controlled, and a chronic abscess involving the fallopian tubes and ovary is formed. This *tubo-ovarian abscess* requires surgical relief.

Salpingitis is often accompanied by inflammation of the adjacent pelvic structures, including the peritoneum and bowel. It then forms a component of a more widespread *pelvic inflammatory disease*. When this disease is acute, because of the peritonitis there are manifestations of an acute abdomen. When chronic, the condition causes painful intercourse (*dyspareunia*), painful menstrual periods (*dysmenorrhea*), and intestinal obstruction secondary to the formation of fibrous adhesions. The *sterility* that results is due to the closure of the fimbriated ends of the fallopian tubes; partial blockage of the tubes by adhesions leads to an increased incidence of ectopic pregnancy. The most common type of pelvic inflam-

matory disease used to be gonococcal, but other sexually transmitted infections, such as with chlamydia and mycoplasma, are also common. Regardless of the initial infection, other organisms are often involved, being secondary invaders. These include staphylococci, streptococci, and coliform organisms. Pelvic inflammatory disease is now encountered principally as a postpartum or a postabortal infection. The nongonococcal types of infection tend to involve the whole wall of the fallopian tubes rather than merely affect the mucosa as is typical of the gonococcal cases. Hence, thickening of the tubes and dense adhesions to adjacent structures are more common.

Tuberculous salpingitis was once a disease to consider as a cause of sterility. The disease, fortunately, is now rare.

THE OVARY

The ovaries develop, as do the testes, in the mesoderm of the posterior abdominal wall. Each ovary has three components: (1) a covering of *germinal epithelium* that is modified peritoneal mesothelium; (2) a *stroma* derived from mesoderm; and (3) *germ cells* that later mature into ova. Stromal cells form each *graafian follicle*, and after the release of the ovum, they also form the *corpus luteum*. Both these structures manufacture sex hormones, as previously described. It should be noted that the primitive gonad is asexual, being neither male nor female. The primordial germ cells, which are sequestered early in the formation of an embryo and are probably of endodermal origin, migrate to the gonad and there develop into either ova or sperm.

Cysts

Cysts derived from unruptured graafian follicles or from corpora lutea are extremely common. Since they rarely exceed 3 cm in diameter, they seldom cause trouble.

Polycystic Ovaries. This condition affects young women and may be associated with various syndromes either alone or in combination. There may be excessive secretion of estrogens leading to endometrial hyperplasia associated with abnormal bleeding. Occasionally, endometrial carcinoma develops. An association with amenorrhea and sterility is called the Stein-Leventhal syndrome. Finally, there may be hirsutism and virilism. The pathogenesis of these various syndromes is not known, and indeed it is probable that several entities are included under the umbrella term of polycystic ovaries. Surgical resection of a wedge of ovarian tissue is sometimes curative in the Stein-Leventhal syndrome. The effect is not mechanical, leading to release of ova, but is related to a reduction of ovarian mass and hence abnormal ovarian secretion.

Neoplasms of the Ovary

The ovary is a common site for neoplasia. Early diagnosis is difficult because the organs are situated deep in the pelvis and symptoms do not appear until there is pressure on adjacent structures, such as nerves or the bladder. Malignant tumors have often spread throughout the peritoneal cavity, making the prognosis poor.

Neoplasms of the Germinal Epithelium

Like the germinal epithelium of the ovary, the müllerian ducts also develop from the celomic epithelium. It is therefore not surprising that germinal epithelial tumors tend to show differentiation into epithelium that resembles that of the fallopian tube, the endometrium (rare), or the endocervix. The tumors tend to form cystic spaces with papillary epithelial ingrowths. They are therefore called papillary cystadenomas or papillary cystadenocarcinomas.

Benign Neoplasms. For practical purposes, there are two groups—mucinous and serous.

Mucinous Cystadenoma. These cystic tumors are usually unilateral and can reach enormous size, filling the pelvis and causing abdominal distention. The cystic spaces are filled with a mucinous fluid and are lined by an epithelium that resembles that of the lining of the endocervix. Malignant change may occur but is uncommon. A rare complication is rupture: the whole peritoneum is flooded with mucin, and multiple tumor implants take root on the peritoneal surface, with the result that all the abdominal viscera become bound together. This produces a surgeon's nightmare if a laparotomy is required for a complication such as intestinal obstruction. The condition is called *pseudomyxoma peritonei* and is generally regarded as local metastasis from a low-grade, well-differentiated carcinoma. A similar condition can complicate the neoplastic type of mucocele of the appendix.

Serous Cystadenoma. This type of tumor is more common than is the mucinous variant. In about one third of patients, the tumor is bilateral. The cystic spaces are lined by an epithelium that resembles that of the lining of the fallopian tubes. Malignant change is quite common.

Malignant Neoplasms. *Papillary cystadenocarcinoma* is the most common primary malignancy of the ovary and is the malignant counterpart of the cystadenoma, usually the serous type. As with papillomatous neoplasms of the bladder, it is difficult to draw a line between benign and malignant lesions. There is a gray area between the two extremes, and in this area, individual pathologists will differ in their opinions. The malignant ovarian tumors show profuse papillomatous projections both into the cystic cavities and from the surface. Since peritoneal seeding is common, the other ovary is often involved (Fig. 27–2). Abdominal swelling due to *ascites* may be a prominent and distressing clinical manifestation. The presence of malignant cells in ascitic fluid is a helpful diagnostic finding. Lymph node and widespread blood-borne metastases occur, as with other carcinomas.

Neoplasms of the Germ Cells

The common benign teratoma is a germ-cell neoplasm and has been described in Chapter 12. Malignant teratomas are rare. Occasionally they differentiate predominantly in one direction and produce such oddities as squamous-cell carcinoma, carcinoid tumor, or choriocarcinoma.

Neoplasms of Ovarian Stroma

The gonadal stroma in the male forms the sex cords (that produce the Sertoli cells and Leydig

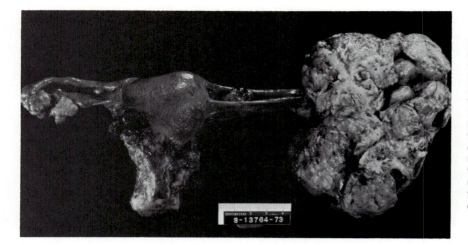

Figure 27–2 Carcinoma of the ovary. The specimen consists of the uterus with both ovaries. The left ovary is enormously enlarged by tumor; the right ovary shows a white area that also contains tumor. Numerous peritoneal nodules of metastatic growth are present in this specimen. Note the asymmetry of the body of the uterus. When the uterus was opened, a septum was found dividing the cavity into two unequal parts as a result of imperfect fusion of the two müllerian ducts.

cells) as well as adult type stromal cells, fibroblasts, and so on. It is therefore not surprising that tumors arising from ovarian stromal cells can be fibrous or epithelial in nature, or that they can produce steroid hormone of either male or female type. The description of this complex group of tumors is beyond the scope of this book, but the possibility of an ovarian tumor should always be considered if a woman shows definite signs of masculinization or excessive endometrial hyperplasia.

Secondary Neoplasms

The ovary is involved in metastatic growth more often than is any other pelvic organ. The common primary sites are the large intestine, the stomach, and the breast.

COMPLICATIONS OF PREGNANCY

Hyperemesis Gravidarum

Nausea and morning sickness are common in early pregnancy, but the origin of these symptoms is not understood. Occasionally the vomiting becomes severe enough to cause dehydration, starvation, and death. Wernicke's encephalopathy can develop in severe cases.

Toxemia of Pregnancy

Although the term "toxemia" is in common use, no specific toxin has ever been identified. The condition occurs during the last 3 months (trimester) of pregnancy, and its early stages are characterized by three features:

1. *Hypertension.* This is the most constant feature.
2. *Albuminuria.* This occurs in severe cases.
3. *Edema.* Some degree of water and salt retention resulting in edema of the legs is common in normal pregnancy and is of no significance. However, edema of the face or arms and any marked weight increase due to water accumulation immediately suggest toxemia.

Severe toxemia (termed *pre-eclampsia*) is characterized by headache, visual disturbances (ranging from flashes of light to blindness), abdominal pain, and vomiting. It is a serious condition because it can be followed by *eclampsia*. This is the most severe manifestation of toxemia and is characterized by seizures that start with twitching of the face, are followed by a *tonic phase* lasting 1 to 2 minutes, and terminate in a *clonic phase* with violent, convulsive movements during which the pregnant woman may damage herself.

Toxemia is sometimes familial; it is associated with abruptio placentae, twin pregnancies, and the presence of a hydatidiform mole. It is most common in primigravidae (women who are pregnant for the first time). Vascular spasm appears to be the cause of the headaches, cerebral edema, visual disturbances, and convulsions. Necropsy findings include glomerular changes and liver necrosis together with evidence of disseminated intravascular coagulation. Rarely, bilateral renal cortical necrosis results in renal failure (see Chapter 19 and Fig. 19–6).

These observations have done little to shed any light on the etiology of toxemia. The disease that causes an appreciable fetal and maternal mortality has no known cause other than that it is associated with pregnancy. Nevertheless, with early diagnosis, the condition responds well to simple medical remedies such as bed rest and salt restriction. For this reason, good antenatal care always includes *routine examination of the patient for hypertension, albuminuria, edema, and excessive weight gain.*

Ectopic Pregnancy

By the time the ovum, which is fertilized in the fallopian tube, reaches the uterus, it is at the correct stage for implantation. If its passage is delayed, implantation occurs in the tube; this is the most common type of ectopic pregnancy. The fetus grows for a time, but its growth usually causes the tube to rupture by the sixth week. Pain and severe intra-abdominal hemorrhage are the result. When the fetus dies, the endometrium is shed, and vaginal bleeding occurs. This sign helps distinguish a ruptured ectopic pregnancy from other abdominal catastrophes.

Abortion

The expulsion of a nonviable fetus* is termed *abortion* or *miscarriage.* Approximately 10 to 15 per cent of all pregnancies terminate in this way, usually between the ninth and the thirteenth week of gestation. Many causes, both fetal and maternal, have been described. Chief among them is fetal abnormality; spontaneous abortion is an important mechanism by which defective

---

*The age at which a fetus becomes viable is arbitrarily set at 20 weeks' gestation by some authorities and at 28 weeks' by others.

fetuses are eliminated, for 50 to 60 per cent of all spontaneous abortuses have a severe karyotypic abnormality.

Bleeding During Pregnancy

Bleeding from the genital tract during pregnancy not only is alarming for the patient but also is often a warning of a serious abnormality. The types of bleeding may be divided into two groups.

Bleeding in Early Pregnancy (before 28 weeks' gestation). Three important causes should be noted and are considered elsewhere in this chapter: (1) abortion, (2) ectopic pregnancy, and (3) hydatidiform mole.

Bleeding in the Later Months of Pregnancy. Bleeding that occurs after the twenty-eighth week of gestation and before delivery is called *antepartum hemorrhage.* Two causes are of paramount importance.

Placenta Previa. In this condition, part or all of the placenta is attached to the lower uterine segment. This part of the uterus stretches and thins out in late pregnancy and especially during labor. The more rigid placenta becomes detached, and this provokes external bleeding. The initial bleeding is often slight and painless; it can be followed by massive bleeding that endangers the life of both mother and child. Urgent hospital treatment is necessary, and often cesarean section is required.

Abruptio Placentae. In this condition, there is premature separation of a normally situated placenta. Bleeding occurs between the placenta and the uterine wall, and there may or may not be external bleeding. The condition is most common in primigravidae and in patients with toxemia. Abruptio placentae is characterized by abdominal pain, tenderness of the uterus, and the development of shock. Death sometimes results, usually because of hemorrhagic shock. As with placenta previa, urgent hospital treatment is necessary.

Gestational Trophoblastic Neoplasms

Tumors derived from trophoblastic (placental) tissue secrete human chorionic gonadotropin

(HCG), and the level of this hormone is increased in the blood and urine. This is useful in diagnosis and also for follow-up after the removal of the tumor; levels are particularly high in choriocarcinoma. The tumors fall into three groups.

Hydatidiform Mole

The mole resembles a bunch of grapes and is formed by marked edema of the chorionic villi (Fig. 27–3). No fetus is present. The disease is very common in the Far East and occurs about once in every 2000 pregnancies in North America.

The cells of the mole have a 46,XX karyotype, and both X chromosomes are derived from the father. The explanation of this remarkable fact is uncertain, but possibly the maternal chromosomal constituents of the ovum are lost, and the haploid sperm duplicates its chromosomes after meiosis.

Clinical Features. The mole is suspected when the uterus enlarges more rapidly than in a normal pregnancy and yet no fetus can be demonstrated. The early onset of toxemia of pregnancy is another feature. Bleeding at about the third month and passage of vesicles of the mole is another mode of presentation. Elevated HCG levels in blood and urine are present.

Hydatidiform moles can be spontaneously delivered, but sometimes surgical treatment is necessary for their complete removal. Occasionally there is secretion of thyrotropic hormone and the patient has hyperthyroidism.

In most cases of hydatidiform mole, removal of the mole is followed by no complications. However, in about 20 per cent of cases, an invasive mole develops; in 2 to 3 per cent, there is progression to choriocarcinoma. These complications should be suspected if there is vaginal bleeding, persistent uterine enlargement, and failure of the HCG levels to drop.

Invasive Mole (Chorioadenoma Destruens)

As its name suggests, this type of mole invades the myometrium. Penetration of the uterine mus-

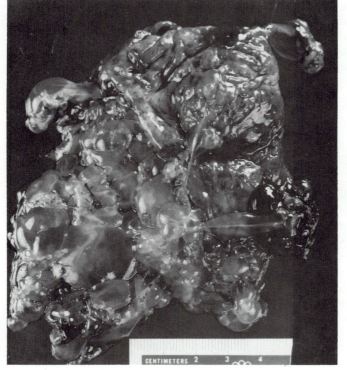

Figure 27–3 Hydatidiform mole. The normal placental tissue has been largely replaced by the mole. Note the presence of numerous fluid-filled cysts, from which the lesion gets its name. *Hydatis* is from the Greek, meaning "a drop of water."

cle can lead to extensive hemorrhage. Occasionally there are metastases to the vagina, vulva, or lung, but the deposits do not show progressive growth and eventually regress. Response to chemotherapy is good.

Choriocarcinoma

Choriocarcinoma, the most malignant trophoblastic tumor, complicates about one in 2500 pregnancies in the United States and up to ten times that number in some other countries. It arises in a hydatidiform mole in half to one third of cases. The remainder are divided almost equally between abortion and a preceding normal pregnancy. The tumor is highly invasive and metastasizes widely. The tumor is characterized by very high levels of HCG in blood and urine. This forms the basis for a useful test both in initial diagnosis and in follow-up. As with hydatidiform mole, thyrotropic hormone secretion may cause thyrotoxicosis. The tumor responds well to chemotherapy, and in many cases cure can be expected with this one lethal tumor.

Summary

- The vulva can be affected by many skin diseases. Particularly important infections are gonorrhea, candidiasis, herpes simplex, and condylomata acuminata.
- In vulval dystrophy, there are white lesions that may show cellular atypia.
- Lesions showing atypia are grouped as vulvar intraepithelial neoplasia, a precursor of squamous-cell carcinoma.
- Carcinoma is the most important lesion of the cervix uteri. Frequent sexual intercourse with commencement at an early age is an important cause. The tumor is preceded by increasing grades of atypia termed cervical intraepithelial neoplasia. This state can be detected by colposcopy. Infection by herpes simplex virus type 2 and human papillomaviruses is a probable causative factor.
- Endometrial hyperplasia is associated with abnormal estrogen stimulation; it causes abnormal bleeding and infertility. If associated with atypia, it is a precursor of endometrial carcinoma.
- Benign leiomyoma is the most common tumor of the body of the uterus.
- Salpingitis is the most important disease of the fallopian tubes with sterility as its sequel. Pelvic inflammatory disease is an important complication.
- Common tumors of the ovary are benign cystadenomas, either mucinous or serous, derived from the germinal epithelium. Their malignant counterparts, papillary cystadenocarcinomas, are the most common malignant tumor. The prognosis is poor.
- The most common germ-cell tumor is the benign teratoma (dermoid).
- Complications of pregnancy are severe vomiting (hyperemesis gravidarum), toxemia (terminating in eclampsia), ectopic pregnancy, abortion, and gestational trophoblastic tumor. Bleeding is an important warning of serious trouble—abortion, ectopic pregnancy, or hydatidiform mole if early in pregnancy, placenta previa or abruptio placentae if late.

Selected Readings

Brunham, R. C., et al.: Mucopurulent cervicitis: The ignored counterpart in women of urethritis in men. N. Engl. J. Med. *311*:1, 1984.

Fox, H., and Buckley, C. H.: Current concepts of endometriosis. Clin. Obstet. Gynaecol. *1*:279, 1984.

Herbert, A. L.: Diethylstilbestrol exposure—1984. N. Engl. J. Med. *311*:1433, 1984.

Howley, P. M.: On human papillomaviruses. N. Engl. J. Med. *315*:1089, 1986.

Hulka, B. S.: Replacement estrogens and risk of gynecologic cancers and breast cancer. Cancer *60*:1960, 1987.

Kurman, R. J. (ed.): Blaustein's Pathology of the Female Genital Tract. 2nd ed. New York, Springer-Verlag, 1987.

Lavery, H. A.: Vulval dystrophies: New approaches. Clin. Obstet. Gynaecol. *11*:155, 1984.

Leading article: Colposcopy today. Lancet *1*:486, 1987.

Syrjänen, K. J.: Human papillomavirus (HPV) infections of the female genital tract and their association with intraepithelial neoplasia and squamous cell carcinoma. Part I. Pathol. Annu. *21*(part I):53, 1986.

Vaitukaitis, J. L.: Polycystic-ovary syndrome: What is it? N. Engl. J. Med. *309*:1245, 1983.

Wilkinson, E. J.: Pathology of the Vulva and Vagina. New York, Churchill Livingstone, 1987.

28

Breast

After studying this chapter, the student should be able to:

- Describe the structure and development of the female breast.
- Describe the main features of acute mastitis, plasma cell mastitis, fat necrosis of the breast, and fibrocystic disease.
- List the groups of women who are especially susceptible to carcinoma of the breast and relate this to the factors thought to be involved in the etiology of the disease.
- Classify the types of carcinoma of the breast.
- Give an account of the early detection, the prognosis, and the treatment of carcinoma of the breast.
- Describe the routes of spread of breast cancer.
- Define gynecomastia and give three examples of this condition.

STRUCTURE AND DEVELOPMENT

The human breast is not a single gland but, on the contrary, consists of about 20 separate glands or *lobes*, each with its own duct opening separately onto the surface of the nipple. The lobes develop, as do the sweat glands, by ingrowths from the surface epidermis; during infancy, they consist only of rudimentary branching ducts surrounded by cuffs of connective tissue that are an extension of the papillary dermis. In the male, this state persists throughout life; but in the female, during the 3- to 4-year period before the onset of menstruation, the breasts enlarge and the ducts and the specialized loose periductal stroma that is a characteristic feature of the breast tissue proliferate. During adolescence, stromal growth continues, and buds form at the end of the ducts. These are the *lobules,* and they are the beginnings of the secretory gland structure that develops later if pregnancy occurs.

In the adult female, the breast shows cyclic changes that parallel those of the endometrium during the menstrual cycle. Under the influence of estrogen, there is epithelial proliferation during the first half of the cycle; this proliferation continues and there is abortive secretory activity as progesterone is added during the second half of the cycle. This causes the breasts to enlarge and feel tense.

The breast attains its maximum development during lactation. The epithelial proliferation and secretory gland formation are such that the organ closely resembles other secretory glands, such as the pancreas.

In the normal resting breast, the epithelial component constitutes about 15 per cent of the organ. The remainder consists of lobules of fat contained by fibrous septa that stretch from the dermis to the fascia overlying the pectoral muscles. These septa play a large part in giving the female breast its firmness and configuration. The septa also form an avenue for the spread of carcinoma to the skin and pectoral muscles.

The lymphatic drainage of the breast has been intensively studied, mainly with the aim of devising radical operations for the treatment of cancer of the breast. Lymph drains into the axillary, supraclavicular, internal mammary (within the chest), and abdominal lymph nodes. As explained later in this chapter, radical operations designed to remove these nodes do not seem to have influenced the prognosis of this form of cancer. Hence, a detailed knowledge of the lymphatic drainage of the breast has not proved to be of any great practical value.

Developmental Anomalies

Supernumerary Breast Tissue. Most mammals develop breast tissue along a milk line. In humans, this extends from the anterior axillary fold to the groin; occasionally, accessory nipples are found along this line. When associated with accessory breast tissue in the female, these enlarge and cause pain at puberty and particularly during pregnancy.

Enlargement of the Breast. It is common to find some enlargement of the breasts in newborn infants in whom some secretion ("witch's milk") may be formed. This enlargement lasts for 1 to 2 weeks and is due to the action of maternal hormones. On rare occasions, enlargement of one or both breasts takes place during childhood if there is excessive estrogen produced as a result of a functioning tumor of the ovary, adrenal, or pituitary.

The most common type of enlargement of the breast (generally called *virginal hypertrophy*) is seen in girls at adolescence. One or both breasts become so enlarged that partial surgical removal (*reduction mammoplasty*) is required.

ACQUIRED DISEASE OF THE BREAST

Inflammation

Acute Mastitis. Acute bacterial mastitis is generally encountered in the breast during the first few weeks of nursing a firstborn child. The offending organism, *Staphylococcus aureus*, gains access through a crack in the nipple. Suppuration requiring surgical drainage generally follows unless early antibiotic treatment is instituted.

Plasma-Cell Mastitis. This is an uncommon condition and generally affects women about 40 years of age. There is often a history of difficult nursing due to inverted nipples, cracked nipples, or infection. In one quadrant of the breast, an area of thickening is found that extends beneath the nipple to cause some distortion. There is usually pain and tenderness and sometimes a discharge from the nipple. The affected area contains dilated ducts with a creamy liquid containing many macrophages with vacuolated cytoplasm. Rupture of this inspissated material into the surrounding stroma causes a chronic inflammatory reaction with many plasma cells and sometimes with tuberculoid granulomas, a picture that mimics tuberculosis. Tuberculosis of the breast is, in fact, very rare.

Fat Necrosis. This condition is generally encountered in fat, pendulous breasts. In about half the patients, a history of trauma is obtained. On histologic examination, there is necrosis of fat cells with an associated inflammatory reaction, at first acute and then progressing to chronicity with a granulomatous reaction containing foreign body giant cells. The lesion presents as a lump in the breast, and the histologic picture must be differentiated from that of tuberculosis.

Fibrocystic Disease (Mammary Dysplasia)

This common condition has been given many names in the past, the most misleading being chronic mastitis, for the condition is not inflammatory and appears to be the end result of the hormonal changes that take place during women's reproductive life. As noted previously, the breast undergoes cyclic changes of hyperplasia and regression during menstruation. The combined effect of these changes over many years is to produce in some women imbalance between the amount of epithelium and the specialized fibrous tissue. The disease may affect one segment of one breast, commonly the upper and outer quadrant, and produce a relatively localized mass, or it may affect much of the tissue of both breasts, producing a widespread lumpiness. A characteristic feature that helps distinguish these lesions from carcinoma is that the lumps tend to increase in size and to become more tender before each menstrual period. Several types of fibrocystic disease have been described, but they represent aspects of a single disease rather than constituting separate entities.

On microscopic examination, fibrocystic disease exhibits fibrosis, cyst formation, or epithelial hyperplasia, either separately or in combination. Fibrosis alone is most common in women 30 to 40 years of age; it gives the affected areas a firm, rubbery consistency. *Cystic change* can lead to the formation of a solitary cyst; more commonly, multiple, bilateral cysts are present. Women of menopausal age are most commonly affected. There may be intracystic papillary ingrowths, and the epithelium can show apocrine metaplasia. *Epithelial hyperplasia* can affect the lobular epithelium (*lobular hyperplasia or adenosis*), which, if associated with fibrosis, is termed *sclerosing adenosis* and produces a histologic picture that can easily be mistaken for carcinoma, particularly on a small biopsy specimen. In *ductular epithelial hyperplasia* (*epitheliosis*), the hyperplastic epithelium can show cellular atypia; progression to carcinoma is thought to be a complication of this uncommon variant of fibrocystic disease.

Relationship to Carcinoma. Views on the relationship of mammary dysplasia to the subsequent development of carcinoma have varied considerably during the last few decades. At one time it was fashionable to regard the condition as premalignant. Many simple mastectomies were performed with a view to averting the development of cancer.

Most patients with fibrocystic disease are at no increased risk for carcinoma. However, if proliferative lesions are present, particularly if there is cellular atypia, there is a risk of development of malignancy. This is particularly true if there is a positive family history of breast cancer.

The importance of fibrocystic disease is that it presents as one or more lumps in the breast; these lumps must be distinguished from cancer, generally by biopsy.

Benign Neoplasms of the Breast

Fibroadenoma. Fibroadenoma is the most common tumor of the breast, occurring in women younger than 30 years of age. Although it may be regarded as a focal form of fibrocystic disease, since it is so localized and encapsulated, it is generally classified as a benign tumor. Nevertheless, it responds to hormonal stimulation like the normal breast. The tumor enlarges during pregnancy and regresses after the menopause.

Papilloma. One or more intraductal or intracystic papillomatous growths are sometimes found in women at or shortly before the menopause. The lesions appear as raspberry-like nodules filling a duct or growing from the wall of a cyst. The lesions frequently bleed and lead to a blood-stained discharge from the nipple. The relationship to carcinoma is disputed, but undoubtedly a number of papillomas do progress to carcinoma, and their removal is a wise precaution.

Malignant Neoplasms of the Breast

Carcinoma

Until recently, carcinoma of the breast has been the most common malignant tumor in women in North America and has been responsible for more deaths than has any other individual tumor. The incidence of the tumor has not declined, but in some populations it has been overtaken by carcinoma of the lung; this is attributed to the popularity of cigarette smoking. In women under the age of 25 years, breast cancer is rare; it attains its maximum incidence at about the menopause. The disease is much less frequent in Japan and the Far East.

Cause of Breast Cancer. A vast amount of

research has been carried out on this subject, and three factors appear to be important.

Inheritance. The incidence of cancer of the breast varies greatly in different strains of mice. In humans, it has been found that if a sister or mother has had cancer of the breast, a woman's chances of developing a similar tumor are increased—up to 50 times is one estimate.

Viruses. The Bittner virus causes cancer of the breast in female mice of suitable strains (Chapter 12). The virus is passed from mother to offspring in the milk, and the high incidence of tumors in a strain, although appearing to be hereditary, is in fact due to neonatal infection. Evidence is steadily accumulating to incriminate an RNA virus as a factor in the cause of human breast cancer. Whether it is a crucial factor or merely one of many agents acting in concert to cause cancer remains to be discovered.

Hormones. Prolonged exposure of breast tissue to the action of estrogen may be important as a factor in causing breast cancer. This would explain the increased incidence associated with advancing age, an early menarche, and a late menopause and in those who have not been pregnant.

Obesity is a risk factor because adipose tissue synthesizes estrogens. Likewise, there is an increased incidence in patients given estrogens for menopausal symptoms. However, the small quantity of estrogen in the birth control pill does not pose a hazard.

Types of Breast Cancer. Cancer can arise either in the lobules or more frequently in the ducts.

Case History I

The patient had noticed a lump in the right breast 1 year before consulting her doctor. A discharge from the nipple finally convinced her of the need to seek medical advice. On examination, the right breast was found to be smaller than the left. A hard mass could be felt deep to the nipple. The nipple itself was indrawn and adherent to the mass. Mobile, enlarged axillary lymph nodes contained secondary deposits of tumor (see Fig. 28–1).

Ductal Carcinoma. In *in situ ductular carcinoma*, the duct becomes filled with malignant cells. This lesion is difficult to feel but may be detected radiographically. In due course, tumor cells invade the surrounding connective tissues and form one of the varieties of infiltrating carcinoma.

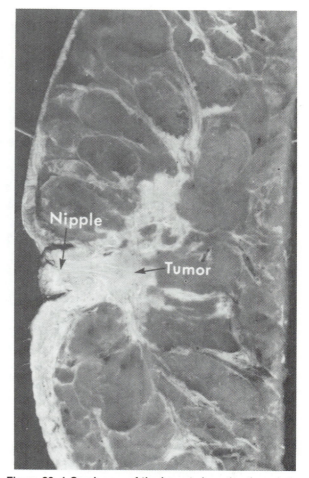

Figure 28–1 Carcinoma of the breast. A section through the breast is shown. The carcinoma is deep to the nipple, to which it is firmly attached. Note how the tumor extends along the fibrous septa in the breast. The tumor is not encapsulated; by gross examination, it is impossible to tell how far the growth has extended. This is an example of an advanced tumor that on clinical examination would be found to be attached to the nipple and to deeper structures.

Scirrhous Carcinoma. This type accounts for about 75 per cent of all cancers of the breast. The tumor is *stony hard* and nonencapsulated (Fig. 28–1). On microscopic examination, these tumors are adenocarcinomas with varying degrees of differentiation (Fig. 28–2). An outstanding feature is the dense fibrous tissue stroma, which accounts for the hardness of the tumor. Clinically, this common type of cancer presents as a hard lump in the breast. As the tumor infiltrates the fibrous septa of the breast, it reaches the skin

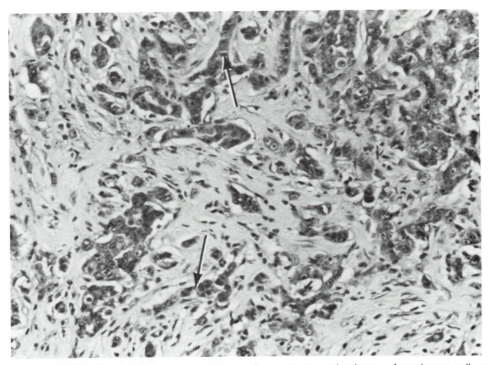

Figure 28–2 Carcinoma of the breast. This photomicrograph shows groups and columns of carcinoma cells embedded in a dense fibrous stroma. In some areas, single columns of cells can be seen (arrows); elsewhere there is the beginning of tubule formation. The tumor is therefore a poorly differentiated adenocarcinoma. The gross appearance of this tumor was that of a typical scirrhous carcinoma similar to the one depicted in Figure 28–1. The name is derived from the Greek *skirrhos*, meaning "hard" (×300).

and pectoral muscle. The lump then becomes *fixed* to both these structures. Contracture of the stroma causes skin dimpling and retraction of the nipple. Invasion of lymphatics and lymphedema give the skin an orange rind appearance *(peau d'orange)*, whereas actual invasion of the dermis converts the skin into a hard mass of tumor like a shield or cuirass *(cancer en cuirasse)*.

Medullary or Encephaloid Carcinoma. This tumor is a very cellular adenocarcinoma with a lymphoid stromal infiltrate but little fibrous reaction. It is therefore bulky and soft. The prognosis is better than that of the usual infiltrating ductal carcinoma.

Mucoid Carcinoma. This uncommon variant is characterized by slow growth and the formation of a bulky, gelatinous, soft tumor.

Lobular Carcinoma. The early stage in the development of this cancer is an *in situ* carcinoma. It is only when the malignant cells invade the surrounding tissues *(infiltrating lobular carci-*

noma) that a mass can be felt clinically. Lobular carcinoma can produce a hard mass similar to that produced by the common scirrhous ductal type carcinoma. Some tumors are less distinct and form a rubbery mass. The characteristic microscopic feature is the appearance of small cells lying in single file between fibrous tissue.

Lobular carcinoma accounts for about 10 per cent of the total number of patients with carcinoma; the tumor is of importance because it often arises multifocally. Since about 20 per cent of patients have a tumor in the opposite breast, it is a common practice to take blind biopsies of the other breast when the mastectomy is performed.

Metastatic Spread of Breast Carcinoma. Embolic spread is the feature that causes carcinoma of the breast to be so lethal.

Lymphatic Spread. Lymphatic permeation and embolism are so common in cancer of the breast that lymph node metastases are present in over

50 per cent of patients when the tumor is first diagnosed. The axillary group are the nodes most frequently involved, particularly from cancers of the upper and outer quadrant. This is the most common site for cancer. Intrathoracic nodes are involved, especially from tumors in the medial quadrants. The supraclavicular nodes are the third common site for metastases.

Case History II

At the age of 53 years, the patient underwent a modified right radical mastectomy for carcinoma of the breast. Seven months later, she experienced shortness of breath and pain in the right side of the chest. Radiographs revealed evidence of metastases in the lungs and in the spine. Nodules of tumor next appeared in the scalp, and a biopsy of one of them confirmed the diagnosis of metastatic adenocarcinoma consistent with breast origin. She died shortly afterward; necropsy disclosed metastatic tumor in the lungs (Fig. 28–3A), bones (Fig. 28–3B), adrenals, thyroid, and brain. The liver contained multiple masses of tumor similar in appearance to those depicted in Figure 12–9.

Blood-Borne Metastases. Hematogenous spread leads to involvement of the lungs, liver, adrenals, ovaries, and bone (Fig. 28–3). These secondary growths are not often detectable at the time of initial diagnosis, but they make their presence known sometimes years later, even after apparently successful treatment. These dormant tumors are common.

Diagnosis of Breast Cancer. Cancer of the breast usually presents as a *painless mass in the breast* discovered by the patient herself or during a routine physical examination.

Any lump in the breast must be presumed to be malignant until proven otherwise. Usually this determination involves biopsy or local excision. It is useless to rely on detecting the classic signs of cancer—fixation to skin, retraction, and elevation of the nipple, among others. Tumors diagnosed by these signs are often already incurable.

Early Detection. One would think that the ease with which the breast can be examined and removed would make early diagnosis and effective treatment easy; such is not the case. It seems that spread has often occurred by the time a lump is palpable. Routine physical examination, either by the woman herself or by a medical attendant, might improve the prognosis, but there is no proof of this. Radiography, or mammography, detection of hot spots by thermography (tumors tend to be vascular and hot), ultrasonic studies, and other methods have been introduced, but their value is unproved and their cost is considerable. Undoubtedly, small lesions can be detected, but a small lesion is not necessarily an early one. Prognosis depends on factors other than mere size.

Management of Breast Cancer. The introduction of radical mastectomy (removal of breast, pectoral muscles, and axillary contents with lymph nodes) by Halsted did much to improve the prognosis of breast cancer. Unfortunately, the appearance of late metastases was not influenced by local surgery, and alternative, less mutilating procedures have been introduced. Radiotherapy (alone or combined with simple excision of the tumor), removal of the breast alone (simple mastectomy), and simple removal of the tumor ("lumpectomy") all have their advocates. The results of treatment seem to be about the same with each of these methods, and there is no agreement as to which is the best. The present trend is to avoid the radical surgery that was once practiced, *e.g.*, radical mastectomy and radical mastectomy combined with removal of intrathoracic lymph nodes (super-radical mastectomy).

Hormone therapy has its uses as a palliative treatment of metastatic disease. It includes the removal of the ovaries, adrenals, or pituitary in premenopausal women; the administration of the estrogen antagonist tamoxifen; and, somewhat surprisingly, the administration of estrogens in older patients. Normal breast tissue has estrogen receptors, which can be detected by their uptake of tritiated estradiol. Breast cancers also have estrogen receptors, and those tumors with the highest receptor content appear to respond more favorably to hormone treatment than do those that lack such receptors.

Prognosis of Breast Cancer. About 50 per cent of patients have lymph node involvement at the time of initial diagnosis, and about 25 per cent are inoperable. The overall 5-year survival rate is 35 to 40 per cent, but of those treated by radical surgery, about 50 to 55 per cent are alive 5 years

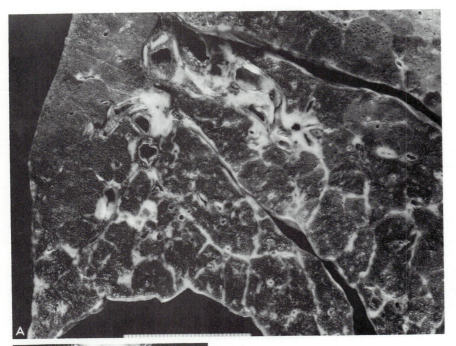

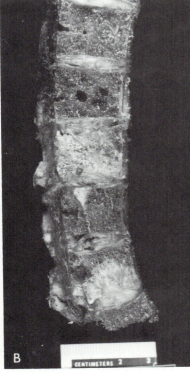

Figure 28–3 Metastatic carcinoma of the breast. *A*, The specimen shows the cut surface of parts of the three lobes of the right lung. Carcinoma has invaded the lymphatics of the septa as well as the region around blood vessels and bronchi. This reticulated appearance resulting from extensive lymphatic involvement is common in metastatic breast cancer; it contrasts with the multiple nodular appearance presented by pulmonary metastases from other primary tumors and from the deposits of growth found in the liver in this case. See Case History II for clinical details. *B*, A segment of the bisected thoracic vertebral column of the same patient. The bodies of two vertebrae show obvious white tumor.

later. The prognosis depends on many factors, including the following:

1. Pregnancy, which sometimes adversely affects prognosis.

2. Histologic grade of tumor. Poorly differentiated tumors do poorly, compared with well-differentiated ones. Mucoid and medullary carcinomas have a relatively good prognosis.

3. The type of tumor in terms of the size of the primary tumor (T), the presence and extent of lymph node involvement (N), and the presence of distant metastases (M). This is the TNM system of classification. A patient with stage 1 tumor (tumor less than 5 cm in diameter with no lymph node or distant metastases) has an 80 per cent 5-year survival rate and a 62 per cent 10-year survival rate, but the tumor can recur even after 10 years, even though the chances diminish with each passing year. For a stage 2 tumor, the 5- and 10-year survival rates are 36 per cent and 22 per cent, respectively; for stages 3 and 4, the outlook is even worse. The overall 5-year survival rate for breast cancer is about 50 per cent, and this figure has apparently not changed for over 40 years.

The spread and prognosis of breast cancer have been described in some detail because they illustrate the difficulties in assessing the effects of therapy. There are so many types and stages of the disease that unless each medical center uses a similar and comprehensive classification, it is not possible to compare the results of different treatments or even the same treatment at different centers.

Paget's Disease of the Breast

This is a chronic eczematous condition involving the nipple, which microscopically shows invasion of the epidermis by large malignant Paget cells (Fig. 28–4). There is almost invariably an underlying ductal carcinoma. Opinions are divided as to whether Paget's disease represents an intraepithelial spread of a breast cancer or whether epidermis and ductal epithelium are both involved simultaneously in a primary malignant process.

Case History III

A 74-year-old woman presented with an oval, red, scaly area of "eczema" centered on the nipple of the

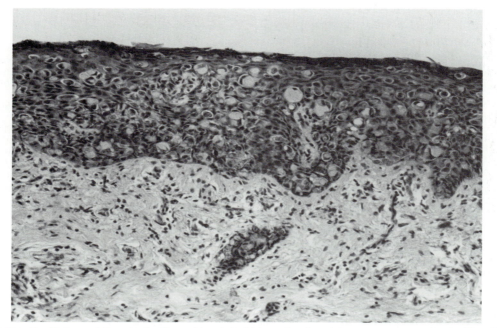

Figure 28–4 Paget's disease of the nipple. The epidermis is thickened and contains numerous round cells (Paget's cells) with cytoplasm that stains palely because of their mucin content.

left breast. She was seen by her family physician, who took a scraping of keratin for fungal examination. The direct examination of the specimen for mycelia was negative, as was the culture; a diagnosis of eczema was made. This lesion was quite unresponsive to treatment, but not until more than 1 year later was it appreciated that a simple eczema should have responded. A 3-mm punch biopsy was performed and showed Paget's disease (Fig. 28–4). Palpation revealed no mass in the breast, but mammography showed an area highly suggestive of carcinoma. Mastectomy was performed, and the presence of carcinoma was confirmed.

Other Malignant Neoplasms

Fibrosarcoma, angiosarcoma, and other malignant tumors occur, but they are rare.

THE MALE BREAST

The diseases of the female breast can also occur in the male, but they are rare. Carcinoma is about 100 times less common in men than in women, but it has a poorer prognosis. Gynecomastia deserves separate consideration.

Gynecomastia is the name given to enlargement of the male breast. As a transient phenomenon, it is not uncommon during adolescence and old age, presumably because it is related to hormonal imbalance during these periods of sexual development and decline. Other causes of gynecomastia include Klinefelter's syndrome (Chapter 3), heavy dosage of estrogens (*e.g.*, for carcinoma of the prostate), cirrhosis of the liver, the effects of certain drugs (*e.g.*, digitalis), and estrogen-secreting tumors of the adrenal, the testis, or other site.

Summary

• Developmental anomalies include accessory nipples and breast tissue and virginal hypertrophy.

• Infections of the breast are unimportant except during breast feeding. Plasma-cell mastitis may be an aftermath of infection.

• Fibrocystic disease of the breast, also called chronic mastitis, is extremely common and is characterized by lumpy, sometimes painful breasts. It is probably related to repeated hormonal fluctuations. Fibrosis, cysts, and epithelial hyperplasia are present, but only if there is epithelial atypia is carcinoma a complication.

• Benign tumors of the breast include the common fibroadenoma and intraductal or intracystic papilloma.

• Carcinoma of the breast is the most important lesion of the breast; it affects about one in 11 women in North America. A family history of the disease, obesity, and excess estrogen stimulation are known predisposing causes. The common type is the ductal carcinoma; lobular carcinoma is important because it can arise multifocally and be bilateral. An RNA retrovirus is involved in the pathogenesis of cancer of the breast in mice and possibly also in humans. Early detection of the tumor, surgery, radiotherapy, and hormonal therapy have influenced the prognosis; even so, only about 50 per cent of patients are alive 5 years after diagnosis. Lymph node metastases appear, later to be followed by blood-borne spread to liver, lungs, bone, and elsewhere.

Selected Readings

Azzopardi, J. G.: Benign and malignant proliferative epithelial lesions of the breast: A review. Eur. J. Cancer Clin. Oncol., *19*:1717, 1983.

Carlson, H. E.: Gynecomastia. N. Engl. J. Med. *303*:795, 1980.

Consensus statement of the Cancer Committee of the College of American Pathologists: Is "fibrocystic disease" of the breast precancerous? Arch. Pathol. Lab. Med. *110*:171, 1986.

Hutter, R. V. P.: Goodbye to "fibrocystic disease." N. Engl. J. Med. *312*:179, 1985.

Kalache, A., and Vessey, M.: Risk factors for breast cancer. Clin. Oncol. *1*:661, 1982.

Mirecki, D. M., and Jordan, V. C.: Steroid hormone receptors and human breast cancer. Lab. Med. *16*:287, 1985.

Mueller, C. B.: Surgery for breast cancer: Less may be as good as more. N. Engl. J. Med. *312*:712, 1985.

Rosai, J.: Breast. *In* Ackerman's Surgical Pathology. 7th ed. St. Louis, C. V. Mosby, 1989.

29

Endocrine Glands

- Describe the main actions of each of the hormones secreted by the adenohypophysis.
- Describe the common manifestations of hyperpituitarism and hypopituitarism. Give at least two causes of each condition.
- List the hormones produced by the adrenal glands.
- Describe the manifestations of Addison's disease.
- Describe the syndromes produced by adrenal cortical hypersecretion.
- Indicate the value of glucocorticoid therapy and list the important complications.
- Define goiter and give four examples of a condition that may cause it.
- Compare hyperthyroidism with hypothyroidism.
- Describe Graves' disease, Hashimoto's disease, and de Quervain's thyroiditis.
- Outline the types of thyroid carcinoma.

After studying this chapter, the student should be able to:

- Describe the mode of action of hormones.
- List the hormones that are manufactured in the hypothalamus.
- Give examples of the common manifestations of hypothalamic disorders.
- Describe the components of the neurohypophysis and the adenohypophysis. Indicate how each part develops.
- Outline the features of diabetes insipidus.
- List the types of endocrine cells of the adenohypophysis, indicate how they have been identified, and list the hormones that are manufactured by each cell type.

Although the nervous system exerts the major controlling influence over the activities of the higher animals, there is an additional mechanism by which one type of cell can influence another—hormone secretion. By the secretion into the blood stream of potent chemicals called *hormones*, cells can exert influence at a distant site. Secreting cells that perform this endocrine function may be grouped together, to form one of the well-known endocrine glands, such as the thyroid gland, or they may be scattered more diffusely in the tissues, such as the cells in the pylorus that secrete the hormone *gastrin* when stimulated by the presence of food in the stomach. Gastrin stimulates the fundus of the stomach to secrete hydrochloric acid.

Mode of Action of Hormones. Hormones act by binding to specific receptor sites on their target organs. This explains the highly specific action of hormones as well as their variable action on target organs. For instance, a lack of insulin effect in some types of diabetes mellitus is due not to a lack of insulin, but to insulin resistance secondary to a diminution of specific receptors. The water-soluble hormones, such as epinephrine and glucagon, act on receptors on the cell membrane; cyclic AMP is formed, and it acts as a second messenger to stimulate or depress a characteristic biochemical activity. The lipid-soluble steroid hormones act on receptors within the cell, and the hormone-receptor complex enters the nucleus and then acts by affecting the expression of the cell's genetic material.

THE HYPOTHALAMUS

Although the pituitary gland has been called the "leader of the endocrine orchestra," many of its activities are themselves controlled by the hypothalamus, which, although part of the brain, also has many endocrine functions (Fig. 29–1).

The hypothalamus consists of a complex collection of nerve cells and fiber tracts that participate in, and help regulate, many functions of the body. These include regulation of the autonomic nervous system, temperature, blood pressure, plasma osmolality, hunger, thirst, emotions, sexual drive, and sleep. The hypothalamus controls body rhythms; a specific *cycling center* is responsible for controlling the menstrual cycle.

Hypothalamic Hormones. The hypothalamus may be regarded as an endocrine organ, because its cells synthesize two groups of hormones.

Oxytocin and Vasopressin. These are discussed later in this chapter.

Releasing and Inhibiting Hormones or Factors. These are polypeptides of low molecular weight that pass to the adenohypophysis via a short portal vein and stimulate or inhibit it.

The following releasing factors are recognized:
Corticotropin-releasing hormone (CRH).
Thyrotropin-releasing hormone (TRH).
Gonadotropin-releasing hormone (GnRH).
Growth hormone–releasing hormone (GHnRH).
Prolactin-releasing factor (PRF).

The action of these hormones may be understood by an examination of the action of CRH. This hormone leads to the release of corticotropin (also known as adrenocorticotropic hormone, ACTH) from the adenohypophysis. ACTH acts on the adrenal cortex to cause the release of cortisol (hydrocortisone). ACTH inhibits the release of CRH, cortisol inhibits the release of both CRH and ACTH. This inhibition is an example of negative feedback, which is a mechanism encountered in the regulation of other hormone secretions.

The releasing factors are produced in picogram (10^{-12}) quantities, the pituitary hormones are produced in nanogram (10^{-9}) quantities, and the target cells (*e.g.*, the thyroid) produce hormone in microgram (10^{-6}) quantities. Thus, the chain reaction shows a considerable amplification effect.

In addition to forming releasing factors, the hypothalamus also forms *inhibiting factors*. The varying release of prolactin-inhibiting factor is the mechanism whereby prolactin secretion is regulated. Inhibitors of the release of thyroid-stimulating hormone (TSH), prolactin, melanocyte-stimulating hormone (MSH), and growth hormone have been described. The growth hormone release–inhibiting factor or *somatostatin*, in addition to being a powerful inhibitor of growth hormone secretion by the pituitary, also inhibits the release of other hormones (*e.g.*, insulin) throughout the body. Indeed, the account given here of the various releasing and inhibiting factors is a simplified version of the facts. Thus, pure TRH causes release of both TSH and prolactin.

Diseases of the Hypothalamus

Many pathologic processes (*e.g.*, encephalitis, vascular lesions, head injury, hamartoma, and tumor) can affect the hypothalamus. The effects differ widely, depending on which function is deranged the most. Occasionally there is increased secretion of a hypothalamic hormone, but usually destruction of a particular area of the hypothalamus leads to impaired hormone secre-

HYPOTHALAMUS

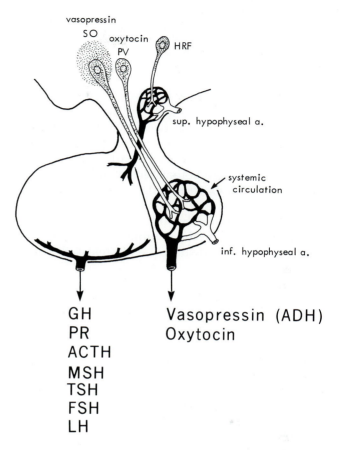

Figure 29–1 The relationship between the hypothalamus and the pituitary gland. Vasopressin (antidiuretic hormone, ADH) and oxytocin are manufactured in nerve cells in the supraoptic (SO) and paraventricular (PV) nuclei of the hypothalamus. These hormones are not released into the circulation until they have reached the neurohypophysis. The shaded area surrounding the SO cell body represents the "osmoreceptor" that is responsive to changes in osmolality of the fluid perfusing it. HRF represents an ill-defined group of cells that secrete a series of releasing factors into the primary capillary network of a portal vein. This vein passes in the pituitary stalk to the adenohypophysis, where cells manufacture the seven hormones of this lobe of the pituitary: growth hormone (GH), prolactin (PR), adrenocorticotropic hormone (ACTH), melanocyte-stimulating hormone (MSH), thyroid-stimulating hormone (TSH), follicle-stimulating hormone (FSH), and luteinizing hormone (LH). (Drawn by Margot Mackay, University of Toronto, Faculty of Medicine, Department of Surgery, Division of Biomedical Communications, Toronto. After a drawing by E. Blackstock in Ezrin, C., Godden, J. O., Volpé, R., and Wilson, R. [Eds.]: Systematic Endocrinology. New York, Harper & Row, Publishers, 1973.)

tion; another mechanism is interruption of the flow of hormone to the pituitary by a pituitary stalk lesion.

The effects of hypothalamic disease include the following:

1. Obesity due to overeating.
2. Somnolence or increased restless activity.
3. Failure to maintain body temperature.
4. Diabetes insipidus that is due to lack of vasopressin, also known as the antidiuretic hormone (ADH).
5. Hypothalamic hypogonadism due to a failure to form gonadotropin-releasing hormone. When combined with obesity, this condition is known as *Fröhlich's syndrome.*
6. Precocious, or premature, puberty.
7. Visual disturbances due to pressure on the optic chiasma.
8. Hypothyroidism and hypoadrenocorticism.

9. Hypoprolactinemia related to lack of prolactin-inhibiting factor. It causes amenorrhea, galactorrhea, and decreased libido in females.

The regulation of the hypothalamic-pituitary function is complex, for apart from the gross lesions mentioned, hypothalamic function is also influenced by impulses emanating from other parts of the brain. Some specific examples illustrate this. Psychological stress, even mild, can lead to amenorrhea in young women. Failure to grow in childhood can be due to severe emotional trauma (*maternal deprivation syndrome*). A return of close emotional support leads to increased growth hormone secretion.

THE PITUITARY GLAND (HYPOPHYSIS)

Although small, the pituitary gland, or hypophysis, secretes an amazing variety and number of hormones. The gland and its stalk consist of two parts: the *neurohypophysis*, which develops as an outpouching from the primitive brain; and the *adenohypophysis*, which originates as a diverticulum from the primitive foregut (Fig. 29–1).

The Neurohypophysis

The neurohypophysis consists of the posterior lobe of the pituitary, part of the pituitary stalk (the *infundibular stem*), and part of the brain adjacent to the hypothalamus (the *median eminence of the tuber cinereum*). Two peptide hormones, oxytocin and vasopressin, are manufactured by cells in the hypothalamus and pass via the cells' axons into the neurohypophysis, where they are stored and subsequently released when needed.

Oxytocin. This hormone causes uterine contraction during labor and is responsible for milk ejection when an infant is breastfed. The act of suckling initiates a reflex that causes oxytocin release.

Vasopressin (Antidiuretic Hormone). This hormone acts on the distal and collecting tubules of the kidney and causes water to be retained. Its release is governed by the action of "osmoreceptors" in the hypothalamus. An increase in plasma osmolality associated with dehydration leads to a release of vasopressin and water retention.

Diabetes Insipidus

This disease is caused by a failure in the development of the neurohypophysis or its destruction by a tumor or inflammation. Huge quantities of very dilute urine are passed (*polyuria*), leading to excessive thirst and drinking (*polydipsia*).

The Adenohypopysis

The adenohypophysis consists of the pars anterior, or anterior lobe, of the pituitary, the pars intermedia (which barely exists in humans), and the pars tuberalis in the pituitary stalk.

Early attempts to delineate the types of cell present in the anterior pituitary gland were based on staining with hematoxylin and eosin and a variety of empirical stains. Three types of cell were recognized: acidophils, basophils, and chromophobes. The chromophobe group stain poorly and are regarded as resting forms of other cell types. Electron microscopy and immunostaining for specific hormones have revealed that there are at least five cell types, each named according to its secretion:

1. *Thyrotropes.* These cells secrete *thyrotropin*, which is also called *thyroid-stimulating hormone* or TSH.

2. *Lactotropes.* The secretion *prolactin* acts on the breast to initiate and maintain lactation. Before this can happen, the breast must have been developed by the action of other hormones— estrogens, progesterone, and so forth.

3. *Gonadotropes.* These cells produce the two pituitary gonadotropins:

Follicle-stimulating hormone or *FSH*, which stimulates follicle development in the ovary and gametogenesis in the testis.

Luteinizing hormone or *LH*, which promotes the formation of the corpus luteum in the ovary. In the male, it stimulates the interstitial cells of the testis to produce testosterone.

4. *Corticotropes.* These cells form a large precursor prohormone from which two compounds are formed by proteolysis:

Corticotropin, or adrenocorticotropic hormone (ACTH). This hormone stimulates the adrenal cortex to produce cortisol, but it also acts on some other tissues directly, *e.g.*, the liver. Alpha-melanocyte–stimulating hormone can be formed from ACTH.

Beta-lipotropin. Beta-melanocyte–stimulating hormone (MSH) and endorphins can be formed from this large molecule. The various types of MSH are formed in amphibians because these hormones enable them to change color rapidly. Little MSH is formed in humans under normal circumstances, but in some diseases it is responsible for darkening of the skin. Endorphins are polypeptides that act as analgesics with a morphine-like action. They resemble the *enkephalins*, which are central nervous system transmitters.

5. *Somatotropes.* Somatotropes secrete somato-

tropin, or growth hormone. This acts on the liver, and perhaps other tissues, and leads to the secretion of somatomedins. These insulin-like polypeptides antagonize the action of insulin and act on many tissues, particularly skeletal tissues, to stimulate growth.

Disorders of the Adenohypophysis

Hyperplasia or neoplasia of the anterior lobe of the pituitary gland may be associated with hypersecretion of one, or several, of the pituitary hormones. On the other hand, non–hormone-secreting tumors of the pituitary, or tumors arising in surrounding areas, may press on and destroy the parenchyma, leading to a diminished hormonal secretion. This also occurs when the pituitary is destroyed by other lesions, *e.g.*, infarction or inflammation. Because the clinical picture may be complex, only the common types are outlined. Tumors in the pituitary region give rise to two additional characteristic effects owing to their anatomic situation: *compression of the optic chiasma*, which causes loss of the temporal visual fields of both eyes (bitemporal hemianopsia); and *enlargement of the sella turcica*, which is detectable radiologically.

Hyperpituitarism. Adenomas of the pituitary produce varying effects, depending on the type of cell involved. The *prolactinoma* is the most common, and the excess prolactin that it secretes causes amenorrhea and sometimes inappropriate secretion of milk (*galactorrhea*). In males, the effects are less striking, but impotence can occur. An *adenoma of the somatotropes* demonstrates the effects of excess growth hormone production. If the condition arises in childhood, the result is *gigantism*: the individual is well proportioned, but huge. If the tumor arises in an adult after the epiphyses have fused, the result is *acromegaly*, in which the hands, feet, and lower jaw are enlarged. There is coarsening of the facial features (Fig. 29–2) and a high incidence of impaired glucose tolerance (see Chapter 16). Clinical diabetes occurs in 10 to 15 per cent of patients.

An *adenoma of the corticotropes* leads to excess ACTH production and is the cause of *Cushing's disease*, which is described later in this chapter. If the disease is treated by adrenalectomy, the pituitary is stimulated to even greater activity, and the excess ACTH production leads to marked hyperpigmentation of the skin. This can mimic Addison's disease, and the condition is called Nelson's syndrome; this emphasizes the MSH-like activity of ACTH.

Adenomas of other cell types of the adenohypophysis are known but are rare. In some cases of hyperpituitarism, the lesion may best be regarded as hyperplastic rather than neoplastic. Sometimes several hormones are secreted, so that mixed syndromes occur. Occasionally the pituitary lesion is frankly carcinomatous.

Hypopituitarism. In children, deficiency of growth hormone causes severe retardation of growth, resulting in midgetism. The unopposed action of insulin can lead to attacks of hypoglycemia (Chapter 16).

Hypopituitarism with lack of gonadotropins leads to lack of testicular or ovarian maturation. Puberty does not take place. Fusion of the epiphyses, normally produced by the sex hormones, is delayed. If growth hormone production is normal, these eunuchoid patients develop abnormally long limbs—their span exceeds their height (normally they are equal). Gonadotropin deficiency can occur in adults. Males exhibit testicular atrophy and loss of libido; females develop amenorrhea and regression of secondary sexual characteristics.

In adults, anterior pituitary insufficiency can manifest itself as hypothyroidism; often this is combined with evidence of adrenal cortical and gonadotropic deficiency.

Acute pituitary insufficiency sometimes occurs after parturition and is due to infarction of the gland. The condition is then called *Sheehan's syndrome*. When destruction of the adenohypophysis is complete, the condition, called *Simmonds' disease*, is characterized by extreme wasting. The patients are apathetic; without treatment, they ultimately die of adrenal insufficiency (see discussion later in this chapter). Simmonds' disease must be distinguished from *anorexia nervosa*.

THE ADRENAL GLANDS

The Adrenal Medulla

The adrenal medulla is derived from the neural crest and contains both ganglion cells of the

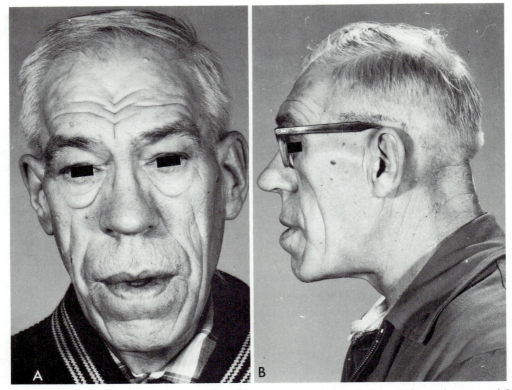

Figure 29–2 Acromegaly. Note how the thickening of the skin has exaggerated the facial wrinkles and coarsened the features. The ears, nose, and lips are prominent. Prominence of the lower jaw (termed prognathism) is particularly characteristic of acromegaly and is best seen in the lateral view (*B*). The patient died of a myocardial infarction; at necropsy, an acidophilic adenoma was found. (Courtesy of Dr. L. F. W. Loach, Department of Medicine, Toronto General Division of the Toronto Hospital, Toronto.)

sympathetic nervous system and pheochromocytes, cells that can secrete epinephrine and norepinephrine into the blood. These hormones cause a rise in blood glucose, a rise in blood pressure, and a redistribution of blood such that the individual is better adapted for fight or flight. A rare tumor, the *pheochromocytoma*, secretes these agents in excess and leads to systemic hypertension. The other important tumor of the adrenal medulla is the *neuroblastoma*, which is derived from the precursor cells that normally mature to ganglion cells. The neuroblastoma is one of the common tumors of childhood and ranks with leukemia, Wilms' tumor, and medulloblastoma of the brain as a principal form of lethal cancer in the young. The tumor has some remarkable properties. When it appears at birth or in patients under 1 year of age, the prognosis is relatively good because often either the tumor

undergoes spontaneous regression or its cells differentiate into ganglion cells and then behave in a benign manner. Such a tumor is then called a *ganglioneuroma*. When the tumor occurs after the age of 1 year, it behaves in a very malignant fashion.

The Adrenal Cortex

Three major groups of hormones (corticoids) are secreted:

Glucocorticoids, *e.g.*, hydrocortisone (cortisol). In physiologic concentrations, these steroids accelerate the synthesis of glucose from noncarbohydrate precursors and inhibit the actions of insulin. These hormones also have a mild salt-retaining activity.

Mineralocorticoids, *e.g.*, aldosterone, which primarily affects electrolyte metabolism. It causes sodium retention and increases potassium loss in the urine. Aldosterone production is stimulated by angiotensin II and is therefore regulated by the renal blood flow (Chapter 19).

Sex hormones, *e.g.*, estrogen, androgens, and progesterone.

Adrenal Cortical Insufficiency

Primary Adrenal Cortical Insufficiency (Addison's Disease). Idiopathic atrophy, perhaps mediated by an autoimmune process, and destruction of the glands, usually by tuberculosis, are the two common causes of Addison's disease (Fig. 29–3). Extreme weakness, loss of appetite, loss of weight, a low blood pressure, and eventual death are the main features. As would be expected, hypoglycemia, a fall in serum sodium (hyponatremia), and a rise in potassium (hyperkalemia) are among the clinical findings. The skin and mucous membranes, including the oral mucosa, show increased melanin pigmentation. This is because the low plasma hydrocortisone level stimulates the pituitary to produce excess ACTH and beta-lipotropin, both of which cause a darkening of the skin by an effect on the melanocytes. Diagnosis is not easy in the early stages, but it is important to diagnose Addison's disease because substitution therapy is lifesaving. The normal maintenance dose of prednisone is 7.5 mg (1½ tablets) daily. This is equivalent to the output of cortisol by the normal adrenal. An acute exacerbation of the disease (acute adrenal insufficiency or addisonian crisis) may occur at any time, particularly when the patient is subjected to any type of stress, *e.g.*, trauma or an infection. The crisis is characterized by extreme weakness, hypotension, hypoglycemia, epigastric pain, vomiting, diarrhea, coma, and death.

Secondary Adrenal Cortical Insufficiency. Adrenal cortical insufficiency may be secondary to pituitary hypofunction in which there is a decreased output of ACTH. It differs from Addison's disease in that the blood level of ACTH is low, skin hyperpigmentation is absent, and aldosterone secretion is unaffected. As in Addison's disease, acute life-threatening crises may occur if the patient is subjected to stress and is not given increased doses of glucocorticoids.

Adrenal Cortical Hypersecretion

Adrenal overactivity may be secondary to pituitary hypersecretion of ACTH. Usually, however, the overproduction of corticoids is due to idiopathic adrenal hyperplasia, adenoma, or (rarely) a carcinoma. The clinical picture is often mixed, but three main patterns may be discerned.

Adrenogenital Syndrome. In boys, puberty may occur prematurely, even as early as 4 years ("infantile Hercules"). In girls, male characteristics may develop. In adult women, this masculinization, called virilism, is manifested as atrophy of the breasts, enlargement of the clitoris, cessation of menstruation, growth of a beard, and deepening of the voice.

Conn's Syndrome. Excess aldosterone secretion, usually by an adenoma, produces a low serum potassium with sodium and water retention as well as hypertension.

Cushing's Syndrome. Obesity is the most common feature and is particularly evident in the face, trunk, cervicodorsal region, and supraclavicular area. The limbs are relatively thin owing to muscular wasting. Typically there is a round "moon face" (Fig. 29–4) and a dorsal "buffalo" hump. Other features are systemic hypertension, osteoporosis, acne vulgaris, and increased growth of body hair in women. Psychiatric disturbances are common, and over 50 per cent of patients with Cushing's disease have emotional disorders, particularly of the depressive type.

Cushing's "disease" was originally described as being due to a pituitary adenoma. However, the same clinical picture (Cushing's "syndrome") is encountered under other circumstances:

1. With hypersecretion of ACTH due to hypothalamic-pituitary dysfunction.

2. With adrenal hyperplasia or neoplasia.

3. With ectopic ACTH syndrome. An ACTH-like hormone can be produced by some tumors, *e.g.*, oat-cell carcinoma of the lung.

4. With glucocorticoid therapy. The syndrome, or mild forms of it, is commonly seen

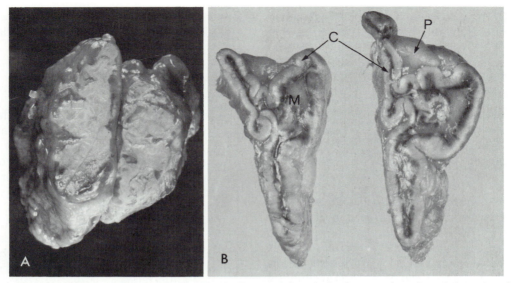

Figure 29–3 Histoplasmosis of the adrenal glands. *A,* The two adrenal glands are enlarged, and the cut surface shows complete replacement of the normal tissue by necrotic, caseous material. *Histoplasma capsulatum* was identified in this specimen. The gross appearance of these specimens is identical with that of tuberculosis, a disease that once accounted for most cases of Addison's disease (idiopathic atrophy is now more frequently encountered as a cause of Addison's disease). See also Figure 25–9 and Case History I, Chapter 25, for details of this case. *B,* Normal adrenals for comparison. C, cortex; M, medulla; P, periadrenal fat.

when glucocorticoids are administered in massive doses. Rounding and swelling of the face ("moon face") are particularly characteristic (Fig. 29–4).

Glucocorticoid Therapy

Replacement glucocorticoid therapy is logical and useful in patients with adrenal insufficiency. However, when used in massive (pharmacologic) amounts, the glucocorticoids have two additional actions that can be useful.

1. *Anti-inflammatory action.* The glucocorticoids (*e.g.,* prednisone) have a suppressive effect on the inflammatory reaction; for this reason they are used in many diseases, *e.g.,* rheumatoid arthritis, herpes zoster, and polyarteritis nodosa. They may be used to advantage when bacterial inflammation might produce serious damage, but antibiotics must also be administered so that the infection does not spread.

2. *Lymphoid atrophy and depression of the immune response.* This may be used to advantage in treating acute lymphatic leukemia, autoimmune dis-

eases, and hypersensitivity states, such as bronchial asthma. The immunosuppressive action of prednisone is of great use in suppressing the graft rejection reaction, such as in patients with kidney grafts.

Complications. The administration of large doses of glucocorticoids over a prolonged period can have serious consequences. Indeed, these may be more serious than the disease for which the treatment was initiated. Important complications are the following.

Cushing's Syndrome. See earlier discussion.

Susceptibility to Infection. Infections of many types are common in patients on glucocorticoid therapy, and this is related to the immunosuppressive effect of the compounds. Attacks of bronchopneumonia and urinary tract infections can be troublesome. Fungal and viral infections can be devastating (Fig. 29–4). A quiescent tuberculous focus can be reactivated and then lead to miliary tuberculosis.

Osteoporosis. Severe and widespread osteoporosis can lead to fracture formation after trivial injury. Collapse of vertebrae is common.

Inhibition of Wound Healing. Wound contrac-

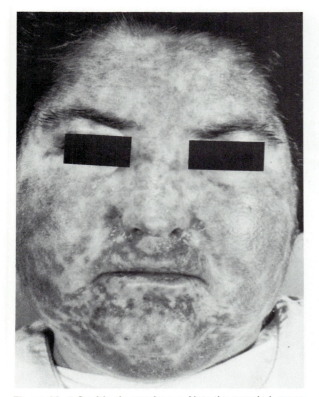

Figure 29–4 Cushing's syndrome. Note the rounded, moon-shaped appearance of the face that is characteristic of this condition. The patient first presented with a severe autoimmune hemolytic anemia. No definite cause for this was found, and it was decided to treat her with prednisone. Doses of up to 100 mg per day were needed to control the anemia, and she became markedly cushingoid. Unfortunately, she developed a widespread infection with *Cryptococcus neoformans* and subsequently died of this superinfection. The erythematous, blotchy eruption seen on the face is an unusual manifestation of generalized cryptococcosis, but it was biopsy of similar lesions on the thigh that led to the diagnosis.

tion, granulation tissue formation, and collagen formation are inhibited.

Peptic Ulcer. Peptic ulceration, if present, is adversely affected; perforation and bleeding may be precipitated.

Cataract Formation. (See Chapter 32.)

Diabetes Mellitus. (See Chapter 16.)

Mental Effects. An acute mental breakdown (psychosis) may be precipitated. Suicide is an occasional cause of death during glucocorticoid drug therapy.

Systemic Hypertension. The development of hypertension or the accentuation of existing dis-

ease appears to be due to the salt-retaining activity of most glucocorticoids.

Acute Adrenal Insufficiency. This emergency, characterized by hypotension, shock, and sudden death, occurs if steroid therapy is suddenly withdrawn. It may also occur if a patient who is taking a steroid develops a severe infection or is subjected to severe injury such as a major surgery and does not have the dose increased. *It is vital that all patients on glucocorticoid therapy as well as their medical attendants be aware of this possibility.*

The Waterhouse-Friderichsen syndrome is often cited as an example of acute adrenal cortical insufficiency. The syndrome most commonly occurs during the course of an overwhelming meningococcal septicemia and is characterized by bleeding into the skin and in internal organs. The adrenals in particular are the site of massive bleeding. Death occurs rapidly and is probably attributable to septicemia associated with disseminated intravascular coagulopathy rather than to any acute adrenal insufficiency. It should be noted that adrenal insufficiency does not occur until over 90 per cent of both glands has been destroyed. Hence, clinically apparent effects are rarely seen with tumors involving the adrenal glands, *e.g.*, the common metastatic carcinoma that is seen in cases of carcinoma of the lung and breast.

THE THYROID GLAND

The thyroid gland has the unique ability to trap iodine from the blood and incorporate it as thyroglobulin in the colloid of its vesicles (Fig. 29–5). By the action of a proteolytic enzyme on thyroglobulin, the iodine-containing thyroid hormones thyroxine (T_4) and triiodothyronine (T_3) are released. This occurs when the gland is stimulated by TSH from the pituitary. TSH secretion is itself stimulated by a low blood level of thyroid hormone both directly and indirectly via TRH. Both T_3 and T_4 are carried in the blood bound to protein and in a free form, the free form being the active state. T_4 is the most avidly bound to protein; in the peripheral tissues, some is converted into T_3, the most active compound. Estimation of the serum levels of T_3 and T_4 and

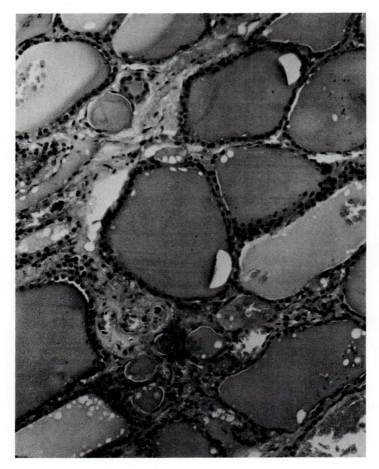

Figure 29–5 Normal thyroid. The gland consists of follicles of varying size, lined by a simple flattened or cubical epithelium and filled with homogeneous colloid. The colloid contains thyroglobulin ($\times 250$).

the total protein binding power are tests commonly employed to assess thyroid function.

The inconspicuous C cells of the thyroid secrete calcitonin. They are the cells of origin of medullary carcinoma of the thyroid. So far, no syndrome has been described in relation to an excess or deficiency of this hormone.

Action of the Thyroid Hormones. In spite of much research, the precise mode of action of the thyroid hormones is not known. However, much has been learned by comparing the normal individual (who is described as *euthyroid*) with those who suffer from excessive or diminished secretion (*hyperthyroid* and *hypothyroid*, respectively).

A *deficiency* of the thyroid hormones causes any or all of following conditions: a reduction in metabolic rate; impaired mental and physical growth (most marked in childhood); and anemia, which is less constant.

A hypersecretion of thyroid hormones causes an increase in the metabolic rate and the other changes encountered in thyrotoxicosis that are described later.

Goiter

Any enlargement of the thyroid is called a goiter; to a minor extent, this occurs at times of stress, *e.g.*, during puberty and pregnancy. A more potent cause is a diet deficient in iodine. The reason is that the thyroid, being unable to manufacture its hormone, cannot check the secretion of TSH that stimulates it to activity. Before iodine was added to table salt, goiters were common in many parts of the world (*e.g.*, the Great Lakes area of North America, the Andes, the Himalayas, and Derbyshire, England) because the soil carried insufficient iodine for foodstuffs to contain even minute quantities of iodine. Repeated phases of hyperplasia followed by involution led to the formation of large, nodular goiters containing many colloid-filled areas, some of which showed necrosis and dystrophic calcification (*nodular colloid goiter;* Fig. 29–6).

The goiters associated with hyperthyroidism, Hashimoto's disease, and neoplasia are described later in this chapter.

Hypothyroidism

Hypothyroidism was once frequent in areas of endemic goiter due mainly to iodine deficiency. Goitrogenic substances in the diet can also block thyroid function and lead to hypothyroidism. The effects of hypothyroidism in the child differ from those in the adult.

Cretinism. An insufficiency of thyroid hormone in the infant leads to cretinism. The child has a bloated face, protruding tongue, and a vacant expression and becomes mentally defective. There is a retardation of growth, and dwarfism results (Fig. 29–7).

Endemic cretinism is usually due to a lack of iodine in the diet but is occasionally caused by a dietary goitrogenic substance. A similar effect is seen if the mother is taking a drug that blocks thyroid function, *e.g.,* thiourea or one of its derivatives. *Sporadic cretinism* occurs in nongoitrogenic regions and is caused by agenesis of the thyroid or a congenital absence of one of the enzymes necessary for T_3 and T_4 synthesis.

Myxedema. This condition is the manifestation of hypothyroidism in the adult. There is a reduction in mental and physical activity, and the patient exhibits a characteristic bloated appearance because of a curious edema of the skin. This disease is associated with an excessive accumulation of mucoprotein.

Patients with myxedema are intolerant of cold and may develop hypothermia in cold climates. The patient may then pass into a coma and die (*myxedema coma*). Muscle weakness, a hoarse voice, and an increase in body weight are other features of the disease. Myxedema may occur as an end result of toxic goiter, nodular colloid goiter, or Hashimoto's disease or after surgical removal or irradiation of the gland. Under these circumstances, the serum levels of T_3 and T_4 are low, but the TSH level is high. Myxedema that accompanies pituitary or hypothalamic hypofunction also exhibits low serum T_3 and T_4 level, but the serum TSH level in reduced.

Case History I

Nodular colloid goiter (see Fig. 29–6). The patient was a 45-year-old woman who complained of a swelling in the neck. The swelling moved when she swallowed and had the features of an enlarged thyroid (goiter). The patient had had seven pregnancies; it was during the last two that she had noticed some swelling of the neck. However, it was only after the last delivery (1 year previously) that the goiter had rapidly become obvious. On examination, several nodules could be felt in the enlarged thyroid. An echogram revealed that one of them was cystic; radioactive studies showed no uptake by this "cold" nodule. T_3 and T_4 levels in the blood were normal. Although a diagnosis of nodular colloid goiter seemed obvious, the fact that the thyroid enlargement had occurred soon after delivery rather than during the pregnancy raised the possibility of malignancy. Cold nodules should always be viewed with suspicion. The left lobe of the thyroid and one nodule in the right lobe were removed.

Hyperthyroidism

This condition is also known as *thyrotoxicosis* and occurs in two forms.

Graves' Disease (Primary Hyperthyroidism). This disease is characterized by a diffuse enlargement of the thyroid gland (goiter) due to a marked hyperplasia of its epithelial elements (Fig. 29–8). There is a raised metabolic rate that manifests itself as a persistent increase in the heart rate; in elderly patients, this may lead to atrial fibrillation and heart failure. The individual is typically jumpy, nervous, and intolerant of hot weather. The hands are warm and sweaty; they are seldom at rest and exhibit a fine tremor when the fingers are stretched out. In spite of a good appetite, there is weight loss. Muscular weakness, which is a common symptom, can be severe. If left untreated, Graves' disease often terminates in heart failure. The eyes have a characteristic appearance: the eyelids are retracted, giving the patient a staring expression; in severe cases, the globe is actually pushed

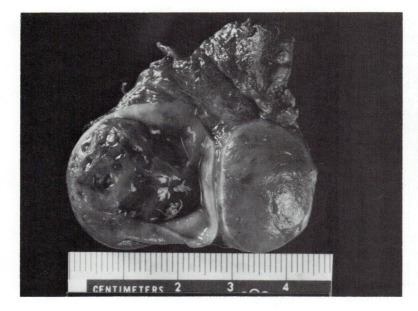

Figure 29–6 Nodular colloid goiter. The specimen consists of the left lobe of the thyroid and shows two nodules, both encapsulated. One is solid, whereas the other is cystic and contains dark, altered blood. Hemorrhage into this degenerate nodule accounts for the sudden swelling experienced by this patient. For further clinical data, see Case History I.

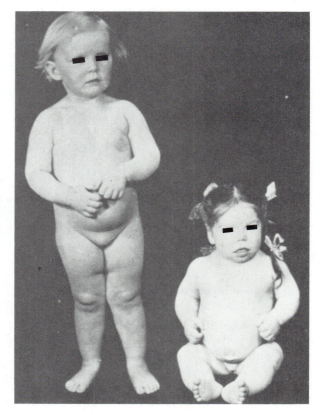

Figure 29–7 Cretinism. Note the dwarfed appearance of the cretin, compared with a child of like age on her right. Other distinctive features are the torpid expression, round face, eyes set widely apart, enlarged protruding tongue, and umbilical hernia. (Courtesy of Mr. G.S. Hoggins and the Department of Clinical Illustration, University of Birmingham, Birmingham, England.)

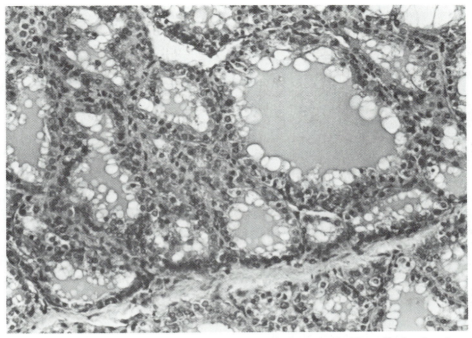

Figure 29–8 Graves' disease. This section shows that the thyroid gland is hyperplastic. The epithelium is columnar, and in some small follicles where colloid is deficient, it encroaches on the acinar spaces. In the large follicles, the colloid shows vacuolation where it abuts on the epithelium (×250).

forward to produce *exophthalmos* (Fig. 29–9). This is produced by edema and lymphocytic infiltration of the contents of the orbit. If severe, these changes can cause loss of sight (*malignant exophthalmos*).

Some patients with Graves' disease have *pretibial myxedema*, a localized pretibial, indurated plaque produced by accumulation of mucopolysaccharide in the dermis.

Patients with thyrotoxicosis may experience sudden exacerbations of their symptoms with hyperactivity, hyperpyrexia, coma, and death.

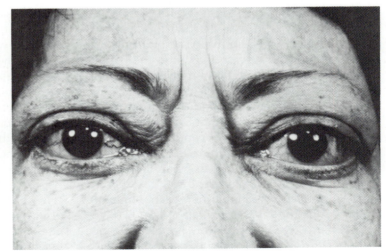

Figure 29–9 Ocular manifestation of Graves' disease. This patient noted the development of prominence of both eyes at the same time as the appearance of other symptoms of Graves' disease. The eyelids and periorbital tissues are swollen; the conjunctiva is congested and moist because of excessive lacrimation. The globe itself is pushed forward (*proptosis*) by an accumulation of mucoprotein in the orbital tissues. A similar change is sometimes encountered in the skin of the lower leg and is called *pretibial myxedema*. Note that this occurs in Graves' disease. (Courtesy of Dr. N. Pairaudeau, North York General Hospital, Willowdale, Ontario.)

This is termed a *thyroid storm* and demands rapid and energetic treatment if life is to be saved.

The thyroid gland in Graves' disease is stimulated by an IgG autoantibody, called *thyroid-stimulating immunoglobulin (TSI)*, that is directed against TSH receptor protein. The antibody has the property of displacing TSH from its binding site and stimulating the gland to activity. It is possible that the basic defect in Graves' disease is an abnormality in T-cell function such that TSI formation is permitted. In addition, a genetic factor is implicated; there is an increased incidence of the disease in subjects with HLA DR3. The exophthalmos and pretibial myxedema do not seem to be related to TSI, and their pathogenesis is not known.

Toxic Nodular Goiter (Secondary Hyperthyroidism). This occurs as a secondary phenomenon in a patient who is already suffering from a goiter from some other cause, such as iodine deficiency. The condition is less severe than Graves' disease, and exophthalmos and other ocular manifestations do not occur. Sometimes a solitary nodule ("toxic adenoma") is present, and the remainder of the gland is suppressed.

Hashimoto's Disease

Like most thyroid disease, this is more common in women than in men. The gland is diffusely enlarged, showing atrophy of its epithelial elements and a massive infiltration by lymphocytes and plasma cells (Fig. 29–10). Clinically, the outstanding feature is the development of a goiter; there may be mild hyperthyroidism in the early stages of the disease, but soon the patient becomes euthyroid; hypothyroidism generally develops in due course.

There are many autoantibodies present in the blood in patients with Hashimoto's disease. They are directed against TSH receptor protein and thyroid antigens, *e.g.*, thyroglobulin, microsomes, and DNA. The disease has features in common with Graves' disease, but the antibodies appear to destroy cells rather than stimulate them. Antibody-dependent cell-mediated cytotoxicity and T-cell destruction have been suggested. The disease is sometimes associated with

other autoimmune disease and is more common in subjects with HLA DR5 and HLA B5.

Subacute Thyroiditis (de Quervain's Thyroiditis)

This is less common than Hashimoto's disease and is suspected of being a viral infection, although a specific agent has yet to be identified. The disease commonly follows 2 to 3 weeks after an upper respiratory infection. The clinical course is that of fever, tender enlargement of the thyroid gland, and spontaneous resolution within a few weeks. On microscopic examination, the gland shows nonspecific inflammatory changes that later develop a granulomatous component with the presence of many giant cells. For this reason, the disease is also sometimes called giant-cell thyroiditis.

Neoplasms

Benign encapsulated nodules in the thyroid gland are common, but the majority are probably focal areas of hyperplasia. These are usually multiple (nodular colloid goiter).

Carcinoma was apparently not uncommon in goitrous districts, but today it is distinctly rare. Carcinoma does not usually take up radioactive iodine and appears as a "cold" nodule on a thyroid scan. The most common type of carcinoma of the thyroid gland is papillary adenocarcinoma, which has a good prognosis (Fig. 29–11). Other well-differentiated tumors more closely resemble normal thyroid tissue. Anaplastic tumors are uncommon but have a poor prognosis. Hence, with carcinoma of the thyroid, the histologic features are important when the outlook for the patient is assessed. As noted previously, the uncommon *medullary carcinoma* has several features that set it apart from other neoplasms of the thyroid. Its cell of origin is the C cell, its stroma frequently contains an abundance of amyloid, and the tumor can secrete a variety of hormones (calcitonin and ACTH) as well as histamine and prostaglandins.

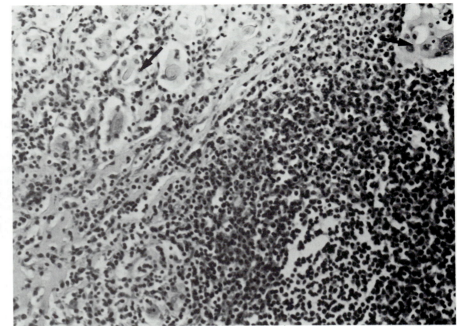

Figure 29–10 Hashimoto's disease. Much of the thyroid parenchyma has been replaced by lymphocytes; remnants of thyroid follicles can still be seen (arrows). In the early stages of Hashimoto's disease, the patient may be hyperthyroid, but by the time the gland shows the degree of destruction depicted in this illustration, the patient is hypothyroid (×250).

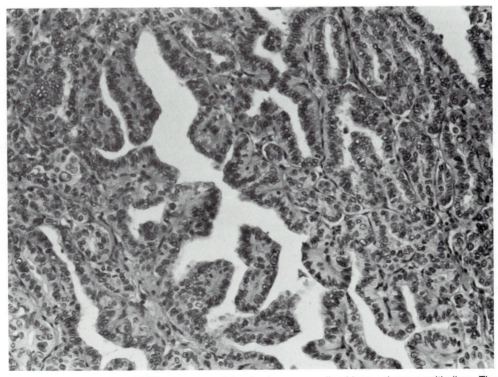

Figure 29–11 Carcinoma of the thyroid. The tumor consists of acinar spaces lined by a columnar epithelium. The spaces vary greatly in size and do not contain colloid. Papillary projections fill the larger acini, and the overall pattern differs markedly from that of the hyperplastic gland (compare with Figure 29–8). The cells of the tumor are uniform in appearance, and mitoses are not in evidence. On the basis of histologic findings, it is tempting to label this tumor a papillary adenoma. However, careful search will generally reveal invasion of its capsule; the tumor also regularly metastasizes to lymph nodes. Hence, it should be called a *papillary adenocarcinoma* (×250).

THE DIFFUSE ENDOCRINE SYSTEM

The concept of a widely dispersed system of cells derived from the neural crest has been proposed, and the term *APUD cells* has been applied to them. The term is derived from the initial letters of their properties, namely, the high content of amines, the capacity for *amine precursor uptake*, and the presence of amino acid *decarboxylase*. The original concept that all members of this group of cells are derived from the neural crest had not been generally recognized, but the term *apudoma* is still sometimes applied to tumors derived from them. Nevertheless, the concept of a diffuse system of endocrine secreting cells is valid. They are characterized by possessing characteristic dark cytoplasmic granules seen on electron microscopy and secreting either amines or polypeptides. At present, the following cells are included in the group: the chromaffin cells (*e.g.*, the pheochromocytes of the adrenal medulla), nonchromaffin paraganglia cells (*e.g.*, of the carotid body), the pancreatic islet cells, the C cells of the thyroid gland, some cells of the adenohypophysis, and a group of cells in the gastrointestinal tract, liver, lung, and elsewhere. Some of the cells (particularly in the intestine) in this last group stain by a silver impregnation (argentaffin) method and have been termed *argentaffin cells*.

Tumors of the diffuse endocrine cells have been given a variety of names. If the site of origin was obvious, they have been called adenomas or carcinomas, for instance, adenoma or carcinoma of the anterior lobe of the pituitary or islets of Langerhans. In the intestine, they have been called *argentaffinomas*; more commonly, the term *carcinoid tumor* is applied. Such tumors tend to invade locally but have a limited capacity to metastasize. Now that specific immunoperoxidase stains are available, the tumors are categorized according to their secretion (*e.g.*, gastrinoma) and their behavior.

Tumors of the diffuse endocrine system may secrete the same hormone as does the parent cell of origin. A good example is a tumor of the B cells of the islets of Langerhans that secretes insulin and causes attacks of hypoglycemia. Sometimes the tumor secretes a different hormone, as when an islet cell tumor secretes an ACTH-like hormone with Cushing's syndrome. This syndrome may occur in association with a diffuse endocrine tumor of the lung (oat-cell carcinoma) or thyroid (medullary carcinoma) or a carcinoid tumor of the lung.

Summary

- The specific action of hormones is due to their action on specific hormone receptors on target cells.
- The hypothalamus controls many body functions such as sleep, body temperature, and the autonomic nervous system. It also forms oxytocin and vasopressin and a group of releasing and inhibiting hormones that act on other endocrine glands.
- The pituitary gland has two parts: the neurohypophysis, which releases oxytocin and vasopressin; and the adenohypophysis, which has five cell types and secretes five groups of hormone.
- Diabetes insipidus is the most important disease of the neurohypophysis.
- Hyperprolactinemia, gigantism, and acromegaly are important examples of hyperpituitarism.
- Sheehan's syndrome and Simmonds' disease are examples of hypopituitarism.
- Pheochromocytoma and neuroblastoma are important tumors of the adrenal medulla.
- The adrenal cortex secretes three groups of hormone: glucocorticoids, mineralocorticoids, and sex hormones. Hypersecretion leads to Cushing's syndrome, Conn's syndrome, or the adrenogenital syndrome. Hyposecretion leads to Addison's disease.
- Glucocorticoid therapy has many severe complications.
- Diseases of the thyroid gland often produce goiter, hypothyroidism, or hyperthyroidism.
- Hypothyroidism causes cretinism or myxedema. Hyperthyroidism occurs in Graves' disease and nodular toxic goiter.
- Hashimoto's disease has an autoimmune basis. Subacute thyroiditis (de Quervain's thyroiditis) is suspected of being a viral infection.
- Tumors of the thyroid, like most thyroid disease, are more common in women. One type, the medullary carcinoma, is derived from calcitonin-secreting C cells.
- The diffuse endocrine system is a widely distributed system of cells that give rise to important tumors, *e.g.*, carcinoid tumors, small cell carcinoma of the lung, and tumors of the islets of Langerhans.

Selected Readings

Bloodworth, J. M. B. (ed.): Endocrine Pathology: General and Surgical. 2nd ed. Baltimore, Williams and Wilkins, 1982.

De Lellis, R. A., et al.: Carcinoid tumors: Changing concepts and new perspectives. Am. J. Surg. Pathol. *8*:295, 1984.

Kovacs, K., and Asa, S. L.: Functional Endocrine Pathology. Boston, Blackwell, 1990.

Kovacs, K., and Howath, E.: The Pituitary Gland: Atlas of Tumor Pathology, Fascicle 21, Series 2. Washington, D. C., Armed Forces Institute of Pathology, 1986.

Leading article: Thyroid autoimmune disease: A broad spectrum. Lancet *1*:874, 1981.

Lefkowitz, R. J., Wessels, M. R., and Stadel, J. M.: Hormones, receptors, and cyclic AMP: Their role in target cell reactiveness. Curr. Top. Cell. Regul. *17*:205, 1980.

Lewin, K. J., et al.: The endocrine cells of the gastrointestinal tract. I: The normal endocrine cells and their hyperplasias. II: Tumors. Pathol. Annu. *21*:1 and 181, 1986.

Melmed, S.: Acromegaly. N. Engl. J. Med. *322*:966, 1990.

Moore-Ede, M. C., Czeisler, C. A., and Richardson, G. S.: Circadian timekeeping in health and disease. N Engl. J. Med. *309*:469, 1983.

Werner, S. C., and Ingbar, S. H. (eds.): The Thyroid: A Fundamental and Clinical Text. 5th ed. Philadelphia, J. B. Lippincott, 1986.

Wilkin, T. J.: Receptor autoimmunity in endocrine disorders. N. Engl. J. Med. *323*:1318, 1990.

30

Musculoskeletal System

**After studying this chapter, the student
should be able to:**

- Describe the formation of bone in the human
embryo and distinguish between membrane bone
and that formed by endochondral ossification.
- Distinguish woven bone from lamellar bone.

- Give an account of the forms in which calcium
occurs in the plasma; describe the actions of
parathyroid hormone and calcitonin.
- Give an account of the various forms of vitamin D,
their metabolism, and their actions in relation to
calcium metabolism and bone formation.
- Describe the pathogenesis of acute staphylococcal
osteomyelitis and chronic osteomyelitis.
- Outline the features of tuberculous infection of the
spine.
- Describe the causes of localized osteoporosis.
- Classify the causes of fracture.
- Describe the stages in fracture healing, and list the
causes of fibrous union, nonunion, and delayed
union.
- Lists the causes of ischemic necrosis of bone.
- Give a brief account of each of the following
conditions:
(a) osteogenesis imperfecta;
(b) achondroplasia;
(c) osteopetrosis;
(d) fibrous dysplasia.
- Classify the causes of hyperparthyroidism and
indicate the main bony and renal lesions that ensue.
- Compare rickets with osteomalacia.
- Classify the causes of generalized osteoporosis.
- Describe the main features of Paget's disease.
- Describe the main features of hypertrophic
osteoarthropathy and list the common causes of this
condition.
- Give an account of the common tumors of bone.
- Describe multiple myelomatosis.
- Describe Ewing's tumor.
- Describe the structure of a synovial joint.
- Differentiate between a sprain, a subluxation, and a
dislocation.
- List three organisms that commonly cause an acute
suppurative arthritis and indicate the end result.

- Contrast rheumatoid arthritis with osteoarthritis.
- Describe how ankylosing spondylitis differs from the classic form of rheumatoid arthritis.
- List the causes of muscle atrophy.
- Give a brief account of
  (a) muscular dystrophy;
  (b) myasthenia gravis;
  (c) malignant tumors of muscle.

During normal embryonic development, condensations of primitive *mesenchyme* are laid down at the sites of future bone, and by the end of the second month, ossification commences. In the development of some bones, notably the vault of the skull, there is a direct conversion of the membranous sheet of mesenchyme to bone. Mesenchymal cells differentiate into osteoblasts, and the bones formed in this way are therefore called *membrane bones*. The long bones develop in a different way: in these, the mesenchyme first differentiates into cartilage, which is subsequently *replaced* by bone. The cartilage cells swell up and die, and the intervening cartilaginous matrix calcifies. This acellular calcified cartilage is eroded by multinucleate osteoclasts, and at the same time osteoblasts lay down lamellar bone (see later). The osteoblasts, once they are embedded in the bone, become *osteocytes*. This process, which is called *endochondral ossification*, continues at the epiphyseal ends of the long bones until adult stature is achieved. Proliferation of cartilage at the epiphyses and its subsequent ossification is therefore the way in which the long bones grow in length.

STRUCTURE OF BONE

Bone is composed of calcified osteoid tissue, which consists of type I collagen fibers embedded in a specialized ground substance. Although the precise composition of bone salts is not known, they are generally considered to be composed of hydroxyapatite, a complex molecule of calcium phosphate and calcium hydroxide. Bone also contains small quantities of magnesium, sodium, and potassium as well as carbonate and citrate ions.

Depending on the arrangement of the collagen fibers, two histologic types of bone may be recognized.

Woven Bone. This type shows an irregular arrangement of collagen bundles and is the type of bone that is formed under the following three circumstances: during the initial stages of the formation of membrane bones; when bone forms in the midst of differentiating granulation tissue, as in fracture healing; and in certain bone disorders and tumors.

Lamellar or Mature Bone. In this type of bone, the collagen bundles are arranged either in parellel sheets or in concentric laminae around a central vessel, thereby forming haversian systems (Fig. 30–1).

In the outer dense cortex of the long bones, haversian systems predominate, whereas flat plates are seen under the periosteum and endosteum. This type of bone is called *compact bone*.

The central portion of the long bones is hollowed out to form the medullary cavity, which contains marrow. Thin struts of bone remain, which are constructed of flat bundles of collagen with few haversian systems. The central trabeculated part of the bone is called *cancellous*; like compact bone, it is composed of lamellar bone.

Lamellar bone is formed when bone is laid down on a previous scaffolding. This may consist of the following: calcified cartilage, as in normal endochondral ossification; woven bone, as in growing membrane bones; and lamellar bone itself, as in the circumferential growth of all long bones.

In the normal adult, the entire skeleton is composed of lamellar bone. Although bone appears rigid and inert, it is as susceptible as are the soft tissues to adverse circumstances. Indeed, the effects on bone are often more severe and permanent.

The osteocytes play an important role in bone homeostasis. If they die (as in ischemic necrosis), the bone crumbles and is removed. Osteocytes are able to demineralize the bone adjacent to them and also remove its osteoid matrix. This process is called *osteolysis* and is probably of great importance in the hour-to-hour regulation of the plasma calcium level (see later). There is a continuous process of remodeling of bone throughout life, with bone resorption not only by osteolysis but also by the action of *osteoclasts*, which

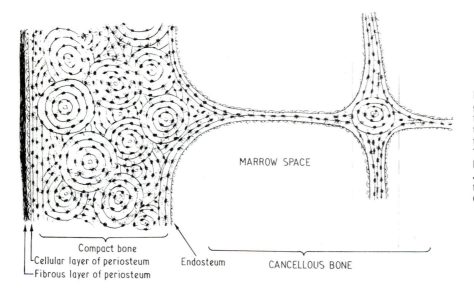

MARROW SPACE

Compact bone
Cellular layer of periosteum
Fibrous layer of periosteum
Endosteum
CANCELLOUS BONE

Figure 30–1 Lamellar bone. Diagrammatic representation of a transverse section through part of the shaft of a long bone to show the arrangement of lamellar bone. The cortex is composed mainly of haversian systems. (From Walter, J.B., and Israel, M.S.: General Pathology. 6th ed. Edinburgh, Churchill Livingstone, 1987.)

are large multinucleate cells that remove both the bone salts and the protein matrix of bone. This destructive osteoclastic activity is probably of great importance in the general remodeling of bone that is continually taking place. After the removal of bone, osteocytes differentiate into osteoblasts and lay down more osteoid, which subsequently calcifies to form bone. It is evident that the integrity of bone is maintained by the delicate balance between bone destruction and bone formation. If either predominates, osteoporosis or osteosclerosis results. *Osteoporosis*, also called *osteopenia*, is a condition in which the organic matrix (*osteoid*), although reduced in amount, is normally mineralized. Osteoporosis is therefore defined as a condition in which there is a decrease to below normal in the amount of bone tissue per unit volume of anatomic bone. On microscopic examination, osteoporotic bone shows normal structure and calcification, but there is too little of it; the cortex of an osteoporotic bone is thin, and the trabeculae in the cancellous portion are attenuated. Hence, as a whole, the bone is fragile and liable to fracture or, in the case of a vertebra, crushing. The radiographic appearance of osteoporotic bone is one of rarefaction. The condition may be brought about either by excessive destruction of bone or by defective formation.

In *osteosclerosis* there is excessive formation of osteoid, which being calcified, makes the bone appear dense on a radiograph. In spite of its density, osteoporotic bone is brittle and also liable to pathologic fracture (described later).

Osteoblasts manufacture the enzyme *alkaline phosphatase*, but the precise role of this in bone formation is not understood. Some of the enzyme escapes into the blood, and the serum level is a good index of the overall osteoblastic activity within the body. For example, in Paget's disease it is high. The enzyme produced by bone differs from that formed in the liver. The two isoenzymes can be separated and identified. Hence, the high alkaline phosphatase level of obstructive jaundice can be differentiated from that due to excessive osteoblastic activity.

METABOLIC FUNCTIONS OF BONE: CALCIUM METABOLISM

Bone serves as a reserve of both calcium and phosphate, containing 99 per cent of the total body calcium and 90 per cent of the total body phosphorus. Nevertheless, the remaining 1 per cent of calcium is a vital fraction because it is available to the soft tissues and it is necessary for proper neuromuscular activity, cardiac rhythm, and enzyme activities, such as in blood coagulation.

Calcium in the blood exists in three forms: (1) *ionized calcium*, which is diffusible and constitutes 65 per cent of the total plasma calcium; the normal level is about 1.2 mmol/L (4.8 mg/dl); (2) *protein-bound calcium*, which is nondiffusible, since it is attached to albumin; (3) *nonionized diffusible calcium*, which is the smallest fraction and exists as citrate. The ionized calcium is the most important fraction and is in equilibrium with the calcium salts in bone.

In spite of a varying diet, the amount of calcium absorbed from the intestine, the amount excreted in the urine, and the amount deposited or withdrawn from bone are so regulated that *the level of plasma ionized calcium remains constant*. The actions of parathyroid hormone, vitamin D, and calcitonin are vitally concerned in this homeostatic mechanism.

Parathroid Hormone. There is a continuous secretion of hormone from the parathyroid glands; the rate of secretion is influenced by the plasma ionized calcium level. A fall in calcium level stimulates parathyroid secretion, whereas a rise in calcium level inhibits it. The major effect of parathyroid hormone is on bone. It promotes osteolysis by osteocytes and stimulates osteoclasts, which proliferate and cause bone destruction with both removal of osteoid and release of its contained minerals. The net effect is release of calcium salts from bone, so that the plasma calcium level rises. Parathyroid hormone appears to be the major factor in regulating the level of plasma ionized calcium.

Vitamin D. Various forms of vitamin D exist. The first apparently pure compound was called D_1 but was in fact a mixture. The radiation of ergosterol produces an active substance called D_2, and this is present in the diet containing artificially fortified foods. Natural vitamin D is produced in the skin by the ultraviolet radiation of 7-dehydrocholesterol and is called D_3 or cholecalciferol. Both vitamins D_2 and D_3 are hydroxylated in the liver to 25-hydroxy compounds ($25[OH]D_2$ and $25[OH]D_3$). These compounds are subsequently further hydroxylated in the kidney to form the final active metabolites ($1,25[OH]_2D_2$ and $1,25[OH]_2D_3$). This final hydroxylation is promoted by a number of factors, including a low blood calcium level and parathyroid hormone.

The main action of vitamin D is to aid the absorption of calcium from the gut. The vitamin also has a mild parathyroid hormone–like action on bone, but this is probably unimportant. Very large doses of the vitamin given therapeutically can, however, lead to hypercalcemia and hypercalciuria. A deficiency of vitamin D results in imparied absorption of calcium from the intestine and subsequent hypocalcemia. There is a *diminution, or even complete cessation, of calcification in cartilage and osteoid*. In the growing child, this results in *rickets*, whereas in the adult there is *osteomalacia*. Both of these conditions are described later in this chapter.

Although parathyroid hormone and vitamin D both play important roles in maintaining calcium homeostasis, the action of vitamin D is the more vital. Patients with hypoparathyroidism can be maintained on vitamin D therapy and additional calcium. On the other hand, the absence of vitamin D leads to severe skeletal disease, and no substitute for the vitamin will prevent it.

Calcitonin. This hormone is secreted by the C cells of the thyroid and has the action on bone of reducing bone resorption by inhibiting osteoclastic activity. The precise role of this hormone in calcium homeostasis has yet to be determined, but it could clearly complement parathyroid hormone, since the stimulus for its secretion is hypercalcemia.

The normal plasma calcium level is 2.2 to 2.6 mmol/L (8.8 to 10.4 mg/dl) and in healthy persons is remarkably constant because of the efficiency of the regulating mechanisms. The serum calcium and phosphate together tend to maintain a reciprocal relationship. Thus, if there is a rise in the serum level of either calcium or phosphate, there is a corresponding fall in that of the other. However, if the level of one substance is low, the other does not necessarily rise.

INFECTIONS OF BONE

Pyogenic Infections

The term "osteomyelitis" is applied to pyogenic infections because both bone marrow cavity and the bone itself are involved. The infection may be blood-borne or result from direct extension either from a nearby focus (*e.g.*, an ulcer of the foot in a diabetic subject) or by contamination of a compound fracture.

Acute Suppurative Osteomyelitis

This infection occurs most often in childhood; generally it develops at the end of one of the long bones of the lower limbs. The explanation for this localization is that this is an area commonly traumatized; furthermore, if an injury occurs during the course of a bacteremia associated with a skin infection, the organisms, commonly *Staphylococcus aureus*, become localized and set up a metastatic lesion. An acute inflammatory reaction ensues, and this is accompanied by rigors, fever, and acute tenderness of the region. Owing to the rigidity of the bone, the increased tension produced by the exudation leads to compression of blood vessels and ischemia. Necrosis of marrow and bone consequently follows; pus is formed, and it tracks under the periosteum, thereby further imperiling the blood supply to the cortex. In this way, quite extensive necrosis of bone can occur; indeed, the whole shaft can eventually become involved. During the early stages, however, no necrosis may be evident on radiography, and if a child has an illness suggestive of acute osteomyelitis, treatment is begun before enough time has passed to produce radiographic changes.

With modern therapy, acute osteomyelitis frequently resolves. This was not so in the preantibiotic days. The dead bone, called a *sequestrum*, acts as a foreign body and provides a focus for continued growth of organisms. Together with the trapped collections of pus, the conditions are ideal for the development of chronic inflammation.

Chronic Suppurative Osteomyelitis

Pus ruptures through the periosteum into the muscular and subcutaneous tissues and ultimately escapes to the skin surface through one or more sinuses. The vascular periosteum attempts to re-form the shaft of bone by producing new bone that encases the sequestrated shaft

and is called an *involucrum* (Fig. 30–2). Osteoclasts slowly erode the sequestrum and detach it at each end, but this process may take many months or years to accomplish; in practice, spontaneous healing does not occur. If the condition is not treated, it may lead to death as a result of pyemia, toxemia, or amyloid disease.

Chronic suppurative osteomyelitis is fortu-

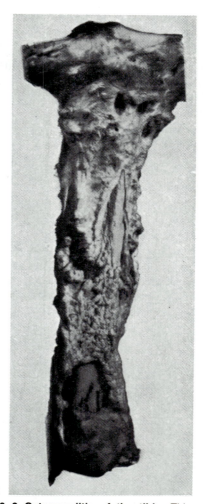

Figure 30–2 Osteomyelitis of the tibia. This amputation specimen shows the typical appearance of extensive chronic osteomyelitis. The dead shaft of the bone forms a sequestrum and is surrounded by thick, irregularly shaped new bone that constitutes the encasing involucrum. The sequestrum can be seen through a hole in the involucrum at the lower end of the specimen. (Reproduced by kind permission of the President and Council of the Royal College of Surgeons of England. Hunterian Museum specimen HS44.1. From Walter, J.B., and Israel, M.S.: General Pathology. 4th ed. Edinburgh, Churchill Livingstone, 1974.)

nately very rare these days. However, a description of it is useful because it illustrates the typical features of a chronic suppurative inflammation. It demonstrates the combination of the following factors: (1) *acute inflammation* with fluid exudation and pus formation; (2) *demolition* by macrophages and osteoclasts; (3) *regeneration* of bone by osteoblasts; and (4) *repair* with granulation tissue and extensive scar tissue formation.

Other types of chronic osteomyelitis are known but are uncommon. *Brode's abscess* is a localized chronic suppurative lesion that causes pain and may simulate a bone tumor. *Salmonella osteomyelitis* can affect several bones simultaneously. It is most common in children, particularly those with sickle cell disease.

Nonsuppurative Infections

Tuberculosis

Unlike pyogenic osteomyelitis, tuberculosis of bone is generally insidious in its onset and is characterized by bone destruction with very little reactive new bone formation. One of the common sites of infection is the vertebral column (*Pott's disease*). The affected vertebrae frequently collapse and produce an angulation of the spinal column; forward deviation is called a *kyphosis* and lateral deviation is called a *scoliosis*. The combination is called *kyphoscoliosis*; if severe, this can interfere with the act of breathing to the extent of causing respiratory acidosis, pulmonary hypertension, and eventually right-sided heart failure (Chapter 20). As with tuberculosis elsewhere, caseous tissue is formed. When this softens, it becomes a "cold abscess" that tracks along the line of least resistance and is ultimately discharged to the exterior. In tuberculosis of the spine, the pus tends to enter the psoas sheath, track down in it beneath the inguinal ligament, and present as a fluctuating mass that subsequently discharges to the surface. Fortunately, tuberculosis of bone is now a rarity.

Syphilis

Syphilis of bone is now extremely uncommon. It is generally seen in the later stages of the disease, with periostitis predominating. The bone tends to become osteosclerotic, in contrast to becoming osteoporotic in tuberculosis.

ISCHEMIC BONE DISEASE

The blood supply to certain bones is precarious and can easily be interrupted by traumatic damage, such as that caused by an adjacent fracture. Well-recognized sites are the head of the femur and the carpal scaphoid bone. *Ischemic necrosis (infarction)* is also called *avascular necrosis* and can occur under other circumstances:

1. *Thromboembolism*, from the heart or elsewhere.
2. *The decompression syndrome*, when nitrogen bubbles block small vessels.
3. *Sickle cell anemia*, when packed abnormal red blood cells occlude small vessels. The necrosis may predispose to *Salmonella* infection, as noted earlier in this chapter.
4. *Fat embolism*. Fat emboli from a fatty liver are the suggested cause of the ischemic necrosis observed in *alcoholism* and as a complication of *glucocorticoid therapy*.
5. *Idiopathic condition*. There are a number of conditions affecting growing children in which an epiphysis undergoes ischemic necrosis without apparent cause. The best known example is *Legg-Perthes disease*, which affects the head of the femur.

Infarction of bone causes no immediate problem to the patient, and healing occurs slowly by the process of *creeping substitution* (Chapter 6). However, if the bone is subjected to pressure, it may crumble; this is particularly important in weight-bearing areas. Thus, with ischemic necrosis of the head of the femur (after fracture of the neck of the femur or in Legg-Perthes disease), the bone collapses, the head becomes flattened, the joint is distorted, and osteoarthritis later develops.

BONE DISORDERS CAUSED BY PHYSICAL DISTURBANCES

Localized Osteoporosis

Whenever a joint is immobilized, either by a cast or by disease, the neighboring bones develop osteoporosis. This effect is a form of disuse atrophy—the greater the degree of immobility, the more marked the osteoporosis. Thus, if there is paralysis of a whole limb (*e.g.*, in poliomyelitis), osteoporosis affects all the bones of that limb.

Pressure Atrophy

Any expanding lesion that exerts pressure on bone causes local ischemia and pressure atrophy. Recall that cartilage, being avascular, does not show this pressure atrophy. Thus, an aneurysm of the aorta that presses on the vertebral column causes pressure atrophy of the vertebrae, but the intervening disks remain unaffected.

Benign tumors arising in bone cause pressure atrophy; the adjacent periosteum responds by producing new bone around the lesion. Thus, a benign tumor gives the appearance of expanding the bone.

Fractures

Causes
Excessive Mechanical Force
Direct Violence. A good example is a blow that causes a depressed fracture of the skull or a broken scapula.

Indirect Violence. A fracture of the clavicle caused by falling on an outstretched arm is an example.

Muscular Action. Sudden, unexpected strains during violent exercise can cause fractures in normal bones (*spontaneous fractures*).

Fractures of Abnormal Bone. A fracture in a diseased, weakened bone that has been subjected to a normal strain is called a *pathologic fracture*. Secondary carcinoma must always be borne in mind as a cause of this. Indeed, a pathologic fracture may be the first indication of malignancy, *e.g.*, carcinoma of the lung.

Stages in Fracture Healing. The stages in fracture healing are illustrated in Figure 30–3. Notice that the hematoma between the bone ends is organized and that the granulation tissue so formed matures to either woven bone or cartilage. This hard material, which initially unites the bone ends, is called *callus*. The woven bone or cartilage of which it is composed is gradually replaced by mature lamellar bone. Thus, during regeneration of bone, the two embryologic methods of bone formation—endochondral and intramembranous—are faithfully repeated in later life.

Abnormalities of Fracture Healing
Repair or Fibrous Union. Although the cells of the granulation tissue of a healing fracture are called osteoblasts, they are capable of differentiation along several lines. If immobilization is not satisfactory, the cells behave like fibroblasts, and the bone ends become united by ordinary fibrous scar tissue that cannot be converted into bone.

Fibrous union is particularly common in situations in which the blood supply is impaired or immobilization is difficult. Thus, it occurs in fractures of the carpal scaphoid bone; when fibrous union has occurred, surgical intervention is necessary to remove the fibrous tissue and to create thereby a new fracture in which bone formation can occur.

Nonunion. Complete lack of union between the fracture ends results from the interposition of soft parts. Muscle or fascia can separate the two bone ends, and because there is no continuous hematoma between them, union of any sort is impossible. This phenomenon is sometimes utilized deliberately in order to form a new false joint.

Delayed Union. In the presence of a continuous hematoma, any cause of delayed healing retards bone regeneration. In practice, the following causes are most important.

Movement. Movement of any sort is harmful to the healing process because it excites an inflammatory reaction, damages the delicate granulation tissue, and inhibits the formation of bone. In surgical practice, every effort is made to reduce movement to a minimum. If the bone ends are impacted, union is usually rapid; indeed, one method of treating a fracture is to bring the ends of the broken bone together under high compression. This provides rigid immobilization and speeds healing. If the bone ends are not impacted, the fracture is stabilized either by external splints or by casts. Alternatively, an operation is performed, and then screws, nails, or plates are inserted to minimize movement between the ends of the broken bone.

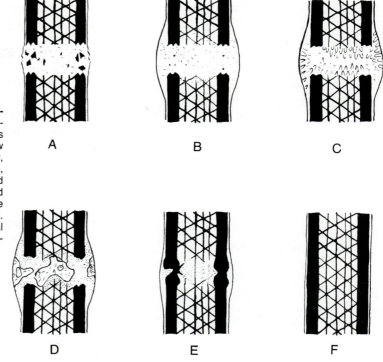

Figure 30–3 Stages in the healing of a fracture. *A,* Hematoma formation. *B,* Acute inflammation followed by demolition. Loose fragments of bone are removed, and the bone ends show osteoporosis. *C,* Granulation tissue formation. *D,* The bone ends are now united by woven bone, cartilage, or a mixture of the two. This hard material is called *callus. E,* Lamellar bone is laid down; calcified cartilage and woven bone are progressively removed. *F,* Final remodeling. (From Walter, J.B., and Israel, M.S.: General Pathology. 6th ed. Edinburgh, Churchill Livingstone, 1987.)

Infection. Infection produces osteomyelitis and can lead to extensive ischemic necrosis with sequestrum formation. Infection is particularly liable to occur if the failure is *compound, i.e.,* if one of the bone ends has penetrated the skin and is exposed to the exterior.

Poor Blood Supply. Whereas complete loss of blood supply results in necrosis of bone, poor blood supply leads to slow granulation tissue formation and to slow healing. Certain sites (*e.g.,* fractures of the neck of the femur, the shaft of tibia, and the carpal scaphoid bone) are notorious for this complication. In these situations, it is particularly important to avoid other possible causes of delayed healing, such as movement. For example, a pin is passed into the head of the femur so that rigid immobilization is immediately obtained. This technique is particularly useful in old people. If an elderly person falls and fractures the neck of the femur, the injury can be treated by external immobilization in a plaster cast. Unfortunately, the patient is confined to bed for many weeks and is liable to develop many complications: venous thrombosis, pulmonary embolism, bronchopneumonia, and urinary tract infection. Pinning the head, on the other hand, can allow the person to get up immediately and to escape these hazards of recumbency.

Myositis Ossificans. If there is an extravasation of fracture hematoma into surrounding muscles, its subsequent organization and ossification results in the condition called *traumatic myositis ossificans.* Sometimes the large masses of bone formed around a joint can seriously interfere with movement.

GENERALIZED BONE DISORDERS

There is no satisfactory classification of generalized bone disorders, but in practice they can be considered under three headings: (1) *developmental anomalies;* (2) *abnormalities due to metabolic disorders;* and (3) *abnormalities occurring in the adult;* these are generally of unknown cause.

Developmental Abnormalities

Many developmental abnormalities of bones are known, but these are rare, for the most part. Four examples are considered.

Osteogenesis Imperfecta

In this condition, the bones are thin and brittle. The cortex is thin, and there is a decrease in the amount of cancellous bone. The fragility results in frequent fractures that occur either spontaneously or as a result of trival injuries. The fractures heal well, but their multiplicity generally leads to severe deformities.

Six types of osteogenesis imperfecta are recognized, but they tend to fall into one of two groups. In the congenital type, which is usually inherited as an autosomal recessive trait, multiple fractures occur *in utero* or during birth, and the prognosis is poor. In the *tarda form*, the disease is less severe; if the child survives, the tendency to sustain fractures decreases after puberty. This form is generally inherited as an autosomal dominant trait and is an illustration of the dictum that dominant traits tend to be less severe than recessive ones (Chapter 3).

Osteogenesis imperfecta appears to be a condition with widespread hypoplasia of the mesenchyme. Affected subjects are of short stature; have lax ligaments, leading to hypermobility of the joints; and have thin sclerae of the eyes, allowing the pigment of the choroid to give them a blue color.

Achondroplasia

This disease is transmitted as an autosomal dominant trait. The essential feature appears to be defective endochondral bone formation, and the long bones of the limbs are therefore short. A person with this condition is called an *achondroplastic dwarf*. The trunk and head are of normal size, although the middle of the face tends to be depressed because the base of the skull is formed of cartilage and is therefore affected. The person with this condition has normal intelligence, is very muscular and agile, and is frequently seen in the circus ring.

Osteopetrosis (Albers-Schönberg Disease)

In this condition, bone formation exceeds bone removal so that the skeleton is hard and inelastic. In some forms of the disease, the defect appears to lie with bone marrow–derived macrophages and osteoclasts. As with osteogenesis imperfecta, there is a severe infantile form of the disease inherited as a recessive trait, and a benign form with dominant inheritance. In the severe form, bones are liable to fracture because of their inelasticity. Bone encroaching on the marrow cavity can result in leukoerythroblastic anemia. The benign form is usually asymptomatic and found by chance in adult life.

Fibrous Dysplasia

Fibrous dysplasia of bone is characterized by the appearance of areas of bone resorption and their replacement by fibrous tissue in which there are thin trabeculae of woven bone. The marrow space is obliterated in the area affected. Any bone may be affected, and the etiology is unknown. In the common type of the disease, young people (median age 14 years) are affected and only one bone is involved (*monostotic fibrous dysplasia*). Polyostotic fibrous dysplasia usually manifests itself in early life, is of insidious onset, and affects many bones. Sometimes only one limb or one side of the body is affected. If the skull and facial bones are involved, there is much disfigurement.

Abnormalities of Bone due to Metabolic Disorders

Endocrine Disturbances. Skeletal changes associated with pituitary and thyroid disease are considered elsewhere. By far, the most important hormone in relation to bone metabolism is parathyroid hormone, which is derived from the four parathyroid glands.

Hyperparathyroidism

Hyperparathyroidism can be divided into two groups.

Primary Hyperparathyroidism. This condition is due to the excessive production of parathyroid hormone, usually by a parathyroid *adenoma*, occasionally by *idiopathic hyperplasia*, and rarely by a *carcinoma* of a parathyroid. The effects of hyperparathyroidism are to increase bone resorption by osteolysis and to promote osteoclastic proliferation and activity. The blood calcium level is raised, and there is increased urine loss of calcium (hypercalciuria). As bone is destroyed, it is replaced by fibrous tissue; the end result is osteitis fibrosa cystica (see later).

Secondary Hyperparathyroidism. Hyperplasia and hypersecretion of the glands can be induced by a persistently *low level of serum ionized calcium.* This is seen most frequently in two groups of conditions: (1) *rickets and osteomalacia*, which are described later in this chapter; and (2) *chronic renal disease.*

The relationship between chronic renal disease and parathyroid function is complicated. In chronic renal disease, there is retention of phosphate and a raised serum level (hyperphosphatemia). There is also a depression in the level of serum calcium, which in its turn acts as a stimulus to the parathyroids, leading to their hyperplasia and hypersecretion. Calcium is mobilized from the bones, which become progressively demineralized. The calcium is excreted by the kidney, but this excretion can lead to further renal damage by metastatic calcification and stone formation. Furthermore, in chronic renal disease, there is impaired hydroxylation of vitamin D to yield the active dihydroxy compound. Hence, there is in effect vitamin D deficiency and defective calcium absorption from the intestine. Chronic renal disease produces its most severe effects on the growing skeleton of children. Growth is stunted (causing renal dwarfism), and the bones show the combined changes of rickets and osteitis fibrosa cystica (*renal osteodystrophy*).

Osteitis Fibrosa Cystica* (von Recklinghausen's Disease of Bone). In the early stages of

*The term is a poor one, because the disease is not inflammatory, and the cysts are not always present.

this disease, there is generalized bone involvement. The outstanding features are pains in the bones and weakening of the bones that can result in bending, deformity, and spontaneous fracture. Because there is an increased excretion of calcium via the kidneys, renal stones are common and can be responsible for the initial symptoms — hematuria, pain, and urinary infection. Metastatic calcification is common (see following). In the late stages of hyperparathyroidism, the bones contain tumorlike masses composed of osteoclasts together with localized blood-filled cysts. These *brown tumors*, as they are called, closely resemble histologically the giant cell tumors of bone but are considered to be merely focal areas of hyperplasia.

Metastatic Calcification

Metastatic calcification is the deposition of calcium salts in normal tissues other than osteoid or teeth; it is due to a derangement of calcium or phosphate metabolism. Often there is hypercalcemia, and hyperparathyroidism is one cause. The most common cause, however, is malignancy. Sometimes there is extensive bone destruction *e.g.*, multiple myelomatosis or widespread metastatic carcinoma, and the hypercalcemia may be related to this. More likely the tumor releases an agent that stimulates osteoclastic activity. Osteoclast-stimulating factors have been demonstrated in some tumors (*e.g.*, lymphoma), whereas others release a prostaglandin or a parathyroid-like hormone. Hyperparathyroidism with metastatic calcification is also a feature of chronic renal disease.

Calcification can occur in many sites, but in the kidney the results are the most serious, because combined with the effects of calculi, progressive renal damage leads to progressive renal failure.

Vitamin D Deficiency: Rickets and Osteomalacia

The metabolism of vitamin D has already been discussed earlier in this chapter. Vitamin D deficiency may be caused by deficient dietary intake, malabsorption, or lack of sunlight. In addition, there are a number of uncommon metabolic disorders of calcium metabolism that may be responsible; for example, in hereditary rickets, there is defective hydroxylation of vitamin D.

The main effects of vitamin D deficiency are impaired absorption of calcium from the gut and defective calcification of cartilage and osteoid. The result is rickets in children or osteomalacia in adults.

Rickets. In rickets, there is a failure of the calcification of cartilage that normally occurs at the growing epiphyses. Cartilage is therefore neither removed nor replaced by osteoid. Continued growth of the cartilage causes a considerable enlargement of the bone ends. Similarly, the costochondral junctions are enlarged, producing the clinical deformity called the "rachitic rosary." Because the overall growth of bone is diminished, the child becomes dwarfed. Even the osteoid that is formed is poorly calcified, and the weakened bones are liable to bend and become deformed. Knock-knees, kyphosis, and other deformities are common.

Osteomalacia. The counterpart of rickets in adults is osteomalacia. It is most common in women, because pregnancy imposes an additional drain on the supplies of calcium and vitamins.

The normal adult bone is continually being remodeled; as bone is removed by osteoclasts, it is replaced by osteoid laid down by osteoblasts. In healthy persons, the osteoid promptly calcifies; but in people with vitamin D deficiency, this calcification fails to occur and the bones ultimately consist largely of osteoid. This is the condition of osteomalacia (softening of the bone): although there is an abundance of osteoid, it is poorly calcified. In osteoporosis, by contrast, the matrix is normally calcified but is reduced in quantity.

All bones are affected in osteomalacia, but it is in the weight-bearing areas that the effects are most severe. Gross pelvic distortion occurs and causes complications in subsequent pregnancies. Collapse of the vertebrae gives rise to pain resulting from compression of the spinal nerves as they leave the intervertebral foramina.

Abnormalities of Bone Occurring in the Adult

Generalized Osteoporosis

Disuse Osteoporosis. Prolonged recumbency leads to increased osteoclastic activity and resorption of bone. There is excessive mobilization of calcium, resulting in hypercalciuria and a tendency for renal stones to form. The blood calcium level remains normal, since the process is gradual.

Idiopathic Osteoporosis. Some degree of bone loss is a normal process of aging and results from a slight imbalance between bone formation and bone destruction. The process is slow and continues over many years so that the blood levels of calcium and alkaline phosphatase are normal. In some patients, the process is more marked and the condition becomes pathologic. This is termed *senile osteoporosis* and affects particularly the pelvis, spine, and ribs. The vertebrae are compressed, and this causes backache, which can be severe (Fig. 30–4). There is also some diminution in height, but since the condition occurs so slowly, the patient rarely notices this. Osteoporosis is particularly common in women past the menopause (*postmenopausal osteoporosis*); this condition has been attributed to lack of estrogens. Treatment with estrogens and additional calcium in the diet has been recommended, but the effects are controversial. Osteoporosis occasionally occurs in a younger age group for no obvious reason.

Other Types of Osteoporosis. Osteoporosis also occurs when collagen formation is impaired, as in (1) scurvy; (2) Cushing's syndrome; this includes prolonged administration of glucocorticoids, such as prednisone; and (3) impaired supply of protein, *e.g.,* in starvation and in the malabsorption syndrome.

Paget's Disease of Bone (Osteitis Deformans)

This disease is not an inflammatory one, although it was so considered by Sir James Paget in the nineteenth century. The cause is not known, and the disease seems to be more com-

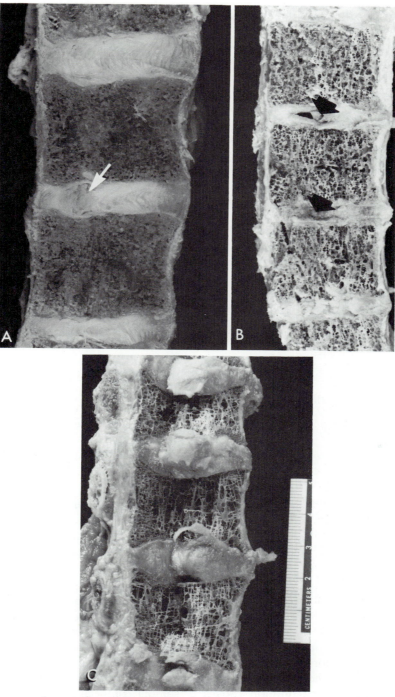

Figure 30–4 Normal versus osteoporotic vertebral bodies. *A*, Normal vertebral bodies. *B*, Moderate osteoporosis. *C*, Severe osteoporosis. The vertebral bodies have been sectioned to show their internal structure. Note the well-formed cancellous bone of the normal vertebral bodies in *A* as well as the structure of the intervertebral disks. One small focus of degeneration can be seen (white arrow). In *B*, the specimen shows well-developed osteoporosis, but the overall shape of the vertebrae is preserved. The disks show severe degenerative changes (black arrows). In *C*, the specimen shows severe osteoporosis. The vertebrae have been compressed by the bulging disks.

mon in males, particularly those over the age of 40 years.

In the early stages of the disease, the bones become softened because of osteoclastic resorption, and the weakened bones tend to bend. Since this is particularly noticeable in the weight-bearing bones, bowing of the femora is characteristic. In the later stages of the disease, irregular subperiosteal bone formation occurs, causing bones to become thicker and hardened. Serum calcium and phosphate levels remain within normal limits, but the serum alkaline phosphatase is greatly raised because of the rapid turnover of bone.

The skull is frequently affected, and as it becomes increasingly thickened, the patient notices a need for an increased hat size. Blindness, deafness, headaches, and facial paralysis are complications that may result from compression of nerves in their bony canals. An occasional complication is the development of osteosarcoma, a tumor that is uncommon in adults except in association with this disease.

Hypertrophic Osteoarthropathy

In its fully developed form, this syndrome has three components:

1. Clubbing of the fingers and toes. The nails of the fingers and toes are curved, and the angle between the nail plate and nail bed is flattened to 180° or more instead of the normal 160°. The nail fold is swollen and spongy.

2. Subperiosteal bone formation (periostitis). This affects the distal ends of the long bones.

3. Swelling and pain of the joints (polyarthritis). This commonly affects the hands and feet and, when acute, can closely mimic early rheumatoid arthritis.

The importance of hypertrophic osteoarthropathy is that it is a complication of a wide variety of underlying diseases. Indeed, it is sometimes the presenting symptom. The common causes are carcinoma of the lung and chronic intrathoracic infection such as lung abscess, bronchiectasis, empyema, and tuberculosis. Clubbing of the nails is the most common manifestation of hypertrophic osteoarthropathy and occurs as a sole finding in cyanotic congenital heart disease, bacterial endocarditis, biliary cirrhosis, ulcerative colitis, Crohn's disease, and a number of other disorders.

The pathogenesis of hypertrophic osteoarthropathy is not understood, but if the underlying disease can be removed or cured (*e.g.*, pneumonectomy in the case of lung cancer), its manifestations abate.

NEOPLASMS

Neoplasms of Bones

The tumors of bone form a complex group in spite of the apparent simplicity of bone structure. Indeed, the histogenesis of some of the tumors is quite obscure. The occurrence of tumors arising from the marrow and the frequency of skeletal metastases add further to the confusion.

It is noteworthy that *pain is often the first symptom of a bone tumor*, and this is due no doubt to the pressure exerted by the dividing abnormal cells on the rigid, unyielding surrounding bone. It will be recalled that in most situations, pain is a late symptom of neoplasia.

Osteoma, chondroma, fibroma, and other tumors all occur but are uncommon.

Giant-Cell Tumor of Bone

This tumor characteristically occurs in the ends of the long bones in young adults. Pain is the predominant symptom, and its onset is followed by swelling. The radiograph generally shows a characteristic appearance; because the tumor destroys areas of bone, these appear as a series of translucent areas that have been likened to a mass of soap bubbles (Fig. 30–5). On microscopic examination, the tumor consists of fusiform cells and abundant multinucleate giant cells that resemble osteoclasts. On this account, the tumor has also been called an *osteoclastoma*, but since the precise nature of the cells is not settled, *giant-cell tumor* is now the current name.

The behavior of giant-cell tumors is generally that of a benign tumor. Nevertheless, local in-

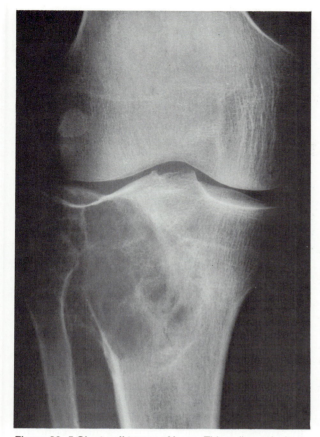

Figure 30–5 Giant-cell tumor of bone. This radiograph shows the "soap bubble" appearance of a tumor that occupies the upper end of the tibia. Note how the joint space is not encroached upon by the growth. Cartilage cannot exhibit pressure atrophy because it is avascular. (Courtesy of Dr. D.E. Sanders, Department of Radiology, Toronto General Division of the Toronto Hospital, Toronto.)

vasion can occur, and between 10 and 15 per cent of the tumors metastasize.

Chondrosarcoma

This tumor is composed of atypical cartilage cells and it is often difficult to distinguish histologically from a benign chondroma. Local invasion and later metastasis to the lungs are the main features.

Osteosarcoma

Osteosarcoma is the most common and most malignant of this rare group of primary bone tumors. It affects males more frequently than females, and it is most commonly seen in persons between the ages of 10 and 25 years. Pain is the usual presenting symptom (Chapter 1, Case History I). In older patients, osteosarcoma may complicate Paget's disease.

The tumor is composed of malignant osteoblasts that exhibit considerable pleomorphism; giant cells are often abundant. In well-differentiated tumors, there is a considerable amount of osteoid produced, which may or may not calcify to form bone. When there is much bone formation, the tumor is described as *osteosclerotic*. Tumor spreads beneath the periosteum, elevates it, and produces a fusiform swelling. Spicules of new bone radiate from the periosteum (Fig. 30–6). On radiography, this gives a characteristic "sun ray" appearance. In tumors producing little calcified material, the lesion is described as *osteolytic*; the radiograph shows an irregular bony defect and a surrounding soft tissue shadow as growth elevates the periosteum and finally penetrates it.

The outlook for a patient with osteosarcoma is extremely poor because pulmonary metastases appear early.

Neoplasms of Bone Marrow

Myeloma

This tumor is derived from cells that show a marked tendency to differentiate into plasma cells. Because the neoplasia is usually multicentric, the condition is known as *multiple myelomatosis*. It occurs predominantly in persons over 40 years of age and produces multiple osteolytic, punched-out lesions of bone, particularly in the bones in which red marrow is normally found, *i.e.*, the skull, the vertebrae, and the ribs (Fig. 30–7). This widespread involvement of the skeleton can produce so much demineralization that hypercalcemia, metastatic calcification, and renal failure occur. The bony lesions often produce severe pain; a pathologic fracture is sometimes the first evidence of the disease.

The tumor cells are monoclonal and form large amounts of homogeneous immunoglobulin called myeloma protein. In addition, some tu-

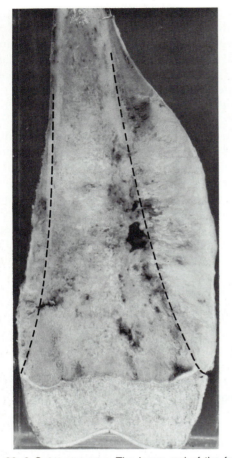

Figure 30–6 Osteosarcoma. The lower end of the femur is greatly expanded by this malignant tumor. The original cortex of the shaft, which can still be discerned, is indicated by the dotted lines. Tumor, in addition to replacing the marrow cavity, has extended beneath the periosteum.

mors produce an excess of light chains, and the peptide produced (Bence Jones protein), having a molecular weight of about 22,000, is excreted by the kidney and can be recognized in the urine. Bence Jones protein may precipitate in the tubules of the kidney, cause obstruction, and lead to renal failure. Metastatic calcification, renal stone formation, and amyloidosis add their quota to kidney damage.

Ewing's Tumor

This uncommon tumor occurs in young children and most often affects the shaft of a long bone. It is composed of small, undifferentiated round cells and is osteolytic. The raised periosteum may produce layers of new bone around the tumor, leading to an onionlike appearance radiologically. The nature of the tumor is obscure. It appears to be a distinct entity, but it can be closely mimicked by metastatic neuroblastoma, a neoplasm that also occurs at the same age. Ewing's tumor is radiosensitive, but the prognosis is poor because it usually metastasizes to other bones and viscera.

Metastatic Tumors

Secondary tumors of bone are much more common than the primary ones. They develop from blood-borne metastases of carcinoma, and the primary site is generally the prostate, breast, bronchus, kidney, stomach, or thyroid (Fig. 30–8). Metastatic tumors are generally multiple and destroy bone locally to produce rarefaction on radiography (*osteolytic secondaries*). Exceptions to this tendency to destroy bone occur with carcinoma of the prostate and occasionally carcinoma of the breast or other site (Fig. 30–8). In these instances, the tumor stimulates new bone formation, and the tumors are hard and radiopaque (*osteosclerotic*). A pathologic fracture or pain is the usual presenting symptom. In addition, if the disease is extensive, a leukoerythroblastic anemia can result.

DISEASES OF JOINTS

A synovial joint consists of two or more opposing *cartilage-covered bone ends* that are united by a sleeve of connective tissue called the *capsule*, the innermost layer of which is modified into a secreting membrane called the *synovium*. The synovium consists of one or more layers of flattened or cubical cells that secrete a clear, pale, viscid fluid (*synovial fluid*) containing mucoprotein. The synovial fluid not only lubricates the joint but is also the main, if not the only, source of nourishment of the hyaline cartilage covering the bone ends.

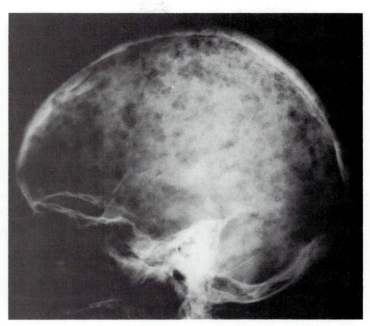

Figure 30–7 Multiple myelomatosis. This radiograph of the skull shows numerous osteolytic tumor deposits that produce a typical moth-eaten appearance resulting from numerous punched-out areas where bone has been destroyed. An appearance similar to this can sometimes be seen in secondary carcinoma. (Courtesy of Dr. D.E. Sanders, Department of Radiology, Toronto General Division of the Toronto Hospital, Toronto.)

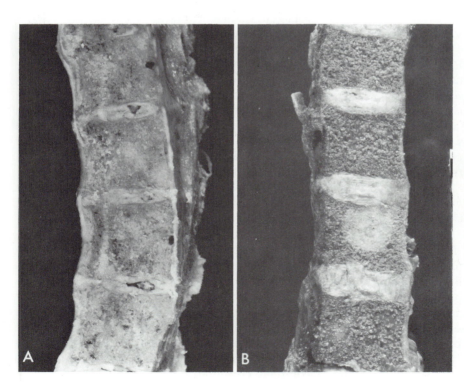

Figure 30–8 Secondary carcinoma in bone. *A,* This section of bone is from a patient who died of carcinoma of the prostate. The cancellous bone in the vertebral bodies shows patchy white tumor deposits that are densely hard because of new bone formation. *B,* Solitary osteolytic metastasis from a carcinoma of the kidney.

Arthritis

Arthritis is an inflammation of a joint. There is usually an increased amount of synovial fluid present because of a concomitant inflammation of the synovial membrane (*synovitis*). Arthritis may be traumatic, as after the forcible twisting, hyperextension, or hyperflexion of a joint. Such an injury may lead to a minor tear (called a *sprain*) in the capsule, but if the injury is more severe, the capsule may rupture and allow partial or complete displacement of the bone ends to occur. A partial displacement is called a *subluxation*, and a complete one is called a *dislocation*. Simple sprains heal well, but the weakness that follows capsular rupture predisposes to recurrent dislocation. Arthritis may be infective in nature. It may follow a penetrating joint injury when the infection is introduced from outside. The infection may be blood-borne; thus, a suppurative (septic) arthritis may complicate gonorrhea, lobar pneumonia, or staphylococcal septicemia. Unless energetically treated in the early stages with antibiotics, infective arthritis leads to rapid destruction of the articular cartilage; the whole joint cavity fills with inflammatory exudate that organizes and obliterates the joint space. In this way, the joint is destroyed, and the bone ends are united first by fibrous tissue (*fibrous ankylosis*) and later by bone (*bony ankylosis*).

Tuberculous arthritis may occur as an isolated lesion or may complicate an adjacent tuberculous osteomyelitis. The disease is now uncommon.

The common types of chronic arthritis are rheumatoid arthritis and osteoarthritis.

Rheumatoid Arthritis

This disease occurs most frequently in young women, characteristically affects many joints, and is symmetric. The small joints of the hands and feet are most severely affected, but the elbows and knees also suffer badly. Rheumatoid arthritis is a systemic disease; in its active phase, there are malaise, anemia, pyrexia, weight loss, and bouts of sweating. The onset of the disease is occasionally acute, but usually it is insidious as swelling, pain, and stiffness of the joints develop.

The affected joints are swollen, tender, and painful. In the early stages, the synovial membrane is acutely inflamed; later, there is proliferation of its connective tissue component together with a heavy infiltration by lymphocytes and plasma cells. The proliferating synovium steadily encroaches upon the articular margins, and a layer of inflamed granulation tissue, called a *pannus*, spreads over the cartilage of the joint surface and destroys it. The joint space is gradually obliterated by fibrous adhesions, and eventually fibrous ankylosis occurs. In this late stage, there is severe disuse atrophy of the adjacent bones and muscles, and the overlying skin is smooth and shiny. The results of advanced rheumatoid arthritis are tragic to see: progressive contractures lead to flexion deformities that are found in particular in the hands, which have a characteristic ulnar deviation of the fingers (Fig. 30–9). The flexed, ankylosed larger joints render the patient immobile and bedridden.

The nature of rheumatoid arthritis is unknown, but the basic lesion seems to be fibrinoid necrosis of collagen. It has therefore been classified as a collagen disease (Chapter 6). The widespread nature of the process is evidenced by the development of lesions in places other than the joints. The most characteristic of these is the subcutaneous nodules that develop over pressure points. They consist of a large area of necrobiotic collagen surrounded by a palisaded layer of fibroblasts and epithelioid cells. Similar nodules are encountered elsewhere; thus, in the sclera of the eye, a rheumatoid nodule can break down and cause perforation of the globe.

Visceral lesions occur in ankylosing spondylitis; they include an aortitis resembling syphilitic aortitis and uveitis. Involvement of the pericardium is a well-recognized type of *chronic pericarditis*. Occasionally the lungs are affected, particularly in miners with silicosis. The lesions resemble rheumatoid nodules. Generalized enlargement of the lymph nodes and splenomegaly may also be present. Amyloidosis is an important complication; indeed, it is the only significant fatal lesion in rheumatoid arthritis, which may otherwise smolder for many years and produce complete crippling.

The sera of most patients with rheumatoid arthritis contain an autoantibody that reacts with

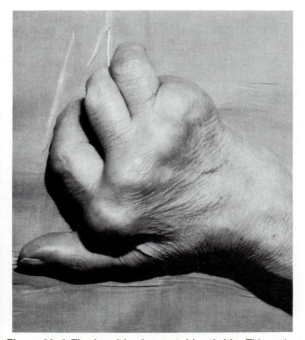

Figure 30–9 The hand in rheumatoid arthritis. This patient had had rheumatoid arthritis for many years and was severely incapacitated. The hand shows marked swelling of the metacarpophalangeal joints and extreme deviation of the fingers toward the ulnar side. Apart from movement of the thumb, very little movement was possible. The hollowed appearance between the metacarpal bones is due to atrophy of the small muscles of the hand. This patient was in a hospital because a rheumatoid nodule had developed in the sclera of her left eye. To prevent perforation of the globe and loss of the eye, a fascia lata graft was applied and was successful in saving her sight.

human immunoglobulin. This antibody is called the *rheumatoid factor*. Although its detection is useful in diagnosis, its significance in the pathogenesis of the disease is not known. The rheumatoid factor is not present in psoriatic arthritis; this is a useful distinguishing point between the two diseases, which in other respects closely resemble each other.

Ankylosing Spondylitis

Ankylosing spondylitis differs in many respects from rheumatoid arthritis; it occurs in young adults, particularly males, and generally affects the sacroiliac and vertebral joints first. Later the large peripheral joints such as the hips are involved, but the small distal joints of the hands and feet are spared. There is bony ankylosis of the affected joints in the later stages of the disease. The spinal ligaments of the intervertebral disks undergo ossification and combine with bony ankylosis of the spinal joints to convert the spinal column into a rigid bony mass, the *bamboo spine*.

The pathogenesis of ankylosing spondylitis is not understood; there is an association with chronic ulcerative colitis and Crohn's disease, particularly in subjects who are of tissue type HLA B27.

Osteoarthritis

Osteoarthritis, despite its name, is not an inflammatory but rather a degenerative disease of joints. Osteoarthrosis is an alternative name that is sometimes used. It is one of the most common human afflictions because it is essentially an accentuation of the inevitable aging process of articular cartilage. The nourishment of the hyaline cartilage of joints is normally rather precarious and depends on the synovial fluid. The constant wear and tear of the joints after many years' activity leads to a gradual deterioration of the central part of the articular cartilage. This process is greatly aggravated by injury; thus, a joint injured in some athletic activity can be complicated by osteoarthritis several years later, even when the patient is still young. Nevertheless, osteoarthritis is generally a disease of later life and affects the spine and large weight-bearing joints, especially the hips. The smaller joints, however, do not escape entirely.

Osteoarthritis, unlike rheumatoid arthritis, is not a systemic disease. The general health remains unaffected, and life is not shortened.

Osteoarthritis begins with softening and fraying of the articular cartilage, which becomes progressively thinner. Ultimately, the underlying bone is exposed, and its surface becomes hard, worn, and polished (a change called *eburnation*). Meanwhile, there is proliferation of the cartilage cells at the margin of the articular area. This new cartilage soon ossifies. The result is that the periphery of the articular cartilage is raised and bossed (a process called *lipping*); this is an important radiologic finding. The projecting nodules of new bone at the margins of the joint are called *osteophytes*. These not only interfere with the range of the joint's movement but also may become nipped off to form *loose bodies* ("joint mice"). These loose bodies are a constant nuisance because they tend to be caught between the opposing bone ends during movement. The result is locking of the joint, which can be excruciatingly painful if a fringe of synovium is also included. A prominent site for osteophytes is the terminal interphalangeal joints of the fingers of elderly people. These painless bony swellings are extremely common and are called *Heberden's nodes*.

The joints do not become ankylosed in osteoarthritis, but the destructive process and the osteophyte formation seriously limit movement. Pain is often a major complaint, and it is in such cases that replacement of the joint by a metallic or plastic prosthesis is so successful.

DISEASES OF SKELETAL MUSCLE

Skeletal muscle constitutes 45 per cent of the mean body weight and is afflicted by remarkably few diseases. It is composed of muscle fibers, each of which is an elongated multinucleate cell containing contractile protein in the form of myofilaments. Two types of muscle fiber are described: The *type 1* fibers (red fibers), which contain an abundance of myoglobin and mitochondria, are adapted to slow, repetitive contractions over long periods of time. The *type 2* fibers (white fibers) contain more myofilaments and are designed for rapid contraction; they show fatigue relatively quickly. The distinction between red and white fibers is obvious in birds but is not evident in humans. The proportion of each type of fiber in any particular muscle depends on the age and sex of the subject, its anatomic site, and use to which the muscle has been put. Muscle is remarkably adaptable, a fact that supports the value of physical training. Exercise can increase the number of myofibrils, cause mitochondria to increase in size and number, and improve the microvascular bed so that is more efficient in sustaining the contractile elements. The proportion of type 1 fibers to type 2 fibers can change.

There is indeed a firm basis for the physical therapists' efforts to retain and build up muscular activity and bulk. It should be noted that the number of muscle fibers present in a muscle is fixed and that any increase in size of the muscle is brought about by hypertrophy of each individual fiber only.

If muscles are not used owing to lack of exercise, whether due to habit, pain, or disease, disuse atrophy occurs. There is diminution in size of muscle fibers, and ultimately some are lost. Loss of motor nerve supply has a similar effect, but the atrophy tends to be in groups of fibers within the area of affected muscle. Whether the muscle as a whole becomes small depends on whether adjacent fibers undergo hypertrophy.

Muscular Dystrophy

Muscular dystrophy encompasses a group of uncommon inherited conditions in which there is progressive degeneration of muscle fibers. On microscopic examination, the fibers show varying stages of degeneration, culminating in complete destruction. Various types of muscular dystrophy have been described, based largely on the mode of inheritance and the clinical picture.

Duchenne's Muscular Dystrophy. This type is inherited as an X-linked trait and therefore affects males only. The disease commences at birth, initially affects the muscles of the pelvic girdle, and later spreads to the shoulder girdle. A striking feature is enlargement of the calf muscles due to an infiltration of fat cells that accompanies the degeneration of muscle fibers. The child with Duchenne's muscular dystrophy has difficulty in walking, has a waddling gait, eventually becomes bedridden, and dies by the age of 30 years.

Facioscapulohumeral Muscular Dystrophy. This type is inherited as an autosomal dominant trait and, as its name implies, affects the muscles of the shoulder girdle and face. The onset is in adolescence, and the disease progresses slowly, so that life expectancy is normal.

Limb-Girdle Dystrophy. This type of dystrophy is probably not a separate entity but rather a group of disorders that do not fit readily into the preceding two types of muscle dystrophy.

Myotonic Muscular Dystrophy. This type of muscular dystrophy is characterized by *myotonia*, a term that describes the difficulty the patient has in relaxing the grip. Limb weakness is initially most marked distally so that there is weakness of the hands. Facial muscles show weakness often evident as drooping of the eyelids (*ptosis*). The disease has several other characteristic features. *Cataracts* (Chapter 32) develop sooner or later in all patients, and males suffer from *testicular atrophy* and *premature baldness*. The disease is inherited as an autosomal dominant trait.

Enzymes in the Diagnosis of Muscular Dystrophy

Several enzymes are characteristic of muscle, and their blood level is increased when muscle fibers are degenerating. The highest levels are seen in the Duchenne type of muscular dystrophy. The most characteristic enzyme is creatine phosphokinase, but this is so sensitive a test that it may give false-positive results. Other enzymes that are elevated are aspartate aminotransferase and lactic dehydrogenase.

Myasthenia Gravis

Myasthenia gravis is a disease characterized by muscular weakness and pronounced muscle fatigability that is associated with the presence of a circulating antibody to acetylcholine receptors.

The disease generally starts at about the age of 20 years and affects females more frequently than males. The weakness characteristically affects the ocular and cranial muscles, leading to ptosis, double vision (*diplopia*), and difficulty in chewing and in swallowing. The limb muscles can also be affected. The disease fluctuates in intensity, and its course is unpredictable. During crises, the respiratory muscles may be affected, and the patient can die of respiratory failure. The ready fatigability of the muscles can be temporarily overcome by the administration of anticholinesterase drugs.

Pathogenesis. Skeletal muscular contraction is initiated by acetylcholine, which is released from motor nerve terminals and acts on acetylcholine receptors of the muscle motor end plates. In myasthenia gravis, the number of receptors is reduced because of an IgG autoantibody that destroys the receptor protein. Virtually all patients have circulating antibodies to acetylcholine receptor protein. In about three quarters of patients, there is enlargement of the thymus. Usually there is simple hyperplasia, but in older patients there may be a neoplasm (*thymoma*). Removal of the thymus generally improves the myasthenia, and this is the common form of treatment, particularly if the gland can be demonstrated to be enlarged and if the myasthenia does not respond adequately to the administration of anticholinesterase drugs, glucocorticoids, or other immunosuppressive drugs.

Myositis

The myositis of dermatomyositis (Chapter 6), trichinosis (Chapter 10), and gas gangrene (Chapter 8) has been described. Other types are uncommon.

Neoplasms of Muscle

Primary Tumors. Most examples of benign *rhabdomyomas* occur in the heart and are probably malformations rather than neoplasms. *Rhabdomyosarcomas* are highly malignant tumors of striated muscle and fortunately are rare. They may occur at any age, and various types are described. One type is seen in children and young adults and can involve the orbit of the eye or the genitourinary tract, particularly the *vagina*.

Metastatic Tumors. In spite of the bulk of muscle present in the body, metastatic tumors are rare.

Summary

- In the normal adult, all bone is lamellar. Woven bone is present only during development or in abnormal conditions.
- The ionized blood calcium is regulated by parathyroid hormone secretion and vitamin D. The active form of vitamin D is formed by hydroxylation of vitamin D first in the liver and then in the kidneys.

- Acute osteomyelitis is usually staphylococcal and readily progresses to chronic infection with pus and involucrum formation.
- Ischemic bone disease may follow small vessel occlusion or occur as an idiopathic condition, *e.g.*, Legg-Perthes disease.
- The callus formed during fracture healing repeats the process of endochondrial and intramembranous ossification. Movement, infection, and poor blood supply are the chief causes of poor healing.
- The developmental abnormalities described (osteogenesis imperfecta, achondroplasia, osteopetrosis, and fibrous dysplasia) are groups of diseases of similar phenotype but differing in genotype.
- Hyperparathyroidism may be primary or secondary (commonly to renal disease). Osteitis fibrosa cystica, metastatic calcification, and renal stones often with infection and renal damage are the chief effects.
- Vitamin D deficiency impairs calcium absorption and leads to impaired calcification. Rickets or osteomalacia is the result.
- Osteoporosis results from disuse or pressure if it is localized and accompanies aging (particularly after the menopause) if it is generalized.
- Hypertrophic osteoarthropathy commonly indicates intrathoracic disease.
- Giant-cell tumor of bone is benign or of intermediate malignancy; osteosarcoma is the most common malignant tumor affecting young adults unless it complicates Paget's disease. Myeloma affects the bone marrow; Ewing's tumor, affecting young children, is of unknown cell origin. Metastatic tumors are commonly from breast, prostate, or lung.
- Arthritis may be of traumatic or infective origin, but the cause of the common rheumatoid arthritis is not known. It is a generalized disease affecting other organs, *e.g.*, skin, eye, blood vessels, and pericardium. It differs from ankylosing spondylitis, which affects large joints, occurs in young subjects, and is associated with chronic bowel disease and HLA B27.
- Osteoarthritis, a disease of wear and tear, causes pain and disability.
- Muscular dystrophy includes a number of distinct entities of genetic origin. Myasthenia gravis is an autoimmune disease associated with loss of acetylcholine receptors on muscle cells.

Selected Readings

Gardner, D. L.: The nature and causes of osteoarthritis. Br. Med. J. *286*:418, 1983.

Heath, D. A.: Hypercalcaemia in malignancy. Br. Med. J. *298*:1468, 1989.

Hosking, D. J.: Paget's disease of bone. Br. Med. J. *283*:686, 1981.

Jamieson, M. J.: Hypercalcaemia. Br. Med. J. *290*:378, 1985.

Krane, S. M., and Simon, L. S.: Rheumatoid arthritis, clinical features and pathogenetic mechanisms. Med. Clin. North Am. *70*:263, 1986.

Mastaglia, F. L., and Walton, J. (eds.): Skeletal Muscle Pathology. Edinburgh, Churchill Livingstone, 1982.

Raisz, L. G., and Kream, B. E.: Regulation of bone formation. N. Engl. J. Med. *309*:29 and 83, 1983.

Reichel, H., Koeffler, H. P., and Norman, A. W.: The role of the vitamin D endocrine system in health and disease. N. Engl. J. Med. *320*:989, 1989.

Revell, P. A.: Pathology of Bone. New York, Springer-Verlag, 1986.

Riggs, B. L., and Melton, L. J.: Involutional osteoporosis. N. Engl. J. Med. *314*:1676, 1986.

Schmidt, N.: Hyperparathyroidism, a review. Am. J. Surg. *139*:657, 1980.

Smith, R.: Osteoporosis: Cause and management. Br. Med. J. *294*:329, 1987.

31

Skin

After studying this chapter, the student should be able to:

- Define the following words: erythematous, macule, patch, papule, plaque, vesicle, bulla, pustule, squamous, telangiectasia, excoriation, and pruritic.
- List the clinical types of dermatitis and describe the outstanding features of each type.
- Describe the main features of psoriasis, pityriasis rosea, urticaria, toxic erythema, and erythema multiforme.
- Describe the types of skin reaction that drugs can cause.
- Classify the vesiculobullous diseases and describe the main features of each type.
- Describe the pathogenesis and lesions of acne vulgaris; compare the disease with acne rosacea.
- Describe the common melanocytic and vascular nevi.
- Describe the dysplastic nevus syndrome.
- Classify the types of squamous-cell papilloma of skin.
- Describe squamous-cell carcinoma of the skin and list the lesions that may precede its development.
- Classify the types of malignant melanoma and relate the types to the prognosis.

It has been estimated that between 15 and 20 per cent of patients who consult their doctor do so because of some skin disorder. Nevertheless, the teaching of dermatology is usually sadly neglected in medical education. Perhaps this is due to the complexity of the subject, because the

573

number of diseases of the skin described far exceeds that of any other individual organ. There are several reasons for this. First, the skin is exposed to many insults from the external environment. Second, it is a complex composite organ, because in addition to having a surface epithelium called the *epidermis*, it has associated *hair follicles* with their *sebaceous glands, eccrine* and *apocrine sweat glands*, and a specialized connective tissue called the *dermis*, itself composed of dense collagenous bundles and elastic fibers. Third, the skin can be examined and biopsied easily. Fourth, throughout the ages, people have considered the appearance of skin to be very important; this fact has added to the complexity of dermatology. This chapter describes some of the common skin diseases and also a few that, although uncommon, are so serious that they must be recognized early if effective treatment is to be given.

TERMINOLOGY

There are few areas in medicine that can compete with dermatology for hiding truth with complex names. Nevertheless, with some basic facts and a minimal knowledge of Latin, it is possible to master this terminology.

An area of skin that is altered, usually red (*erythematous*), flat, and not palpable (*i.e.,* cannot be felt) is called a *macule* if it is less than 1.0 cm in diameter; if it is larger, it is called a *patch*. Similar areas that are palpable are called *papules* if they are small (less than 1.0 cm in diameter) and *plaques* if they are over that size. A blister is called a *vesicle* if small and a *bulla* if large. *Pustules* contain pus. In due course, the inflammatory fluid in a vesicle, bulla, or pustule dries to form a *crust*. If flakes of keratin are seen obviously adherent to a lesion, this lesion is called *squamous*. Since most such lesions can be felt, they are called *papulosquamous*. The presence of visible, abnormally dilated vessels is called *telangiectasia*. Shallow ulcers or erosions are termed *excoriations* if they are produced by scratching. The observation and description of each individual skin lesion is important, because certain types are characteristic of certain diseases. For example, psoriasis is characteristically papulosqua-

mous and is occasionally pustular but is never vesicular.

The distribution of the lesions seen in any skin disease is equally important. A localized rash often indicates a localized cause. Thus, a dermatitis on only one wrist is probably due to sensitivity to a wrist band or a watch strap. In a consideration of any skin disease, it is important, therefore, to include the distribution of the rash and the individual characteristics of its lesions.

The presence of itching is characteristic of certain skin diseases, such as scabies, neurodermatitis, and atopic dermatitis. The term *pruritus*, which is commonly used, is synonymous with itching. Note that the presence or absence of itching is as dependent on the individual as it is on the nature of the lesions. Some people itch easily, and others do not.

DERMATITIS AND ECZEMA

Dermatitis and *eczema* are synonymous terms used to describe a particular skin reaction pattern that primarily involves the epidermis. On the basis of their clinical appearances and the histologic pattern of reaction, three types are recognized: acute, subacute, and chronic.

Morphologic Types of Dermatitis

Acute Dermatitis. Clinically, acute dermatitis is characterized by erythema, swelling, and the formation of blisters, which can vary from small vesicles to large bullae (Figs. 31–1 and 31–3). If the vesicles rupture, the surface becomes wet or "weeping," and as the exudate dries, the lesion become crusted. On histologic examination, the epidermis shows intercellular edema (*spongiosis*) that terminates in the separation of epidermal cells and in the formation of vesicles or bullae (Fig. 31–1). The dermis shows an acute inflammatory reaction with edema and, surprisingly enough, a perivascular lymphocytic infiltrate. The absence of polymorphs is noteworthy.

Chronic Dermatitis. Clinically, chronic dermatitis appears as scaly papules or plaques, and the skin markings tend to be accentuated (Fig. 31–4); this feature is known as *lichenification*. On

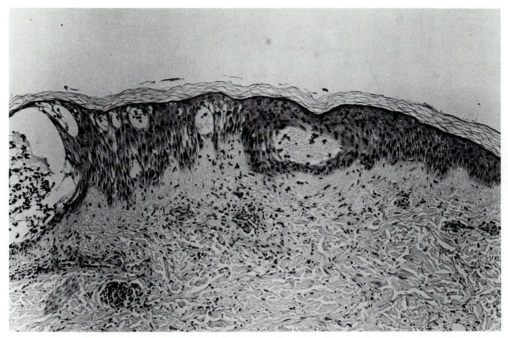

Figure 31–1 Acute dermatitis. The epidermis is thickened (acanthosis) owing mainly to the separation of cells by edema (*spongiosis*). In several places, the cells have torn apart to produce intraepidermal vesicles. The largest of these spongiotic vesicles is on the left-hand side and contains coagulated exudate. There is a sparse infiltrate of the dermis by lymphocytes. The biopsy was taken from a patient with acute allergic contact dermatitis due to exposure to poison ivy (×240).

histologic examination, the epidermis is thickened; this is termed *acanthosis* and is associated with an increased mitotic activity of the epidermal cells. Keratinization is disturbed, for not only is the keratin layer increased in thickness (*hyperkeratosis*), but in places the nuclei are retained. This condition is called *parakeratosis* (Fig. 31–2). Foci of spongiosis may be present, but vesicle formation is absent.

Subacute Dermatitis. The clinical picture of subacute dermatitis has features midway between acute and chronic dermatitis. The lesions are papulosquamous, but small vesicles can be detected. There is acanthosis and hyperkeratosis on histologic examination, but this is less marked than in chronic dermatitis. Parakeratosis and spongiosis, on the other hand, are more marked, and in places small vesicles are evident.

It should be noted that there is no sharp distinction among the three grades of dermatitis. Vesiculation is marked in acute dermatitis, inconspicuous in subacute dermatitis, and absent in chronic dermatitis. Acanthosis and hyperkerato-

sis are marked in chronic dermatitis, less obvious in the subacute stage, and absent in acute dermatitis.

Clinical Types of Dermatitis

The clinical types of dermatitis are many and various. They cannot be distinguished from each other histologically but differ in their causes and clinical presentation.

Primary Irritant Dermatitis. Externally applied chemical irritants are a frequent cause of dermatitis (*contact dermatitis*): a common example is the chronic lichenified hand eczema seen in housewives whose hands are brought repeatedly into contact with water, detergents, and other household agents. Likewise, medical and dental personnel who are involved in direct patient care and are obliged to wash their hands frequently between procedures are liable to suffer from chronic hand eczema. Alkalis, acids, and many industrial chemicals can act as primary irritants;

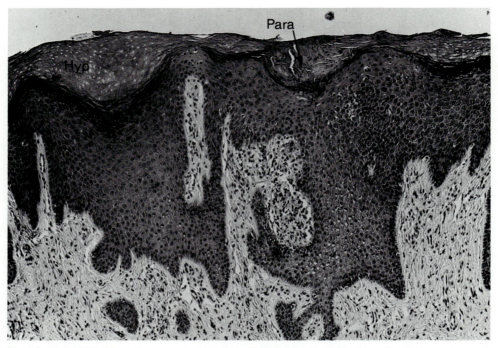

Figure 31–2 Chronic dermatitis. There is marked acanthosis with hyperkeratosis (Hyp) together with one focus of parakeratosis (Para). These changes should be compared with the normal skin present on the right-hand side of the specimen in Figure 31–1 (×240).

if applied over a long period, they lead to a refractory chronic dermatitis. Laboratory technologists are particularly at risk through the use of chemicals and stains, particularly those lipid solvents, such as xylol, that remove the protective lipid covering of the skin. *Elderly individuals* with dry skin may develop a dermatitis that is due to exposure to agents such as water, soap, and detergents that would be harmless in a younger person. These agents may also affect *atopic individuals* whose skin tends to be dry, especially during the winter months in those who live in inadequately humidified houses.

Allergic Contact Dermatitis. The development of cell-mediated hypersensitivity to chemicals results in the production of *allergic contact dermatitis.* Iodine, formaldehyde, dyes, plants (*e.g.,* poison ivy), and nickel (used in costume jewelry) are among the many agents that can act as haptens and cause this type of dermatitis (Fig. 31–3). It is noteworthy that certain parts of the skin are more sensitive to contactants than are others. Thus, allergic contact dermatitis is more common on the backs of the hands than it is on the palms.

Likewise, the face is particularly sensitive and may react to agents that elsewhere cause little trouble. Dermatitis around the eyes can be due to nail polish, which causes little trouble to the hands or feet.

Photodermatitis. Ultraviolet light can act on chemicals (either applied topically or taken systemically) present in the skin and so alter them that direct irritant effects (*phototoxic dermatitis*) or new antigen formation and subsequent sensitization (*photoallergic dermatitis*) result. Agents well known to cause this sensitizing effect when applied topically are perfumes, coal-tar derivatives, and halogenated salicylanilides (used in deodorant soap).

Many drugs taken internally can have a similar effect. Common examples are chemotherapeutic agents such as sulfonamides and tetracyclines, diuretics (*e.g.,* chlorothiazide), and tranquilizers (*e.g.,* chlorpromazine), to name a few.

Atopic Dermatitis. Atopic dermatitis occurs in atopic (allergic) individuals, but the pathogenesis is obscure, for although the associated respiratory diseases such as hay fever and bronchial

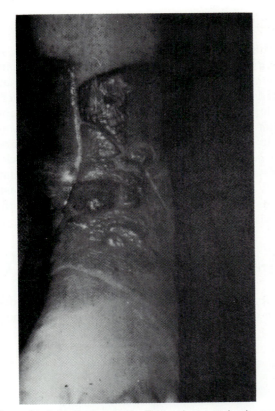

Figure 31–3 Acute dermatitis. This patient sustained a sprain of the left ankle, and adhesive tape was applied for support; 36 hours later, an acute vesicular dermatitis appeared and subsequently became bullous. Note how the rash is limited to the region previously covered by tape (lines of demarcation are obvious). Areas where the skin was folded are spared.

asthma appear to be mediated by IgE sensitization, the skin lesions are more complex and the damage is probably cell-mediated.

The distribution of the rash varies with the age of the patient. In the *infantile phase* (3 to 18 months), the *face* and other exposed parts of the skin are commonly affected. Atopic dermatitis at this age is also called *infantile eczema.* In the *childhood phase* (over 18 months), the *elbow and knee flexures* are characteristically involved. In the *adult phase,* the flexures are again involved, but the rash can be widespread and involve other areas — hands, upper limbs, and trunk. Atopic dermatitis is *intensely itchy,* so that lichenification, excoriations, and areas of crusting are common. Atopic disease has been stressed because it is extremely common, although just how common is difficult to state because estimates range from 2 to 25 per cent of the population. Probably about 5 per cent are afflicted with atopic dermatitis, and although for some it is a mere annoyance in the winter months, for others it is a lifelong illness of itching and scratching that demands constant medication and causes anguish to both patient and therapist alike. Fortunately, the disease tends to remit as age advances.

Nummular Eczema. This condition tends to occur in atopic individuals and is characterized by the formation of localized, coin-shaped plaques of subacute or chronic dermatitis. Itching is usually marked.

Stasis Dermatitis. Stasis dermatitis occurs on the legs and is related to chronic venous stasis. It occurs after venous thrombosis in the lower limbs and in patients with varicose veins. In addition to the usual features of a dermatitis, stasis dermatitis is characterized by a brown discoloration of the skin. This is produced by hemosiderin secondary to petechial hemorrhages. The poor blood supply to the skin causes atrophy with loss of hair follicles and thinning of the epidermis. Chronic ulcers are a common complication and are usually initiated by trauma, caused either accidentally or by scratching. Such *stasis ulcers* (see Fig. 5–16) are often situated over the medial malleolus and heal slowly because of the poor blood supply to the skin. After many years of repeated ulcerations, low-grade bacterial cellulitis, and chronic edema (the result of both venous and lymphatic obstruction), there is overgrowth of the dermal connective tissues, so that the leg becomes chronically swollen and woody hard to the touch. Occasionally, the tissue overgrowth, accompanied by papillomatous epidermal overgrowth, is so marked that the term *elephantiasis* is applied.

Seborrheic Dermatitis. A type of chronic dermatitis is frequently seen in the scalp and results in the formation of greasy scales or dandruff. This condition is termed *seborrheic dermatitis;* although it is extremely common, its precise nature is not understood. The dermatitis can extend beyond the scalp and affect the face. There is occasionally involvement of the trunk, particularly the front of the chest, and the flexural regions such as the axilla or under the breasts. This type of dermatitis can be encountered in all age groups, ranging from infants (cradle cap) to old people. It is particularly common in the acquired immunodeficiency syndrome (AIDS).

Neurodermatitis. A feature of some forms of dermatitis, including the atopic variety, is marked itching. This leads to scratching and self-perpetuation because of the continued physical trauma. The condition is then referred to as *chronic neurodermatitis* (Fig. 31–4). Localized plaques of chronic neurodermatitis are often called lichen simplex chronicus.

PAPULOSQUAMOUS ERUPTIONS

A group of diseases, of widely differing origins, is characterized by papulosquamous lesions. Common examples are chronic dermatitis, psoriasis, pityriasis rosea, secondary syphilis, and ringworm.

Psoriasis

This is a chronic disease that fluctuates in intensity both spontaneously and under the influence of treatment. It occurs as sharply demarcated erythematous plaques with a dry, silvery scale. Common sites are the elbows, knees, and other extensor surfaces. The palms, soles, and scalp are also frequently affected (Figs. 31–5 and 31–6). Psoriasis is not usually itchy, and vesicles are never formed. This distinguishes it both clinically and histologically from dermatitis. Psoriasis tends to be common in certain families, but the precise mode of inheritance is unknown.

Pityriasis Rosea

Pityriasis rosea is a common, self-limiting disease of young adults. The first lesion to appear

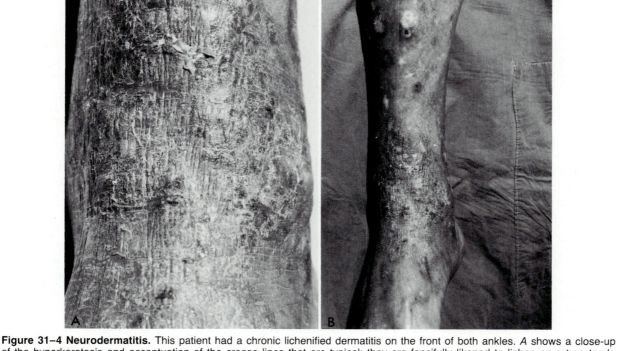

Figure 31–4 Neurodermatitis. This patient had a chronic lichenified dermatitis on the front of both ankles. *A* shows a close-up of the hyperkeratosis and accentuation of the crease lines that are typical; they are fancifully likened to lichen on a tree trunk. Constant scratching and rubbing, often with the opposite heel, perpetuate the condition. The nodules shown higher on the leg in *B* are also self-induced. They consist of dense scar tissue with overlying acanthosis and hypopigmentation. The lesions are called prurigo nodularis (from the Latin *prurigo*, meaning "to itch") and are produced by the patient's continually picking at them.

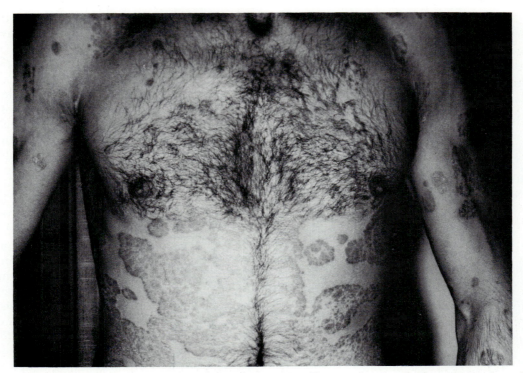

Figure 31-5 Psoriasis. The patient has widespread psoriatic lesions. They consist of well-demarcated scaly erythematous papules and plaques.

is an oval, sharply defined, erythematous, scaly plaque 2 to 5 cm in diameter (the *herald patch*). It may easily be misdiagnosed clinically as ringworm. About 1 week later, a widespread eruption of pink macules or scaly papules develops; on the trunk, the lesions tend to follow the lines of the ribs to give a "Christmas tree" pattern on the patient's back. The rash of pityriasis rosea can easily be confused with that of secondary syphilis, and it is a wise precaution to perform a VDRL in all cases.

Pityriasis rosea clears spontaneously in 6 to 8 weeks and does not recur. Its cause is unknown, but the pattern of the disease suggests that it is a viral infection. To date, no virus has been isolated.

THE SUPERFICIAL MYCOSES

Ringworm, or Tinea

Ringworm is caused by a group of fungi that are termed the *dermatophytes* and have the property of digesting the keratin of skin or hair. The dermatophytes are molds that grow as a mycelium and reproduce by the formation of spores.

Ringworm, which is due to invasion of keratin by one of the dermatophytes, can affect the scalp (causing *tinea capitis*, in which involvement of hair shafts causes a bald patch), the body skin (causing *tinea corporis* with its variant *tinea cruris* affecting the inguinal region), the foot (causing athlete's foot, or *tinea pedis*), the hands (causing *tinea manuum*), and sometimes the nails (causing *tinea unguium*). Clinically, each type of ringworm has its own particular characteristics, but in general the lesions are erythematous, scaly, and sometimes vesicular and tend to have a sharp red spreading border that gives the lesions a ringlike shape from which the disease acquires its name. Diagnosis is easy. Scrapings of keratin can be examined by direct microscopy for hyphae, and from the culture one can readily identify the particular strain of mold responsible. Local treatment with antifungal agents is effec-

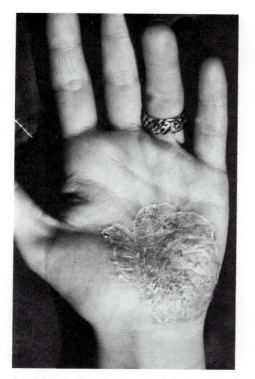

Figure 31–6 Psoriasis. The characteristic psoriatic plaque is sharply delineated, red, and covered by a silvery scale. The lesions, particularly when on the soles of the feet, can easily be misdiagnosed as ringworm.

tive, except in the case of ringworm of the nails, for which the only effective treatment is prolonged oral administration of griseofulvin, one of the few antibiotics that are effective against these fungi.

Not all ringlike lesions are ringworm. Psoriasis and nummular eczema can mislead the unwary; vigorous, ill-advised treatment can lead to contact dermatitis. Most patients who complain of ''ringworm'' and ''athlete's foot'' do not have a fungal infection.

Candidiasis

Infection with *Candida* species is one of the most frequent fungal infections in humans. The organism most commonly involved is *Candida albicans*, a yeastlike fungus that reproduces by budding but sometimes elongates to form pseudohyphae. The yeast form is characteristic of superficial candidal infections, whereas the pseudomycelial growth is found when the organism invades deeper tissues. *C. albicans* is a common commensal in the *oral cavity, alimentary tract*, and *vagina*. Infection occurs when general or local conditions become suitable. Superficial infections of the mucous membrane appear as white patches called *thrush*. In the mouth, this is very common in infants, especially premature ones, and it may be accompanied by perianal lesions. Oral candidiasis can occur at any age during the course of any debilitating disease. It is extremely common in AIDS. Vaginal thrush is common during pregnancy, in women using the birth control pill, and in patients with diabetes mellitus. Cutaneous candidiasis can occur in moist intertriginous areas, such as in the groin, under the breasts, and in the nail folds (chronic paronychia) of those whose occupations bring their hands repeatedly into water. Candidiasis constitutes one type of *diaper rash*; at the other extreme of age, *Candida* may cause *angular stomatitis*. This occurs because elderly subjects with dentures suffer from loss of vertical height between the mandible and the maxilla secondary to atrophy of the alveolar bone after the extraction of teeth. The moist folds at the corners of the mouth form a ready site for a troublesome *Candida* infection.

Generalized infection with *C. albicans* is occurring more frequently and is a serious and often fatal opportunistic infection (see Chapter 6). Steroid therapy, the presence of lymphomas, the administration of cytotoxic drugs, and indeed any disease in which cell-mediated immunity is impaired are predisposing factors for widespread invasion by the organism. Disseminated lesions affect many internal organs.

Less extensive candidal infections are seen under particular circumstances. Endocarditis occurs in addicts who inject themselves intravenously with narcotics. Mouth lesions can spread to produce extensive gastrointestinal infections after the prolonged oral administration of a broad-spectrum antibiotic that upsets the balance of the local bacterial flora. Finally, there is an inherited type of immunologic T-cell deficiency in which there is a selective susceptibility to *Candida* infection. These patients have persistent widespread skin and mucous membrane infections with *Candida* that defy all treatment. Nevertheless, despite the distressing skin lesions, dissemination to the internal organs does not occur.

DISEASES CHARACTERIZED BY A DERMAL INFLAMMATORY REACTION

An inflammatory reaction in the dermis is present in many skin diseases, including those that affect primarily the epidermis (*e.g.*, dermatitis, psoriasis, and pityriasis rosea). A localized area of dermal inflammation is a feature of many infections (*e.g.*, tuberculosis and erysipelas), but there is a group of conditions in which the primary event is a widespread vascular inflammatory reaction within the dermis. The most mild example of this group is urticaria.

Urticaria

Urticaria, or *hives*, is a common disease that affects many individuals at some time or another in their life. Symptoms include an acute inflammatory reaction in the dermis that is characterized by vasodilation, scanty polymorph accumulation, and marked edema. Clinically, urticaria commences with marked itching, which is followed by the appearance of erythema and swelling. The lesions tend to develop a pale center, or *wheal*, surrounded by an erythematous edge. They thereby resemble the common mosquito bite and the triple response (Chapter 5).

Acute urticaria is sometimes a type I hypersensitivity reaction mediated by IgE, but it is also seen in immune-complex reactions. It may follow the ingestion of a particular food or drug, and as in other hypersensitivity reactions, small quantities of the agent are sufficient to induce an attack. Thus, the menthol in a cigarette or toothpaste can precipitate acute urticaria in a sensitized person.

Each urticarial lesion lasts only a few hours, but repeated attacks of urticaria may occur over a period of many months or even years (*chronic urticaria*). In patients having such attacks, the cause is rarely found.

Urticaria affects the dermis. When the subcutaneous tissues are involved, the condition is termed *angioedema*. In both urticaria and angio-edema, the mucous membranes (including that of the tongue) can be involved. In one type of hereditary angioedema, there is a deficiency of C_1-esterase inhibitor. This is a serious condition, because lesions occur not only in the intestine, causing colic, but also in the larynx, in some cases leading to death from asphyxiation (the lesions obstruct the passage). In some families, many members ultimately die in this way.

Toxic Erythema

This general term is applied to many conditions in which the epidermis is normal, at least in the early stages, but in which there is a dermal inflammatory reaction showing vasodilation and a perivascular accumulation of cells, particularly lymphocytes. Viral exanthems (*e.g.*, measles) fall into this group. Toxic erythema is one manifestation of an adverse drug reaction.

DRUG ERUPTIONS

Drug eruptions are so common and produce such a wide variety of lesions that they must be considered in the differential diagnosis of any skin eruption. Any patient with a skin eruption must be asked what drugs are being taken, specific enquiry being directed to medications such as laxatives, headache pills, vitamin preparations, and others that are not always regarded as ''drugs'' by the patient. Likewise, the patient should be asked what local medications have been applied, for the original lesion may well have been overshadowed by a contact dermatitis. Some ''over-the-counter'' preparations, *e.g.*, medications for sunburn, contain potent sensitizers.

The common type of drug eruption is erythematous, papular, of widespread distribution, and very itchy (Fig. 31–7). Severe cases become vesicular and constitute one variety of erythema multiforme. Petechial lesions are not uncommon, and severe cases exhibit a definite vasculitis and lead to the formation of hemorrhagic and necrotic lesions. Sometimes the lesions closely resemble well-recognized dermatoses, such as measles and lupus erythematosus. The pathogenesis of drug

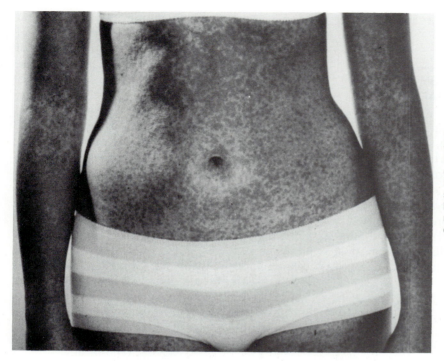

Figure 31–7 Drug eruption. The patient developed a widespread, very itchy, erythematous maculopapular eruption as a consequence of taking Dilantin for epilepsy. In places, for instance, on the right arm, the lesions have become confluent. A more severe reaction could have evolved into a generalized erythroderma.

eruptions varies. Those of an urticarial nature appear to be IgE-mediated. Others are mediated by immune complexes. In most, the pathogenesis is obscure.

VESICULOBULLOUS DISEASES

The formation of vesicles or bullae is an outstanding feature of this group of diseases. For accurate diagnosis, a biopsy of an early lesion is often necessary, because the situation of the vesicle is of vital importance in differential diagnosis. Some vesicles are formed within the epidermis, whereas others are formed beneath the epidermis.

Intraepidermal Vesicles

The superficial subcorneal vesicles and pustules of impetigo and candidiasis can generally be diagnosed so easily clinically that a biopsy is not necessary. Likewise, the spongiotic vesicles of acute and subacute dermatitis rarely need histologic confirmation. There are, however, two groups of intraepidermal vesiculating diseases in which biopsy is often useful. These are pemphigus and the vesiculating viral diseases.

The Pemphigus Group of Diseases. Pemphigus vulgaris is a chronic blistering disease that tends to occur in middle and old age, particularly in Jews of eastern European ancestry. Blisters frequently involve the mouth and lead to soreness, inability to eat, and great incapacity. The blisters are generally flaccid and on pressure can be made to extend laterally. They break easily, leaving eroded, painful surfaces. On microscopic examination, the epidermal cells above the basal cell layer are seen to lose their cohesiveness and separate from each other so that vesicles are formed. This process is termed *acantholysis* (Fig. 31–8), and the free or acantholytic cells are found lying in the fluid of the vesicle. Pemphigus vulgaris is regarded as an autoimmune disease. The blood contains an autoantibody directed against the intercellular substance of epidermis; the titer of this antibody parallels the activity of the disease. The antibody can be demonstrated on skin biopsy (Fig. 31–8), and the free or acantholytic cells are found lying in the fluid of the vesicle. Pemphigus vulgaris is regarded as an autoim-

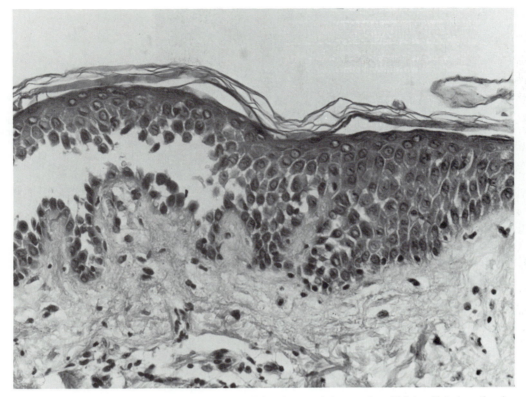

Figure 31–8 Pemphigus vulgaris. Acantholysis has produced the characteristic suprabasal blister. Note how the dermal papillae are covered by a row of basal cells still adherent to the basement membrane. These have been likened to a row of tombstones. Compare this acantholytic vesicle with the spongiotic vesicles of acute dermatitis (×500).

mune disease. The blood contains an autoantibody directed against the intercellular substance of epidermis; the titer of this antibody parallels the activity of the disease. The antibody can be demonstrated on skin biopsy (Fig. 31–9), and this is a useful confirmatory test.

A number of other acantholytic blistering diseases are known; some are variants of pemphigus, but others are rare and will not be considered.

The Vesicular Viral Diseases. The vesicles formed in zoster, chickenpox, and herpes simplex closely resemble each other histopathologically. The invaded epidermal cells show intranuclear inclusion bodies and swelling of the cytoplasm (ballooning) followed by degeneration. Some epithelial cells fuse together to form multinucleate giant cells, and as intercellular edema develops, the cells show *acantholysis*. The intraepidermal vesicle so formed contains degenerate and multinucleate acantholytic cells.

Distinction between the various types of virus vesicles is difficult histologically, but the clinical features combined with electron microscopy of vesicle fluid and other virologic investigations can distinguish one disease from the other.

A biopsy of the lesions of a typical case of chickenpox, herpes simplex, or zoster is not generally warranted. Sometimes, however, atypical cases are encountered, and if a virologic service is not available, a biopsy is useful in distinguishing such cases from other localized vesiculating diseases, such as a patch of acute contact dermatitis or a bullous drug reaction.

Subepidermal Vesicles

Subepidermal vesicles are formed in severe erythema multiforme, in certain drug eruptions, and in bullous pemphigoid.

Erythema Multiforme. This is an acute disease

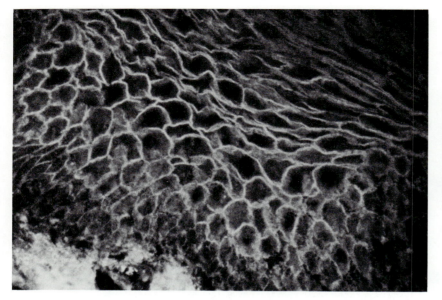

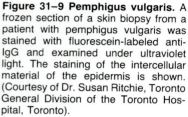

Figure 31–9 Pemphigus vulgaris. A frozen section of a skin biopsy from a patient with pemphigus vulgaris was stained with fluorescein-labeled anti-IgG and examined under ultraviolet light. The staining of the intercellular material of the epidermis is shown. (Courtesy of Dr. Susan Ritchie, Toronto General Division of the Toronto Hospital, Toronto).

of unknown etiology, although in about 50 per cent of cases it may follow some precipitating factor, *e.g.*, sun exposure, herpes simplex infection (cold sore), vaccination, x-ray therapy, drug intake, pregnancy, or the presence of some malignancy of an internal organ. The onset is usually sudden, and the patient rapidly develops symmetrical lesions of varying types—urticarial, erythematous macular, papular, vesicular, or, in the severe form of the disease, bullous (Fig. 31–10). The characteristic lesion is an erythematous papule with a central hemorrhagic area, so that the lesion tends to resemble a *target* or an *iris*. The dermal inflammatory reaction is sometimes so marked that fluid accumulates beneath the epidermis, and a *subepidermal vesicle* forms. The dermal reaction causes secondary degeneration of the epidermis. The severity of the dermal inflammatory reaction and the degenerate appearance of the epidermal roof serve to distinguish the lesions from those of bullous pemphigoid, which is described later. The lesions of erythema multiforme may occur on any part of the body, but they tend to be most common on the extremities. Severe erythema multiforme is associated with marked constitutional upset and high fever. Bullous lesions occur not only on the skin but also on the mucous membranes, where the bullae soon rupture to form painful ulcers.

This type of the disease with mucosal involvement is called the *Stevens-Johnson syndrome.* Ulcerations in the mouth and hemorrhagic crusting of the lips are characteristic. Oral feeding becomes impossible. Involvement of the conjunctiva can lead to blindness. Genital lesions can also occur in this severe form of erythema multiforme. There is no specific treatment for erythema multiforme, and recovery is the rule. However, in severe cases of the Stevens-Johnson syndrome, death can occur, generally from pneumonia.

Erythema multiforme tends to recur, particularly if the precipitating cause is itself recurrent, *e.g.*, recurrent herpes simplex.

Bullous Pemphigoid. Bullous pemphigoid is a chronic blistering disease that resembles pemphigus vulgaris clinically but has a much better prognosis. Unlike the lesions of pemphigus, the vesicles and bullae of this condition are usually tense rather than flaccid. Mucous membrane involvement is less common and less severe.

The vesicles are found to be subepidermal on microscopic examination. A useful diagnostic test is the demonstration of autoantibodies to skin basement membrane, both free in the serum and fixed in the skin. Patients with pemphigus vulgaris also produce an autoantibody, but its specificity is directed against epidermal intercellular

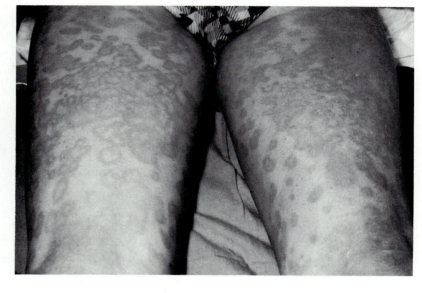

Figure 31–10 Erythema multiforme. The lesions have a bright red border and a pale center produced by subepidermal edema. In places, the papules have joined together to produce plaques with an arcuate border.

substance. Hence, the two diseases are quite distinct from each other both histologically and immunologically.

ACNE

Acne is a general term for inflammatory disease of the pilosebaceous follicles of the skin. Two types are described.

Acne Vulgaris

This familiar disorder of teenagers affects those areas in which sebaceous glands are plentiful—face, back, and upper chest. The primary lesions are due to the plugging of pilosebaceous follicles with adherent keratin. Oxidation of the surface of the plugs produces a dark-colored substance and results in the familiar *"blackhead,"* or *comedo.* The affected follicles dilate and become filled with the lipid secretions of sebaceous glands. The anaerobic saprophyte *Propionibacterium acnes* proliferates and splits the lipids to produce irritating fatty acids. The inflammation that results leads to pustule formation. If the follicle ruptures into the dermis, a large abscess is formed (*cystic acne*). Tetracycline therapy, which is now so much in vogue, is designed to inhibit the growth of *P. acnes.*

Acne Rosacea (Rosacea)

This is a common disorder that affects the central area of the face and has many features in common with acne vulgaris but occurs in an older age group, generally in persons over the age of 30 years. Three types of lesion occur:

1. *Papules, pustules,* and *cystic nodules* resembling those of the common type of acne. The pathogenesis is presumably similar in both conditions, for both respond to tetracycline therapy.
2. *Periodic flushing* and finally permanent *telangiectasia.* Ingestion of alcoholic beverages and spicy foods accentuates this component of the disease.
3. *Sebaceous gland hyperplasia,* particularly of the nose, where it produces the "W. C. Fields nose" or *rhinophyma.* Plastic surgery offers the best hope to these patients.

HAMARTOMAS OF THE SKIN

The hamartomas of the skin are termed *nevi.* The common examples are the melanocytic and angiomatous varieties.

Melanocytic Nevi

Melanocytic nevi are commonly called moles. Almost every person has at least a dozen or more of them. The parent cell is the melanocyte, which develops from the neural crest and migrates to the epidermis with the peripheral nerves. The melanocytes become incorporated into the basal layer of the epidermis and appear as cells with clear cytoplasm (Fig. 31–11). A focal abnormal proliferation of these cells leads to a mass that

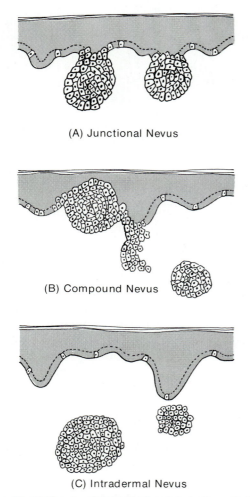

(A) Junctional Nevus

(B) Compound Nevus

(C) Intradermal Nevus

Figure 31–11 The development of melanocytic nevi of the skin. The only cells drawn are melanocytes or nevus cells. *A*, Junctional melanocytic nevus. Focal proliferation of melanocytes in the basal layer of the epidermis produces groups or nests of cells that become nevus cells. *B* Compound melanocytic nevus. Some nevus cells have invaded the dermis. *C*, Intradermal melanocytic nevus. The junctional nevus cells have disappeared, and all the nevus cells are in the dermis. The epidermis is normal and contains scattered melanocytes that, unless specifically stained, appear as clear cells in the basal layer of the epidermis. (Drawn by Margot Mackay, University of Toronto, Faculty of Medicine, Department of Surgery, Division of Biomedical Communications, Toronto.)

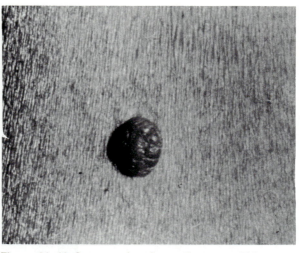

Figure 31–12 Compound melanocytic nevus. This nevus had been present on a 56-year-old woman's back for many years. The lesion has a lobulated, smooth surface, is uniformly pigmented, and is not ulcerated. It appears benign, but the patient had detected a slight increase in size over the preceding year; excision was performed for cosmetic reasons.

soon invades the dermis. The proliferating cells lose their ability to produce melanin and are then termed nevus cells. Early in the formation of a nevus, melanin-producing cells are formed at the dermoepidermal junction, and the lesion is called a *junctional nevus*. This is deeply pigmented and barely palpable. As the nevus develops, a dermal portion is formed, and ultimately a nonpigmented intradermal nevus results (Fig. 31–12). Nevi are seldom present at birth, but they develop during childhood.

Melanocytic nevi occasionally become malignant. *Any change, such as an increase in size, bleeding, ulceration, or change in degree of pigmentation, should suggest the possibility of malignancy.* Excision or biopsy is then indicated.

Spindle and Epithelioid Cell Nevus of Spitz. The Spitz nevus is a type of nevus, usually compound. It usually occurs in young people; in the past, it has been called a juvenile melanoma because its rapid growth and histologic appearance closely imitate a malignant melanoma. Nevertheless, the lesion is entirely benign.

Dysplastic Nevi. The lesion called a dysplastic nevus has recently attracted much attention because of its possible relationship to malignant melanoma. The dysplastic nevus is usually over

1 cm in diameter and has an irregular outline, a central pigmented, often elevated area, and a surrounding flat zone with a varying depth of pigmentation. This appearance is produced by the junctional pigmented component extending far beyond the intradermal component. The junctional component is made up of plump, often spindle-shaped nevus cells that show some degree of atypia. Occasionally, individuals are encountered who develop numerous dysplastic nevi and have a family history of malignant melanoma. Such individuals have a high incidence of melanoma also. This familial incidence of atypical nevi and melanoma constitutes the *dysplastic nevus syndrome.* Many individuals are now being identified who have one or several dysplastic nevi but have no family history of melanoma. They are probably not at risk of malignancy. Hence, the use of the term "dysplasia" in this context is unfortunate because it implies in many people's minds the tendency of such a lesion to be premalignant, as are dysplastic lesions in the cervix uteri. There is no definite evidence that dysplastic nevi are liable to become malignant, although it may well be that an individual who has a large number of nevi of any type is at a greater risk of developing malignant melanoma than is one who has few. Likewise, a family history of melanoma increases the risk.

Vascular Nevi of Skin

Various types of vascular anomalies are encountered in the skin. Sometimes at birth or shortly afterward, a red, vascular, spongy nodule develops in the skin; this grows rapidly for a while, but regresses after a few years and leaves an area of scarring. This type of nevus is composed of capillary-sized blood spaces and is often called a *capillary hemangioma* or strawberry nevus. Another type of nevus is composed of a few dilated capillary channels. Such a lesion appears as a flat, erythematous patch that is colloquially called a *port-wine stain.* Vascular nevi are of little importance apart from their cosmetic appearance. Sometimes they are multiple, and on occasion they are associated with similar lesions in deeper organs. When vascular nevi involve the face, for instance, angiomatous lesions of the

central nervous system or eye are sometimes found, and a number of characteristic syndromes can be recognized. Small hemangiomas commonly develop in elderly people and appear as bright red papules, 2 to 4 mm in diameter, on the trunk (*cherry angiomas*).

BENIGN NEOPLASMS OF THE SKIN

Squamous-Cell Papilloma

This is used as a descriptive term that indicates a number of separate entities. The common types are described.

Epithelial Nevus. This type of papilloma is generally present at birth and appears as a warty lesion, sometimes of linear distribution. It tends to recur after simple curettage.

Seborrheic Keratosis. Papillomas, frequently with considerable melanin pigmentation and overlying hyperkeratosis, are extremely common on the backs of the hands, on the trunk, and on the face of elderly people. The lesions seem to be stuck onto the surface of the skin and appear as flat or roughened pigmented warty nodules or plaques (Fig. 31–13). Such lesions are easily eliminated by curettage. The lesions never become malignant, but when heavily pigmented, they are liable to be confused with other pigmented lesions of the skin, such as melanocytic nevus, pigmented basal-cell carcinoma, or malignant melanoma.

Verruca Vulgaris. The *common wart* is a type of papilloma that is due to an infection by one of the human papillomaviruses (Fig. 12–3). Indeed, there are over 40 serotypes of the virus, and each tends to infect different areas. Unfortunately, the virus has never been grown in tissue culture, and this has greatly hindered research. The development of a successful vaccine would be of inestimable value, for although warts are rarely serious, they are unpleasant to look at and their treatment is tedious and sometimes painful — particularly to children, who are their most frequent victims. On the soles of the feet, the epidermal overgrowth and hyperkeratosis produce a painful lesion known as a *plantar wart.* Sometimes the virus produces multiple small, flat lesions called *plane warts.* In moist

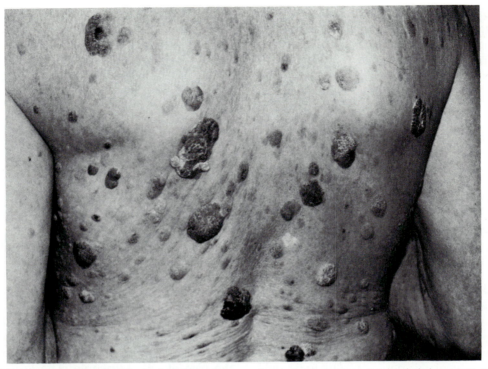

Figure 31–13 Seborrheic keratoses. The back of this elderly man is covered by numerous seborrheic keratoses, some of which are deeply pigmented. The large lesions have the characteristic stuck-on appearance, and they can be easily removed by curettage. This process involves scraping the skin for removing the epithelial element of the tumor; relatively little dermal damage is caused. Hence, scarring is minimal; excision by a scalpel leads to unnecessary scarring.

areas, such as on the penis and in the female genital region, pedunculated cauliflowerlike lesions are produced and are known as *condylomata acuminata.*

MALIGNANT NEOPLASMS OF THE SKIN

Basal-Cell Carcinoma

The most common malignant tumor of the skin in whites is the basal-cell carcinoma. This is illustrated in Figure 31–14 and is described fully in Chapter 12. As with squamous-cell carcinoma, the major predisposing cause is prolonged exposure to ultraviolet light.

Squamous-Cell Carcinoma

This tumor commonly arises on the sun-exposed skin in a pre-existing actinic keratosis.

Actinic keratoses are areas of epidermal dysplasia caused by prolonged exposure to ultraviolet light. They appear as scaly, erythematous areas on the face, ears, backs of hands, or forearms. In contradistinction to seborrheic keratoses, they must be regarded as precancerous. Squamous-cell carcinoma arising in an actinic keratosis is invasive, but metastases are late and the prognosis is relatively good. It should be stressed that the transition to malignancy frequently takes many years, and quite simple treatment is adequate for the cure of most actinic keratoses.

Squamous-cell carcinoma may also arise in burn scars, in chronic ulcers, and in the sinus of a chronic draining osteomyelitis. Occasionally it arises in Bowen's disease; this is a type of carcinoma *in situ* that can occur on any part of the body and appear as a circumscribed, erythematous, slightly indurated scaly plaque. Squamous-cell carcinoma is also more common in immunosuppressed patients, *e.g.,* those having a renal transplant. This group of squamous-cell carcino-

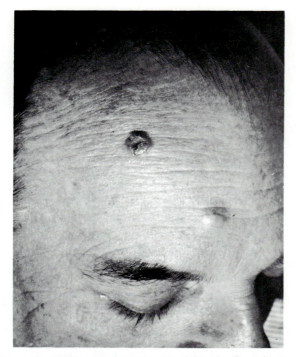

Figure 31–14 Basal-cell carcinoma. A basal-cell carcinoma of the right side of the forehead of this 56-year-old man is shown. The tumor has a typical appearance, having a depressed center and a raised, rolled edge over which dilated blood vessels (telangiectases) are coursing. The dome-shaped swelling just above the medial aspect of the right eyebrow is an epidermoid cyst, commonly called a sebaceous cyst or wen. It is formed by cystic dilation of a plugged pilosebaceous follicle.

mas not arising from a pre-existing actinic keratosis behave more aggressively and metastasize more frequently than do the sun-induced lesions.

Squamous-cell carcinoma must be differentiated both clinically and pathologically from a keratoacanthoma, which it closely resembles and which also occurs on the sun-exposed skin.

Keratoacanthoma. In this lesion, there is a localized exuberant overgrowth of atypical squamous epithelium that appears to invade the dermis and to surround a central keratotic plug. Around the lesion is an inflammatory reaction. Keratoacanthoma has been regarded by some as a type of self-healing carcinoma. The shape of the lesion is characteristic clinically, because it appears as a volcano-like lesion with a central keratotic depressed plug. The natural history also is quite characteristic: the lesion grows rapidly for 2 or 3 months, remains stationary, and then

involutes spontaneously. Healing results in considerable scarring, and the treatment of choice is therefore simple excision because this gives a good cosmetic result as well as provides material for pathologic examination.

Malignant Melanoma

The incidence of malignant melanoma, commonly now called simply melanoma, is increasing in frequency owing apparently to excessive exposure to sunlight. The tumor, derived from melanocytes, commences as an *in situ* lesion; its prognosis is related to the type of tumor and its spread (Fig. 31–15). Three types of melanoma *in situ* can be recognized.

1. *Superficial spreading melanoma in situ*. This lesion is the most common, occurs at any age (commonly 20 to 40 years), and may affect non-exposed skin. The back, especially in men, and the lower legs, especially in young women, are common sites. The lesions have an irregular border and variable pigmentation. On microscopic examination, there is proliferation of atypical melanocytes in the basal layer of the epidermis, and the malignant cells migrate superficially into the epidermis to produce a pagetoid appearance. Invasion of the dermis occurs within a year or two.

2. *Lentigo maligna (Hutchinson's freckle)*. This lesion occurs on the face of elderly subjects as a patch of uneven pigmentation. Atypical melanocytes are present in the basal layer of the epidermis, but there is no dermal invasion. The lesion gradually extends peripherally, and after many years, an invasive melanoma may develop.

3. *Acral lentiginous melanoma in situ*. This resembles lentigo maligna microscopically but appears as an area of pigmentation on the hairless skin—palms, soles, the nail bed, or the nail folds. The lesion is dangerous because invasive malignant melanoma soon develops.

Invasive Malignant Melanoma

In invasive malignant melanoma, the malignant cells invade the dermis as well as the epi-

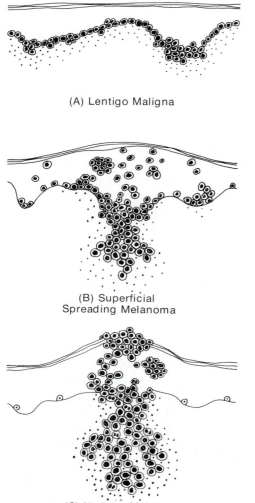

(A) Lentigo Maligna

(B) Superficial
Spreading Melanoma

(C) Nodular Melanoma

Figure 31–15 Types of malignant melanoma. *A*, Lentigo maligna. Proliferation of atypical melanocytes in the basal cell layer of the epidermis is accompanied by a lymphocytic response in the papillary dermis. This is a type of melanoma *in situ*, and at some stage dermal invasion can occur. *B*, Superficial spreading melanoma. Proliferation of atypical melanocytes occurs over a wide area of the basal layer of the epidermis. The melanoma cells invade the epidermis to produce a pagetoid appearance. At one point, there is dermal invasion. *C*, Nodular melanoma. The lesion is more localized than in the superficial spreading type. Melanoma cells invade the epidermis but also soon extend deeply into the dermis. (Drawn by Margot Mackay, University of Toronto, Faculty of Medicine, Department of Surgery, Division of Biomedical Communications, Toronto.)

dermis (Fig. 31–15). Four main types of malignant melanoma of the skin may be recognized.

1. *Superficial spreading melanoma.* This appears as a flat, variably pigmented lesion. The outline is irregular, and the color varies from black to brown together with areas of erythema in addition to white areas where local tumor regression has occurred. There is radial growth as well as vertical growth into the dermis to produce a nodule (Fig. 31–16).

2. *Nodular melanoma.* This commences on normal skin and appears as a nodule because vertical growth predominates over radial growth (Fig. 31–17).

3. *Lentigo maligna melanoma.* This arises in a lentigo maligna as a late event.

4. *Acral lentiginous melanoma.* This melanoma has a poor prognosis.

How often melanoma arises in a pre-existing nevus has been argued for years. A pre-existing nevus is seen in about 35 percent of malignant melanoma, but whether the melanoma arises in the nevus cells or in melanocytes in the adjacent epidermis is difficult to assess. The incidence of malignancy is greatest in congenital nevi and is particularly high if the nevus is large, for instance, the giant hairy nevus that can occupy a large area of skin such as the bathing trunk area.

Prognosis of Malignant Melanoma

Prognosis is related to stage of the tumor. Stage I, with no clinical evidence of metastasis, has a better prognosis than does stage II (regional lymph node metastases) or stage III (disseminated metastases). For stage I lesions, the single most important factor affecting prognosis is the thickness of the tumor as measured on the stained slide by a micrometer in the eyepiece of the microscope. Tumors less than 0.75 mm have a good prognosis; those over 1.5 mm often metastasize to nodes.

Malignant Neoplasms of Connective Tissue

Malignant tumors of fibrous tissue, nerve sheath, fat, and muscle are uncommon. The two most frequently encountered are a peculiar vascular tumor termed Kaposi's sarcoma and mycosis fungoides, a T-cell lymphoma.

Kaposi's Sarcoma

Kaposi's sarcoma is a malignant tumor of vascular endothelial cells. Two types of disease can

Figure 31–16 Superficial spreading type of malignant melanoma. Two black nodules of tumor are surrounded by superficial, barely palpable radial growth. Some areas are pigmented, whereas others are erythematous. The pale areas of depigmentation are due to tumor regression. Features leading to a diagnosis of malignancy in this pigmented lesion are the irregular shape, the nodules, the irregular pigmentation, the erythema, and the changing clinical appearance. (Courtesy of Dr. Wallace H. Clark, Jr.)

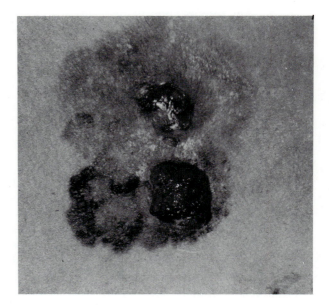

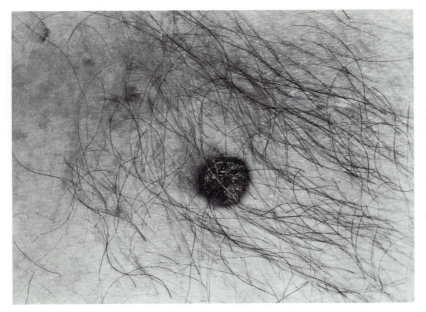

Figure 31–17 Nodular malignant melanoma. This black lesion had recently appeared and ulcerated. The clinical diagnosis was malignant melanoma. Before radical treatment of such a lesion, it must be biopsied or preferably totally removed if it is small. Histopathologic confirmation of the diagnosis is essential before there is definitive treatment of any malignant lesion. (Courtesy of Dr. Wallace H. Clark, Jr.)

be recognized. The type that occurs in eastern Europe runs a slow course evolving over many years. It generally first affects the legs and appears as areas of blue discoloration, first of one ankle and then the other. Later lesions appear on the skin at the wrists and elsewhere. Finally there is involvement of internal organs.

Kaposi's sarcoma that occurs in black Africans differs in many respects; it runs a more rapid course. Skin tumors, lymph node involvement, and generalized visceral spread soon bring the disease to a fatal termination. This is the type of Kaposi's sarcoma that is encountered in immunosuppressed patients such as those with AIDS (Fig. 31–18).

Mycosis Fungoides

Mycosis fungoides is a disease of later life. It is a primary T-cell lymphoma of the skin. Occasionally, the appearance of tumor masses is the first indication of the disease, and the course is rapidly downhill. More usually, the disease has a prolonged course lasting many years. At first the skin lesions are flat and closely resemble a dermatitis. Gradually the lesions become more indurated, and tumor masses develop. Involve-

ment of lymph nodes and internal viscera in this type of mycosis fungoides is a late event.

Other Neoplasms of the Skin

Many different types of tumors are known, but they are described in detail in specialized texts. Their diagnosis depends on histologic examination, a fact that emphasizes the necessity for submitting all excised tissue for pathologic examination. The experienced clinician is not surprised to find that an occasional lesion that is "typical" of a wart or mole turns out to be something quite different. Likewise, if a lesion worries a patient, a doctor, nurse, or physical therapist is usually ill-advised to reassure the person that there is nothing to worry about. The lesion should be examined carefully and treated appropriately. When there is doubt, it is better to have a small scar in 6 months' time than to have multiple metastases.

THE EFFECT OF SUNLIGHT ON THE HUMAN SKIN

Although a deep suntan is regarded by many as a status symbol indicative of health and

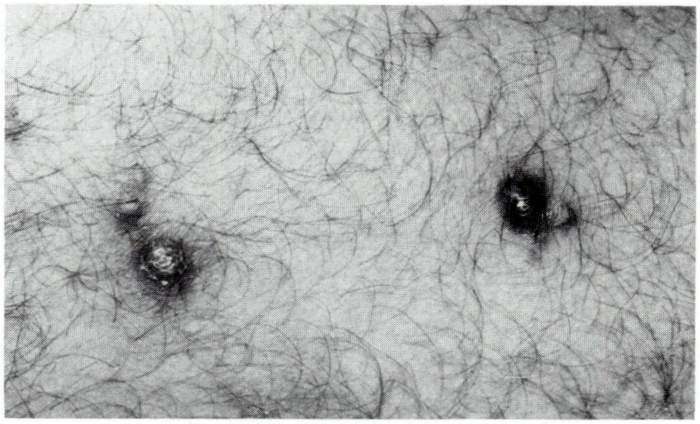

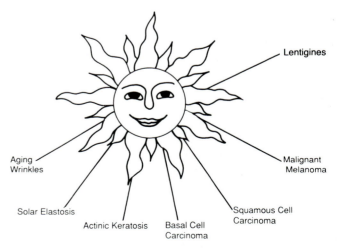

Figure 31–18 Kaposi's sarcoma. The patient had AIDS with widespread cutaneous deposits of Kaposi's sarcoma, here shown as purple nodules on the thigh.

wealth, the effect of sunlight on human skin is predominantly detrimental (Fig. 31–19). Prolonged exposure leads to dermal damage with deposition of elastic material. This contributes to the wrinkled appearance of aging skin; the accompanying lentigines (liver spots) are also an effect of sun exposure. A lentigo is a pigmented area of skin produced by an increase in the number of pigment-containing melanocytes. Epidermal damage leads to actinic keratoses, basal-cell carcinoma, squamous-cell carcinoma, and malignant melanoma. These effects are most marked in individuals with fair skin. They have blue eyes and are of northern European stock.

There are many effective sun-blocking lotions on the market, although there is still room for improvement because not all damaging wavelengths are filtered out. It is to be hoped that their use will lead to a decrease in the incidence of skin cancer. Nevertheless, the best advice is that if you want to look young, stay out of the sun!

Summary

- Diseases of the skin are grouped and classified on the basis of type of primary lesions: macule, patch, papule, papulosquamous, vesicle, bulla, pustule, ulcer, nodule, or tumor; distribution of lesions (localized, generalized, flexural, extensor, sun-exposed, other); and cause (familial, inherited, infective, hamartoma, neoplasm, other).
- Eczema or dermatitis is primarily an epidermal reaction; it may be due to a primary irritant or be immunologically mediated, be associated with atopy or sun exposure, or be idiopathic.
- Psoriasis and pityriasis are examples of papulosquamous eruptions.

Figure 31–19 The effect of sunlight on the human skin. Drawn by Susie Shin.)

Lentigines

Aging Wrinkles

Malignant Melanoma

Solar Elastosis

Actinic Keratosis

Basal Cell Carcinoma

Squamous Cell Carcinoma

- Ringworm (tinea) and candidiasis are common superficial fungal infections.
- Urticaria is a transient area of dermal inflammation and usually of a type I or type III immunologic reaction.
- Drug eruptions are very common and are of many types.
- Intraepidermal vesicles occur in acute dermatitis, herpes simplex, herpes zoster, and a group of acantholytic diseases, notably pemphigus.
- Erythema multiforme and bullous pemphigoid are subepidermal vesiculating diseases.
- Autoimmune antibodies are important in the pathogenesis and diagnosis of pemphigus and bullous pemphigoid.
- Nevi are hamartomas of the skin; melanocytic, vascular, and epidermal are the common types.
- Spitz and dysplastic nevi are important types of melanocytic nevi.
- Squamous-cell papillomas of the skin include seborrheic keratoses and common warts (verruca vulgaris).
- Malignant epidermal tumors are basal-cell carcinoma (which invades but does not metastasize) and squamous-cell carcinoma (which commonly arises in an actinic keratosis and ultimately metastasizes).
- Malignant melanoma starts as an *in situ* lesion and later becomes invasive. The prognosis is related to its location, its pattern of growth, its thickness, and its stage.
- Kaposi's sarcoma is a type of angiosarcoma that occurs in two forms; one type evolves very slowly, the other progresses rapidly. The latter type is found in patients with AIDS.

Selected Readings

Fitzpatrick, T. B., Poland, M. K., Suurmond, D., and Johnson, R. A.: Color Atlas and Synopsis of Clinical Dermatology. New York, McGraw-Hill, 1989.

Greene, M. H., et al.: Acquired precursors of cutaneous melanoma. The familial dysplastic nevus syndrome. N. Engl. J. Med. 312:91, 1985.

Koh, H. K.: Cutaneous melanoma. N. Engl. J. Med. 325:171, 1991.

Organs of Special Sense

After studying this chapter, the student should be able to:

- Describe the receptors for the sense of smell and taste.
- Describe the development of the eye.
- List the common causes of conjunctivitis.
- Define cataract and give six causes of this condition.

- Classify the types of glaucoma and describe the outstanding clinical and pathologic features of each type.
- Describe the pathogenesis and effects of retinal detachment and indicate the treatment.
- Classify the types of uveitis and describe the main features of acute iritis.
- Describe the important features of malignant melanoma of the choroid and retinoblastoma.
- List the common diseases of the external ear.
- Describe the clinical features, pathology, and complications of acute otitis media and chronic otitis media.
- Describe otosclerosis and Ménière's disease.
- Compare and contrast conductive deafness with sensorineural deafness.

The evolution of the organs of special sense has proceeded hand in hand with the adaptation of the cranial nerves to supply them. The sense of smell is served by special olfactory receptor cells present in the olfactory mucosa, an area of mucosa that lines the upper part of the nasal cavity. The olfactory receptor cells are bipolar neurons that have their short processes projecting from the surface of the mucosa; their long processes run with other axons to form a network and then are collected into branches that traverse the cribriform plate of the ethmoid bone and terminate in the olfactory bulb. Each branch has a pia-arachnoid sheath and a space that is continuous with the subarachnoid space. In fractures involving the anterior cranial fossa, the branches of the olfactory nerves can be torn, and because they do not regenerate, loss of the sense of smell (anosmia) results. There may also be a leakage of cerebrospinal fluid into the nose, and the pathway opened up provides an avenue of infection to the meninges. The sense of smell is difficult to test objectively; minor variations in ability to detect certain smells is inherited. The sense of smell is diminished if the nasal mucosa is swollen and covered by a thick layer of mucus that obstructs access of the processes of the receptor cells to the air in the nasal cavity. The

effect is usually temporary, as any sufferer from the common cold will testify. With chronic rhinitis, the loss may be permanent. The patient, in fact, usually complains of a loss of the sense of taste, because taste as ordinarily perceived is a combination of aromatic smells and impulses from the taste buds. Taste itself, comprising the sensation of salty, sweet, bitter, and sour, is detected in the mouth by specialized structures, the taste buds, supplied by the seventh, ninth, and tenth cranial nerves. The taste buds have a limited life span (about 10 days) and are continually being replaced.

The major organs of special sense, the eye and the ear, are described in more detail.

The Eye

A knowledge of the complex structure of the eye and the manner of its formation is essential for a proper understanding of ocular disease. This information is summarized in Figures 32–1 and 32–2.

Many human eye disorders are poorly understood because they are difficult to investigate adequately. Because it is not practicable to take biopsies of the eye, the early morphologic changes of disease cannot be examined. Sight is

so valuable an asset that the eye is preserved at all costs, and its removal is considered only when there is the threat of malignant disease, or when advanced disease has destroyed all useful function.

DEVELOPMENT OF THE EYE

A hollow bud of the forebrain (the primary optic vesicle) develops at the future site of the

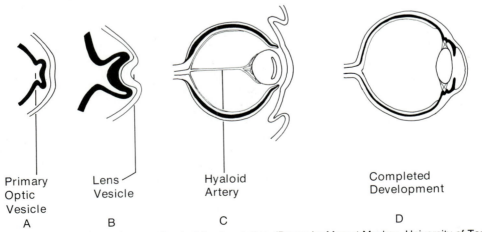

Primary
Optic
Vesicle

A

Lens
Vesicle

B

Hyaloid
Artery

C

Completed
Development

D

Figure 32–1 Development of the human eye. See text for description. (Drawn by Margot Mackay, University of Toronto, Faculty of Medicine, Department of Surgery, Division of Biomedical Communications, Toronto.)

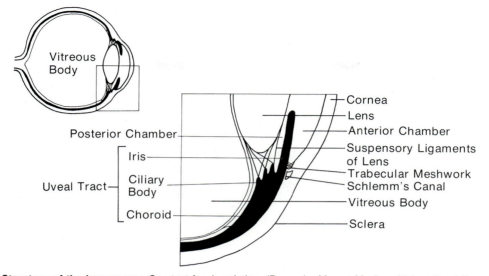

Figure 32–2 Structure of the human eye. See text for description. (Drawn by Margot Mackay, University of Toronto, Faculty of Medicine, Department of Surgery, Division of Biomedical Communications, Toronto.)

eye, and as it approaches the surface ectoderm, the vesicle becomes invaginated to form the optic cup (Fig. 32–1A and B). The outer layer of this cup remains thin and forms the pigment layer of the retina; the inner layer thickens to form the sensory layer. This complex structure contains the highly specialized rods and cones, which are sensitive to light, as well as nerve cells, whose long axons converge on the optic disk and constitute the optic nerve. It will be appreciated that the retina and the optic nerve are really part of the central nervous system, and if they are damaged in humans, regeneration is impossible.

The two layers of the retina never fuse firmly; it is in the plane between these layers that separation can occur in the condition known as *retinal detachment*. The optic vesicle induces the overlying ectoderm to thicken, invaginate, and form a vesicle that matures to form the lens (Fig. 32–1B and C). Meanwhile, mesoderm around the globe differentiates to form the choroid, which is a vascular connective tissue coat containing pigmented melanocytes and helps to nourish the retina. Anteriorly, mesoderm contributes to the formation of the ciliary body and the iris. The ciliary body, the iris, and the choroid are conjointly called the *uveal tract* (Fig. 32–2). The ciliary body contains muscle that is attached via the suspensory ligaments to the lens. Contraction of

this muscle changes the shape of the lens and therefore alters its focal length. The ciliary body has one other important function: its epithelium-covered processes secrete a clear fluid, the *aqueous humor*.

The ectoderm and mesoderm overlying the developing eye form the cornea. The bulk of this structure consists of orderly, parallel bundles of collagen embedded in a specialized ground substance and so arranged that the cornea is transparent. It forms the major lens component of the eye because refraction of light is greater at a tissue-air interface than at a tissue-fluid interface. The anatomic lens of the eye, surrounded by fluid, is of lesser importance in this regard. However, because the lens can change its shape under the influence of the muscles of the ciliary body, it provides a fine-adjustment mechanism by which one can focus quickly from distant to close objects. With advancing age, the lens becomes more rigid and less capable of adjustment; the person with this lens rigidity finds it difficult to focus on close objects and requires simple eyeglasses in order to read. This condition is called *presbyopia*.

The formation and disposal of aqueous humor are important because derangements of the mechanisms involved are a major cause of glaucoma and therefore of blindness. The fluid is secreted into the posterior chamber, flows forward between the iris and the lens, and then flows through the pupil and into the anterior chamber (Fig. 32–2). This cavity is bounded anteriorly by the cornea and posteriorly by the iris. Absorption of aqueous humor occurs at the angle of the anterior chamber. Fluid passes through a meshwork of connective tissue bundles, termed the *trabecular meshwork*, and ultimately drains into the canal of Schlemm, which encircles the globe at the corneosclerotic junction. From this canal, aqueous humor passes into the venous plexuses at the corneosclerotic junction.

DISEASES OF THE EYE

Conjunctivitis

Acute conjunctivitis can occur as a result of many irritants. Dust and chemicals can cause an acute primary irritant effect. There may be an allergic reaction, such as in patients who are hypersensitive to components of eyedrops (*e.g.*, atropine). A mild conjunctivitis is commonly associated with rhinitis in patients with hay fever. Acute inflammation may be a component of the exanthem of an acute viral disease such as measles, or it may be caused by a direct infection—bacterial, chlamydial, or viral (*e.g.*, herpes simplex and zoster). Mild attacks of acute conjunctivitis show a typical catarrhal inflammation, but severe infections are purulent and more serious, because there is a constant danger of corneal involvement (keratitis), ulceration, and subsequent scarring. Infections by streptococci, staphylococci, and gonococci are usually purulent. Ophthalmia neonatorum (acute conjunctivitis occurring during the first 10 days of life) is generally gonococcal.

Injuries and ulcerations of the cornea heal by scar tissue formation, and although the scar is made of collagen, it does not resemble the normal cornea because it is not transparent. Hence, involvement of the pupil area leads to blindness. Allografts from the eyes of cadavers are useful in treating this type of blindness. Similarly, they are of value in replacing the distorted, deformed corneas that are grouped as the *corneal dystrophies*.

Cataract

If the lens changes its physical characteristics and becomes opaque, the condition is called a *cataract*. The lens is a unique structure; it is of epithelial origin and is completely surrounded by a capsule that is in fact a basement membrane, and it has no blood supply. The hyaloid artery that nourishes it during development does not persist. Ionizing radiation, systemic administration of glucocorticoids, uveitis, trauma, hypocalcemia, galactosemia, and diabetes mellitus are among the numerous factors that can adversely affect the metabolism of the lens and result in its degeneration and opacification. Nevertheless, the most common cause of cataract formation is old age, and some degree of senile cataract is present in all persons over 70 years of age. Removal of these cataracts produces a welcome return of sight. Plastic lens inserts are being used with increasing frequency. Glasses can compensate for the loss of accommodation.

Glaucoma

The term *glaucoma* is applied to any condition in which the intraocular pressure is increased. It is an important condition because it causes blindness. The raised intraocular pressure impairs the blood supply to the sensory retina; in particular, the sensitive nerve cells and their long processes that form the optic nerve undergo degeneration. Two major types of glaucoma are recognized: primary and secondary.

Primary Glaucoma

This disease is typically bilateral and is not accompanied by any other obvious intraocular disease. Two types can be distinguished.

Open-Angle or Chronic Simple Glaucoma. This form of glaucoma is a slowly progressive disease of the elderly and is usually painless and symptomless until late in its development. An observant patient may notice a reduction in peripheral vision, but often the person's only complaint is that of difficulty in reading. The patient probably seeks eye care simply to request a stronger pair of reading glasses. For this reason, it is imperative that all patients older than middle age should have tests to detect glaucoma during the course of periodic examinations for a change in glasses. The intraocular pressure can be measured quite simply, and an ophthalmoscopic examination will often reveal another sign of glaucoma called *optic nerve cupping*. This is a name given to enlargement of the central depression normally seen in the optic disk. It is due to the pressure-induced atrophy of the optic nerve fibers. Untreated, this type of glaucoma results in blindness, whereas a patient whose glaucoma is detected early has a good prognosis for retaining vision. The pathogenesis of open-angle glaucoma is not known. The filtration angle of the anterior chamber is open, and subtle abnormalities in the trabecular meshwork have been described and are assumed to be the cause.

Angle-Closure Glaucoma. This disease typically affects women between 40 and 60 years of age. The anterior chamber is shallow, and this anatomic variation is responsible for the obstruction of the outflow of aqueous fluid at the angle of the anterior chamber.

This form of glaucoma is characterized by a series of episodes of raised intraocular pressure. An attack can be precipitated by dilating the pupil with eyedrops containing a mydriatic drug, *e.g.*, phenylephrine hydrochloride (Neo-Synephrine). In a subacute attack, there is blurring of vision; the patient sees *rainbow-colored halos around lights* because of the edema of the cornea. Later, if an attack of acute glaucoma occurs, there is *pain* (so severe that it can cause vomiting), edema and congestion of the eyelids and conjunctiva, clouding of the cornea, and rapid loss of vision. Vision may be saved if an acute attack is treated early, but persistent high pressure leads to a state of absolute glaucoma, a term used to describe the end result of any type of uncontrolled glaucoma. The eye is painful, blind, and stony hard. The eye ultimately shrinks and softens when the ciliary body stops producing aqueous fluid.

Secondary Glaucoma

In secondary glaucoma, which is usually unilateral, the increased pressure occurs as a complication of some other disease and results in mechanical obstruction of the flow of aqueous fluid from the ciliary body to the venous channels into which it ultimately drains. Generally, the obstruction is in the trabecular meshwork, which may become blocked by inflammatory exudate, fibrin, blood, or degenerate tumor. Uveitis, trauma (particularly if it is accompanied by bleeding), advanced cataracts, and tumors are causes of secondary glaucoma. Glaucoma may occur as a complication of glucocorticoid therapy, either when applied locally or when given systemically.

RETINAL DISEASE

Retinal Detachment. A retinal detachment is the result of a separation of the sensory retina from the pigmented layer; it can be produced by inflammatory exudate, hemorrhage, or tumor, *e.g.*, a malignant melanoma (Figs. 32–3 and 32–4). Nevertheless, the most common type of retinal detachment occurs in elderly persons, particularly those who are nearsighted. Thinning of the retina leads to the formation of a hole that is usually situated anteriorly and is identified by careful ophthalmoscopic examination. Often, the first symptoms of a detachment are flashing lights and "floaters," followed by the appearance of a dark shadow in the visual field. It is essential for the physician to make a correct diagnosis, to locate the site of the tear, and subsequently to seal this tear, either by directing a photocoagulating beam into the eye or by applying diathermy to the scleral surface. If the hole is sealed, the retina reattaches, and usually no further trouble occurs. However, if the hole is not sealed, the detachment will extend. Since the retina loses its blood supply from the underlying choroid, it soon undergoes degeneration and irreversible loss of function.

Retinopathy Due to Small-Vessel Disease. The sensory retina, which is the most important functional part of the eye, derives its major blood supply from the central artery of the retina. Disease of this vessel and its branches leads to degenerative changes in the retina itself.

Hypertensive Retinopathy. In systemic hypertension, there is thickening of the small retinal arterioles. As these vessels become occluded,

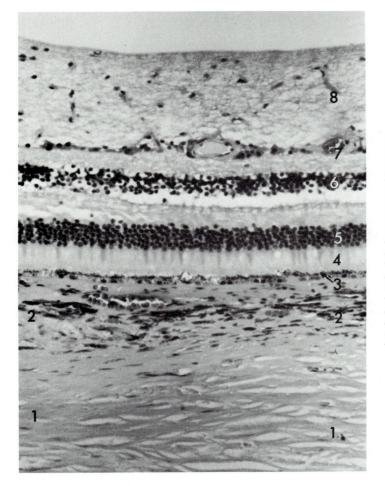

Figure 32–3 Normal retina, choroid, and sclera. Many layers have traditionally been described, but it must be appreciated that these are not layers in the sense that they can be separated from one another. They refer to zones with a different microscopic appearance. The following layers are shown: (1) Sclera, composed of dense collagen. (2) Choroid, more cellular and containing many blood vessels. (3) Pigment epithelium, formed from the outer layer of the optic cup. (4) Rod and cone layer consisting of rod- or cone-shaped light-sensitive processes of the photoreceptors. (5) Layer containing the nuclei of the rod and cone photoreceptors. (6) Nuclei of the bipolar cells; processes of these cells connect with the photoreceptors externally and with the ganglion cells internally. (7) Ganglion cell layer; the long axons of these cells enter the layer of nerve fibers and ultimately form the optic nerve. (8) Layer of nerve fibers (×250).

areas of the retina become infarcted. These lesions are called cotton-wool spots because of their fluffy appearance. Because the weakened vessels rupture, hemorrhages are frequent; in the acute malignant phase of hypertension, there is edema of the optic disk (*papilledema*) owing to raised intracranial pressure.

Diabetic Retinopathy. Diabetic retinopathy is the second leading cause of adult-onset blindness in North America. This form of retinopathy, along with the renal lesions, constitutes the most important change produced by small-vessel disease in diabetes mellitus. Diabetic retinopathy usually occurs in diabetics whose disease began in youth and who have been treated for many years with insulin. Now that these diabetics are able to survive into middle age, diabetic retinop-

athy is becoming much more common than in the days when the patients died while still young. The characteristic finding is saclike aneurysmal dilation of some of the capillaries. The abnormal vessels proliferate and bleed. Vision is lost because of vitreal scar tissue formation, which leads eventually to retinal detachment. As in hypertensive retinopathy, areas of infarction and inflammation also occur.

Retinoblastoma. This is the most common intraocular tumor of childhood. It is often present at birth and invariably manifests itself before the age of 4 years. In some patients, the disease is inherited as a mendelian dominant trait; this is one of the few human malignant tumors in which heredity has been proved to be important. Inherited cases are often bilateral.

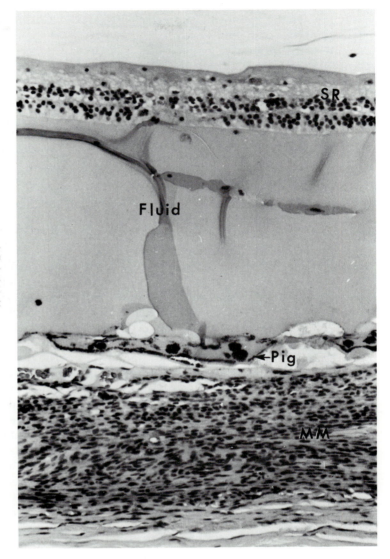

Figure 32–4 Retinal detachment in melanoma. The sensory retina (SR) is atrophic (compare with layers labeled 4 to 8 in Figure 32–3) and is separated from the pigment epithelium (Pig) by coagulated protein-containing fluid. The choroid is invaded by spindle-shaped cells of malignant melanoma (MM) (×250).

THE UVEAL TRACT

The uveal tract, which is the principal vascular connective tissue component of the eye, is the part most severely affected by inflammatory disease. The iris, ciliary body, or choroid may be affected separately (termed *iritis*, *cyclitis*, and *choroiditis*, respectively) or in combination. Iridocyclitis, or anterior uveitis, is a common combination. Choroiditis, or posterior uveitis, often occurs alone.

Both acute and chronic uveitis may be caused by known infective agents—bacterial, viral, pro-tozoal, and helminthic. Nevertheless, many examples have no known cause and present a grave problem in both diagnosis and treatment.

Acute Uveitis

Acute Suppurative Iridocyclitis. This disease is usually a complication of a penetrating injury; rarely, pyogenic organisms reach the eye during the course of a septicemia or a pyemia. The condition is serious because the infection can easily involve the entire eye (*panophthalmitis*) and can lead to loss of sight.

Acute Nonsuppurative Iridocyclitis. This is a poorly understood condition. Probably it is not caused by simple infection but rather results from some immune mechanism. It is a complication of many systemic diseases, *e.g.*, syphilis, sarcoidosis, lupus erythematosus, rheumatoid arthritis, and particularly ankylosing spondylitis.

Effects. In acute iritis, the eye becomes painful and red, and there is hyperemia of the deep vessels of the conjunctiva. The pupil is contracted, and the iris may be difficult to see clearly because of inflammatory exudate in the anterior chamber. This response causes the aqueous fluid to become hazy or milky and to produce a "flare" in the narrow beam of light from a slit lamp. Clumps of white cells and fibrin stick to the posterior surface of the cornea as white *keratic precipitates*. Fibrinous adhesions, which later organize to fibrous tissue, form between the iris and the lens posteriorly and between the iris and cornea anteriorly. These anterior adhesions (called *synechiae*) obliterate the filtration angle and can lead to glaucoma. To prevent these adhesions from forming and to break down any that are already present, atropine drops are used to dilate the pupil. Note that this treatment is diametrically opposite to that of angle-closure glaucoma, in which the pupil is made to constrict by the application of pilocarpine drops. Therefore, it is of vital importance to be able to distinguish between acute glaucoma and acute iridocyclitis.

Chronic Uveitis

This is a condition that may be caused by a known infective agent, *e.g.*, *Treponema pallidum* or *Mycobacterium tuberculosis*, but it is often idiopathic. Visual defects are also a feature, because with choroiditis, the sensory retina undergoes degeneration.

Neoplasms of the Uveal Tract

The important tumor of the uveal tract is the *malignant melanoma* derived from the melanocytes that are normally present. It is a disease of white adults and is therefore rare in most parts of Africa and in the Orient.

More than 80 per cent of ocular melanomas arise in the choroid, and they are often symptomless in the early stages. Elevation and detachment of the retina occur when the tumor breaks through the pigment epithelial layer of the retina and causes subretinal fluid to accumulate (Fig. 32–4). The patient's seeing a flash of light may be the first indication of an underlying tumor. A large tumor may cause glaucoma or may bleed into the vitreous. Malignant melanoma of the choroid is known to metastasize widely; but after the eye has been removed, about 60 per cent of the patients survive longer than 10 years. Even so, it is not uncommon for metastases to appear many years later. The classic, but uncommon, picture is that of a man with an artificial eye, who 30 years after enucleation presents with an enlarged liver that is due to secondary deposits from an intraocular melanoma.

The Ear

The sense of hearing is comparable to the sense of sight in that it is of immense practical and psychological value to humans. The vital sensory component of the ear in the cochlea, like the retina of the eye, is highly specialized; it cannot regenerate and cannot be biopsied without irreparable damage to the sense organ. Even at necropsy, the ear is technically extremely difficult to examine. Both the cochlea and the vestibular apparatus, which subserves the functions of balance and positional sense of the head, are deeply embedded in one of the hardest bones of the human body. It is therefore of little wonder that our knowledge of the pathology of these sense organs is fragmentary.

The ear is conveniently divided into three separate parts: external, middle, and internal. (Fig. 32–5).

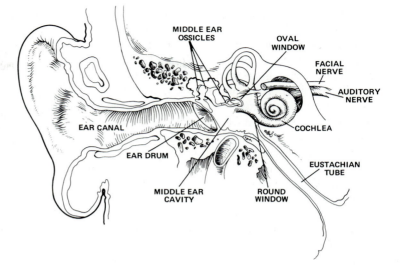

Figure 32–5 Diagrammatic section through the human ear. The ear canal terminates at the eardrum. From the eardrum, vibrations are transmitted by the three ossicles to the oval window. The round window is covered by a membrane and is designed to equalize pressures between the middle ear and the inner ear. Thus, when the stapes is pushed inward, the membrane in the round window bulges outward into the middle ear. (From Beadle, K.R.: Communication disorders: speech and hearing. *In* Bleck, E.E., and Nagel, D.A. [Eds]: Physically Handicapped Children. New York, Grune & Stratton, 1975. Reproduced by permission of Allyn & Bacon, Inc.)

THE EXTERNAL EAR

The external ear, with its pinna and external auditory meatus, terminates medially at the eardrum, or tympanic membrane. In general, diseases of the external ear closely resemble those of the skin. Inflammation, called *otitis externa*, is common and has many causes. It may be a component of seborrheic, atopic, or contact dermatitis. Mechanical irritation by the overzealous use of cotton swabs, hairpins, matchsticks, and other foreign bodies introduced by the patient is a common cause, because itching is a frequent symptom. The chemical irritation produced by an accumulation of earwax is another cause; disease is sometimes perpetuated by the ill-advised use of prescription ear drops containing irritating or sensitizing chemicals (*e.g.,* neomycin). Bacterial, viral, and fungal infection, particularly by *Aspergillus* species, can sometimes be incriminated. A chronic otitis externa should also lead to the suspicion of an underlying chronic otitis media associated with a perforated drum.

The specialized ceruminous glands can produce so much secretion that the earwax blocks the auditory canal. This is a common cause of conductive deafness and one that can be easily relieved with gratifying results.

Neoplasms

Squamous-cell carcinoma is the most common malignant tumor of the external ear and generally begins with an actinic keratosis. Basal-cell carcinoma is not uncommon; occasionally, tumors of the ceruminous glands are encountered.

THE MIDDLE EAR

The middle ear is a cavity filled with air and lined by respiratory type epithelium. The vibrations of the eardrum in its lateral wall are relayed by the *malleus* and *incus* to the *stapes* (these are the three auditory ossicles), which fits into the oval window and transmits impulses to the inner ear. Anteriorly, the cavity of the middle ear communicates with the pharynx via the *eustachian (pharyngotympanic) tube*, whereas posteriorly there is connection with the air spaces in the mastoid process of the temporal bone.

Acute Otitis Media

Acute infections of the middle ear (acute otitis media) are usually bacterial in origin, with *Streptococcus pyogenes*, the pneumococci, *Haemophilus influenzae*, and *Staphylococcus aureus* being the common causative organisms. The disease is most frequent in children and is often a complication of an upper respiratory streptococcal or viral infection. At this age, the shortness of the eustachian tube and blockage produced by swelling of the nasopharyngeal lymphoid tissue ("adenoids") are factors that encourage organisms in the nasopharynx to ascend into the middle ear and cause infection. Lack of IgA in the secretions has been suggested as another predisposing factor. The disease is characterized by severe pain in the ear combined with conductive hearing loss. The inflammatory exudate that collects in the cavity of the middle ear is at first clear but can later become purulent. The eardrum becomes inflamed and may rupture. This event is often averted by surgical incision of the tympanic membrane (a procedure called *myringotomy*), because a well-placed surgical wound heals better than one produced by spontaneous perforation.

Acute otitis media usually resolves with modern chemotherapy aided by surgical drainage, but the following complications should be noted:

1. *Adhesions.* These can affect the tympanic membrane and form between the three ossicles. Fibrinous at first, they are later replaced by scar tissue.
2. *Chronic otitis media.*
3. *Spread of infection.* Involvement of meninges, brain, and mastoid air cells is described later.

Chronic Otitis Media

This condition may occur insidiously or may follow an acute attack, especially if the treatment has been inadequate. Persistent ear discharge and deafness are the main features of chronic otitis media.

The chronic inflammatory reaction in the mucosa is sometimes characterized by the formation of inflammatory granulation tissue containing cholesterol crystals surrounded by foreign body giant cells. The condition is called a *cholesterol granuloma*. Fibrous adhesions can form in the cavity of the middle ear, and by involving the eardrum and the ossicles, these adhesions can lead to conductive deafness.

Complications of Otitis Media

Spread of Infection. In both acute and chronic otitis media, infection can spread to involve adjacent structures. The conditions resulting are described.

Mastoiditis. Involvement of the mastoid air cells is a particularly serious condition, since suppuration occurs and further spread of infection is a danger. The disease is characterized by generalized signs of an acute suppurative process (causing malaise and fever) together with pain, redness, and swelling of the bony mastoid prominence behind the ear.

Sigmoid Sinus Thrombosis. The sigmoid sinus, which is one of the large venous sinuses within the skull, lies in close proximity to the mastoid air cells. Thrombosis itself is serious, but when a thrombus is invaded by pyogenic organisms, the result is *pyemia*. Infected thrombi break off and lead to pulmonary pyemic abscesses.

Meningitis. Organisms either from the mastoid air cells or from the middle ear can penetrate the thin bone to reach the meningeal space and lead to meningitis.

Brain Abscess. If infection reaches the meninges, adhesions may limit the spread of infection and yet allow bacteria to continue their onward march into the brain, causing either a cerebellar or a temporal lobe abscess.

Seventh Nerve Paralysis. The seventh, or facial, nerve pursues a tortuous course through the middle ear and can be damaged either by otitis media or by surgery performed on a diseased ear.

Labyrinthitis. Infection can spread to involve the inner ear.

Epidermoid Cholesteatoma

This misleading name is applied to a cyst within the middle ear that is filled with keratin and lined by epidermis. The cyst is thought to be derived from squamous epithelium that migrates into the middle ear through a perforated eardrum. This condition is a serious complication of otitis media, because the cyst enlarges and produces local pressure effects as well as perpetuates a chronic infection. Surgical treatment is necessary for its cure.

Middle Ear Effusions

A persistent middle ear effusion can have many causes. In adults, it may follow obstruction to the eustachian tube, e.g., by a tumor in the nasopharynx. It can follow sudden pressure changes, as may occur during diving or air flight.

Mucoid otitis media, also called *glue ear*, is the most common cause of conductive hearing loss in children. It is the result of a previous otitis media in which partial resolution has left the middle ear filled with a thick, tenacious, gluelike fluid. Myringotomy, aspiration of the fluid, and insertion of a ventilation tube may be necessary if the fluid does not spontaneously resolve.

Otosclerosis

In this disease of unknown cause, parts of the petrous temporal bone are replaced by woven bone. The disease is probably quite common, but it becomes clinically apparent only if the stapes is involved. When this bone becomes ankylosed in the oval window, deafness ensues. The disease is particularly distressing because it is generally bilateral. It has been estimated that approximately 2 per cent of all white persons suffer from deafness from this cause. The plight of these victims of otosclerosis has indeed been the inspiration for the development of microsurgery in which the surgeon operates by using a binocular microscope.

Conductive Deafness

This term is applied to any form of deafness in which there is a failure of conduction of sound impulses from the external environment to the internal sensory organ of the inner ear. Blockage of the external auditory meatus, lesions in the middle ear, and otosclerosis are the main causes. Congenital abnormalities of the middle ear are a cause of congenital deafness (see later).

THE INNER EAR

This region of the ear is situated in the dense, petrous temporal bone and consists of a bony labyrinth containing the intercommunicating channels of the membranous labyrinth—the cochlea with its complex sensory auditory organ, and the semicircular canals, whose main function is concerned with balance and sense of position of the head. The cochlear nerve arises from the sensory end organs in the cochlea, joins with the vestibular nerve, and transmits to the brain stem impulses that are then relayed to the cortex.

Sensorineural Deafness

Deafness due to a defect of the sensory organ or the cochlear nerve is termed *sensorineural*. It is beyond the scope of this chapter to describe this in any detail, but the following causes are noteworthy.

Lesions in the Receptor Sensory Organ in the Labyrinth. The most common cause of degeneration of the sensory hair cells of the cochlea is old age (presbycusis). Likewise, loud noise, whether from an industrial source or from rock music, is capable of causing permanent damage. It is well recognized that certain drugs can damage the organ of hearing; the most important are aminoglycosides, *e.g.*, streptomycin and gentamicin. Other causes are fractures, vascular occlusion, and inflammatory lesions, which may be viral, *e.g.*, mumps. Intrauterine rubella is an important cause of *congenital deafness;* other causes include hypoxia (associated with hemolytic disease of the newborn and difficult deliveries) and hereditary factors. The diagnosis of hereditary deafness rests on obtaining a positive family history. It is important to recognize congenital and neonatal deafness early, because otherwise the child may be misdiagnosed as being mentally retarded and appropriate education will not be provided.

Nerve Damage. Schwannoma of the vestibulocochlear (eighth cranial, or auditory) nerve is an important cause.

Brain Damage. Diseases that involve the nerve cells and tracts that relay impulses from the cochlear nerve to the temporal lobe cortex may produce defects in hearing. These defects are not usually noted by the patient and can be detected only by special tests.

Ménière's Disease

The auditory component of the inner ear is closely connected with the organ of balance. This association is illustrated by the symptoms of *Ménière's disease*. The disease affects the membranous labyrinth as a whole and is characterized by paroxysmal attacks of intense giddiness (*vertigo*) associated with unilateral deafness and tinnitus (buzzing in the ears).

Summary

- Defects of smell and taste are difficult to investigate and are poorly categorized.
- Conjunctivitis can be caused by physical and chemical irritants, hypersensitivity reactions, and infection.
- In cataract, the lens becomes opaque; many causes are known, but the common type is associated with advanced age.
- Glaucoma is characterized by an increase in intraocular pressure and, unless relieved, can terminate in blindness. In the primary type, the angle of the anterior chamber of the eye may be open (chronic simple glaucoma) or shallow and obstructed (angle-closure glaucoma). Secondary glaucoma is a complication of some other intraocular disease.
- Retinal detachment involves separation of the sensory retina from the pigment layer.
- Retinopathy due to small-vessel disease is a feature of hypertension, particularly the malignant type, and diabetes mellitus.
- Uveitis is inflammation of the uveal tract; it has many causes.
- Common tumors of the eye are retinoblastoma in childhood and melanoma in adults.
- Acute otitis media is a bacterial infection common in children. Spread of infection can have serious consequences—mastoiditis, sigmoid sinus thrombosis, pyemia, meningitis, brain abscess, and labyrinthitis. Persistence of infection causes chronic otitis media and glue ear.
- Deafness may be conductive owing to blockage of the external auditory meatus, middle ear disease, or otosclerosis.
- Sensorineural deafness is due to damage to the auditory nerve, the cochlea, and rarely the brain. Cochlear damage or degeneration occurs with old age, Ménière's disease, exposure to loud noise, drugs, and infections, particularly rubella *in utero*.

Selected Readings

Hawke, M., and Jahn, A. F.: Diseases of the Ear. Philadelphia, Lea & Febiger, 1987.

Perkins, E. S., Marsh, R. J., and Hansell, P.: An Atlas of Diseases of the Eye. 3rd ed. Edinburgh, Churchill Livingstone, 1986.

Vaughan, D., Asbury, T., and Khalid, F. T.: General Ophthalmology: A Lange Medical Book. 12th ed. Norwalk, Conn., Appleton and Lange, 1989.

Central Nervous System

After studying this chapter, the student should be able to:

- Describe the overall structure of the central nervous system and the meninges.
- Distinguish between neurons and neuroglia.

- Describe the formation and fate of cerebrospinal fluid (CSF).
- Describe the effects of a raised intracranial pressure and list the common causes.
- Distinguish between subdural and extradural hemorrhage in terms of these factors:
  (a) site of bleeding;
  (b) source of bleeding;
  (c) causes;
  (d) clinical effects.
- Describe the cause and effects of subarachnoid hemorrhage.
- Outline the causes and effects of cerebral hemorrhage, cerebral thrombosis, and cerebral embolism; describe the differences between these three types of stroke.
- Define the following terms:
  (a) hemiplegia;
  (b) Babinski sign;
  (c) pseudobulbar palsy.
- Describe pyogenic meningitis with respect to the following factors:
  (a) causes;
  (b) clinical effects;
  (c) CSF findings;
  (d) Complications.
- List the causes of cerebral abscess.
- List the agents that cause aseptic meningitis and encephalitis.
- Discuss the pathology of multiple sclerosis and describe its clinical features.
- Give examples of poisons that cause permanent central nervous system damage.

- List the neurologic complications of the following
  conditions:
  (a) thiamine deficiency;
  (b) pellagra;
  (c) pernicious anemia;
  (d) alcoholism and liver disease.
- Outline the important features of
  (a) Alzheimer's disease;
  (b) Parkinson's disease;
  (c) Huntington's chorea;
  (d) motor neuron disease.
- Describe the outstanding features of the following:
  (a) psychomotor epilepsy;
  (b) petit mal epilepsy;
  (c) grand mal epilepsy;
  (d) jacksonian fit.
- List the causes of symptomatic epilepsy.
- Describe the types and effects of the common
  tumors that arise in the brain and in the meninges.

STRUCTURE AND FUNCTION

The central nervous system consists of nerve cells (*neurons*) and a supporting matrix of neuroglia in which they are embedded. It is richly supplied by blood vessels and is formed as a hollow tube during development, lined on the inside by *ependyma*, and covered on the outside by a layer of *pia mater*.

The neurons are the essential cells of the nervous system. They are formed by the differentiation of primitive neuroblasts during embryonic life and are unable to divide at a later time. Neurons possess the specialized property of excitability. They may be excited by a variety of stimuli to produce an impulse that is propagated throughout the cytoplasm of the cell. Since the axon of a nerve cell is often several inches or even feet in length, the impulse is conducted from one part of the body to another. *Excitability and conduction* are thus two characteristic properties of the nerve cells. Under abnormal circumstances, there may be changes in their excitability and conductibility. In the case of motor neurons, the effects may be obvious enough and may take the form of paralysis or convulsions. With sensory neurons, the equivalent effects can be anesthesia or pain and paresthesia (abnormal spontaneous feeling such as tingling).

The brain cannot be regarded as a simple organ comparable to the liver. Each cell is not equivalent to its neighbor and cannot be regarded as

performing a similar function. In fact, the brain acts as a series of systems, and the elaborate interrelationship between the vast number of neurons is responsible for the complex function and behavior of the nervous system of the higher animals. Not only is the nervous system responsible for receiving and transmitting all sensory stimuli from its peripheral receptor organs, but also its central organization is designed for interpreting all stimuli. At its highest level, the nervous system is responsible for consciousness, memory, and intelligence. Abnormalities in function in these areas produce diseases that at present are mainly in the realm of the psychiatrist and have no known morphologic features. This aspect of the abnormalities of the nervous system cannot be dismissed lightly, since it has been estimated that approximately one half of all patients occupying hospital beds do so because of psychiatric disease.

With regard to its efferent properties, the nervous system controls or influences all muscular activities in the body, including beating of the heart, contraction of the walls of blood vessels, function of skeletal muscle, ventilation of the lungs, and motility of the gastrointestinal tract. Furthermore, much glandular secretion is influenced by the nervous system. Indeed, there is scarcely any body structure or function that is not in one way or another under nervous control. It is therefore of little wonder that abnormal nervous function can produce many diverse effects. When no obvious structural change is present, these effects are classified as functional disease. Two examples of such diseases may be quoted. First, hysterical hyperventilation can be so marked that it causes respiratory alkalosis and tetany. Second, impotence in the male and frigidity in the female are most commonly related to psychological causes. Whether abnormal nervous function can produce structural abnormalities in other organs is a much debated point. Anorexia nervosa in humans and pseudocyesis (false pregnancy) in animals are good examples. In the first instance, individuals (usually young women) refuse to eat, become emaciated, and may ultimately die of starvation or one of its complications. In the second instance, the animal's hormonal balance is so changed that pregnancy is closely simulated. Whether a psychosomatic explanation is responsible for other disease states is less well substantiated. Nevertheless, diseases such as primary thyrotoxicosis, peptic ulcer, urticaria, and psoriasis seem to be aggravated by mental stress.

To understand the behavior of the nervous system in disease, one must first have knowledge of its normal structure and function. The student is therefore advised to consult the standard texts on neuroanatomy and physiology. It is necessary to have an overall picture of the organization of the major motor tracts before many diseases can be understood.

The Motor System

The large neurons of the frontal cortex give rise to long axons that constitute the corticospinal, or pyramidal, tract. This tract crosses to the opposite side in the medulla, and its axons control the anterior horn cells of the spinal cord. Damage to the pyramidal tract results in an *upper motor neuron paralysis*. Voluntary movement is lost, but the muscles retain their tone. The arms assume a flexed position, whereas the legs are extended. The tendon reflexes are brisk, and there is a Babinski sign.* If the anterior horn cells (or their cranial equivalents) or their axons in the peripheral motor nerve are damaged, a *lower motor neuron lesion* results. There is paralysis, but the muscles are flaccid, and the reflexes are absent.

The Meninges

There are three coverings, or meninges, of the central nervous system: (1) the *pia mater*, (2) the *dura mater*, and (3) the *arachnoid*. Their functions are described briefly.

1. The *pia mater* closely envelops the brain and spinal cord.
2. The *dura mater* is closely adherent to the bony and ligamentous protective housing provided by the skull, vertebral column, and con-

---

*A Babinski sign means that when the sole of the foot is stroked, the big toe dorsiflexes and there is fanning of the toes. Normally all the toes move down (plantarflex).

necting ligaments. The *falx cerebri* forms an extension of the dura mater that assumes a sickle shape and separates the two cerebral hemispheres. A similar extension of the dura mater forms the *tentorium*, which separates the cerebrum above from the cerebellum below.

3. The third layer of the meninges is the *arachnoid*, which forms a thin, translucent covering like a spider's web lying between the pia mater and the dura mater.

The space between the arachnoid and the pia mater is called the *subarachnoid space* and contains cerebrospinal fluid (CSF). This fluid originates in the choroid plexuses of the ventricles and finally escapes through the foramina in the roof of the fourth ventricle to reach the subarachnoid space. Ultimately, the fluid is absorbed in the arachnoid granulations of such major sinuses as the superior sagittal sinus.

INCREASED INTRACRANIAL PRESSURE

Effects

The rigid, bony enclosure of the brain is a necessary protective shield; its presence, however, has some attendant disadvantages. Any lesion that causes the brain to expand tends to cause a rise in intracranial pressure, which in turn increases the pressure in the veins. Initially, CSF and venous blood are displaced; but in due course, there is a marked rise in intracranial pressure and a rise in CSF pressure. The increased venous and capillary pressure combined with hypoxia leads to cerebral edema, which further increases the volume of the brain. The rise in intracranial pressure tends to reduce cerebral blood flow, but it activates reflexes that counteract this effect by raising the systemic blood pressure. An increase—sometimes to very high levels—in blood pressure is an important sign of raised intracranial pressure. In its turn, it reflexly slows the heart rate. *Routine care of a patient with a suspected intracranial lesion therefore involves monitoring of the blood pressure and the heart rate.*

Raised intracranial pressure is characterized by

headaches, often severe, that are probably caused by stretching of the meninges. *Vomiting* is common and is due to stimulation of the medullary centers. Progressive mental impairment may also occur. Pressure around the optic nerve impedes the venous return and causes edema of the optic nerve. The result is swelling of the optic disk, termed *papilledema*, which can be seen with an ophthalmoscope. Papilledema is an extremely important sign of increased intracranial pressure; it is also serious because, if allowed to persist, it causes atrophy of the optic nerve and ultimately blindness.

Causes

Edema of the Brain. Generalized edema of the brain is a feature of a raised arterial Pco_2, water intoxication (page 320), and encephalitis. Localized edema is a feature of injury and infarction of the brain.

Obstruction of the Flow of CSF. Any obstruction of the flow of CSF from the choroid plexuses in the ventricular system to the superior sagittal sinus causes an increase in the intracranial pressure. Blockage of the aqueduct of Sylvius, obstruction of the foramina in the roof of the fourth ventricle, and adhesions in the subarachnoid space (such as may occur after meningitis) are examples of such obstruction.

Meningitis. Any form of meningitis causes an increase in exudation of fluid into the CSF. In addition, there is obstruction due to the formation of fibrinous and subsequent fibrous adhesions, particularly at the base of the brain.

Space-Occupying Lesions. *Hemorrhage* into the brain, the formation of a *hematoma* (whether within the brain, subdural space, or extradural space), and the formation of an *abscess* or *tumor* are all examples of space-occupying lesions that ultimately cause an increase in intracranial pressure.

Apart from the generalized consequences of raised intracranial pressure, space-occupying lesions have additional effects. A lesion of one cerebral hemisphere causes such swelling that part of the hemisphere is pushed beneath the falx cerebri to the other side. *This is an example of herniation* (see Fig. 33–6). Furthermore, in such a

supratentorial lesion, the expanded brain pushes downward through the orifice of the tentorium cerebelli in such a way that the midbrain is forced downward and part of the cerebrum (the unci of the temporal lobes) herniates. This uncal herniation has several effects, which are described in the following paragraphs.

1. There is pressure on the third nerve. The nerve affected first is on the same side as the lesion, and this leads to dilation of the pupil. A *fixed, dilated pupil is an important sign of the herniation and occurs first on the same side as the cerebral lesion. Careful and frequent examination of the eyes is therefore an important part of the care of patients with suspected cerebral lesions, e.g.*, a head injury.

2. Downward movement of the brain stem tears small blood vessels. Compression of, or bleeding into, the midbrain and pons causes serious effects. When the upper brain stem is affected, there is loss of consciousness. With lower brain stem damage, there is respiratory arrest and death.

3. An expanding lesion of one cerebral hemisphere may force the midbrain to one side in such a way that a cerebral peduncle is pressed against the tentorium. This causes damage to the pyramidal fibers on the side opposite the cerebral lesion; since these fibers cross over in the medulla, there is an upper motor neuron paralysis of the body on the same side as that of the cerebral lesion.

Increased intracranial pressure can force the medulla and herniated cerebellar tonsils into the foramen magnum. The herniated tissue is cone-shaped, being molded by the conical foramen magnum. Hence, the common clinical term "coning" is used. The condition is serious because compression of the vital centers in the medulla causes respiratory arrest and death. *Coning can be precipitated by performing a lumbar puncture on a patient with a markedly raised intracranial pressure.* This procedure is therefore contraindicated under these circumstances.

TRAUMATIC LESIONS OF THE CENTRAL NERVOUS SYSTEM

An injury involving the jaws is sometimes accompanied by a much more important injury to the brain. Blows on the head produce damage to the region beneath the injury and to the brain at the opposite pole; this is the so-called *contre-coup injury*. Minor injuries cause petechial hemorrhages and traumatic inflammatory edema, whereas more severe injuries may actually tear (*lacerate*) the brain, and hemorrhage may be of sufficient magnitude to cause death.

Subdural Hemorrhage. Sometimes after an injury, one of the poorly supported bridging veins that pass from a venous sinus to a cerebral vein is torn, and a subdural hematoma forms. Less commonly, a venous sinus itself is disrupted, as when there is a fracture of the base of the skull. The hematoma tends to enlarge, partly because of repeated bleeding and partly because it imbibes fluid. The *chronic subdural hematoma* so formed acts as a space-occupying lesion. The injury that causes this type of lesion is often relatively mild, and in an elderly or alcoholic patient, it may be completely overlooked. Headaches and other signs and symptoms of raised intracranial pressure develop several weeks later.

Extradural Hemorrhage. This form of hemorrhage occurs when the *middle meningeal artery* is torn; it is usually in association with a fracture of the skull involving the temporal region. Unconsciousness may occur immediately after the injury, but the patient often recovers and feels well for a few hours. This *lucid interval* is deceptive. Presently, as the bleeding proceeds, increasing signs of raised intracranial pressure appear; this is followed by coma and death. It is evident that all persons who have sustained a head injury, except the most trivial, should be carefully examined and kept under observation for 24 hours. Even if they smell of alcohol, they should not be left unattended or allowed to die either at home or in a prison cell.

NONTRAUMATIC CEREBROVASCULAR DISEASE

Subarachnoid Hemorrhage. This condition is not uncommon in persons between the ages of 20 and 50 years. The hemorrhage usually stems from a ruptured aneurysm of one of the major cerebral arteries in the area of the circle of Willis. The aneurysms lie in the subarachnoid space and are from 0.5 to 1.0 cm in diameter; because of this size, they are often called *berry aneurysms* (Figs. 33–1 and 33–2). They are thought to arise at the site of congenital defects in the elastic coat of the arteries. Sometimes they are multiple. Subarachnoid hemorrhage may also result from the rupture of a congenital arteriovenous malformation.

Cerebral Hemorrhage, Thrombosis, and Embolism. Atherosclerosis and hypertension both predispose to *cerebral hemorrhage* (sometimes called *cerebral apoplexy*). Commonly, the site is from a branch of the middle cerebral artery. The area of brain affected is in the region of the basal ganglia, the external and the internal capsule. The immediate effects of hemorrhage tend to be more severe than are those produced by thrombosis. In both, there is the clinical picture commonly called a "stroke."

With *hemorrhage*, there is usually sudden loss of consciousness. As blood disrupts the substance of the brain, coma deepens and death ensues. This course is not inevitable, however, and the bleeding may stop.

With *thrombosis*, the patient may experience prodromal or warning signs (*e.g.*, transient hemiplegia, blindness in one eye, speech defect, or confusion) before the onset of the stroke. The stroke itself often occurs during sleep; although consciousness may be lost, this effect is not invariable. Sometimes evidence of progressive damage may be apparent over a period of several days. Apparently, this is due to spread of the thrombosis and hence is called a *thrombotic stroke in evolution*. Thrombosis causes *infarction*, which can itself lead to later hemorrhage in the damaged area (Fig. 33–3). There is considerable edema surrounding the infarct, so that the initial functional effects are greater than the area of infarction would indicate. The infarct caused by thrombosis is usually pale; in those patients who survive, the area softens (a process called *colliquative necrosis*). The microglial cells enlarge, become phagocytic, and appear as large, foamy macrophages. The damaged nerve fibers are not replaced, and the area heals by proliferation of astrocytes, which produces a *glial scar*. The area of brain thus collapses, and sometimes a central cyst remains where once there was brain tissue.

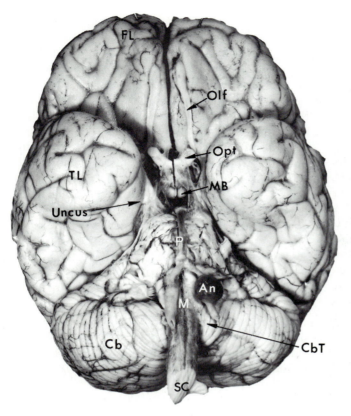

Figure 33–1 Berry aneurysm. An unruptured aneurysm (An) is seen to be arising from the left vertebral artery. Note the following normal structures: FL, frontal lobe; TL, temporal lobe; Olf, olfactory nerve; Opt, optic nerve; MB, mamillary body; P, pons; M, medulla oblongata; SC, spinal cord; Cb, cerebellum; CbT, cerebellar tonsil; and uncus. (Courtesy of Dr. N.B. Rewcastle, Chairman, Department of Pathology, University of Calgary, Alberta, Canada.)

Note that any nerve cells destroyed are not replaced.

Infarcts are sometimes found in the absence of detectable thrombosis of a cerebral artery. The explanation is generally to be found in the extracranial arterial supply to the brain—the carotid and vertebral arteries. Severe stenosis of these vessels can seriously imperil the blood supply to the brain. Under these circumstances, infarction is to be found in the "watershed" areas that are at the boundary zones where the vascular territories of two cerebral vessels join.

Cerebral embolism is a common cause of stroke. The embolus generally originates from the heart, and the onset of the stroke is sudden.

Clinical Features of Stroke. In cerebral hemorrhage, thrombosis, and embolism, the clinical picture depends on the size and location of the area of brain affected. With a severe stroke, consciousness is lost, but recovery gradually sets in, and consciousness then returns. At first, speech is often impaired, but as time passes, it returns to normal. The neurologic findings depend on the area of brain affected. Commonly, the long cerebrospinal tracts in the internal capsule are destroyed, and the picture is that of *hemiplegia*—loss of voluntary movement on the side of the body opposite to that of the cerebral lesion (upper motor neuron lesion). Destroyed neurons are never replaced, and lost axons are never regenerated. Nevertheless, considerable clinical recovery can be expected after a stroke, as inflammation and edema associated with the damaged area subside. Good nursing and physical therapy can do much to tide the patient over the severe initial period. For example, during this time, bedsores and urinary tract infections should be prevented. Good oral hygiene and maintenance of adequate fluid and food intake are also important. Finally, encouragement and physical exercises can do much to minimize the effects of the ultimate paralysis or other neurologic losses.

Quite apart from acute episodes of thrombosis

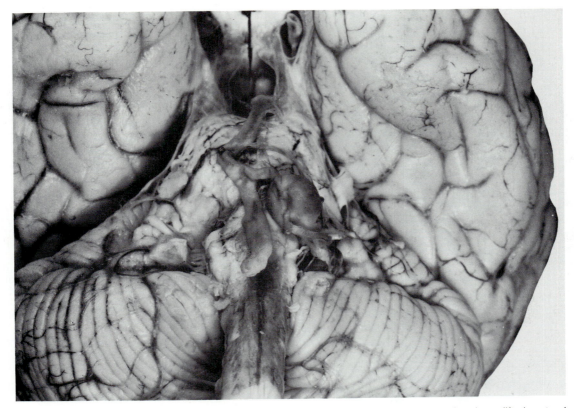

Figure 33–2 Berry aneurysm. This is the same specimen as in Figure 33–1, but the aneurysm has been lifted up to show its connection with the vertebral artery. (Courtesy of Dr. N.B. Rewcastle, Chairman, Department of Pathology, University of Calgary, Alberta, Canada.)

or infarction, cerebral atherosclerosis can lead to multiple, bilateral ischemic lesions in the brain. The characteristic mental deterioration of old age is one effect of the lesions, but if they are extensive, there may be severe bilateral damage to the corticospinal tracts. When bilaterally innervated muscles such as those of the tongue and pharynx are affected, the condition is called *pseudobulbar palsy.*

INFECTIONS OF THE CENTRAL NERVOUS SYSTEM

Pyogenic Bacterial Infections

Pyogenic bacteria may produce a diffuse infection of the subarachnoid space, a condition that is called *meningitis*, or they may produce a local-ized suppuration in the brain substance, a condition called *cerebral abscess.*

Pyogenic Meningitis

Mode of Infection. Two routes are common.
Blood-borne. *Haemophilus influenzae* and the meningococcus gain entry to the blood, presumably from an infection in the upper respiratory tract. The route is probably via the choroid plexuses, where the organisms are filtered out of the blood during the course of a septicemia. The infection spreads through the ventricular system and reaches the subarachnoid space in the region of the basal cisterns. It is here that the most severe effects are seen. The pia mater and the arachnoid are acutely inflamed, and there is a massive neutrophil and fibrinous exudate into the subarachnoid space. With modern chemo-

Right   Left

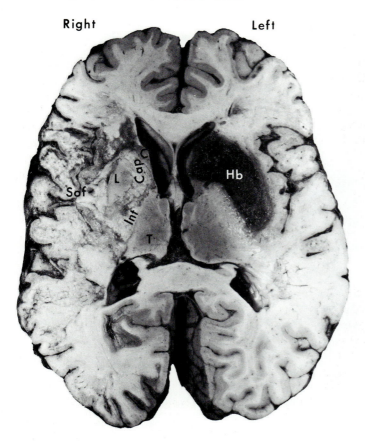

Figure 33–3 Cerebral softening and hemorrhage. The brain has been sectioned horizontally and is viewed here from below. There is severe damage. On the right-hand side, there is extensive softening (Sof). Note the shrunken appearance of the affected area, which extends outward to involve the gray matter of the cerebral cortex. The internal capsule (Int Cap) is severely affected. It lies between the lentiform nucleus (L) and the caudate nucleus (C) anteriorly and between the lentiform nucleus and thalamus (T) posteriorly. Loss of its corticospinal fibers leads to an upper motor neuron lesion of the opposite side of the body. The patient had had a stroke 3 months before death. This attack, which had been attributed to a cerebral thrombosis, left the patient with a left hemiplegia. She subsequently had another stroke involving the opposite side. Note the extensive hemorrhage (Hb) that has occurred into the area of softening on the left side. (Courtesy of Dr. N.B. Rewcastle, Chairman, Department of Pathology, University of Calgary, Alberta, Canada.)

therapy, the patients often survive; but even then, the exudate may undergo organization, and the foramina in the roof of the fourth ventricle may become blocked. Cerebrospinal fluid accumulates in the ventricular system, which expands accordingly; this is one mechanism by which *hydrocephalus* develops. In the young child, the pressure exerted on the developing bones leads to a tremendous enlargement of the vault of the skull.

Local Spread. Meningitis may follow the spread of infection from the middle ear or mastoid air cells, sites of infection that are common in childhood. It is also a complication of a fractured skull in cases in which the wound is exposed to the exterior or to the nasal cavity. Fracture of the cribriform plate of the ethmoid bone is followed by an escape of CSF into the nose (a condition called *cerebrospinal rhinorrhea*). Meningitis may follow.

Clinical Features. Fever, severe headache, disorders of consciousness, and convulsions (particularly in children) are the outstanding symptoms. Stiffness of the neck and resistance to forward bending are the outstanding signs. The diagnosis is made by performing a lumbar puncture (recall the dangers of this procedure in a patient with raised intracranial pressure). The pressure of the fluid is increased, as is its protein content. The glucose level is low, because the organisms ferment the sugar. Numerous polymorphs are present, and organisms can be demonstrated either directly on a smear or by culture.

Cerebral Abscess

Mode of Infection. As with meningitis, there are two modes of infection.

Blood-borne. Patients with chronic chest infections (empyema, lung abscess, and bronchiectasis) sometimes develop a cerebral abscess. Presumably, the infection is blood-borne; an alternative explanation is that spread occurs from an infected nasal air sinus, a common accompaniment of chronic chest suppuration.

Local Spread. As with meningitis, local spread occurs from an infected middle ear or nasal air sinus (Fig. 33–4).

Viral Infections

Viral Meningitis

Many viruses can cause a meningitis, including echoviruses, coxsackieviruses, mumps virus, Epstein-Barr virus, and herpes simplex virus. Sometimes no causative agent can be identified, and the term aseptic meningitis or acute lymphocytic meningitis is used. The symptoms are similar to those of pyogenic meningitis, but they are less severe. The CSF contains lymphocytes rather than polymorphs. An important point of differentiation is that *the glucose level is normal.*

Viral Encephalitis

The syndrome of encephalitis resembles that of aseptic meningitis, but to it is added evidence of cerebral damage: coma, cranial nerve paralysis, and hemiplegia, for example. Viruses causing encephalitis include herpes simplex virus, cytomegalovirus, arboviruses, and human immunodeficiency virus. Polioviruses and rabies viruses cause distinctive diseases. Subacute sclerosing panencephalitis is a slowly progressive disease caused by the measles virus. It resembles the spongiform encephalomyopathies, a group of diseases caused by slow viruses (see also Chapter 9).

DISEASES AFFECTING THE MYELIN SHEATH

The major nerve fibers both within the central nervous system and in the peripheral nervous system have a myelin sheath, which acts as an insulating covering, thereby aiding in transmission of impulses in the axon. Damage to the myelin sheath leads to impaired conduction,

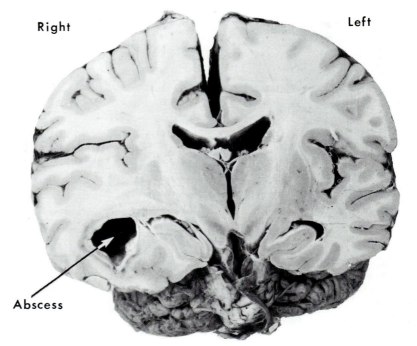

Figure 33–4 Cerebral abscess. Sagittal section of the brain shows a large abscess in the right temporal lobe. When the brain was sectioned, pus drained from the abscess, which now appears to be empty. Owing to chronic otitis media, the patient had a chronic discharge from his right ear. He developed headaches and stiffness of the neck and was moribund by the time he reached the hospital. Necropsy revealed an extradural abscess overlying the roof of the right middle ear. Infection had spread into the brain. (Courtesy of Dr. N.B. Rewcastle, Chairman, Department of Pathology, University of Calgary, Alberta, Canada.)

Right

Left

Abscess

even though the axon itself remains intact. Two groups of disorders are recognized:

1. *The demyelinating diseases*, of which multiple sclerosis is by far the most frequent.

2. The *dysmyelinating diseases* or *leukodystrophies*, in which myelin formation is impaired.

Multiple Sclerosis

Multiple Sclerosis is a chronic disease characterized by exacerbations and remissions that often extend over many years. The brain and spinal cord show the development of well-circumscribed foci (plaques) of demyelination (Fig. 33–5). These plaques occur in all parts of the central nervous system, but they are more frequent in certain areas. During the acute phases, there is an inflammatory reaction and severe impairment

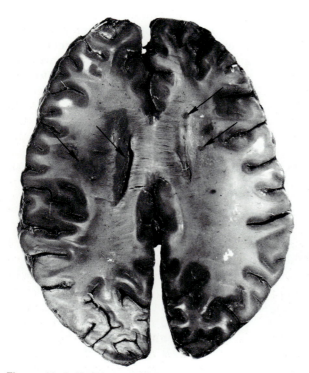

Figure 33–5 Multiple sclerosis. Horizontal section of the brain shows many areas of demyelination (arrows). Since it is the myelin sheaths of nerve fibers that give the white matter its color, areas of demyelination appear gray and superficially resemble the gray matter. (Courtesy of Dr. N.B. Rewcastle, Chairman, Department of Pathology, University of Calgary, Alberta, Canada.)

of nerve conduction. The nerve axons are generally preserved, and a considerable degree of functional recovery occurs after each phase. Depending on the site of damage, multiple sclerosis first manifests itself as sudden impairment of vision, inability to speak clearly (dysarthria), cerebellar dysfunction, or paralysis due to pyramidal tract damage. Alteration in emotional state and bladder dysfunction also occur. Each acute episode is followed by recovery, occasionally complete; but more frequently there is some residual damage, so that with the passage of years, the patient ultimately becomes quite disabled.

Other Demyelinating Diseases

Several diseases are known that resemble multiple sclerosis but are more acute. Demyelination is also a feature of the encephalitis that occasionally follows certain viral infections, such as after vaccination for smallpox and rabies, as well as after certain naturally occurring viral diseases such as rubella.

The Leukodystrophies

The leukodystrophies constitute a group of rare diseases in which there is a defect in the formation of myelin. Usually manifested during infancy or childhood, they are familial.

TOXIC, DEFICIENCY, AND METABOLIC DISORDERS

The brain is a very active metabolic organ. Although it represents about 2 per cent of the body weight, it is responsible for 20 per cent of the body's resting oxygen consumption. It is not surprising, therefore, that it can easily be affected adversely by many agents that interfere with metabolism. A few of these are listed.

Poisons. Lead and mercury are examples of agents that can cause permanent brain damage. Likewise, poisoning by carbon monoxide can cause necrosis of the basal ganglia and can lead to extrapyramidal syndromes, which are described later.

Deficiency of Oxygen (Hypoxia). The brain is extremely sensitive to oxygen deprivation. Even short periods of hypoxia can produce permanent damage.

Vitamin Deficiencies

Vitamin B₁ (Thiamine) Deficiency. In some patients, vitamin B_1 deficiency causes focal areas of necrosis in the brain. In North America, the condition is usually associated with alcoholism. Several syndromes can occur. For example, in *Wernicke's disease*, there is impaired mentation and unsteadiness, which, when severe, makes the patient unable to stand or walk without help. Paralysis of the external eye muscles resulting in double vision (*diplopia*) is common, as is polyneuritis. Wernicke's disease may be combined with *Korsakoff's psychosis*, in which there is grave mental impairment with inability to learn new facts and severe loss of memory (*amnesia*). The patient may fill in memory gaps by fictitious stories, a condition known as *confabulation*.

Pellagra Encephalopathy. This condition is described in Chapter 15.

Subacute Combined Degeneration of the Spinal Cord. This condition is due to vitamin B_{12} deficiency and accompanies pernicious anemia.

Metabolic Encephalopathies

Hepatic Encephalopathy. Degeneration of neurons is responsible for the mental deterioration encountered in chronic liver disease (Chapter 24).

Chronic Alcoholism. The pathetic state of some chronic alcoholics is a combined effect of alcohol, vitamin deficiency, and liver damage.

Hypoglycemia. Poisoning with insulin causes hypoglycemia, coma, convulsions, and death. Permanent neuronal loss can occur in those who survive; the changes resemble those of hypoxia.

DEGENERATIVE NERVOUS DISEASES

There are many diseases of the nervous system in which neuronal degeneration occurs for no known reason. In some of these conditions, there is a strong hereditary factor; in others, the degeneration is probably due to slow virus infection (*e.g.*, in kuru and Creutzfeldt-Jakob disease; see

Chapter 9). A few common examples of degenerative nervous diseases are described.

Alzheimer's Disease. Deterioration of intellectual capacity (called dementia) is one of the great problems facing modern society, since it places a great financial as well as emotional burden on the family, the health services, and society as a whole. Dementia affects one person in every six over the age of 65 years, and the most common cause is Alzheimer's disease. Early signs are inability to learn new material and loss of short-term memory. In due course, there is relentless loss of intellect, mental ability, and physical capability. This results in death from intercurrent infection or other complication of the bedridden state. On pathologic examination, the brain shows loss of neurons and in addition "senile plaques," which include microscopic deposits of amyloid material. The cause of Alzheimer's disease is unknown; among the many suggested possibilities are chronic poisoning with aluminum and infection with some slow virus.

Senile Dementia. Cerebral atrophy with compensatory dilation of the ventricles is a common event in old age and is the second most common cause of dementia. Sometimes it is combined with Alzheimer's disease.

Parkinson's Disease. This common disease is due to selective degeneration of neurons in the substantia nigra. Axons from this part of the brain pass to the basal ganglia and influence them by releasing dopamine. Release of the basal ganglia from this influence results in the symptoms of Parkinson's disease. The patient's muscles become rigid, the face is expressionless, and movement becomes difficult. A fine tremor completes the picture; "pill rolling" movements of the fingers are characteristic. As noted by Parkinson in his original description in 1817, the patient tends to bend forward, so that when walking, he or she has a tendency to change to a running pace. The senses and intellect remain unimpaired. The whole picture is termed the *extrapyramidal syndrome* and is also seen after encephalitis (postencephalitic parkinsonism), vascular ischemic episodes, and poisoning with carbon monoxide.

Huntington's Chorea. Patients with this disease exhibit basal ganglia degeneration as well as cortical neuronal loss. Bizarre grimacing and uncontrolled irregular jerking movements (*chorea*) are combined with progressive dementia in this disease, which is inherited as a mendelian dominant trait.

Motor Neuron Disease. Primary degeneration of the pyramidal tracts, the anterior horn cells, and their cranial equivalents can occur either singly or in combination to produce a variety of syndromes.

EPILEPSY

Epilepsy is a common disease, affecting about 1 per cent of the population. It is characterized by sudden episodes of an abnormal electric disturbance in the brain. Each episode, called a seizure, may affect a localized area of the brain and cause an upset in motor or sensory function of the brain. This is called a *partial or focal seizure.* The disturbance may spread throughout the brain, and the seizure becomes generalized. In some forms of epilepsy, the seizures appear to be generalized from their inception, seemingly without a focal origin (*primary generalized seizures*).

Partial or Focal Seizures

In *simple partial seizures,* the disturbance affects a localized area of brain and the effects are similarly localized. Consciousness is not lost. If a motor area is affected, there is rhythmic twitching of a group of muscles. In *Jacksonian seizures,* the movement commences in the hand and steadily spreads to involve the arm and face on the same side; it may become generalized. If a sensory area is involved in focal epilepsy, there are sensory phenomena, such as tingling in the affected area. Sometimes there are auditory or visual hallucinations. In the *déjà vu* phenomenon, there is a strange feeling of familiarity and of having experienced something similar before.

In *complex partial seizures,* the subject loses contact with the environment and experiences a variety of abnormal feelings—an unusual smell or a sudden emotional disturbance, such as a feeling of *déjà vu.* There may be repeated rhythmic motor activity, such as smacking the lips; even complex activity, such as playing a piano, may take place. This type of epilepsy is often called "temporal lobe" or "psychomotor" epilepsy because the seizure activity is believed to commence in the temporal lobe, commonly the hippocampus or the limbic system. When the seizure ceases, consciousness may not be regained for several hours. Generally, there is complete amnesia for the attack; however, some recollection of the initial events may remain and provide an aura that heralds the next attack.

Secondary generalization of partial seizures may occur and is generally manifested as convulsions and loss of consciousness. The presence of an aura or evidence of a focal lesion, such as twitching of a group of muscles or aphasia, distinguishes this condition from primary generalized seizures.

Primary Generalized Seizures

In the common *tonic-clonic* or *grand mal seizure,* the attack comes on suddenly, although the patient may experience a vague uneasy feeling preceding it. The attack is characterized by generalized tonic muscular spasms, and the patient may fall to the ground and sustain injury; the tongue may be bitten. As air is forced through the glottis, there may be a characteristic cry. Prolonged contraction of the respiratory muscles results in cyanosis. Incontinence of urine and feces is common. After a few seconds, the limbs exhibit rhythmic clonic contractions, and after a variable time, the muscles relax. The patient remains unconscious for minutes or even hours and later has no memory for the event, except perhaps for the aura that preceded it.

Absence seizures or *petit mal* epilepsy commonly commences in children and consists of a very brief period of loss of consciousness or awareness of the surroundings. Multiple, frequent attacks, each lasting a few seconds, are common; the patient does not fall to the ground and makes an instant recovery. Hence, the attacks may be described by the patient as "fainting attacks" or "dizzy spells" and may not be recognized as epilepsy.

Causes of Epilepsy

In the common *idiopathic epilepsy*, no obvious cause is apparent, although some genetic influence may play a part because the disease is more common in certain families.

In *symptomatic epilepsy* some discernible event or local abnormality of the brain appears to trigger the seizures. Seizures can be produced even in normal individuals if a sufficiently strong stimulus is applied, e.g., an electric current applied to the brain or insulin-induced hypoglycemia. Of interest, both of these maneuvers have been used for the treatment of depressive psychoses. The following possible causes of symptomatic epilepsy should be noted:

1. *Generalized and metabolic conditions.* Hypoglycemia, hypocalcemia, uremia, water intoxication, and cerebral hypoxia are associated with seizures. Withdrawal of some drugs, particularly alcohol and barbiturates, is another cause. In infants and young children, fever is a common cause (fever convulsions); in about one third of subjects, the seizures may continue in later life as epilepsy not precipitated by fever.

2. *Localized brain disorders.* A wide range of abnormalities can act as foci for the initiation of epilepsy, and the likely causes depend on the age of the patient. In infancy, asphyxia, birth injuries, and congenital abnormalities are of primary importance. Seizures are a feature of *cerebral palsy.* This is the popular name for a condition that is generally nonprogressive and present since infancy. Spasticity caused by upper motor neuron damage and dysarthria are the main features. Athetosis, characterized by jerky movements, and facial grimacing are common. Cerebral palsy is not a single entity but, rather, is a syndrome caused by a variety of processes, for example, birth trauma, infection, and genetic defects. In childhood, epilepsy is associated with intracranial infections, such as meningitis and encephalitis; in young adults, head trauma predominates, causing epilepsy either during the acute episode or later, when a scar develops. Over the age of 30 years, neoplasms, either glioma or metastatic carcinoma, become an important cause. Tumors should always be considered when epilepsy develops in an adult for the first time. In the over-50 age group, neoplasms are still important. However, cerebrovascular lesions become more frequent; embolism, infarction, or hemorrhage, even when small, can initiate a seizure.

Case History I

The patient had had no previous history of epilepsy; he suffered his first attack at the age of 58 years. It started with twitching of the left foot, and then the involuntary movements spread to involve the whole leg, the left arm, and finally the whole body. With the onset of a generalized convulsion, the patient lost consciousness. This type of focal motor seizure that steadily extends to involve adjacent areas is called jacksonian epilepsy. Examination of the patient at this time revealed no abnormal neurologic signs. Radiography and electroencephalography showed no evidence of a focal brain lesion. Although a diagnosis of carcinoma of the lung was considered, sputum examination was negative for malignant cells, and a chest radiograph was normal. Nevertheless, the epileptic attacks continued. On several occasions, the patient bit his tongue and was incontinent. Three months after the first attack, the patient suddenly developed a left-sided hemiplegia. Carotid artery thrombosis was considered, but arteriography failed to confirm the diagnosis. Radiographs, however, showed deformity of the right lateral ventricle. The patient died suddenly. A necropsy revealed a glioblastoma multiforme (see Fig. 33–6).

NEOPLASMS OF THE CENTRAL NERVOUS SYSTEM

Primary Tumors. The most common type of primary tumor of the central nervous system is derived from glial tissue and is called a *glioma*; several types are described, the one occurring most frequently being derived from astrocytes (Fig. 33–6). Well-differentiated astrocytomas invade slowly, but the poorly differentiated tumors (grade III and grade IV astrocytoma, also called glioblastoma multiforme) are more malignant and kill rapidly. Although all gliomas are locally invasive and may metastasize within the central nervous system, one curious feature of these tumors is that *none of them ever produces distant metastases.* In spite of this, the prognosis is usually poor, because gliomas are difficult to remove surgically.

The *meningioma* is a benign tumor arising from the meninges; it is therefore not a tumor of the

Right   **Left**

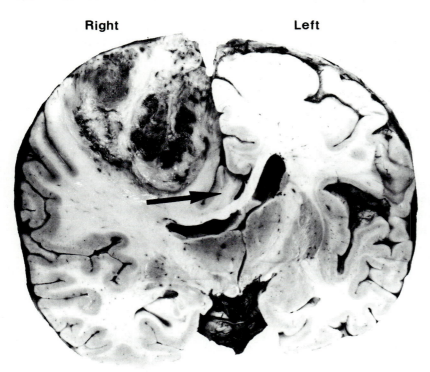

Figure 33–6 Glioma of cerebral hemisphere. Sagittal section through the brain shows a large tumor in the right cerebral hemisphere. The center of the tumor is necrotic, and it shows dark areas that result from bleeding. Note that the tumor is not encapsulated and that its growth has distorted the lateral ventricles, particularly the one on the right-hand side. The expanding tumor has caused herniation of the hemisphere beneath the falx cerebri (arrow). The falx itself has been removed. (Courtesy of Dr. N.B. Rewcastle, Chairman, Department of Pathology, University of Calgary, Alberta, Canada.)

brain itself. It is included here because the effects produced are very similar to those of a cerebral tumor. Meningiomas usually grow slowly and produce pressure atrophy of the underlying brain. They may remain symptomless, and it is not uncommon to encounter a meningioma as an incidental finding in an autopsy performed on a patient who has died of some other disease. Nevertheless, when symptoms occur, the tumor should be removed. Occasionally growth is more rapid, and it may kill the patient by reason of its location or because of increased intracranial pressure.

Secondary Tumors. Secondary tumors are common and may be responsible for the presenting symptoms of a disease. Carcinoma of the lung in males and carcinoma of the breast in females are the common primary tumors to produce cerebral metastases.

Summary

- Increased intracranial pressure occurs with edema of the brain, obstruction of the flow of CSF, meningitis, and space-occupying lesions. Headache, vomiting, papilledema, and brain herniations are important effects. Coning is often fatal.
- Subdural hemorrhage follows minor trauma, is of venous origin, and, if chronic, produces a space-occupying lesion that may mimic tumor.
- Extradural hemorrhage is associated with fracture of the skull, is of arterial origin, and is rapidly fatal.
- Subarachnoid hemorrhage is often due to the rupture of a berry aneurysm.
- A stroke is due to cerebral hemorrhage, thrombosis, or embolism; atherosclerosis and systemic hypertension are common causative factors.
- Pyogenic infections of the brain cause meningitis or brain abscess; viral infections lead to meningitis or encephalitis.
- Multiple sclerosis is the most important demyelinating disease. It has a long relapsing course and affects many parts of the brain.
- Brain damage and dysfunction can be caused by poisons (lead and mercury), vitamin deficiencies (particularly of the vitamin B members), and metabolic disorders (hepatic encephalopathy, alcoholism, and hypoglycemia).
- Alzheimer's disease is a common cause of dementia in subjects aged over 60 years. The cause is unknown.
- Parkinson's disease and motor neuron disease are degenerative diseases of unknown cause. Huntington's chorea is inherited.

- Epilepsy may be focal or generalized — grand mal or petit mal. The disease may be idiopathic; of the symptomatic group, a brain tumor (either primary or metastatic) is an important member of the many known causes.
- Gliomas are the most common primary tumor of the central nervous system. They invade tissue locally, may metastasize within the central nervous system, but almost never produce distant metastases.

- Meningioma arises from the meninges, is generally benign, but can kill by virtue of its situation.

Selected Readings

Leech, R. W., and Shuman, R. M.: Neuropathology: A Summary for Students. Hagerstown, Harper & Row, 1982.

Okazaki, H.: Fundamentals of Neuropathology. Tokyo, Igaku-Shoin, 1983.

Index

Note: Page numbers in *italics* refer to illustrations; page numbers followed by t refer to tables.

Interferon *(Continued)*
    as antigen, 241
    viral interference and, 177
Interferon-gamma, 106, 107
    B-cell stimulation and, 101
Interfibrillary matrix, 61
Interleukin-1, 23, 79, 91, 107
    fever and, 258
    in antigen recognition, 106
    in macrophage, 70, 72
Interleukin-2, 23, 107
    as antigen, 240, 241
    B cell stimulation and, 101
    immune response and, 107
    in antigen recognition, 106
Intermediate filament, 27
Intermittent claudication, 336
Interstitial nephritis, 495–496
Interstitial pneumonia, 393–397, *394, 396, 397*
Intestinal angina, 440
Intestinal bacilli, gram-negative, 147–148, *148,* 148t
Intestine, large. *See* Colon.
    obstruction of, 453–454
Intima of blood vessels, 371–372
    fatty streaks in, 373
Intoxication, 131
Intracellular adhesion molecule 1 (ICAM-1), 66
Intracranial pressure, 609–610
    headache and, 610
Intracytoplasmic filament, 27
Intrahepatic bile duct, 476
Intrahepatic cholestasis, 461
Intraperitoneal hemorrhage, 452
Intrarenal reflux, 498
Intrinsic factor, in gastric juice, 429
Intron, 30, *30*
Intussusception, 453
Inulin clearance, 484, 485, 486
Invasive mole, 524–525
Involucrum, 556
Iodine, amyloid and, 286
    goiter and, 544–545
    in Schiller test, 517
    radioactive isotope of, 67
5-Iodo-2'-deoxyuridine, 178
Ionizing radiation. *See* Radiation, ionizing.
Iridocyclitis, 601–602
Iris, 597
Iritis, 601, 602
Iron, in blood cell formation, 296
Iron deficiency anemia, 298–299
    in Plummer-Vinson syndrome, 425
Irradiation. *See* Radiation.
Irreversible shock, 327–329, *328*
Ischemia, 51, 211–212, 339
    aneurysm and, 378
    in bone disorders, 557
    myocardial, 354–358, *356–358*
Ischemic bowel disease, 440
Ischemic heart disease, 354–358, *356–358*
Ischemic hypoxia, 338
Islets of Langerhans, 478, 481–482
    diabetes mellitus and, 276
    tumors of, hypoglycemia and, 278
Isoenzyme, 59

Isograft, 115, 117
Isoniazid, acute hepatic pattern and, 466
    pyridoxine and, 268
Isospora belli, 114
Isotopes, radioactive, 9–11, *12*
Isotretinoin (Accutane), 206
Itching, 574
Ixodes dammini, 160

Jacksonian epilepsy, 618
Jaundice, 460–461, *462,* 467
    obstructive, gallstones and, 476–477
JC virus, 181
Jenner, E., 181
Joint disease, 566–570
Joint mice, 570
Junctional nevus, 586
Juvenile melanoma, 586
Juvenile-onset diabetes, 274–275, 275t

K cell, 106
Kahn reaction, 162
Kala-azar, 194t, 194–195
Kallikrein, 76, 77, *78*
Kaposi's sarcoma, 591–592, *593*
    in AIDS, 113, 114
Karyolysis, 58
Karyorrhexis, 58
Karyotype, 45, *45,* 46
    tumors and, 241
Katayama fever, 198
Kcal (kilocalorie), 253
Keloid, 88, *89*
Keratin granuloma, *95*
Keratinization, of mobile mucosa, 420
    of uterus, 515
Keratoacanthoma, 210, 589
Keratomalacia, 265
Keratoses, 420
Kernicterus, 461
Ketonuria, 275
Kidney, 483–501. *See also* Renal *entries;* Urinary tract.
    amyloid and, 287–289
    carcinoma of, 499–501, *500*
    disease of. *See* Renal disease.
    functions of, 484–487, *486*
    hyaline droplets in, 54
    infection of, 497–499
    malignant hypertension and, 332
    neoplasms of, 499–501, *500*
    normal, *492*
    protein-losing, 487–488
    regeneration of, 89
    shock and, 328, *328*
    transplantation of, 118
    urinary obstruction and, 502
Kilocalorie (kcal), 253
Kinetoplast, *195*
Kinin, 484
    complement activation and, 105
    in carcinoid syndrome, 443